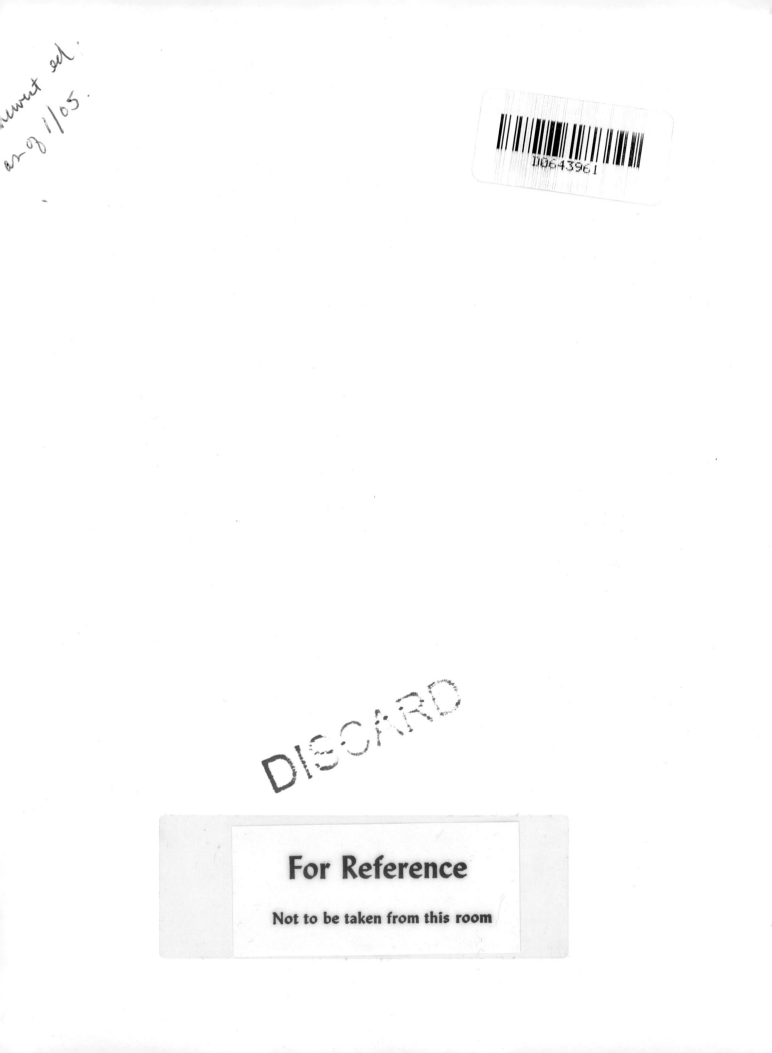

DISCARD

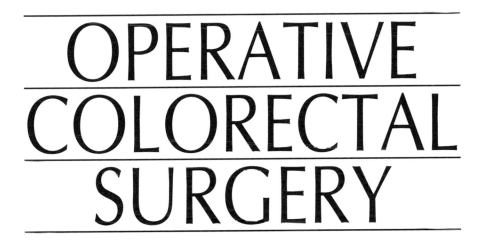

OPERATIVE
COLORECTAL
SURGERY

OPERATIVE COLORECTAL SURGERY

George E. Block, M.D., M.S. (Surg.), F.A.C.S.

The Thomas D. Jones Professor
Department of Surgery
University of Chicago Medical Center
Chicago, Illinois

A. R. Moossa, M.D., F.R.C.S. (Ed.), F.A.C.S.

Professor and Chairman
Department of Surgery
University of California at San Diego
San Diego, California

Illustrations by Kathryn A. Sisson

W.B. SAUNDERS COMPANY
A Division of Harcourt Brace & Company
Philadelphia   London   Toronto   Montreal   Sydney   Tokyo

W. B. SAUNDERS COMPANY
A Division of
Harcourt Brace & Company

The Curtis Center
Independence Square West
Philadelphia, Pennsylvania 19106

Library of Congress Cataloging-in-Publication Data

Operative colorectal surgery / [edited by] George E. Block, A.R. Moossa.

  p. cm.

ISBN 0–7216–3366–8

1. Colon (Anatomy)—Surgery.   2. Rectum—Surgery.
  I. Block, George E.,   II. Moossa, A. R.   III. Operative colorectal
surgery. [DNLM: 1. Colonic Diseases—Surgery.   2. Rectal Diseases—
Surgery.   3. Surgery, Operative.   7WI 520 061]

RD544. 064 1994   617.5′547—dc20

DNLM/DLC   92–48340

Operative Colorectal Surgery   ISBN 0–7216–3366–8

Last digit is the print number: 9   8   7   6   5   4   3   2   1

To our families

To Mary, George, Randy, and Edward, with love

G.E.B.

To Denise, Pierre, Noel, Claude, and Valentine,
whose sacrifices made it all possible

A.R.M.

CONTRIBUTORS

Tommaso Balestracci, M.D.
Research Associate, Department of Surgery, University of Chicago Medical School, Chicago, Illinois.
Special Operations on the Colon and Rectum

P. Balladur, M.D.
Centre de Chirurgie Digestive, Hopital Saint Antoine, Paris, France.
Proctocolectomy

Joel J. Bauer, M.D., F.A.C.S.
Mount Sinai School of Medicine, University of New York, New York, New York.
Intestinal Stomas: Construction and Care

Robert W. Beart, Jr., M.D., F.A.C.S.
Professor of Surgery, University of Southern California School of Medicine, Los Angeles, California.
Anal Incontinence

Scott J. Boley, M.D., F.A.C.S.
Professor of Surgery and Chief of Pediatric Surgical Services, Albert Einstein College of Medicine—Montefiore Medical Center of Yeshiva University, Bronx, New York.
Vascular Diseases of the Colon

David G. Brachman, M.D.
West Michigan Cancer Center, Kalamazoo, Michigan.
Radiotherapy of Colorectal and Anal Carcinomas

Isidore Cohn, Jr., M.D., D.Sc. (M.Ed.) F.A.C.S.
Professor of Surgery, Louisiana State University School of Medicine in New Orleans; Medical Center of Louisiana at New Orleans, New Orleans, Louisiana.
Perioperative Management of Colon, Rectum, and Anus Disorders

Robert E. Condon, M.D., F.A.C.S.
Ausman Foundation Professor and Chairman, Medical College of Wisconsin; Attending Surgeon, Milwaukee County Medical Complex and Froedtert Memorial Lutheran Hospital, Milwaukee, Wisconsin.
Physiology of the Colon, Rectum, and Anus

Ralph Crum, M.D.
Department of Surgery, University of California, San Diego, School of Medicine, San Diego, California.
Large Bowel Obstruction

Jerome J. DeCosse, M.D., F.A.C.S.
Professor of Surgery, Cornell University Medical College; Attending Surgeon, New York Hospital, New York, New York.
Tumors of the Anal Canal

Thomas L. Dent, M.D., F.A.C.S.
Professor of Surgery, Temple University School of Medicine, Philadelphia; Chairman, Department of Surgery, Abington Memorial Hospital, Abington, Pennsylvania.
Lower Gastrointestinal Endoscopy: Diagnostic and Therapeutic Procedures

Charles D. Dietzen, M.D., F.A.C.S.
Clinical Assistant Professor of Surgery, Louisiana State University School of Medicine in New Orleans, New Orleans; Staff Surgeon, Slidell Memorial Hospital and Northshore Regional Medical Center, Slidell, Louisiana.
Perioperative Management of Colon, Rectum, and Anus Disorders

Roger R. Dozois, M.D., F.A.C.S.
Professor of Surgery, Mayo Medical School; Chairman, Division of Colon and Rectal Surgery, Mayo Clinic and Mayo Foundation, Rochester, Minnesota.
Prolapse of the Rectum

Scott A. Dulchavsky, M.D., F.A.C.S., F.C.C.M.
Assistant Professor of Surgery, Wayne State University School of Medicine, Detroit, Michigan.
Trauma to the Colon and Rectum

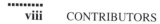

John Dunn, M.D., F.A.C.S.

Assistant Professor of Surgery, University of California at San Diego, School of Medicine; Assistant Professor of Surgery, General Surgery, and Organ Transplantation, University of California at San Diego, Medical Center, San Diego, California.

Surgical Anatomy and Embryology of the Colon, Rectum, and Anus

Harold Ellis, M.D., F.R.C.S.

Professor, Department of Anatomy, Cambridge, United Kingdom.

Colorectal Surgery; Historical Introduction

Kenneth Eng, M.D., F.A.C.S.

Professor of Surgery, New York University School of Medicine; Attending Surgeon, New York University Medical Center, New York, New York.

Abdominosacral Resection

Warren E. Enker, M.D., F.A.C.S.

Professor, Department of Surgery, Cornell University Medical College; Attending Surgeon, Colorectal Service, Department of Surgery, Memorial Sloan-Kettering Cancer Center, New York, New York.

Operative Treatment for Carcinoma of the Abdominal Colon

Constantine T. Frantzides, M.D., Ph.D., F.A.C.S.

Associate Professor, Medical College of Wisconsin; Attending Surgeon, Milwaukee County Medical Complex, Froedtert Memorial Lutheran Hospital, and Columbia Hospital, Milwaukee, Wisconsin.

Physiology of the Colon, Rectum, and Anus

Neill Freeman, M.D., F.R.C.S.

Department of Pediatric Surgery, Royal Hospital, Sultanate of Oman.

Anorectal Malformations in Infants and Children

Irwin M. Gelernt, M.D., F.A.C.S.

Mount Sinai School of Medicine, University of New York, New York, New York

Intestinal Stomas: Construction and Care

Stephen R. Gorfine, M.D., F.A.C.S.

Mount Sinai School of Medicine, University of New York, New York, New York.

Intestinal Stomas: Construction and Care

Nicholas A. Halasz, M.D., F.A.C.S.

Professor of Surgery and Head, Division of Anatomy, University of California at San Diego School of Medicine; Attending Surgeon and Director, Renal Transplant Program, University of California at San Diego, Medical Center, San Diego, California.

Surgical Anatomy and Embryology of the Colon, Rectum, and Anus

Ira M. Hanan, M.D.

Assistant Professor of Clinical Medicine, University of Chicago School of Medicine; Director of Gastrointestinal Endoscopy, University of Chicago Hospitals, Chicago, Illinois.

Diagnostic Approaches to Colorectal Disease

Daniel J. Haraf, M.D.

Assistant Professor, Clinical Director, Radiation and Cellular Oncology, University of Chicago Medical Center, Chicago, Illinois.

Radiotherapy of Colorectal and Anal Carcinomas

Frank J. Harford, M.D., F.A.C.S.

Professor of Clinical Surgery, Loyola University Stritch School of Medicine; Chief of Colorectal Surgery, Foster G. McGaw Hospital; Director of Surgery, MacNeal Memorial Hospital; Maywood, Illinois.

Ileocolectomy, Total Abdominal Colectomy, and Segmental Resections

Stephen G. Harper, M.D.

Clinical Instructor of Surgery, Temple University School of Medicine, Philadelphia; Assistant Surgeon, Abington Memorial Hospital, Abington, Pennsylvania.

Lower Gastrointestinal Endoscopy: Diagnostic and Therapeutic Procedures

Ronald N. Kaleya, M.D.

Assistant Professor of Surgery, Albert Einstein College of Medicine of Yeshiva University, Bronx, New York.

Vascular Diseases of the Colon

John S. Kukora, M.D., F.A.C.S.

Professor of Surgery, Temple University School of Medicine, Philadelphia; Associate Director, General Surgery Residency Program, Abington Memorial Hospital, Abington, Pennsylvania.

Lower Gastrointestinal Endoscopy: Diagnostic and Therapeutic Procedures

S. Arthur Localio, M.D., F.A.C.S.

Johnson and Johnson Distinguished Professor of Surgery Emeritus, New York University School of Medicine; Attending Surgeon, New York University Medical Center, New York, New York.

Abdominosacral Resection

Fabrizio Michelassi, M.D., F.A.C.S.

Associate Professor, Department of Surgery, University of Chicago Medical School, Chicago, Illinois.

Special Operations on the Colon and Rectum

Santhat Nivatvongs, M.D., F.A.C.S.

Mayo Clinic and Mayo Foundation, Rochester, Minnesota.

Prolapse of the Rectum

Roland Parc, M.D.

Centre de Chirurgie Digestive, Hopital Saint Antoine, Paris, France.

Proctocolectomy

Jack Pickleman, M.D., F.A.C.S.

Professor, Department of Surgery, Loyola University Stritch School of Medicine; Chief, Division of General Surgery, Foster G. McGaw Hospital, Maywood, Illinois.

Ileocolectomy, Total Abdominal Colectomy, and Segmental Resections

Elliot Prager, M.D., F.A.C.S.

Director, Colon and Rectal Residency, Sansum Clinic; Attending, Santa Barbara Cottage Hospital, Santa Barbara, California.

Common Ailments of the Anorectal Region

Hernan M. Reyes, M.D., F.A.C.S.

Department of Surgery, Section of Pediatric Surgery, Cook County Hospital, Chicago, Illinois.

Anorectal Disease in Children

Jonathan M. Sackier, M.D., F.R.C.S.

Associate Professor of Surgery, University of California, San Diego, School of Medicine, San Diego, California.

Complications of Colorectal Operations; Laparoscopy for the Diagnosis and Treatment of Diseases of the Colon and Rectum

Theodore R. Schrock, M.D., F.A.C.S.

Professor of Surgery, University of California, San Francisco, School of Medicine, San Francisco, California.

Rectovaginal Fistula

Harvey M. Shapiro, M.D.

Professor of Anesthesia and Chief, Department of Anesthesiology, University of California at San Diego; Chief of Anesthesia and Director of Pain Service, University of California at San Diego Medical Center, San Diego, California.

Anesthesia for Colorectal Operations

Dennis W. Shermeta, M.D., F.A.C.S.

Attending Surgeon, Phoenix Children's Hospital and St. Joseph's Children's Medical Center, Phoenix, Arizona.

Tumors of the Perineum and Perirectal Region

Lewis Spitz, M.D., F.R.C.S.

Department of Paediatric Surgery, Institute of Child Health, University of London, London, United Kingdom.

Hirschsprung's Disease

Takashi Takahashi, M.D.

Department of Surgery, Tokyo Metro Komagome Hospital, Tokyo, Japan.

Operative Treatment for Carcinoma of the Rectum

Joji Utsunomiya, M.D.

Second Department of Surgery, Hyogo College of Medicine, Nishinomiya, Hyogo, Japan.

Total Colectomy, Mucosal Proctectomy, and Ileoanal Anastomosis

Alexander J. Walt, M.B., C.B., F.A.C.S., F.R.C.S.(Eng.), F.R.C.S.(C.)

Distinguished Professor of Surgery, Wayne State University School of Medicine, Detroit, Michigan.

Trauma to the Colon and Rectum

Ralph R. Weichselbaum, M.D.

Harold H. Hines, Jr. Professor and Chairman, Department of Radiation and Cellular Oncology, University of Chicago Medical Center, Chicago, Illinois.

Radiotherapy of Colorectal and Anal Carcinomas

William C. Wilson, M.D.

Assistant Clinical Professor, Cardiothoracic Anesthesia and Critical Care Medicine, University of California at San Diego; Staff Anesthesiologist and Attending, Surgical Intensive Care Unit, University of California at San Diego Medical Center, San Diego, California.

Anesthesia for Colorectal Operations

T. Yamamura, M.D.

Second Department of Surgery, Hyogo College of Medicine, Nishinomiya, Hyogo, Japan.

Total Colectomy, Mucosal Proctectomy, and Ileoanal Anastomosis

F O R E W O R D

Surgery is the primary treatment for many diseases of the large bowel: colon, rectum, and anus. Even though inflammatory diseases and non-neoplastic conditions might be medically treated early, at some point the patient becomes a surgical candidate because the process becomes intractable or chronic or because complications exist; thus, the surgeon and physician must be fully knowledgeable about these conditions and the wide spectrum of surgical procedures available to manage them.

The history of any field of surgery is always pertinent to current discussion of issues related to it. If one searches back in history, there is infrequently anything new. Previously, suggestions have been made or surgical procedures proposed or tried but met with failure because of lack of knowledge or support that is available today. We must respect those preceding us for their contributions, often made under difficult circumstances. For instance, anterior resection was tried at the turn of the century, but it met with failure because of inability to control infection and because of complications occurring primarily with the anastomosis. A stem ileostomy was considered the exchange of one disease (chronic ulcerative colitis) for another (ileostomy dysfunction) and so was used as a last resort. Today the Brooke ileostomy (full-thickness eversion) has resolved the complications of the stem ileostomy. Surgical treatment of inflammatory disease can be initiated earlier, offering the patient a better quality of life without experiencing complications and protracted disease. The evolution of surgical management of chronic ulcerative colitis has also led from the stem ileostomy to the continent ileal reservoir (Kock pouch) to the new ileoanal anastomosis (originally proposed by Ravitch and Sabiston), which offers the patient continence (95%) and evacuation of the bowel through the normal anatomic route. History has led to progress and will continue to do so.

Diagnostic capability has increased. Physical examination of the abdomen and the digital rectal examination were all that was available in earlier years. Since then, we have seen first the rigid proctoscope, then the flexible one, and now the colonoscope. Radiographic diagnosis involved first the barium colon x-ray film, then the air-contrast study, followed by computed tomography and magnetic resonance imaging to delineate colonic disease. The advance of technology and imaging has greatly enhanced the physician's capability to diagnose and treat diseases of the colon and rectum.

Dukes proposed a method of delineating the anatomic extent of cancers of the rectum. Over the years, the classification has been extended to the colon and modified by many surgeons and pathologists. Most recently, the American Joint Committee on Cancer and the TNM Committee of the International Union Against Cancer have proposed a more sophisticated staging scheme that will aid in planning treatment, indicating prognosis, evaluating results of treatment, and facilitating the exchange of information between treatment centers. Other biologic, genetic, and molecular markers are being studied that will probably lead beyond anatomic extent to a more meaningful prognostic index.

What factors have made it possible for our generation to capitalize on the results of the generation before us? Improvements of anesthesia, blood transfusions, availability of antibiotics and other chemotherapeutic agents, and advance of diagnostic capability are among them. Intensive care units, trauma care, and sophisticated monitoring technology are among services now available that contribute to improved results. Also, increased knowledge of biologic behavior of disease and screening for early diagnosis and for asymptomatic conditions have permitted treatment to be carried out at a time when results of management are more likely to be satisfactory. The American Cancer Society Guidelines for early detection of colorectal cancer are leading to earlier diagnosis and treatment with more favorable results. These include sigmoidoscopy in patients 50 years of age and older every 3 to 5 years, fecal occult blood test every year for patients 50 years and older, and digital rectal examination every year in persons 40 years of age and older.

Improved and new technology has added to the scope of surgical treatment for many conditions. Endoscopic and laparoscopic procedures have added a new dimension to the surgical armamentarium. This has increased benefits to the patient in reducing the time spent in the hospital and convalescing and in reducing pain and discomfort. Today, the cost of health care has become another parameter that must be considered in decisions about the method of treatment. It has been said that an appendectomy requires an incision of an inch and a half, an instrument and a half, and a minute and a half. There are reports of appendectomy being done laparoscopically by using sophisticated and costly equipment, taking as long as 90 minutes, and requiring long periods of anesthesia and costly use of the operating room. Hospitalization should be no more than one day postoperatively in either case. Although it is nice to be "out front," the cost effectiveness of the operation must be considered. The potential surgical and pathologic hazards of new technology must also be kept in mind.

When the exterioration procedure was done, seeding of the tumor in the operative wound was not an unusual complication. Carefully handling a colonic tumor in resecting it or using the "no-touch technique" has contributed to the improved results in the treatment of colorectal cancer and the reduction of recurrence. To treat the patient by a closed technique could jeopardize the patient's best chance to get well. This emphasizes the fact that surgeons must use their most sound surgical judgment in the best interest of the patient.

The management of many diseases of the large bowel today requires the use of multiple modalities. The surgeon needs to know not only embryology, anatomy, and physiology but also the essence of radiotherapy, chemotherapy, and other isoteric methods of treating disease. A thorough knowledge of pathology, nutrition, cellular biology, and technology, as well as techniques of the operation, is essential.

The surgeon is no longer (and never should have been) a technician providing a mechanical service but is a physician, in the broadest sense of the word, with operating capability.

A textbook such as this one, with multiple authors who are experts in their fields, provides the broadest perspective to the subject of colorectal surgery. The authors present their own knowledge and experience as well as that of others. Further comments by the editors contribute information and another perspective in many chapters.

Although a textbook such as this brings together current information, there will be new information on topics such as etiology, biologic behavior, and cytopathology of colorectal disease and its management that will require revisions and new editions.

OLIVER H. BEAHRS, M.D.

P R E F A C E

Operative Colorectal Surgery is written for the student of surgery—the surgical resident, the fellows in a surgical specialty, and the experienced surgeon who wishes to review treatment options and their methods of execution. *Operative Colorectal Surgery* is not intended as an exhaustive reference for all diseases of the hindgut; rather, it is primarily a text of operative surgery describing when to choose a particular operation, how to perform it, and how to avoid the pitfalls and complications associated with the procedure.

All of the authors are internationally recognized authorities in their fields, and they present to the reader their preferred operative procedures for the various disease entities under consideration. Not all conceivable operations on the hindgut are presented; rather, authors have chosen their preferred operation(s) for a particular disease and present in detail their methods of performance.

Topics other than the actual performance of operations on the colon, rectum, and anus are presented when they have direct bearing on the care of the surgical patient and the proper and safe performance of the operation. These topics include such specific entities as colonic obstruction, specific considerations of surgical anatomy, perioperative care, anesthesia, an algorithmic presentation of diagnostic and therapeutic options, and adjuvant treatments of hindgut neoplasms.

The editors have made editorial comments where appropriate, emphasizing surgical principles, alternative methods of operative treatment, and, occasionally, their disagreement.

The operative text is generously illustrated, and all illustrations were executed by the same artist for consistency and clarity.

The authors and the editors trust that this book will help students of surgery choose the most appropriate operation for their patient, allowing for a precise and enlightened performance of the operative procedures while avoiding or properly managing their complications.

GEORGE E. BLOCK
A. R. MOOSSA

ACKNOWLEDGMENT

Elizabeth Gramhofer and Rachel Ramiro deserve full recognition and heartfelt thanks for their dedication to the day-to-day work on this book and for coordinating the hectic activities of the contributors and editors.

CONTENTS

SECTION I

GENERAL CONCEPTS

Colorectal Surgery: Historical Introduction

C H A P T E R   1

Harold Ellis

HISTORY OF COLORECTAL SURGERY

Up to a century ago, much of our current knowledge of disease of the colon remained shrouded in mystery, awaiting the development of contrast radiology and endoscopy. Similarly, current approaches to surgery of the colon depended on the introduction of anesthesia and antisepsis. In contradistinction, disease of the anorectum, so obvious to the eye and to the examining finger, and so demanding of the surgeon's attention because of its unpleasant features, has a history that begins in the earliest days of medicine.

The earliest known treatise completely devoted to anorectal disease is a papyrus preserved in the British Museum and dated the twelfth or thirteenth century B.C.[1] This manuscript, known as the *Chester Beatty Medical Papyrus*, comprises eight columns of 14 lines written in the hieratic script and contains 41 remedies. These are prescriptions for drinks, pastes, suppositories, enemas, and dressings for a variety of anal symptoms, including heaviness, sickness, itching, prolapse, painful swelling, and bleeding. No less than ten of the remedies are for pruritus.

Proctology was obviously practiced at the time of the ancient Greeks. Two books in the Hippocratic writings are devoted to this topic.[2] *On Fistulae* clearly describes the use of the seton. A slender thread of lint is wrapped with horsehair. This is threaded through the fistula by means of a director made of tin. The seton is then knotted and tightened when it becomes loose. If the thread rots, then another piece of lint can be pulled through the track by the horsehair, which, unlike the lint, is not liable to rot. Once the fistula has sloughed through, the wound is washed with hot water and dressed with a soft sponge smeared with honey.

On Haemorrhoids, the second short volume, vividly describes the radical Hippocratic technique of treatment in the fifth century B.C.:

> Lay the patient on his back with a pillow below the breech, force out the anus as much as possible with the fingers, and make the irons red-hot, and burn the pile until it be dried up . . . and burn so as to leave none of the haemorrhoids unburnt . . . you will recognise the haemorrhoids, for they project on the inside of the gut like dark coloured grapes, and when the anus is forced out they spurt blood.

The wound is then dressed with a soft sponge covered by a cloth smeared in honey and held in place by means of a girdle. After evacuating the bowel, the parts are washed with hot water, and every third day a bath is taken. Another piece of advice is

> When the cautery is applied, the patient's head and hands should be held so that he may not stir, but he himself should cry out for this will make the rectum project the more.

On the other hand, if the practitioner (and, one imagines, the patient) wishes to effect the cure by suppositories rather than by cautery, Hippocrates advises a mixture of a variety of substances including the shell of the cuttlefish, alum, bitumen, and a small quantity of boiled honey.

Hemorrhoids

Even the names given to the condition of hemorrhoids are ancient. *Haemorrhoids* derives from the Greek *haema*, "blood," and *rheo*, "flow." Variations in the spelling are common in older writings: thus, the Latin *haemorrhoida*, Old French *emoroyde*, Middle English *emerod*, and Late Middle English *emeroidis*. The synonymous term "piles" appeared in Middle English and derives from the Greek work *pila*, "ball," and hence refers to any swelling.

Over the centuries, surgeons also applied various acids (including nitric and carbolic acids), caustic pastes, and other powerful medicaments to burn away the prolapsed pile. Operative procedures included simple excision, ligature of the pile together with the overlying skin, and either excising the mass of tissue or allowing it to slough. Others crushed the pile with clamps or wire. All of these procedures, performed without any form of anesthesia, must have caused agony as well as an unpleasantly painful postoperative period and the serious risk of stricture formation. Deaths from hemorrhage were not infrequent.

Even the great Sir Astley Cooper of Guy's Hospital, London, encountered mortality in his practice. He notes in his lectures:

> *The Earl of S—— applied to me for piles with prolapsus ani. . . . I removed with the scissars one of the largest, and desired his Lordship to keep the recumbent posture. In about 10 minutes he said, "I must relieve my bowels," and he rose from his bed and discharged into the close stool what he thought to be faeces, but which proved to be blood. In 20 minutes he had the same sensation, and evacuated more blood than before . . . and soon became very faint from the free haemorrhage. I, therefore, opened the rectum with a speculum, and saw an artery throwing out its blood with freedom, I therefore requested him to force down the intestine as much as he could, and raising the orifice of the bleeding vessel with a tenaculum, secured it in a ligature . . . his Lordship bled no more. On the following day he was low, his pulse very quick, and he had a shivering; on the next he complained of pain in his abdomen; he had sickness, and tenderness upon pressure, and in 4 days he died. . . . I opened his body and found inflammation of the rectum.[3]*

It was Frederick Salmon, founder of St. Mark's Hospital in London in 1835, who first described the operation on which modern hemorrhoidectomy is based. He made a scissors-cut at the mucocutaneous junction of the haemorrhoid and stripped the mucosa-covered portion to the top of the anal canal, where it was firmly ligated and the pile excised.

The radical operation, in which most of the involved pile-bearing area was excised, was introduced in 1882 by Walter Whitehead; the hemorrhoids were cured but only at serious risk of stricture formation. In 1937 at St. Mark's, Milligan and Morgan described their low-ligation technique, which with all its modifications represents the standard operation of today.[4]

The injection treatment of piles was introduced comparatively late in the history of the subject, because it depended on the invention of the hypodermic syringe. It was first practiced in 1869 by Morgan of Dublin, who used a solution of iron persulfate. The treatment was then employed by Abraham Colles, of Colles fracture fame. It was taken up with great enthusiasm in the United States, where it was pioneered by Mitchell, who used a secret formula of carbolic acid in olive oil. He passed on his secret before his death to a large number of itinerant "pile doctors," who traveled around the country plying their trade. The formula was obtained by Andrews (1879) of Chicago,[5] and the injection treatment of hemorrhoids by using a variety of sclerosing solutions (the most popular appears to be phenol in almond oil) remains part of today's surgical armamentarium.

Fistula-in-Ano

"Fistula" derives from the Latin word for "pipe." Through the ages, anal fistula appears to have been an extremely common disease. Some examples were undoubtedly tuberculous or malignant, but the majority probably resulted from neglected cases of perianal infection. Laurence Heister (1753) writes:

> *It has been an observation made by many of the camp-surgeons and physicians, that troopers, or the riding part of an army, are very frequently troubled with this disorder, especially after long marches in hot weather. An abscess thus formed may degenerate into a fistula, by the neglect and bashfulness of the patient, especially if it be not timely opened and cleansed from its foul contents.[6]*

In 1882, Allingham reported, from St. Mark's Hospital in London, an analysis of 4,000 consecutive cases in his outpatient department.[7] No less than 1208 were examples of fistula-in-ano. The breakdown of his cases, which is of interest in comparison with that of modern proctologic practice, is shown in Table 1–1.

The surgical treatment of fistula has a remarkably long history. We have already quoted a perfectly rational method of treatment in the Hippocratic writings. Instruments used in this operation have been unearthed at Pompeii, and laying open the fistula with the knife is advocated by Celsus in his great encyclopedia of medical practice, *De re Medica* of 30 B.C.

The father of proctology in England was John of Arderne, who flourished in the fourteenth century. He practiced surgery first in Newark, in the Midlands, but later moved to London. His book *Treatises of Fistula in Ano, Haemorrhoids and Clysters* was a notable landmark in surgical history.[8] His operation for fistula consisted of threading a ligature through the fistulous track. This was tightly tied and then the tissue within

Table 1–1. ANALYSIS OF 4,000 CONSECUTIVE CASES OBSERVED BY MR. ALLINGHAM, IN THE OUTPATIENTS' DEPARTMENT OF ST. MARK'S HOSPITAL

Fistula*	1,208
Abscess, 196 (of these 151 became fistulas, the rest probably were cured)	45
Hemorrhoids, internal	863
Hemorrhoids, external	102
Fissure or painful ulcer	446
Syphilitic diseases of the anus and rectum	348
Ulceration (neither malignant nor syphilitic)	190
Constipation	185
Pruritus ani	180
Stricture of the rectum (with or without ulceration)	178
Cancer of the rectum	105
Procidentia	53
Polypus without fissure	16
Haemorrhage (cause not ascertained)	15
Impaction of feces	14
Neuralgia	12
Dysentery	12
Spasmodic contraction of the sphincter (no fissure)	8
Proctitis	7
Foreign bodies in the rectum	5
Necrosis of bone (sacrum, and tuberosity of the ischium)	4
Rodent ulcer	2
Vicarious menstruation from the rectum	2
	4,000

*Of these cases of fistula, 172 presented more or less marked symptoms affecting the lungs: hemoptysis, frequent cough, or want of resonance in some part of the chest.

the ligature boldly cut through to lay open the tract in its entirety. If multiple sinuses were present, they also needed to be opened. His aftercare included simple cleaning of the wound with avoidance of the unnecessary and irritating medications then so often employed. He devised the instruments required for his procedure and advised his readers about the fees they should charge:

> Therefore for the cure of fistula-in-ano, when it is curable ask . . . of a worthy man and a great, a hundred mark or forty pound, with robes and fees of a hundred shilling term of life by year. Of lesser men, forty pound or forty mark ask he without fees; and take he naught less than a hundred shillings. For never in my life took I less than a hundred shillings for cure of that sickness.[8]

John of Arderne was also familiar with the role of perianal abscess in the etiology of fistula and advised early drainage:

> An abscess breeding near the anus should not be left to burst by itself, but the leech should busily for to feel with his finger the place of the abscess, and where so is found any softness, there, the patient not knowing, carefully be it boldly opened with a very sharp lancette, so that the pus and the corrupt blood may go out. . . . If it bursts both within and without, then it can never be cured except

by a surgeon fully expert in his craft. For then may it from the first day be called a fistula.[8]

Later surgeons diverged from simple laying open of the fistula. Some, such as Le Dran of Paris, advised radical extirpation of the diseased parts. Others returned to the use of mercury and escharotics in the dressing of the wound, whereas still others invented all sorts of ingenious probe-pointed scissors and probe razors to divide the tissues. It was Percival Pott (1765), of St. Bartholomew's Hospital in London who, in his *Remarks on the Disease Commonly Called a Fistula-in-Ano*, a monograph of 115 pages, advocated a return to the use of a curved, probe-pointed knife with a narrow blade. The blade was introduced into the fistula with the help of a surgeon's index finger in the rectum and used to divide the fistulous track; the wound was then dressed simply with soft fine lint.[9] "This first dressing should be permitted to continue until a beginning suppuration renders it loose enough to come away easily; and all the future ones should be as light, soft, and easy as possible." This simple technique was modified by Frederick Salmon at St. Mark's by adding to the main incision a further T-shaped cut, which enlarges the wound radially beyond the original external opening. This "Salmon's back-cut" prevents premature healing of the wound, whose saucer shape contributes toward sound healing.

Diverticula of the Colon

In the Western World, diverticula of the colon represent the most common pathologic condition of the large bowel and are present in about 30% to 40% of the elderly population. Although they are easy to recognize post mortem, diverticula were not recorded in medical publications before the mid–nineteenth century, and it was obvious that such great observers as John Hunter (1728 to 1793) never saw an example. Cruveilhier (1849) gave the first satisfactory description of the condition:

> We not infrequently find between the bands of longitudinal muscle fibres in the sigmoid a series of small, dark, pear-shaped tumours, which are formed by herniae of the mucous membrane through the gaps in the muscle coat.[10]

He noted that these sacs could be irritated by fecal matter, leading to inflammation and perforation. Habershon (1857), physician at Guy's Hospital, wrote:

> Pouches of the colon sometimes become of considerable size . . . these pouches are the result of constipation, the muscular fibres become hypertrophied, but their effort to propel onward their contents leads to these minute hernial protrusions.[11]

He notes also that "these pouches do not appear to produce any symptom or lead to dangerous result" and also comments that "appearances of this kind are by no means uncommon in the colon, especially towards its termination."[11]

To the clinicians and pathologists of the nineteenth century, these diverticula were curiosities and, indeed, Sir Arthur Keith (1910) could collect only seven specimens in the museum of the Royal College of Surgeons, London, and the museums of the London medical schools.[12]

Good descriptions of diverticulosis of the colon and its complications were given by Graser[13] and by Maxwell Telling[14] of Leeds, who reviewed reports of 324 examples of colonic diverticula. The first resection of the sigmoid colon for this condition appears to have been performed by Rutherford Morison in 1903.[15] The patient was a male aged 60 years, who was thought to be suffering from obstruction of the colon due to carcinoma. The resected specimen showed what Morison termed "sacculitis." The anastomosis leaked, and the patient died 2 days postoperatively.

The development of the barium enema x-ray examination was of immense value in the investigation of diverticula. In 1926, Spriggs and Marxer published a study of 1,000 barium enema examinations, of which 100 demonstrated colonic diverticula.[16] These authors describe a "prediverticular" phase of sigmoid colon contraction with a "sawtooth" irregularity. Later they reported the subsequent development of diverticula in such affected zones. This formed the basis of our modern concept of etiology.

Ulcerative Colitis

Noncontagious chronic diarrhea has been recognized for some 2,000 years, even though the name "ulcerative colitis" dates only from the middle of the nineteenth century.[17] Early descriptions of what may have been this condition were given by Aretaeus (A.D. 300) and by a physician who was named (most appropriately for a proctologist) Soranus (A.D. 117). Sydenham described the "bloody flux" in 1666, and Prince Charles (the Young Pretender, "Bonnie Prince Charlie") developed bloody diarrhea following his defeat at the Battle of Culloden in 1746.

A good description of the macroscopic appearance of ulcerative colitis was given by Wilks and Moxon (1874) in their *Pathological Anatomy*.[18] They clearly differentiate this condition from febrile epidemic dysentery and write:

> For example, we have seen a case attended by discharge of mucus and blood where, after death, the whole internal surface of the colon presented a highly vascular, soft, red surface, covered with tenacious mucus or adherent lymph, and here and there showing a few minute points of ulceration; the coats, also, were much swollen by exudation into the mucous and submucous tissues. In other examples there has been extensive ulceration, commencing in the follicles, and spreading from them to destroy the tissue around, thus producing a ragged, ulcerated surface.[18]

An excellent clinicopathologic description of an undoubted case of ulcerative colitis was given by Allchin (1885) from my own hospital.[19] This was a female who died at Westminster Hospital after an 11-day illness of bloody diarrhea (with between 17 and 22 stools daily). She had abdominal pain, a temperature of 101°F and a pulse of 112 beats per minute. The postmortem examination was performed by Allchin himself. There were no abnormal findings except in the colon. Externally this showed only slight congestion. However, the mucosa from the ileocecal valve distally showed numerous large ulcers.

Since then, great progress has been made in the detailed clinical description of the condition and its complications, but its cause remains unknown. Specific bacteria have been implicated, such as Bargen's diplococcus (1924), and others have invoked mucolytic enzymes, allergies, hypersensitivity to milk and its products, psychological factors, autoimmunity, and collagen disease.

The early treatment of ulcerative colitis was entirely nonspecific and comprised a wide variety of antidiarrheal medications. The first specific drug treatment was sulfasalazine, a diazo compound of sulfapyridine and salicylic acid. This was developed in Sweden, and its clinical use established by Nanna Svartz (1942) in Stockholm.[20] Corticosteroids were used in the management of this condition soon after their development. Their value was established by one of the first carefully controlled prospective trials carried out by Truelove and Witts[21] of Oxford, which paved the way for modern controlled studies of treatment modalities of all kinds and in a wide variety of conditions.

Toward the end of the nineteenth century, attempts were made to put the colon to rest by means of an ileostomy, performed by Baum in 1879, or cecostomy, performed by Follet in 1885 and Novaro in 1887.[22] Appendicostomy was suggested by Keetley in 1895 as a means of irrigating the colitic bowel and was first performed by Weir of New York in 1902. This procedure was carried out until World War II, by using a wide variety of irrigation fluids. Ileostomy certainly provided total fecal diversion but was associated with a high mortality because it was so often carried out only when the patient was already moribund. Moreover, until Brooke[23] introduced his spout ileostomy and efficient appliances were devised, the life of the ileostomy patient was miserable indeed.

A history of intestinal surgery would be incomplete without the inclusion of Alfred Strauss of Chicago (1881–1971) (Fig. 1–1). Strauss was born in Germany and immigrated alone to America as a boy of 10 years. He crossed the United States to the state of Washington where he eventually attended the University of Washington. At the University of Washington he was a star football player and graduated with honors in 1904. He received his Medical Degree from Rush-University of Chicago, graduating at the top of his class. For 25 years he was Chief of the Gastrointestinal Surgical Group at Michael Reese Hospital and at this institution developed procedures and concepts that were decades ahead of his time. He is putatively credited with operating on approximately 500 patients with ulcerative colitis for whom he performed an ileostomy. These patients were often moribund and Strauss successfully operated upon these unfortunates without the benefit of modern anesthesia, antibiotics, transfusions, or intravenous fluids. Strauss later pioneered the concept of colectomy for ulcerative colitis. Together with Koenig, his patient, Strauss developed the first practical and commercially available stoma appliance.

Strauss's prescience is illustrated by his published description of a "matured" and everted stoma in 1924, one quarter of a century before the advent of the Brooke ileostomy. Nyhus credits Strauss with performing the first gastrectomy for duodenal ulcer in the United States.

Strauss developed the concept of electrofulguration of rectal cancers and first published this thesis in 1913. At age 88 he published a monograph on the subject, which firmly established electrocauterization of rectal cancers as another of the seminal contributions of Alfred Strauss to surgery. In 1951 Strauss's life and contributions were recognized by his alma mater by the designation *Alumnus Summa Laude Dignatus.*

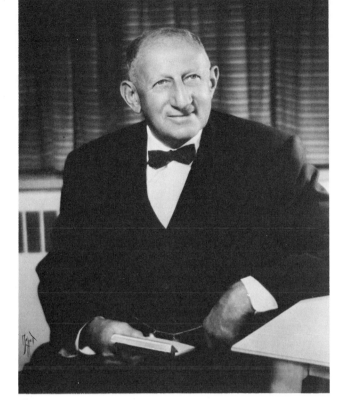

Figure 1–1. Alfred Strauss (1881–1971).

During the 1940s, the concept of resection of the diseased colon, first as a staged and then as a one-stage colectomy, with or without synchronous excision of the rectum, began to be performed.

A wide variety of procedures have been introduced to obviate the need for an incontinent stoma. These include the ileorectal anastomosis, the Koch pouch, and now the ileoanal anastomosis with pouch.

The future must lie with the discovery of the etiology (or etiologies) of ulcerative colitis and its prevention or specific treatment. No doubt, future surgeons will be just as amazed that surgeons of today have to remove the whole of the large bowel because its mucosa is inflamed as present surgeons are amazed by the surgical treatment of pulmonary tuberculosis in the preantibiotic era.

Cancer of the Rectum

Cancer of the rectum, with its vivid local symptoms and its ready detection by the insertion of the finger into the fundament, was well known to the ancients. Celsus, in the first century A.D., even describes the use of caustics and the cautery in its treatment. John of Arderne gave a good description of rectal cancer in the fourteenth century and states, "I never saw nor heard of any man that was cured of cancer of the rectum but I have known many that died of the foresaid sickness."

Once autopsies began to be performed routinely, cancers of the colon were frequently observed. Thus, Matthew Baillie (1793) gave an excellent description of bowel cancer:

> Schirrus is a disease which takes place much more commonly in the great than in the small intestines, but the latter are occasionally affected by it . . . in the great intestine at an advanced period of life, Schirrus is not uncommon; it is not equally liable to affect every portion of this intestine, but is to be found much more frequently at the sigmoid flexure of the colon, or in the rectum, than anywhere else; the reason of this it is, perhaps difficult to determine.[24]

He proceeds to debate whether this condition is attributable to the increased amount of glandular tissue of the mucosa of the distal large intestine, or whether narrowness at the sigmoid makes it more susceptible to damage by the passage of hard fecal material. He describes the ulceration of the mucosa, the progressive obstruction of the bowel lumen with proximal intestinal distention, and ulceration into adjacent viscera. Interestingly, he does not mention secondary deposits in the liver (or "tubercles") as an associated phenomenon.

Treatment of Cancer of the Rectum

Until comparatively recent times, of course, the treatment of rectal cancer was entirely palliative. Warm baths, anodyne and emollient enemas, opium-containing medicines, and dilatations of the malignant stricture with bougies and tents were employed. Because the tumor was thought by some to be of venereal origin, mercurials were sometimes used. In cases in which the tumor was pedunculated, more radical, surgical treatment might be employed. Thus Heister (1753) writes,

> The root of the tumour ought to be divided, if it be not over-large, either by ligature, the scissars or knife; if the root is too large to be conveniently separated by ligature, it may be performed either with the scissars or knife, holding the tumour fast with a hook or pliers. The wound being permitted to bleed in proportion to the strength of the patient, in order to prevent a consequent inflammation, and, after stopping the haemorrhage with proper styptics, the wound may be dressed at first with scraped lint, compress and bandage; but afterwards it may be proper to apply some vulnerary balsam, desiccative ointment, and, lastly, dry lint, in order to cicatrize and heal the part. Care should be taken, in the subsequent dressings, to remove any small part of the tumour that may yet remain behind, either by cutting them off with scissars, or corroding them with blue stone.[6]

The early history of extirpation of the rectum for cancer has been well documented by Gabriel.[25] The first surgeon to amputate the rectum for cancer was Lisfranc in 1826, and 3 years later he had performed nine such operations. His procedure comprised an oval perianal incision, dissection of the distal rectum, and its amputation above the growth. This resulted, of course, in the formation of an uncontrollable perineal colostomy. In 1873, Verneuil improved access by excision of the coccyx. The following year, Theodore Kocher, of Berne, performed preliminary closure of the anus with a pursestring suture in order to prevent fecal contamination of the wound. The extent of the operation was also increased by Kocher, because his aseptic technique allowed the peritoneal cavity to be opened from below with more adequate mobilization of the upper rectum.

In 1885, Paul Kraske introduced his well-known operation of sacral resection of the rectum, exposure being achieved by removal of the coccyx and lower sacrum. The peritoneum was freely opened from below, the pelvic colon mobilized and brought down, and following resection of the growth, an end-to-end anastomosis was carried out to the rectal stump. If this was impossible, a sacral colostomy was established.

The Kraske operation became extremely popular on the continent of Europe but had the disadvantage of a high rate of anastomotic breakdown. Hochenegg developed a pull-through technique, in which the proximal colonic segment was brought out through the anal canal and either sutured to the everted rectal stump or allowed to become adherent after excision of the lining of the anal canal. The Kraske operation and its modifications had the advantages of a relatively low mortality and reasonable survival results. Thus Mandl, in a review of 984 such operations at Hochenegg's clinic in Vienna, was able to show a mortality of 11.6% with 30% of good results after 5 years.

Although it had advocates in both the United Kingdom and the United States, the conservative sacral resection operation never became popular in these countries, probably because of the high risk of the breakdown of the anastomosis, the formation of troublesome fecal fistulas in the sacral region, and the development of stricture.

Lockhart-Mummery (1923), who had been Allingham's assistant and then his successor at St. Mark's Hospital, was responsible for the development of an effective technique of perineal resection of the rectum in the early years of this century.[26] A preliminary laparotomy was performed and a loop colostomy fashioned. The perineal stage could then be performed at once but was more usually delayed for 10 days and carried out in the left semiprone position. The incision started from the base of the sacrum and widely encircled the anus. The coccyx was excised, the levator ani divided well clear of the bowel, the peritoneum opened, the lateral ligaments divided, and the rectum then drawn down so that the superior rectal vessels could be ligated and divided as high as possible. The colon was then divided between crushing clamps in the upper part of the wound, and the blind stump closed. The peritoneum was then sutured with catgut, leaving the sigmoid stump on the wound side of the pelvic diaphragm. The skin wound was then closed with mattress stitches without drainage, but any fluid collection was evacuated by passing dressing forceps between sutures on the first postoperative day. The author states that the operation should not take more than 45 minutes; the patient should be out of bed in 14 days and usually able to return home in 3 weeks. Ordinary solid food is given from the start.

This operation had the disadvantage of leaving a blind sigmoid stump distal to the colostomy, which might leak and give rise to a mucous fistula. However, it was a relatively adequate cancer operation and had the advantage, in the days of fairly primitive anaesthesia and rarity of blood transfusion, of being relatively simple and having a low mortality rate, in the region of 10%. Up to the 1930s it was probably the most commonly employed technique in the United States and the United Kingdom.

Abdominoperineal Excision

Removal of the rectum by a combined abdominal and perineal operation was first performed by Czerny in 1884. Although this was not a planned procedure, it had to be carried out because an attempted sacral excision was impossible to complete from below. A number of other surgeons employed this method, but it was Ernest Miles (1908) who established the definitive abdominoperineal operation.[27] Miles, who was surgeon to the Cancer and the Gordon Hospitals in London, was disturbed by the high rate of early recurrence in his own experience of the perineal method of rectal excision. Careful postmortem examinations convinced him of the importance of wide and extensive excision of the rectum, the anal canal, the levator ani

muscles (in considerable part), the pelvic peritoneum adjacent to the rectum, and the pelvic mesocolon and its contained lymph nodes. He particularly stressed the importance of high ligation of the vascular pedicle below the point where it gives off its uppermost branch to the pelvic colon.

Dr. Harvey White has kindly made available to me the notes of the first such operation performed by Miles at the Cancer Hospital (now the Royal Marsden Hospital). The patient was a house painter, aged 55 years, and the operation was carried out on February 21, 1907. After performing the abdominal part of the operation, the patient was turned on the right side for the perineal procedure. The cavity of the pelvis was packed with gauze and a small tube drain placed in the lower part of the wound. He notes, "The actual removal of the gut and growth through the perineum was quite easily and quickly done, there being little need for rough handling, and haemorrhage was easily controlled. The full time for the operation was 1 hour 45 minutes." The patient was discharged on April 27 and labeled "cured."

Miles was a master technician. He operated in a calm, unhurried manner so that, as Lord Moynihan remarked when he watched him, "the clock stood still"; however, when the clock was consulted, it was often noticed that the entire operation of abdominoperineal excision of the rectum had taken, in many cases, no longer than 30 minutes.

The great disadvantage of this procedure initially was the high mortality. In Miles' first 62 cases there were no less than 22 deaths, although this was reduced

---

EDITORIAL COMMENT

In his *Lancet* 1908 description of the abdominoperineal resection, Miles stated that until 1906 he had relied solely upon the perineal methods of excision of the rectum. He performed 57 such operations, only to have recurrence in 54 patients. From postmortem examination Miles observed that the recurrences were commonly in the pelvic peritoneum, the pelvic mesocolon, and the lymph nodes situated over the bifurcation of the left common iliac artery. With these observations in mind, Miles designed his operation based on four principles: (1) that an abdominal anus was necessary; (2) that the whole of the pelvic colon must be removed; (3) that the whole of the pelvic mesocolon below the point where it crosses the common iliac artery must be cleared away; (4) that the lymph nodes situated over the bifurcation of the common iliac artery are to be removed; and (5) that the perineal portion of the operation should be carried out as widely as possible so that the lateral and downward zones of spread may be effectively extirpated. Miles stated that the operation performed took from 1¼ hours to 1½ hours and that he hoped a future series of cases would show a lower degree of mortality than 41.6%.

in his third 100 cases to 13 deaths. This mortality was greatly reduced, of course, with the introduction of modern anaesthesia, antibiotics, and routine blood transfusion.

The synchronous combined excision was originally suggested by Charles Mayo and practiced by Kirschner of Heidelberg in 1934 and by Devine in Australia in 1937. This two-team approach was popularized by Lloyd-Davies and Clifford Naunton Morgan at St. Mark's Hospital, where it was first performed in 1938, and greatly assisted by the invention of the Lloyd-Davies adjustable leg supports, which allowed the operation to be performed in comfort in the lithotomy-Trendelenburg position.[28] Certainly, this has now become the standard technique for the operation in the United Kingdom.

The penalty of these procedures, of course, is the permanent colostomy, and many surgeons had attempted removal of cancers of the upper part of the rectum without sacrifice of the anal sphincter. Already noted were the Kraske operation and the pull-through procedure of Hochenegg. Operations of this type, however, not only were technically difficult but appeared to contravene the principles of radical surgery laid down by Miles, particularly with regard to the downward spread of the tumor. However, from 1930 onward, further studies on the pathology and spread of rectal malignant disease, particularly by Westhues and by Cuthbert Dukes, showed that the lymphatic spread of rectal cancer is, indeed, mainly in an upward direction. This provided a renewal of interest in the possibility of spinchter preservation. A variety of techniques were employed, including abdominosacral resection and abdominoanal pull-through resection. However, most centers employ anterior resection with anastomosis as low as at the anorectal ring. This procedure was pioneered by Dixon of the Mayo Clinic in the 1930s, and in spite of early opposition, this procedure has stood the test of time.[29] Unquestionably, the introduction of the stapling gun has greatly increased the popularity of this operation.

Colostomy

A splendid account is given by Sir Zachary Cope (1965) of the early history of colostomy, which dates among the earliest of abdominal surgical procedures.[30] Littré suggested the feasibility of opening the colon to relieve large bowel obstruction in 1710, as a result of performing an autopsy in an infant with an imperforate anus. It fell to Pillore of Rouen, France, to perform the first cecostomy in 1776. The patient was a wine merchant with chronic large bowel obstruction due to a scirrhous

tumor of the upper rectum. The distended cecum was exposed through a transverse abdominal incision, opened, and fixed to the margins of the wound with a couple of sutures. The operation produced great relief of the obstruction, but the patient died on the 28th postoperative day owing to necrosis of a loop of jejunum produced by the large amounts of mercury (amounting to 2 pounds in weight), which had been given in the original conservative attempts to overcome the obstruction.

> **EDITORIAL COMMENT**
> The analogy of the unfortunate vintner to his counterparts 200 years later is inescapable: a patient survives the operative procedure only to succumb to the toxicity of doubtful adjuvant therapy.

Pierre Fine, of Geneva, carried out the first successful transverse colostomy in 1797. The patient, a woman aged 63 years, with a rectosigmoid obstructing growth, lived for 3½ months before dying of ascites.

A number of successes were reported of "artificial anus" in infants with imperforate anus, but the next successful case in an adult was reported by Pring in 1820. With regard to the inconveniences of a colostomy, Pring wrote, "she is now at no loss for an interest, and is provided with something to think of for the rest of her life." Small comfort indeed, even for a phlegmatic English woman.

The risk of opening the large bowel in those preantiseptic days was peritonitis from escape of the gut contents. Amussat in 1839 carried out autopsy studies after injecting the colon with air and demonstrated that the dilated left colon could be approached extraperitoneally through a lumbar approach. He carried out the first such operation in 1839, evacuating three wash basins full of fecal material. "This large evacuation and the escape of gas which was greviously distending the abdomen allowed the patient to breathe freely and to express joyfully how relieved she felt."

For the next 40 years, lumbar colostomy remained the operation of choice in patients with obstruction of the lower large bowel and continued to be a palliative procedure in patients with advanced rectal cancers.

The introduction of antiseptic surgery, following Lister's classic papers in 1867, obviated the need for the lumbar approach. It was an operation that was difficult in the obese subject, the exposure of the colon could be awkward, the peritoneum was frequently accidentally opened, and the position of the lumbar colostomy made its management difficult. By 1890, lumbar colostomy had fallen out of use and had been replaced by the iliac approach.

Treatment of Cancer of the Colon

We have already described the earliest contributions to the treatment of colonic cancer, which were directed to the relief of intestinal obstruction by means of the formation of an "artificial anus."

Although Reybard of Lyons, France, performed a successful resection of a sigmoid colon growth in 1823 (the patient, a man of 29 years of age, survived for 1 year), the development of general anesthesia and the introduction of antiseptic surgery were needed before a flood of reports of attempted curative operations on large bowel tumors was reported. Interesting accounts of these are given by Meade,[31] by Rankin and Graham,[32] and by Welch.[33]

In 1879 Czcrny successfully resected a colonic growth with end-to-end anastomosis, and in the same year Billroth performed a colonic resection and brought the proximal end of the bowel out of the abdominal wound as a colostomy. By the end of 1899 the number of reported resections had risen to 57 with 19 operative deaths, a mortality rate of 37%. The majority of these deaths were due to peritonitis, the infection taking place either during the operation or from leakage or necrosis ot the suture line in the colon some 5 to 10 days after operation. It was soon appreciated that resection and anastomosis of the colon, especially its left half, was much more dangerous than the same procedure elsewhere along the alimentary canal, and surgeons turned their attention (as they do today) to the solution of this problem.

An early approach was excision of the tumor with exteriorization. Initially, this involved exteriorization of the loop of bowel containing the tumor, with or without insertion of a tube to drain the proximal limb of the loop. At the second stage the protruding growth was removed, and at a third stage the resulting colostomy was closed, usually by crushing the spur with an enterotome. Successful cases were reported by Heineke in 1884, Maydel in 1886, and Bloch in 1894. The following year, Paul published his technique in which he exteriorized the affected loop, sutured a glass tube into the bowel above and below the site of the tumor, and then immediately excised the growth, thus reducing the operation to a two-stage procedure.[34] Mikulicz of Breslau popularized this procedure on the continent of Europe and was able to show a reduction in operative mortality in his own cases from 43%, when he attempted primary anastomosis, to 12.5%, for the exteriorization technique, which subsequently came to be termed the Paul-Mikulicz operation.

Undoubtedly this represented a considerable advance in making colonic surgery safe. The disadvantages were difficulty of the procedure when applied to bulky tumors or growths in the nonmobile segments of the large bowel, and the fact that adequate resection of the areas of lymphatic drainage was impossible. Indeed, local recurrence in the wound was not uncommon.

Safe modern surgery of primary resection and anastomosis of the large bowel depended first on the development of efficient techniques of bowel anastomosis, with contributions by Lembert, Halsted, the Mayo brothers, Cushing, Connell, Moynihan, and many others. The importance of operating on a decompressed bowel with the risk of primary resection in the event of large bowel obstruction, the importance of adequate blood supply at the anastomosis, and the protective effects of efficient antibiotics (including the need for antibiotic cover during the perioperative period) were all major factors that came to be understood in the development of resection with an immediate anastomosis of elective cases, as practiced today.

In the presence of obstruction, today's surgeon has the choice of preliminary decompression by means of a colostomy or cecostomy, on-table decompression of the bowel, or resection of the entire distended large bowel down to and beyond the growth by means of immediate ileocolic anastomosis.

CONCLUSION

Henry Ford said, "History is bunk." Like so many sayings of the great, the reverse is true. The surgeon of today can learn much from the genius, inventiveness, and imagination as well as the mistakes of his surgical forebears. Moreover, the innovative surgeon is likely to discover, when delving into history, the real truth of another old proverb: "There is nothing new under the sun."

REFERENCES

1. Banov L. The Chester Beatty Medical Papyrus: The earliest known treatise completely devoted to anorectal diseases. Surgery 1965;58:1037–1043.
2. Adams F. The Genuine Works of Hippocrates translated from the Greek. Baltimore: Williams & Wilkins, 1939.
3. Cooper A. The Lectures of Sir Astley Cooper Bart on the Principles and Practice of Surgery. Vol 2. London: Underwood, 1825.
4. Milligan ETC, Morgan C, Naunton Jones LE, Officer R. Surgical anatomy of the anal canal, and the operative treatment of haemorrhoids. Lancet 1937;2:1119.
5. Andrews E. The treatment of haemorrhoids by injection. Med Rec 1879;15:451.
6. Heister L. A General System of Surgery. 5th ed. [English translation]. London, 1753.

7. Allingham W. Fistula, Haemorrhoids, Painful Ulcer, Stricture, Prolapsus and Other Diseases of the Rectum, Their Diagnosis and Treatment. 4th ed. London: Churchill, 1882.

8. Arderne J. Treatises of fistula in ano, haemorrhoids and clysters. In: Power D, Kegan P, eds. London: Trench, Trubner, 1910.

9. Pott P. Remarks on the Disease Commonly Called a Fistula in Ano. London: Hawes, Clarke and Collins, 1765.

10. Cruveilhier J. Traité d'Anatomié Pathologique Général. Paris: Bailliére, 1849, 1:492.

11. Habershon SO. Pathological and practical observations on diseases of the alimentary canal. London: Churchill, 1857, p 296.

12. Keith A. Diverticula of the alimentary tract of congenital and of obscure origin. Br Med J 1910;1:376.

13. Graser E. Über multiple falsche Darmdivertikel in der Flexura sigmoidea. Munch Med Wschr 1899;46:74.

14. Telling WHM, Gruner OC. Acquired diverticula, diverticulitis and peridiverticulitis of the large intestine. Br J Surg 1917; 4:468.

15. Morison R. Surgical Contributions. Bristol: Wright, 1916, p 623.

16. Spriggs EI, Marxer OA. Intestinal diverticula. Br Med J 1926;1:130.

17. Myren J. Inflammatory bowel disease—a historical perspective. In: de Dombal FT, Myren J, Bouchier IAD, Watkinson G, eds. Inflammatory Bowel Disease. Oxford: Oxford University Press, 1986.

18. Wilks S, Moxon W. Lectures on Pathological Anatomy. 2nd ed. London: Churchill, 1875.

19. Allchin WH. A case of extensive ulceration of the colon. Trans Path Soc Lond 1885;36:199–202.

20. Svartz N. Salazopyrin—a new sulfanilamide preparation. Acta Med Scand 1942;110:577–598.

21. Truelove SC, Witts LJ. Cortisone in ulcerative colitis. Br Med J 1954;2:375.

22. Goligher JC, de Dombal FT, Watts JM, Watkinson G. Ulcerative Colitis. London: Bailliére Tindall and Cassell, 1968.

23. Brooke BN. Ulcerative Colitis and Its Surgical Treatment. Edinburgh: Livingstone, 1954.

24. Baillie M. The Morbid Anatomy of Some of the Most Important Parts of the Human Body. London: Johnson, 1793.

25. Gabriel WB. The Principles and Practice of Rectal Surgery. 5th ed. London: Lewis, 1963.

26. Lockhart-Mummary J. Diseases of the Rectum and Colon. London: Bailliére, Tindall and Cox, 1923.

27. Miles WE. A method of performing abdomino-perineal excision for carcinoma of the rectum and the terminal portion of the pelvis colon. Lancet 1908;2:1812.

28. Morgan CN. Carcinoma of the rectum. Ann Roy Coll Surg 1965;36:73–97.

29. Dixon CF. Anterior resection for malignant lesions of the upper part of the rectum and lower part of the sigmoid. Trans Am Surg Assoc 1948;66:175.

30. Cope Z. A History of the Acute Abdomen. London: Oxford University Press, 1965.

31. Meade RH. An Introduction to the History of General Surgery. Philadelphia: WB Saunders, 1968.

32. Rankin FW, Graham AS. Cancer of the Colon and Rectum. 2nd ed. Springfield, IL: Charles C Thomas, 1945.

33. Welch CE. The historical development of surgical treatment of cancer of the colon and rectum. In: Beahrs OH, Higgins GA, Weinstein JJ. Colorectal Tumours. Philadelphia: JB Lippincott, 1986.

34. Paul FT. Colectomy. Br Med J 1895;1:1136.

Surgical Anatomy and Embryology of the Colon, Rectum, and Anus

C H A P T E R   2

John Dunn
Nicholas A. Halasz

COLON AND APPENDIX

The anatomy of the large intestine is relatively constant, especially that of the transverse and descending segments. Variations in the position of the appendix and the mobility of the cecum are related to the region of the primitive gut from which the right colon develops and to the greater complexity of the developmental changes that form the appendix and cecum. These observations become apparent in the following discussion.

Although the colon does not have a continuous mesentery, such as that of the small bowel, the transverse and sigmoid segments do have mesenteries that allow varying degrees of mobility. For example, the transverse colon may remain as high as the epigastrium or may drop as low as the pelvis. The sigmoid colon usually remains in the left lower quadrant, but because of the sigmoid mesentery, it may extend across to the right lower quadrant. Thus, acute diverticulitis may occasionally mimic acute appendicitis.

One can more fully understand these variations by examining how the colon and the appendix develop from the primitive midgut and hindgut during gestation.

Development of the Colon and the Appendix

The Colon

An endodermal tube surrounded by mesoderm forms the primitive gastrointestinal tract. The endoderm de-velops into the epithelial and glandular lining cells of the gut, whereas the mesoderm forms the muscular and connective tissue layers as well as the peritoneum. Three distinct areas form in the primitive gut: the foregut, which develops into the esophagus, stomach, and duodenum; the midgut, which forms the small intestine, right colon, and most of the transverse colon; and the hindgut, which forms the remainder of the colon and rectum. The midgut is defined as the portion of the primitive gut that develops within the extraembryonic coelom between gestational weeks 5 and 10. The hindgut remains within the embryonic coelom proper during its development.

The midgut is attached at its midsection to the yolk stalk (vitelline duct). Just distal to this attachment, a small diverticulum forms on the antimesenteric side of the midgut at a gestational age of about 5 weeks; this will become the cecum. Simultaneously, the midgut begins to elongate so rapidly that it begins to coil on itself and prolapses into the extraembryonic coelom. At about 7 weeks, the midgut begins to rotate counterclockwise, thus positioning the cecum to the right of the cranial portion of the midgut and the transverse colon ventral to the foregut (stomach and duodenum). Shortly thereafter, the hindgut begins to elongate distal to the cecum to form the ascending colon. This elongation, combined with rotation, changes the relationship of the terminal ileum to the cecum, so that the former end-to-end relationship becomes an end-to-side one. These processes also account for the usual C-shaped form of the large intestine enclosing the small intestines.

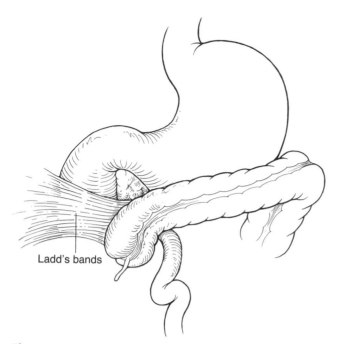

Figure 2–1. Ladd's bands in association with incomplete midgut rotation during development.

At about 10 weeks the abdominal cavity is large enough to accommodate all of the intestinal tract, and the developing midgut begins to move back through the umbilical ring from the yolk stalk. The small intestines retract ahead of the developing cecum and push the descending colon toward the left side of the abdominal cavity, thus establishing the descending colon's characteristically close apposition to the body wall.

In contrast, the cecum has a variable amount of mobility, depending on the degree of the tightness of the fusion between the right colon and the posterior body wall. The cecum does not have a mesentery, because it developed as an outpouching of the anti-mesenteric border of the primitive midgut. When the posterior attachments fail to anchor the cecum to any degree and/or fail to fuse with the posterior body wall, the cecum and ascending colon are particularly mobile ("floppy cecum" syndrome) and may fold cranially and medially upon themselves to cause obstruction (cecal volvulus or bascule) in the adult.

When rotation is incomplete, the cecum remains abnormally high in the abdominal cavity, and peritoneal bands that normally fix the cecum to the lateral body wall may obstruct the duodenum (Ladd's bands) (Fig. 2–1). Furthermore, the usual elongated attachment of the mesenteric root does not develop; thus the root of the midgut mesentery is nearly a single point based on the superior mesenteric vessels, instead of an oblique line from left upper quadrant to right lower quadrant as is normally found (Fig. 2–2). Subsequently, the small bowel may rotate about this point, resulting in midgut ischemia in the newborn.

The Appendix

As the cecum begins to enlarge, the distal end lags behind the more proximal end and remains small, resulting in a slender blind sac of bowel of various lengths (2 to 20 cm in the adult), known as the vermiform appendix. Because the anterolateral portion of the cecum tends to enlarge more than the postero-medial aspect, the appendix appears to originate from the more posteromedial aspect of the cecum, and the cecum is sacculated farther toward the right (Fig. 2–3).

Anatomy of the Colon and the Appendix

The human colon is distinguished by the condensation of the external longitudinal muscle layer into three bands called *teniae coli*. Because the teniae are shorter than the rest of the colon, outpouchings of the colon between the teniae form a series of sacculations, known as haustra (see Fig 2–2), that can usually be visualized

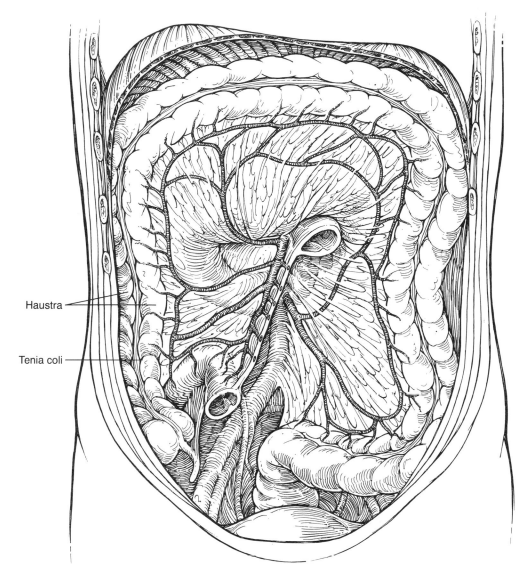

Figure 2–2. Position of the colon in the abdominal cavity.

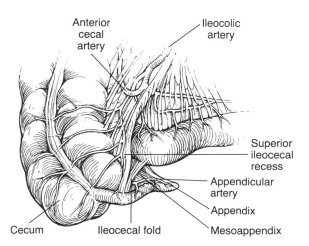

Figure 2–3. The cecum and vermiform appendix.

on plain radiographs of the abdomen. The teniae coalesce at the cecal point where the appendix emerges; thus when the appendix is difficult to find (e.g., if it is retrocecal), one may follow the teniae down to the end of the cecum to locate the base of the appendix. Another distinguishing characteristic of the colon is the presence of fatty appendages from the peritoneally covered teniae called *appendices epiploicae*.

As noted, the colon has no continuous mesentery, but rather the ascending and descending colon segments lie directly on the posterior body wall with peritoneum reflected over the medial, anterior, and lateral walls of the colon (Fig. 2–4). Paracolic gutters are formed laterally by the reflection of the peritoneum between the lateral body walls and the ascending and descending colon segments. The transverse colon has its own mesentery, as does the sigmoid colon, and these are described further on.

The Appendix

The orifice of the vermiform appendix is circular and found about 3 cm distal to the ileocecal valve. Its narrow lumen renders the appendix prone to obstruction, and because it is a blind end, further pathologic conditions ensue readily. Supplied with its own small, triangular mesentery, called the mesoappendix, the appendix is thus completely invested by peritoneum (see Fig. 2–3). It usually projects medially and downward toward or across the pelvic brim. However, about 25% of the time the appendix is retrocecal (fused to either the cecum or the posterior body wall), or, less commonly, the appendix is in a retroileal position.

The visceral innervation of the appendix derives from the superior mesenteric plexus. Thus, the initial pain of acute appendicitis (i.e., visceral pain from gut wall distention) is nearly always referred to the epigastric or periumbilical region of the abdomen. The somatic pain varies, depending on the lie of the appendix. When the appendix is retrocecal, the pain may be principally manifested in the back or flank. When the cecum and appendix are unusually long and the appendix rests in the pelvis, the somatic pain is suprapubic. A retroileal appendix may cause testicular pain in males as a result of irritation of the testicular artery.

The Cecum and Anterior Cecal Artery

The cecum may lie as high as the iliac crest or may lie below the pelvic brim, depending on the degree of elongation of the ascending colon. Most commonly it lies somewhere between the two. The peritoneum becomes thickened between the antimesenteric border of the ileum and cecum as well as the base of the appendix to form the ileocecal fold. Division of this

fold during an appendectomy can usually be performed without ligatures, as it is relatively avascular.

Another fold of peritoneum can often be found between the terminal ileum and the ascending colon, just above the ileocecal junction. It contains the anterior cecal artery and, if present, is called the vascular fold of the cecum. If the fold is prominent, there is a pocket, between it and the mesentery to both the terminal ileum and the ascending colon, called the superior ileocecal recess.

Ileocecal Valve

The ileocecal valve is formed by the circular muscular layer of the terminal ileum. Upper and lower labia form from this muscular layer with lateral and medial frenula covered by the epithelial lining of the colon. The upper lip tends to hang over the lower one, but as a valve, it is not very effective. It is not difficult to demonstrate contrast material flowing retrograde into the terminal ileum during contrast radiography and this technique is used to demonstrate terminal ileitis by the typical "string sign" (Kantor's sign).

Ascending Colon

Approximately 15 cm long, the ascending colon runs cephalad to a bend in the colon, which is known as the hepatic flexure. This portion of the colon is invested with peritoneum medially, anteriorly, and laterally. The posterior surface of the ascending colon rests on the quadratus lumborum proximally and centrally, while the cephalad portion lies in close apposition to the right kidney and right lobe of the liver (see Fig. 2–4). The medial aspect of the proximal ascending colon lies in close proximity to the right ureter and gonadal vessels, which are situated retroperitoneally. The root of the small bowel mesentery also is in close proximity to the proximal ascending colon (see Fig. 2–4). The cephalad portion of the ascending colon and hepatic flexure lies behind the posterior parietal peritoneum, directly over the right kidney and the second portion of the duodenum. Areolar tissue connects this part of the colon to these structures, and during a right hemicolectomy the surgeon must be particularly careful not to injure the duodenum, because it can be lifted into the plane of dissection as the hepatic flexure and transverse colon are elevated during resection (see Fig. 2–4).

The peritoneum covering the ascending colon becomes attached to the posterior body wall and forms the lateral paracolic sulcus. This gutter can conduct infectious material downward from an anterior duodenal perforation or perforated gallbladder, or conduct material upward from an inflamed and perforated appendix, sometimes leading the examiner to an im-

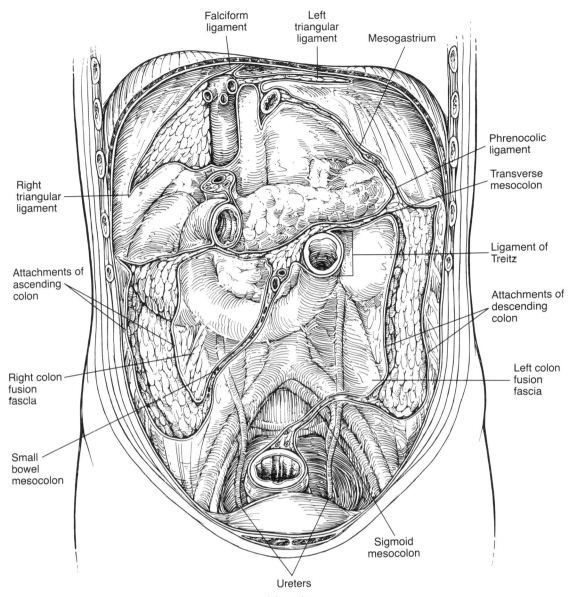

Figure 2–4. Peritoneal attachments and mesenteries of the colon.

proper diagnosis. It is this reflection onto the posterior body wall that the surgeon incises to mobilize the ascending colon. This is a fusion fascia, a relatively avascular tissue plane, and the colon with its blood supply and lymphatics can be lifted upward medially with gentle dissection, thus re-establishing the fetal mesentery.

Hepatic Flexure

The hepatic flexure represents an anteromedial bend in the right colon just below the right hepatic lobe. Behind and superior to the hepatic flexure, one finds the hepatorenal recess (Morison's pouch), which runs superiorly and posteriorly over the right kidney toward the diaphragm (see Fig. 2–4). Abscesses often form in

this space after free visceral perforations because this area is the most dependent portion of the peritoneum above the pelvic brim in the supine patient. Often a fold of peritoneum runs farther to the right than usual to form an attachment of the hepatic flexure to the liver and/or gallbladder; this is known as the hepatocolic ligament. At the hepatic flexure, the colon turns toward a transverse, slightly inferior, and ventral lie in front of coils of small intestine to begin the transverse colon.

Transverse Colon

The fundus of the gallbladder is usually draped over the first portion of the transverse colon; thus when a cholecystocolic fistula forms as the result of a large

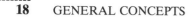

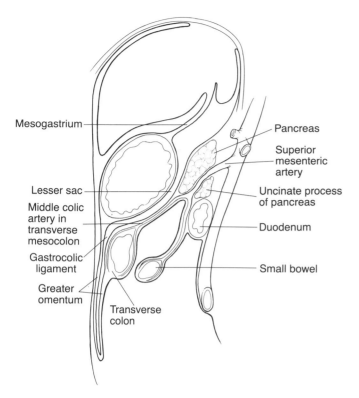

Figure 2–5. The transverse mesocolon and its relationships to the lesser sac and pancreas.

gallstone, it becomes connected to the proximal transverse colon. The transverse colon runs for approximately 45 cm with varying degrees of drop within the abdomen. It may traverse straight across to the splenic flexure, or it may hang as low as the mid portion of the sigmoid colon, depending on the length of the mesocolon.

Most of the transverse colon is completely invested by peritoneum. The mesentery to the transverse colon begins posteriorly and superiorly along the inferior border of the pancreas and forms the lower portion of the lesser sac (see Fig. 2–4; Fig. 2–5). The greater omentum hangs from the greater curvature of the stomach and becomes closely, although loosely, applied to the upper portion of the transverse mesocolon and transverse colon, before dropping to varying degrees over the loops of small bowel. By elevating the omentum, one can sharply dissect it off the colon and mesocolon in a bloodless fashion in order to enter the lesser sac. The surgeon may choose to enter the lesser sac directly through the gastrocolic ligament (the part of the great omentum between the stomach and the colon). In doing so, the surgeon must take care not to penetrate too deeply, because the transverse mesocolon near the colon is in very close apposition to the gastrocolic ligament and because the downward extent of the lesser sac is unpredictable. Thus, one could easily injure the middle colic artery in the process of dividing the gastrocolic ligament. The surgeon who

inadvertently penetrates the transverse mesocolon re-enters the greater peritoneal sac and will miss the lesser sac altogether.

Splenic Flexure

The splenic flexure represents a posterior and superior turning of the distal transverse colon such that this flexure lies higher and more posterior than the hepatic flexure. The apex of the splenic flexure lies at about the level of the middle section of the left kidney (see Fig. 2–4) and is very closely apposed to it, as this is where the transverse mesocolon disappears. The diaphragm and rib cage lie adjacent to the splenic flexure posteriorly and laterally. Peritoneum that covers the front of the splenic flexure thickens into a band that extends laterally to the diaphragm to form the phren-icocolic ligament. This band supports the colon and spleen (see Fig. 2–4). Care must be taken when retracting the splenic flexure downward, because attachments of the phrenicocolic ligament to the lower portion of the spleen, known separately as the lienocolic ligament, may cause a tear in the splenic capsule if retraction is too forceful.

The flexure itself is formed by an acute downward turn of the colon to begin the descending colon. As noted, the colon loses its mesentery as it crosses the left kidney. The narrow descending colon then descends vertically for about 20 cm, where, below the iliac crest, it crosses medially over the iliac vessels and left ureter. Below the iliac crest the colon again acquires a mesentery and becomes the sigmoid colon.

Sigmoid Colon

The sigmoid colon begins where the left colon crosses the medial margin of the left psoas muscle (see Fig. 2–4; Fig. 2–6). It is beyond this point that the mesentery is retained. The base of the mesentery runs superiorly and medially from the medial psoas margin and then vertically downward at or just to the left of the midline. The left ureter is usually located deep to the apex of the inverted V formed by the mesosigmoid (see Figs. 2–4 and 2–6). The sigmoid mesocolon becomes progressively shorter where the bowel begins its vertical descent over the sacrum, until it disappears where the sigmoid colon becomes the rectum near the level of the third sacral segment. The sigmoid loop rests within the pelvis, adjacent to the bladder in males and to the uterus and bladder in females. Both the sigmoid colon and the sigmoid mesocolon are of variable length. When they are particularly redundant, the sigmoid colon may twist upon itself, causing a blind loop obstruction and varying degrees of bowel ischemia (sigmoid volvulus) in the adult. Because the sigmoid colon ends at about 12 to 15 cm from the anal verge, a volvulus may be relieved by the gentle insertion of a sigmoidoscope; one should take care to dodge the explosive release of liquid stool when the point of obstruction is passed.

The teniae coli begin to disappear in the distal sigmoid colon as they spread to become a continuous longitudinal layer of muscle surrounding the rectum. This change in the teniae takes place over a variable distance of 7.5 to 10 cm in the distal sigmoid colon.

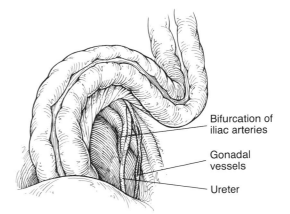

Bifurcation of iliac arteries

Gonadal vessels

Ureter

Figure 2–6. The sigmoid colon and mesosigmoid.

Blood Supply to the Colon

Arterial System

Embryologically, the foregut derives its blood supply from the celiac trunk; the midgut from the superior mesenteric artery (SMA), and the hindgut from the inferior mesenteric artery (IMA). The appendix, cecum, ascending colon, hepatic flexure, and transverse colon are supplied by branches from the SMA (Fig. 2–7). These branches include (in order from their origins from the SMA) the middle colic, right colic, and ileocolic arteries. The middle colic artery runs obliquely toward the right within the transverse mesocolon and then divides into right and left branches, which are components of the marginal artery. If the middle colic artery divides early, the left branch will arch obliquely toward the distal transverse colon.

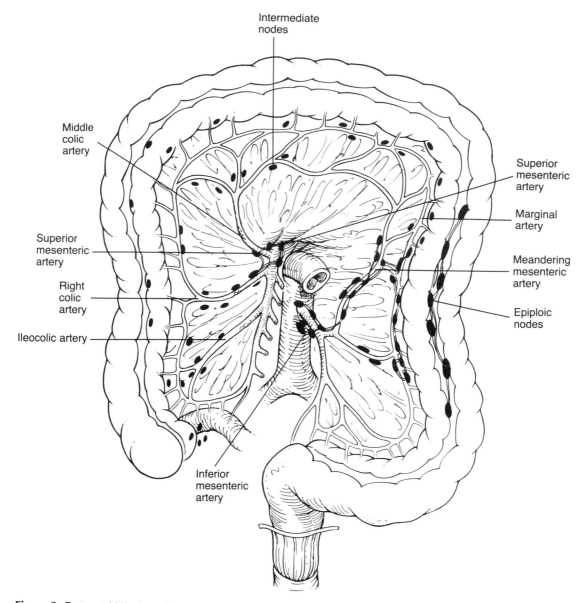

Figure 2–7. Arterial blood supply and associated lymph nodes of the colon.

When creating an opening in the transverse mesocolon (e.g., for a retrocolic gastroenterostomy), the surgeon must search for and avoid injury to the middle colic artery and its branches.

The right colic artery is quite variable, ranging from being a separate branch of the SMA (27%) to being totally absent (13%). It may arise from the middle colic artery or from the root of the ileocolic artery (26%) (see Fig. 2–7). The surgeon who performs a cecectomy must be wary that there is about a 1:3 chance of compromising the vascular supply to the entire right colon. The sigmoid colon, the descending colon, and the splenic flexure are supplied by branches of the IMA. The first branch is the left colic artery, which then divides into ascending and descending branches to supply the left colon. After several sigmoid arteries branch off from the IMA, it continues on as the superior rectal artery.

The marginal artery (already mentioned) represents a continuous vessel from the sigmoid arteries, anastomosing with the descending branch of the left colic artery. The descending branch, in turn, is continuous with the ascending branch of the left colic artery, which runs up the medial aspect of the left colon and around the splenic flexure to anastomose (48%) with the left branch of the middle colic artery, thus providing collateral circulation to the colon between the SMA and the IMA. Likewise, the right branch of the middle colic artery anastomoses with a branch from the right colic artery, and a branch of the ileocolic artery anastomoses with a branch of the right colic artery. Thus, the collateral circulation from the sigmoid colon to the cecum is completed (see Fig. 2–7). The whole anastomotic series of arteries is called the marginal artery (artery of Drummond). The anastomosis between the left branch of the middle colic artery and the ascending branch of the left colic artery is also known as the arch of Riolan. This anastomosis is present in only 48% of the population. Thus, the splenic flexure may be particularly vulnerable to ischemia in low-flow states.

Meandering Mesenteric Artery

A separate collateral artery, described in 1964, was named the "meandering mesenteric artery." The vessel usually originates from the proximal left colic artery and runs in a tortuous course superiorly medial to the ascending branch of the left colic (see Fig. 2–7). By anastomosing with a branch of the middle colic artery, it provides a potential supply of blood from the IMA system to the SMA system, or vice versa, depending on which mesenteric artery has more pressure and flow. If the surgeon encounters a particularly prominent meandering mesenteric artery, the presumption must be that it is an important conduit, and care must be taken to avoid injuring it.

Obviously, the implications of indiscriminately dividing a prominent meandering artery during a left colon resection can be appreciated. If the SMA were occluded and derived its flow through a patent IMA and meandering artery, dividing the meandering artery might cause ischemia in the entire small bowel and right colon. If there is antegrade flow through the meandering artery, such as occurs with an occluded IMA, ligating it may cause necrosis of the sigmoid colon and upper rectum and, possibly, ischemia in the lower extremities, as discussed further on.

Anastomoses

Another mesenteric vascular watershed was described by Sudeck in his study of the collateralization of vessels between the superior rectal and middle rectal arteries. He demonstrated poor anastomoses where the last branch from the superior rectal artery leaves to supply the rectosigmoid junction. Known as the critical point of Sudeck, it is the region of the rectosigmoid that he thought to be vulnerable to ischemia or infarction from low-flow states or occlusion of the IMA or superior rectal artery.

In fact, arteriographic studies have rendered Sudeck's point less critical by demonstrating usually adequate anastomoses between the middle and superior rectal arteries. It was shown how the pelvic organs and lower extremities could receive a blood supply despite total occlusion of the aorta. As long as there is flow in the mesenteric vessels down to the superior rectal artery, anastomoses between it and the middle rectal arteries can supply retrograde flow through the internal iliac arteries to the external iliac arteries. Similarly, if the IMA or superior rectal artery is occluded, these anastomoses could provide blood to the distal sigmoid via the hypogastric and middle rectal vessels.

One can imagine the lower extremities being supplied, through a series of collateral anastomoses, by the celiac artery alone if the SMA and IMA as well as the distal aorta were occluded. The blood would flow through the celiac trunk, common hepatic artery, gastroduodenal artery, pancreaticoduodenal arcade, SMA, middle colic artery, meandering artery, IMA, superior rectal artery, middle rectal artery, internal iliac artery, external iliac artery, and common femoral artery.

Venous Drainage

The venous drainage of the right colon follows the course of the branches of the SMA to form the superior mesenteric vein (SMV) (Fig. 2–8). The middle colic artery also has its associated vein that joins the SMV at the level of the inferior border of the pancreas. Although the sigmoid and left colons are drained by veins following the various arterial branches, these venous tributaries form the inferior mesenteric vein (IMV), which has its own distinctive course, running superiorly and medially in a retroperitoneal position. The IMV can easily be found just to the left of the ligament of Treitz, where it passes posterior to the pancreas to join the splenic vein, the SMV, or their confluence, where the portal vein begins. Portosystemic connections are present between the veins draining the ascending and descending colon and the veins draining the posterior body wall to the inferior vena cava. Other connections occur at the hepatic and splenic flexures between mesenteric veins and renal veins. These connections become prominent with portal hypertension, particularly around the renal veins.

Lymphatic Drainage of the Colon

The lymphatics of the colon follow the vasculature to the colon in the embryonal (lost) mesenteries. Therefore, these mesenteries must be re-established to remove nodes. There are essentially four levels of lymph nodes: epicolic, paracolic, intermediate, and principal, or periaortic, nodes (Fig. 2–9). Lymphatics draining the splenic flexure, the descending colon, and the sigmoid colon run toward the IMA nodes, which drain into periaortic lumbar nodes. SMA nodes are end points for lymphatics draining the remainder of the colon, including the splenic flexure. Lymphatics leaving

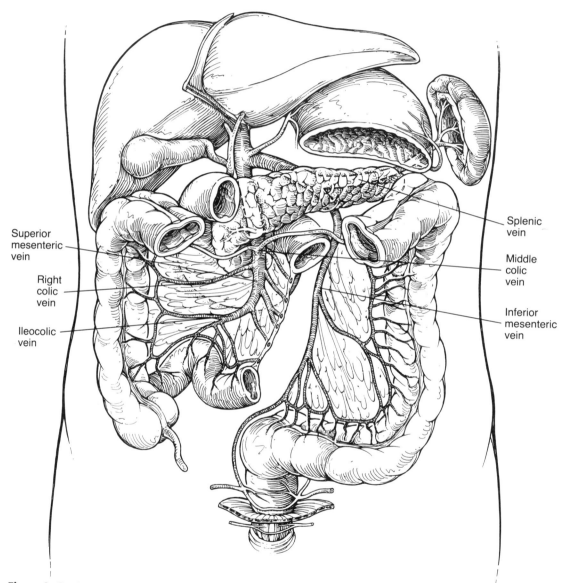

Superior
mesenteric
vein

Right
colic
vein

Ileocolic
vein

Splenic
vein

Middle
colic
vein

Inferior
mesenteric
vein

Figure 2–8. The venous drainage of the colon.

the SMA nodes drain into celiac and upper lumbar nodes, which together give rise to the intestinal trunk that helps form the cisterna chyli. Thus, the splenic flexure lymphatics may drain toward either the SMA or the IMA lymph nodes (see Figs. 2–7 and 2–9).

Innervation of the Colon

Because the autonomic nervous system follows the blood supply to various organs, it follows that the nerve supply to the midgut-derived colon (right and transverse) is different from that of the hindgut-derived left and sigmoid colons (Fig. 2–10). The sympathetic fibers to the right colon or transverse colon arise from T7 to T12 and run down the sympathetic trunks to the celiac plexus via the thoracic splanchnic nerves. Without synapsing in the plexus, the sympathetic fibers course to the superior mesenteric and preaortic plexuses to the colon. The parasympathetic supply to the right and transverse colons arises mainly from the right trunk of the vagus nerve and passes through the celiac plexus.

The left and sigmoid colons obtain their sympathetic nerve supply from L1 and L2 segments via the lumbar splanchnic and preaortic plexus of nerves to the inferior mesenteric plexus. The parasympathetic supply arises from S2, S3, and S4 coming through the anterior sacral foramina and running forward, laterally, and superiorly to join sympathetic fibers along the pelvic side walls. Parasympathetic fibers travel along the presacral nerves up to the inferior mesenteric artery, where they turn sharply to reach the inferior mesenteric plexus and proceed to the left colon.

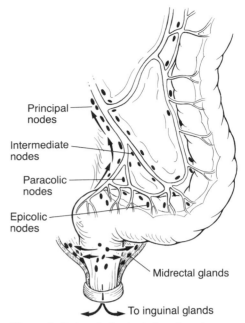

Principal nodes

Intermediate nodes

Paracolic nodes

Epicolic nodes

Midrectal glands

To inguinal glands

Figure 2–9. Level of colonic lymph nodes.

RECTUM AND ANUS

Development of the Rectum and the Anus

At approximately 3 weeks after fertilization, the embryonic gut extends into the tail as the beginning of the hindgut (Fig. 2–11A). The yolk sac opens into the midgut, and the allantois opens into the ventral surface of the hindgut. The gut is apposed to the skin at its distalmost end, where a membrane forms that is composed of entoderm and ectoderm: the cloacal membrane. During the fifth and sixth weeks, a transverse ridge arises at the angle where the allantois joins the cloaca and descends downward (Fig. 2–11B). This, the urorectal septum, meets lateral folds from both sides that permit completion of the separation of the cloaca into an anterior urogenital component and a posterior rectal one (Fig. 2–11C). This separation is complete at

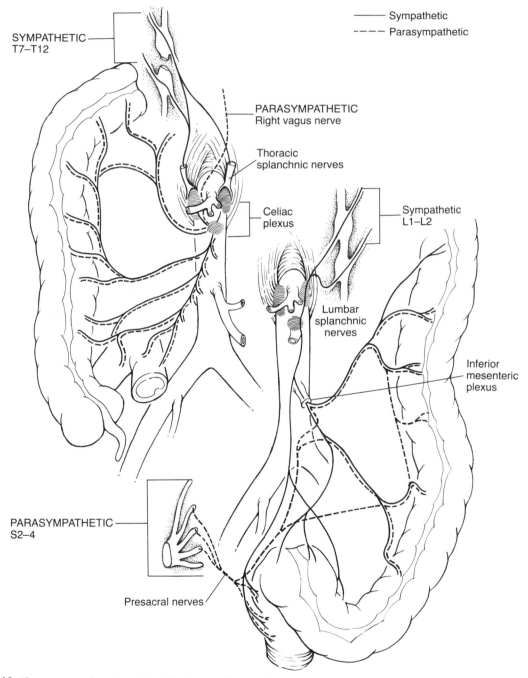

SYMPATHETIC
T7–T12

—— Sympathetic
- - - Parasympathetic

PARASYMPATHETIC
Right vagus nerve

Thoracic
splanchnic nerves

Celiac
plexus

Sympathetic
L1–L2

Lumbar
splanchnic
nerves

Inferior
mesenteric
plexus

PARASYMPATHETIC
S2–4

Presacral nerves

Figure 2–10. The nerve supply to the colon, like the vascular supply, is separate for the right and transverse and the left and sigmoid segments.

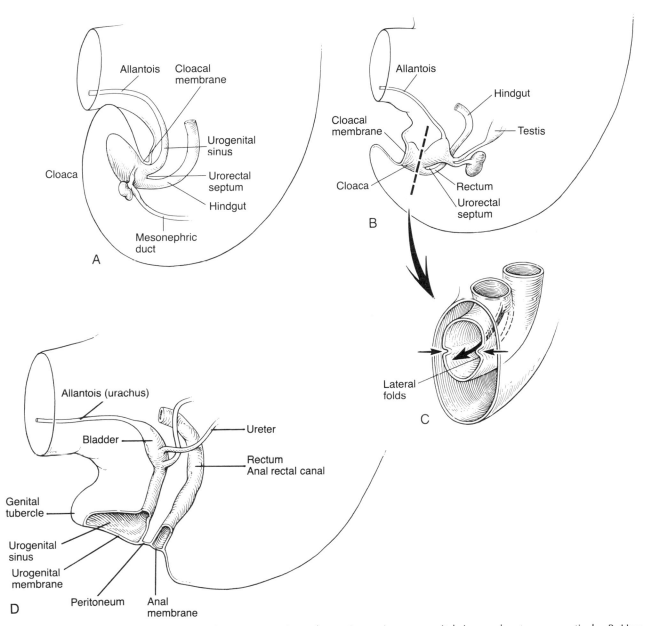

Figure 2–11. *A*, Beginning separation of the cloaca into anterior and posterior portions, urogenital sinus and rectum, respectively. *B*, Here the urorectal septum has descended farther and the lateral folds are beginning to form. The dashed line shows the level of the cross-section shown in C. *C*, Transverse section of the tail of the embryo showing the lateral folds that will ultimately divide the urogenital sinus from the rectum along with the urorectal septum. *D*, At 9 weeks, both openings have broken through to the outside. The mesonephric duct remnant has migrated distally and will become the ductus deferens.

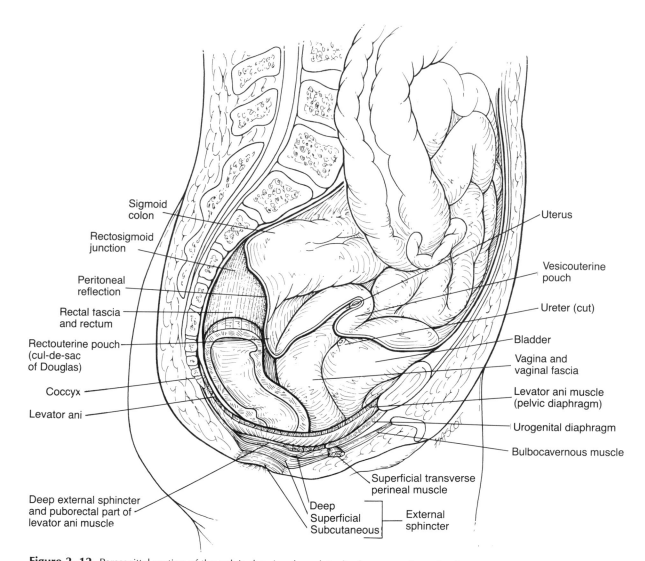

Figure 2–12. Parasagittal section of the pelvis showing the pelvic diaphragm, peritoneal reflections, and recesses.

about 7 weeks of age. The posterior remnant of the cloacal membrane, known as the anal membrane, ruptures usually in the ninth week; by this time the mesenchymal anlagen of the sphincteric apparatus have become apparent (Fig. 2–11*D*).

Anatomy of the Rectum and the Anus

The Rectum

The rectum is the continuation of the sigmoid colon, and it begins at the top of the middle piece of the sacrum, that is, at S3 (Fig. 2–12). At about this level the teniae coalesce to form a continuous longitudinal muscle layer. In spite of its name, the rectum is anything but straight. Its first 12 to 14 cm follow the curve of the sacrum and coccyx, so that at the lowermost end of this portion the rectum points downward

and forward. Below the tip of the coccyx it turns abruptly backward by about 75 degrees, with the puborectal sling acting as the turning point. As a result, there is an angulation in the course of the rectum, comparable to that between the vagina and uterine body but as a mirror image thereof. The lower portion, aimed backward and downward, measures 3 to 4 cm in length and ends at the anus. The rectum also exhibits flexures in the lateral direction. At or just above the sacrococcygeal junction it swings to the left, and at the midcoccyx it swings back to the midline. These lateral flexures give rise to the transverse rectal folds, or valves of Houston.

Peritoneal Relationships

The rectum, being the lower end of the intestinal canal, must pass through peritoneum to gain access to the outside (see Fig. 2–12; Fig. 2–13). Its upper third

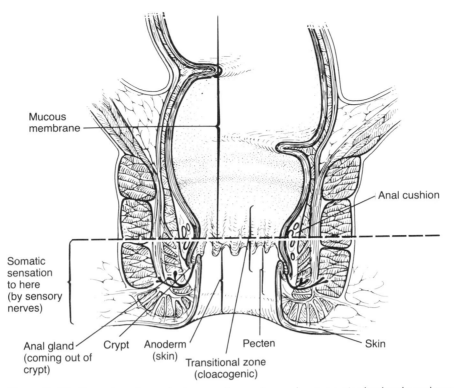

Figure 2–13. Coronal section to the lower rectum and anus showing major landmarks and muscles.

(between the top and middle valves of Houston) is essentially intraperitoneal, attached posteriorly by a short, stout mesorectum. The middle third (between the middle and lower valves) loses its peritoneum as the serosa sweeps forward and thereby creates an oblique transition from being intraperitoneal to retroperitoneal. Finally, the lower third of the rectum, below the inferior valve of Houston, is entirely extraperitoneal. As the peritoneum leaves the anterior surface of the rectum, it sweeps onto the back of the prostate and seminal vesicles in the male, usually 8 to 9 cm above the level of the perineal skin, and this creates the rectovesical pouch. In the female the peritoneum covers the top 1 to 2 cm of the back of the vagina and then extends up onto the back of the uterus. Its lowermost level is usually 5 to 7 cm above the perineum, in the rectovaginal pouch (pouch of Douglas).

Pelvic Fascia

The transversalis fascia sweeps over the pelvic brim and across the top of the pelvic diaphragm (levator ani), where it is known as the superior fascia of the pelvic diaphragm (Figs. 2–14 and 2–15). It is contiguous laterally with the obturator fascia, more posteriorly with the psoas fascia, and in back with the rectosacral fascia. These four components make up the endopelvic fascia. Separate fascial layers cover the inferior surface of the pelvic diaphragm, as well as both the superior and inferior surfaces of the urogenital diaphragm (the last also known as the perineal membrane). Thickenings in the superior fascia of the pelvic diaphragm serve to stabilize pelvic organs. Thus, the transverse cervical or cardinal ligaments (ligaments of Mackenrodt) stabilize the cervix laterally to the pelvic wall, and the uterosacral ligaments posteriorly to the sacrum; the rectosacral ligaments anchor the rectum to the periosteum of the sacrum. The lateral ligaments of the rectum extend in a coronal plane between the bowel and the superior fascia of the pelvic diaphragm, and they carry branches of the middle rectal vessels to the bowel.

The rectum is enveloped by its fascia propria. The sacrum, in turn, is covered by the rectosacral (Waldeyer's) fascia that is continuous with the endopelvic fascial layer. It extends down to the fourth or fifth sacral segment from where a part of it sweeps forward to fuse with the fascia propria. Mobilization of the rectum from above takes place between these two layers, ultimately extending to the anococcygeal ligament. This has to be divided in order to gain entry from below into the supralevator and the retrorectal spaces. The anterior layer of the fascia propria becomes more dense where the rectum is apposed to the prostate and seminal vesicles in the male, and the vagina in the female. This layer is known as Denonvilliers' fascia.

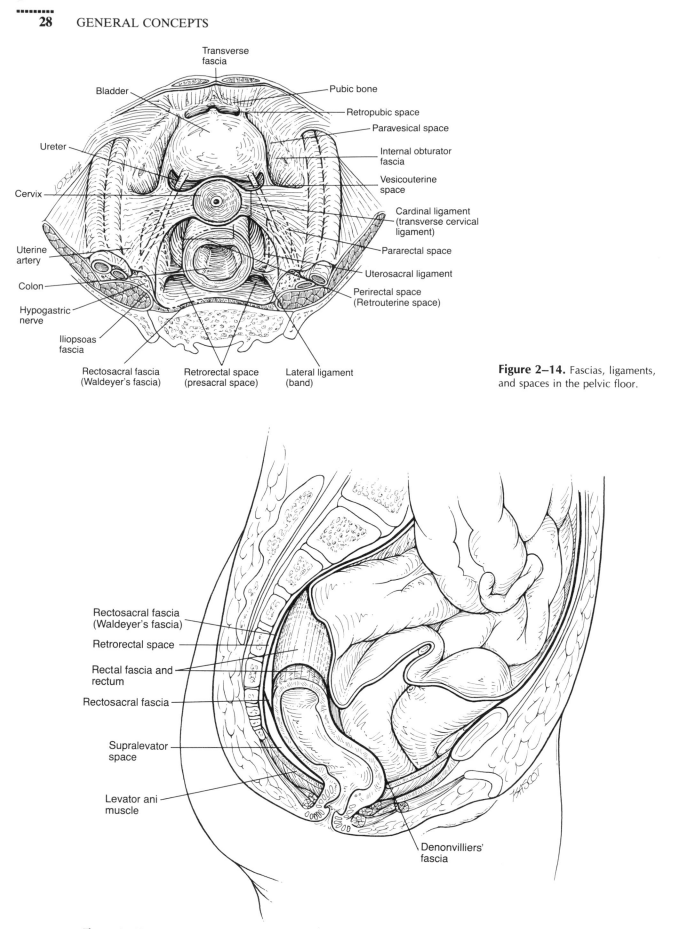

Figure 2–14. Fascias, ligaments, and spaces in the pelvic floor.

Figure 2–15. Sagittal view of spaces and fascias of the pelvis.

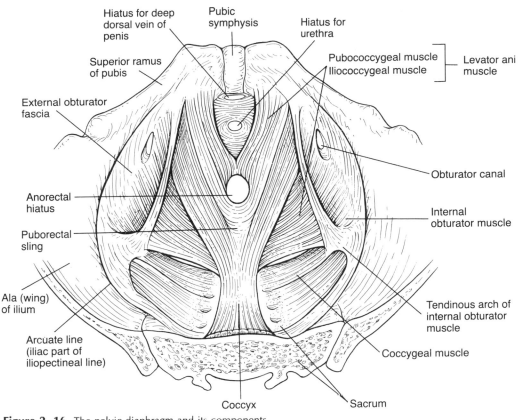

Figure 2–16. The pelvic diaphragm and its components.

The Pelvic Floor (Diaphragm)

Underlying the peritoneum in the true pelvis, there is a variable amount of loose cellular tissue and fat, in which the visceral branches of the internal iliac artery and the ureters run (see Fig. 2–14). Below this layer (deep to it) lies the extension of the transversalis fascia known as the endopelvic fascia. In this layer, as already outlined, various thickenings define the ligaments of the uterus, the prostate, and the rectum. The ligaments also define two spaces that can be utilized to facilitate surgical dissection in the female. These are (1) the paravesical space located anterior to the transverse cervical ligament between the bladder and the obturator fascia and (2) the pararectal space between the uterosacral ligament and the posterolateral pelvic wall. Additional spaces at this level are the retrorectal space between the rectum and retrorectal fascia, and the perirectal space immediately surrounding the anterior two thirds of the rectum.

Inferior to these structures lies the pelvic diaphragm (levator ani) (Fig. 2–16). In anatomic terms, it consists of three components: the pubococcygeal muscle, the iliococcygeal muscle, and the coccygeal muscle proper. However, it is more useful to visualize and discuss these muscles in functional rather than purely morphologic terms. The pubococcygeal muscle is most clearly viewed as the component of the muscle that consists of a series of slings originating on the pubis and looping behind each of the tubular structures passing through the pelvis, that is, the rectum, the vagina or prostate, and the urethra. Thus are derived the puborectal, pubovaginal, puboprostatic, and pubourethral portions. Functionally, by far the most important of these is the puborectal, the most powerful of the muscles responsible for rectal continence. This muscle accounts for the 70- to 80-degree rearward angulation of the distalmost rectum.

The second component of the levator ani, mainly consisting of the iliococcygeal muscle, originates on the iliopubic ramus and the surface of the internal obturator fascia along the tendinous arch extending back to the ischial spine. From these bilateral origins, the fibers of the second component sweep down toward the midline and insert on the raphe in that location and on the tubular structures exiting the pelvis. The muscle thus creates a hammock across the pelvis, contraction of which accounts for the name of the muscle; because its origins lie higher than the insertion, the effect of the muscle is to raise the anus along with the pelvic floor. These two components of the levator function in concert. At rest (in the continent state), both are in a state of tonic contraction (Fig. 2–17). Thus the anus is elevated, and a certain amount of

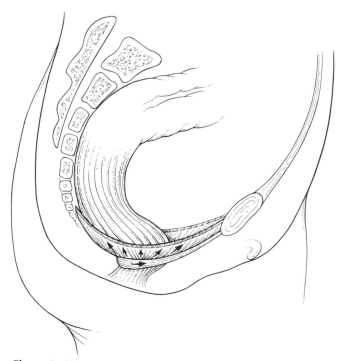

Figure 2–17. Actions of the levator ani complex during continence.

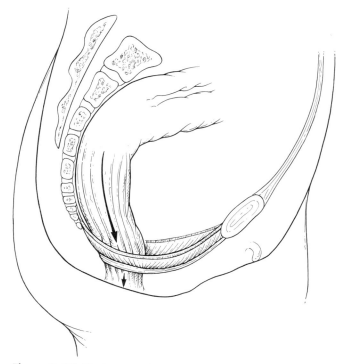

Figure 2–18. The levator ani complex relaxed, during defecation.

slack is created in the rectum by the contraction of the hammock portion. This allows the sling (puborectal muscle) to sharply angulate the lower rectum forward. As a result, intra-abdominal pressure is not transmitted down the length of the rectal canal and continence is maintained. When defecation is about to take place, both components of the muscle relax (Fig. 2–18). This allows the anus and pelvic floor to drop, at the same time as the puborectal muscle relaxes. Thus, the angulation is removed and intra-abdominal pressure can now be transmitted in a straight line through the rectum to the outside, expelling the fecal contents.

Once expulsion is completed, the muscle again contracts, as it were, pulling the rectum back up into the pelvic cavity and leaving the stool column behind. The coccygeal muscle serves to occlude the posterior portion of the pelvic outlet behind the rectum and, other than serving as part of the pelvic diaphragm, has no major functional significance.

The Anus

The dentate (pectinate) line represents the level of the embryonic cloacal membrane, and the anal valves (valves of Morgagni) are thought to be remnants of it (see Fig. 2–13; Fig. 2–19). Below the dentate line, the anal canal is lined by skin, is innervated by somatic sensory nerves, and drains to the systemic circulation and the inguinal lymph nodes. Malignancies found here are usually squamous carcinomas. Above the dentate line, the lining consists of mucosa of the columnar type. The innervation here is autonomic, and the drainage is portal and to the inferior mesenteric nodes. Neoplasms here are typically adenocarcinomas. One to two centimeters on each side of the dentate line there is a transitional zone where the epithelium is variable and where innervation and drainage are unpredictable; neoplasms that arise from this region are often cloacogenic.

About halfway between the dentate line and the anal verge, there often is a circular depression that is the result of fibrous septa attaching the skin to the lower end of the internal sphincter. This is known as Hilton's white line, deep to which lies the intersphincteric groove. The area above this, extending to the dentate line, is often known as the pecten. The mucosa between the dentate and anorectal lines is thrown into longitudinal folds that are known as the rectal columns (columns of Morgagni). At the lower ends of the columns, mucosa bridges the intervening grooves, thus creating the anal valves. Mucosal depressions extending somewhat distally from these are the anal crypts. The anal glands drain into these, and the body of the gland itself extends back to or into the underlying internal sphincter. There are usually four to eight glands present. Therefore, some crypts do not have a

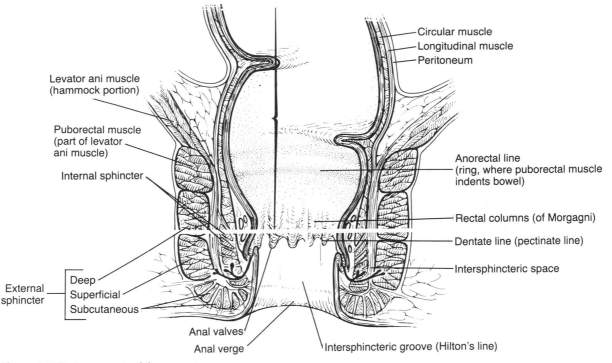

Figure 2–19. Components of the anorectum.

gland draining into them. Some glands are found to extend through the internal sphincter to end in the intersphincteric space.

Above the tops of the rectal columns and extending to the anorectal ring is a slightly raised circular structure elevating the mucosa, known as the anal cushion. This consists of fibrovascular tissue and may make some contribution to continence. Internal hemorrhoids originate here, when the shearing stress of hard stool working against tight surrounding sphincters loosens the moorings of the cushions and they are torn free, to prolapse distally.

The musculature is most clearly understood by following down the usual arrangement of circular and longitudinal coats from the bowel. The internally placed circular muscle layer is thickened for the 2 to 3 cm before its distal termination. This portion is called the internal sphincter, and it is innervated by autonomic nerves as an extension of the bowel musculature. Only the external sphincter is present distal to the termination of the internal sphincter. The space separating these is known as the intersphincteric plane. Where it is evident at Hilton's line, it produces the intersphincteric groove.

The longitudinal muscle layer located externally on the bowel is gradually replaced by fibrous tissue in its distal few centimeters. This fibrous tissue fragments, and it ultimately serves to split the bundles of the subcutaneous portion of the external sphincter, with which it commingles.

The external sphincter muscle (Fig. 2–13), voluntarily innervated, lies distal and peripheral to the internal sphincter. The deep and superficial portions partly surround the lower portion of internal sphincter, thus boosting its activity, and partly extend beyond it, thereby providing the most distal level of sphincteric control that is under voluntary innervation. The deep portion of the sphincter lies uppermost, and it is immediately adjacent to the puborectal sling, with which its fibers intermingle. The superficial portion of the external sphincter is distal to the puborectal sling. The subcutaneous component is, as its names implies, located most superficially and accounts for most of the anal "wink" reflex. Under spinal or muscle relaxant anesthesia, the external sphincter relaxes and retracts laterally, and the first sphincteric layer encountered at the anal verge is the distal (free) edge of the internal sphincter. The puborectal sling is the uppermost of the sphincters, located at the level of the anorectal ring (indeed it creates most of it by compressing and angulating the canal at this level), and it also is under voluntary control. However, it is a tonic muscle, which under normal circumstances is partially contracted. During defecation it is allowed to relax completely; in contrast, during forced continence (e.g., coughing, sneezing, lifting) it is maximally contracted.

Several potential spaces exist in the anorectal region (Fig. 2–20). The perianal space begins at the dentate line and surrounds the anal canal, extending to the subcutaneous sphincter, where it ends by virtue of the

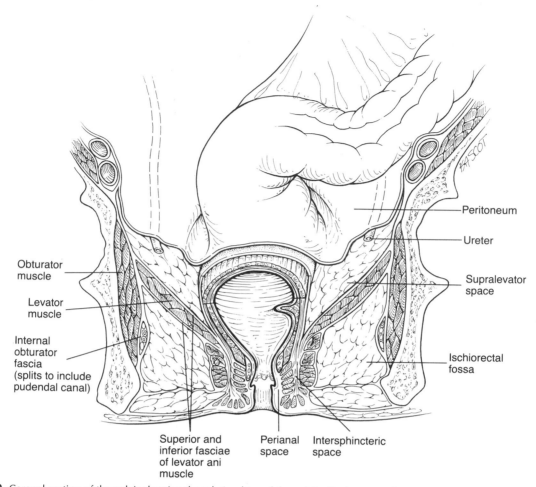

Figure 2–20. Coronal section of the pelvis showing the relationships of the pelvic diaphragm to the anorectum and the pelvic walls.

anchorage of the fibrous continuation of the longitudinal muscle to the dermis. The ischiorectal fossa is bounded by the levator ani above and medially, the obturator fascia and inferior pubic ramus laterally, and the deep fascia (sometimes referred to as the transverse septum) inferiorly. Abscesses arising from the anal glands can remain confined to the perianal space; they can extend peripherally into the intersphincteric space and into the ischiorectal fossa; and, rarely, they can track upward into the supralevator space. These spaces must be visualized as only potential spaces, although they exist as potentially circumferential, doughnut-shaped spaces that can allow pus to surround the anorectum to varying degrees.

Blood Supply to the Rectum and the Anus

The upper rectum receives its arterial supply from the lowermost, terminal branch of the inferior mesenteric artery, namely, the superior rectal (hemorrhoidal) ar-

tery (Fig. 2–21). This vessel travels down with the sigmoidal arteries through the mesosigmoid, and then it passes over the promontory of the sacrum to gain access to the rectum. The rest of the anorectum is supplied by the internal iliac artery, by two different paths. The middle rectal branches of the artery are given off above the pelvic floor and gain access to the midrectum via the lateral bands (stalks). These are the major points of attachment of the rectum to the pelvic diaphragm and must be ligated or clipped when the midrectum is mobilized.

The anus and the anal sphincters are supplied by the internal iliac artery via the pudendal artery. This, the terminal branch of the internal iliac artery, exits the pelvis via the greater sciatic foramen; it then turns forward in the ischiorectal fossa and runs in its lateral wall in a canal created by the splitting of the internal obturator fascia: the pudendal (Alcock's) canal (see Fig. 2–20). Just before or at the point of entering the canal, the pudendal artery gives off one or two medially directed branches, known as the inferior rectal arteries. The triple blood supply to the anorectum is intercon-

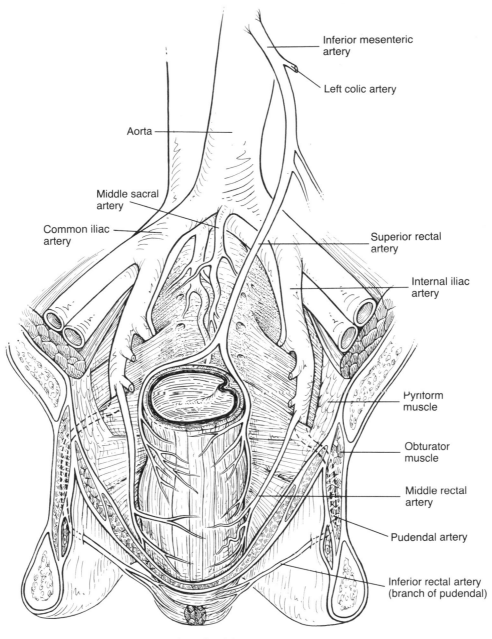

Figure 2–21. Diagram of the arterial supply of the anorectum.

nected within the bowel wall, and there is ample collateralization to the contralateral side. The internal iliac artery often compensates for the lack of inflow from the inferior mesenteric, a vessel frequently compromised by conditions such as arteriosclerosis and aneurysms.

The venous drainage follows the arterial distribution. The superior rectal vein drains into the portal system via the inferior mesenteric vein. On the other hand, the middle and inferior rectal veins, being internal iliac vein tributaries, drain into the systemic circulation. The sacral venous plexus provides yet another outflow. It represents a rich intercommunicating venous net-

work that envelops the sacrum and must be avoided when mobilizing the rectum in the retrorectal space. It intercommunicates freely with the entire perivertebral plexus (plexus of Batson). This is an open, valveless system, which can allow the free passage of bacteria or tumor cells up and down the axial skeleton.

Lymphatic Drainage of the Rectum and the Anus

As in much of the rest of the body, the lymphatics follow the blood supply. The paths of lymphatic drainage from the rectum and anal canal extend upward, and only the perianal skin drains downward into the inguinal nodes. However, on occasion, when the central connections are blocked by tumor, it is possible for cloacogenic tumors at or above the anal verge to spread distally. The lymphatic vessels draining the lower rectum pass upward within its wall, and no clear-cut lymph nodes can be identified until the mesorectum is reached behind the upper third of the rectum. Even here, only small insignificant collections of lymphoid tissue are present, and nodes do not appear until the mesosigmoid is reached. The extent of lateral drainage from the rectum is controversial. Classical teaching clearly denies its existence. However, clinical experience has shown that with bulky, low-lying tumors, obturator and internal iliac lymphatics can be involved. Once again, whether this is the result of central obstruction and an alternate pathway for tumor cells is unclear. Nevertheless, some surgeons think that internal iliac and obturator lymph node dissections should be done in low-lying large tumors, particularly when no preoperative radiatotherapy has been given. The practical implications of regional lymphadenectomy are fully discussed in Chapter 9 in the subchapter by Dr. Takahashi.

Innervation of the Rectum and the Anus

Autonomic innervation extends to the dentate line of the anus. The sympathetic fibers originate from the lowermost thoracic segments and L1 (± L2). They pass down the sympathetic chains and over the aortic bifurcation as the two hypogastric (presacral) nerves. These form a plexus just below the promontory of the sacrum and then split into two pelvic plexuses on the posterolateral side wall of the pelvis. At this point they are joined by parasympathetics from S2, S3, and S4. The sympathetic fibers carry visceral afferent components from the rectum and upper anal canal. Their motor components contribute to activity of the internal sphincter of the anus.

In developing the retrorectal space to mobilize the rectum, it is helpful to elevate the distal mesosigmoid with the superior rectal artery forward and away from the aortic bifurcation, thereby leaving the hypogastric plexus behind and intact. If the dissection is carried out in this slightly more anterior plane, pelvic sensation and ejaculatory function are least likely to be compromised. During operation for benign disease, this midline plane can be followed laterally, allowing division of the rectal stalks close to the rectum, reflecting the pelvic plexuses and the parasympathetic nerves extending to the genitalia laterally. This protects the nerves from injury and preserves parasympathetic function (i.e., erection). The topic of preservation of sexual function during proctectomy is discussed further in Chapter 9 in the subchapter by Dr. Takahashi. The responsible fibers travel at about the level of the prostate. They often need to be sacrificed in the case of low-lying rectal carcinomas when the lateral pararectal tissues must be widely removed in order to provide a secure margin on the neoplasm.

The parasympathetic innervation of the rectum and anus originates in segments S2, S3, and S4. Fibers then join the pelvic plexus. From there some of them ascend along with the hypogastric nerve into the base of the mesentery of the sigmoid. They are ultimately distributed cephalad along this part of the bowel and the left colon to the level of the splenic flexure. The remaining fibers are distributed from the pelvic plexus along with sympathetic branches to the pelvic viscera, providing motor innervation to the rectum and inhibitory fibers to the internal sphincter. Both the sympathetic and the parasympathetic fibers in the pelvis reach the viscera they innervate by way of a direct path, and they do not follow blood vessels, as is often the case in other parts of the body.

Somatic sensory and motor innervation is derived from the lower sacral segments in a concentric fashion: S4 innervates the anal canal distal to the dentate line; S3 innervates the skin immediately below it; and the higher sacral segments innervate the skin of the buttock and perineum. Motor innervation to the external sphincter also is from the lower sacral segments. These nerves reach the anus and perineum via the pudendal nerve (S2, S3, S4), with branches corresponding to (and following) those of the pudendal artery: the inferior rectal nerves and the perineal nerves.

Physiology of the Colon, Rectum, and Anus

C H A P T E R 3

Robert E. Condon
Constantine T. Frantzides

The colon and rectum used to be considered merely a reservoir for the storage of bulk waste. Gradually, it was realized that the colon has important dynamic physiologic functions.[1] In the 1950s, two separate units of the colon became recognized: the right colon, which functions primarily in the absorption of fluids and electrolytes from the lumen, and the left colon, which serves primarily as a storage vessel from which waste is eventually expelled.[2] Although this is the traditional view of colonic activity, it is oversimplified. The large bowel is actually a highly sophisticated organ with myriad complex physiologic interactions.[3] The principal components of colonic and rectal function include secretion, absorption, propulsion, storage of feces, and controlled expulsion. These functions are precisely coordinated by neural, hormonal, and muscular interactions both locally and centrally.

ABSORPTION AND SECRETION

The secretion of mucus by goblet cells occurs throughout the colon. The mucus serves to coat the stool, facilitating its passage and reducing abrasion injury to the mucosa. Mucus secretion is stimulated by bile salts and by irritants, for example, soapsuds, which are commonly used in enemas. The mucosa secretes immunoglobulins into the colon lumen. Whether this occurs with the secretion of mucus, or more directly from other epithelial cells, has not been precisely defined. Considerable speculation surrounds the potential functions of the immunoglobulins secreted into the colon lumen, but a definite physiologic or immunologic role for these substances has not yet been established.

In health, the human colon cannot absorb nutrients but absorbs water, sodium, and chloride very efficiently.[4, 5] Most of the electrolytes and water are absorbed in the proximal colon, but this is probably an opportunity-associated phenomenon, because there are no intrinsic differences in the capacity of different colon segments to accomplish these tasks.[6, 7] Each day, between 2 and 10 liters of electrolyte-rich fluid enters the colon from the ileum. Most of this volume is derived from the secretions of the small intestine and stomach. Because the amount of water lost in stool each day is about 200 ml, with only 5 to 10 mEq of sodium and potassium, nearly all of the water and electrolytes entering the colon is absorbed.[8]

There are no direct studies of water absorption by the human colon, but inferences from our understanding of the processes of small bowel absorption of water and from animal experiments suggest that water absorption is coupled to and dependent on the absorption of solutes. The colon appears capable of absorbing water against an osmolar gradient,[9] and net absorption of water by the colon exceeds that accomplished in any other bowel segment.

In animal experiments, two different transport processes for water and sodium absorption have been identified. In the rat, sodium absorption from the colon lumen occurs primarily via an electrically neutral mechanism coupled to chloride. The chloride absorption is passive, the active force being the sodium pump. Water passively accompanies the electrolytes. In contrast, in the rabbit, electrogenic sodium absorption through a bicarbonate exchange mechanism predominates.[10] The lumen of the colon is electrically negative compared with the colon wall, the potential difference being about 10 to 50 mV. Thus sodium must be absorbed electrogenically against an appreciable electrical gradient.

Whether the human colon is more like that of the rat or the rabbit remains to be determined, because the mechanism of sodium absorption in humans has not been identified. The final concentration of sodium in the colon lumen, however, is very hypotonic with respect to plasma.[9] It is known that the permeability of the apical membrane in the colon mucosa increases as the concentration of sodium in the lumen falls; this enables absorption of sodium from the lumen to be very efficient, and the residual concentration of sodium in stool to be very low.[11] Sodium and chloride absorption are significantly increased by mineralocorticoids and aldosterone. The few studies of ion transport across isolated human colon mucosa do not support neutral coupled sodium absorption,[12, 13] suggesting that the human colon resembles that of the rat and uses an electrogenic process to absorb sodium.

In ulcerative colitis and Crohn's disease, and probably in all forms of colitis, sodium and water absorption is decreased. In animals, a net secretion sometimes has been identified; this extreme state probably does not occur in humans with colitis. Abnormalities of the absorption of bile acids and hydroxy fatty acids, as occur in ileal resection or bypass, lead to entry of these substances into the colon and to consequent diarrhea. Bile acids and hydroxy fatty acids reverse net fluid and electrolyte absorption by the colon mucosa, resulting in the net secretion that is responsible for the diarrhea associated with abnormalities in the distal small bowel.

MOTILITY

Colon Myoelectric Activity

Colon myoelectric activity in many species, including guinea pig, rabbit, pig, cat, dog, and subhuman primates, has been defined reasonably well by investigations over many years. In contrast, human colonic myoelectric activity is less well defined, because the colon, especially the proximal portion of the large bowel, is relatively inaccessible to traditional means of study. Most motility recordings in humans have been obtained from the anal canal, rectum, and sigmoid colon. Furthermore, the complexity of colonic myoelectric recordings compared with those obtained from the small bowel makes interpretation of this colon activity difficult.

The devices that record human colonic myoelectric activity include suction or clip electrodes attached to the colon mucosa and intraluminal balloons. These types of electrodes have several technical limitations: frequently they become detached; even when they remain in situ, they can be used to measure activity only for a relatively short period of time. Replacement at precisely the same site in order to obtain longer duration recordings is not possible. Intraluminal balloons are inappropriate transducers in a chambered organ such as the colon.[14]

It has become possible to attach Teflon-coated, stainless steel electrodes to the serosal surface of the colon during elective surgical procedures.[15–20] This has facilitated continuous, chronic recordings from patients during the period of postoperative ileus and following recovery of normal bowel function. This technique has allowed the beginning of characterization of normal colonic myoelectric activity as well as the evolving colonic myoelectric patterns during recovery from postoperative ileus.

The smooth muscle of the colon, like that of the small intestine and stomach, generates two kinds of electrical signals: slow electrical transients called electrical control activity (ECA), or slow waves, and rapid transients called electrical response activity (ERA), or spike bursts. The origin, frequency, and incidence of ECA in the colon are subject to debate. Some in vivo studies found slow waves to be present intermittently at two or more frequencies.[18, 21] We have shown that slow waves are present continuously in humans.[16] Multiple pacesetters of different frequencies are thought to exist in the colon, with dominance between these pacesetters varying over time.

In general, most investigators agree that ECA is present in two dominant frequency ranges, a lower range of 2 to 9 cycles/min and a higher frequency range of 9 to 13 cycles/min. There is an increase in slow wave frequency from more proximal to distal sites along the colon. The rectal slow wave frequency is approximately 20 cycles per minute, and a gradient is observed between the colon and rectum.

ECA may be phase-locked or -unlocked. When phase-unlocked, smooth muscle cell depolarizations occur randomly. When phase-locked, individual smooth muscle cells generating ECA do so in such a way that depolarizations in adjacent cells occur with a constant time lag and along a directional gradient that permits the related ERA to cause coordinated contractions. The factors that control phase locking are presumed to be neurohumoral but have not been precisely identified. ECA in the colon is poorly coupled compared with the small intestine. Most of the time, the right colon is phase-unlocked and motor activity is random, with twitches and dimpling occurring continuously in an uncoordinated fashion similar to brownian movement. Such nonpropulsive activity serves, however, to permit maximal absorption of fluid and electrolytes by the right colon.

Circumferential phase locking occurs intermittently, resulting either in a standing ring contraction (haustra) or in a migrating contraction that serves to propel stool distally. Migrating contractions are uncommon in the right colon, and when they occur usually are limited to a relatively short distance. Phase locking is seen somewhat more frequently in the left colon, but it is not the dominant state. Phase-unlocked random contractions also predominate in this bowel segment, but phase-locked coordinated contractions do occur more frequently in the left colon compared with the right colon and more frequently are migratory. Contractions usually begin in the transverse colon (sometimes even in the right colon) and rapidly migrate distally to propel stool into the distal sigmoid and rectosigmoid colon.

In vivo studies in both animals[22] and humans[15–19, 23–25] have shown that spike bursts or ERA in the colon occurs as either short phasic bursts (as in the small bowel) or as longer bursts. The dominant ERA in the colon is composed of random phasic spike bursts at different locations in the colon. Both long and short spike bursts may appear in clusters. Long bursts typically are in a series of 2 or 3 bursts/min, whereas the short bursts often are in clusters of up to 12 bursts/min. Individual spike bursts or clusters of spike bursts occasionally migrate in a cephalad or caudad direction.[16] Long spike bursts that migrate rapidly caudad are accompanied by passage of flatus or defecation.[15, 16] Studies in our laboratory suggest that long spike bursts occur when the slow wave frequency is low (2 to 3 cycles/min).[26] Alternatively, shorter spike bursts occur when the slow wave frequency is higher (9 to 12 cycles/min). It is now reasonably clear that phase locking of the ECA in a short segment of bowel usually results in segmentation, whereas phase locking in a long segment results in propulsive movement.

Colonic and Rectal Contractions

Contractions are the physical expression of colon myoelectric activity. Radiographic and manometric measurements, using balloons or open-tipped catheters, provided most of our early understanding of colonic motor activity. As noted, such transducers are inappropriate in a chambered organ such as the colon, because the contraction causing the pressure change registered by the transducer may occur at any point in the chambered segment rather than precisely at the transducer.[14] A strain gauge attached to the bowel is more precise in directly measuring contractions, but it cannot be readily employed in investigations in patients. The solution, in studies in humans, has been to depend on the electrical record. As a result of extrapolating from studies performed in primates, it appears

that there is a 1:1 correlation between spike bursts and contractions.[22, 27]

Early studies in dogs[28] and humans[29] recognized three patterns of colonic motor activity. Type I contractions are simple, monophasic waves of low amplitude and short duration. These contractions create surface dimpling of the wall of the colon and yield intraluminal pressures of 5 to 10 cm H_2O. The duration of each contraction varies from 5 to 10 seconds with a frequency of 8 to 12/min. Type II contractions are similar but of higher amplitude (15 to 30 cm H_2O) and longer duration (25 to 30 seconds). They primarily involve the circular muscle and usually all of the circumference of the colon. When this type of contraction occurs in bursts, the rate is approximately 2 to 3/min. Type I or II contractions function to actively mix the intraluminal contents of the colon. Type III contractions are characterized by a change in basal intraluminal pressure with Type I or II waves superimposed. A fourth type of contraction has been observed in disease processes such as diarrhea and ulcerative colitis and at rare times in patients with a normal colon. Type IV activity is characterized by large-amplitude waves lasting for 2 to 5 minutes. The validity of these descriptions has been called into question, because the measurements from the intraluminal pressure devices utilized to record the motor events do not accurately reflect intrinsic colonic motility.[14, 21]

Colonic contractions can be classified as nonpropulsive, or stationary, contractions and propulsive contractions.[30] Nonpropulsive contractions are isolated phasic or tonic circular muscle contractions that function to mix the colon intraluminal contents and help to ensure uniform exposure of the contents to the colonic mucosal surface. These contractions occur in a random fashion and tend to delay the transit of contents through the large bowel. Nonpropulsive contractions allow more time for intraluminal mixing and absorption of water from the stool.

Contractions that propel the intraluminal contents can be divided into two types: those that travel over short bowel segments and others that migrate rapidly over long lengths of bowel. Short propulsive activity that migrates both caudad and cephalad is seen primarily in the right colon and facilitates the movement of intraluminal contents in a "back-and-forth" manner.[31] The long propulsive contractions have been called "mass movements"[32] and usually involve coordinated activity of the entire colon. They are preceded by relaxation of the colon distal to the contraction. The mass movement contractions are of high amplitude and migrate rapidly from the proximal to the distal colon. They occur three to four times a day, are stimulated by food intake or physical activity, and cause propulsion of the intraluminal contents over long lengths of bowel.[33]

These motility patterns suggest that the right and left colon each have distinct functional activities.[34, 35] The movement of intraluminal contents forward and backward in the right colon ensures complete mixing and facilitates absorption of water and electrolytes. The contents of the right colon are evacuated at intervals into the transverse colon by displacement and by peristaltic action. In the left colon, mass movements are responsible for the propulsion of stool into the sigmoid colon and rectum for storage and eventual expulsion.

The physiologic activity of the anorectum is as complex as that of the colon. Several new techniques allow quantitative analysis of anorectal motility.[36] Based on these new methodologies, the following observations have been recorded. Resting rectal intraluminal pressure is approximately 5 mm Hg. At present three patterns of contractile activity are recognized. Minor contractions have a frequency of 5 to 20 cycles/min. Contractions of 3 cycles/min also have been observed, which have an extremely high amplitude (100 cm H_2O). The third type of rectal contraction is a migrating contraction of high amplitude.[37, 38]

In the anal canal another distinct motility pattern is observed. Contractions occur at 15 cycles/min with a pressure (amplitude) of 10 cm H_2O superimposed on the resting tone. In some normal individuals, a unique wave can be recorded that has a duration of 33 seconds with an amplitude of 30 to 100 cm H_2O.[39] The anal canal demonstrates a pressure gradient that is higher distally. It has been suggested that this gradient serves to keep the anal canal free of contents and ensures continence.[40]

Gastrocolic Response

Eating is one of the main physiologic stimuli of colon motor activity. The gastrocolic response involves extensive propulsive activity in the colon and promotes defecation after eating, usually most urgently after breakfast.[41, 42] The gastrocolic response is characterized by an increase of colon phasic contractions beginning 15 to 30 minutes after ingestion of a meal. The response is not abolished by gastrectomy[33] and can be initiated by the introduction of food directly into the duodenum.[42] The gastrocolic response may not depend solely on entry of food into the stomach or upper small bowel, but it may involve a cephalic phase as well. In support of a cephalic mechanism is the observation that the mere sight of anticipated food resulted in increased colonic activity in experimental animals.[43]

It is uncertain whether the gastrocolic response is mediated by neural or hormonal mechanisms, or by a combination of both. The hormones implicated include gastrin, cholecystokinin, and gastric inhibitory polypeptide. The increase in colonic activity in response to feeding coincides with an elevation of these substances in the circulation.[44] In some studies, however, the duration of increased colonic activity appears to be shorter than the period of elevation of these three hormones.

Some studies have suggested that neural pathways are involved in the mechanism of the gastrocolic response. Following electrical stimulation of the vagus nerve, an increase in colon contractile activity is observed, suggesting involvement of a reflex pathway.[45, 46] The mechanism of this response is thought to include the vagus nerve, central nervous system, and lumbar colonic nerves. Some investigators, however, have observed the same colonic responses mediated through a vagovagal pathway.[47] Colonic excitatory responses similar to those seen after afferent vagal stimulation are reported to occur when the stomach is distended with a balloon; these responses are also believed to be mediated by a vagolumbar colonic reflex pathway.

It is possible that a combination of neural and hormonal mechanisms may be responsible for the gastrocolic response to eating. The initial response is blocked by cholinergic antagonists, whereas the later response is less affected by such drugs. This finding suggests that the initial response is controlled by neural mechanisms, whereas the later response is predominantly under hormonal control.

Other Factors Affecting Motility

The *emotional state* of an individual affects motility. Hostility, anger, anxiety, and fear are known to be associated with colonic motility changes. It is, however, difficult to design an objective study to investigate these phenomena. *Physical activity* has been shown to increase both segmental and peristaltic contractions. In contrast, *sleep* is known to depress colonic activity. *Mechanical distention* of the colon is known to stimulate motility and is the rationale behind such bulk laxatives as polysaccharides and cellulose derivatives. These bulking agents absorb water and distend the colon with soft fecal material, thus stimulating propulsive colonic movements.

Continence and Defecation

The function of the anus and rectum in the important processes of continence and defecation is made possible by the viscoelastic properties of the rectal wall, the rectoanal angle, the rectoanal inhibitory reflex, and the rectoanal contractile reflex. The elastic nature of the rectal wall facilitates the bulk storage of fecal waste. The rectum has the capacity to store a large volume of stool. When the intraluminal volume increases, the rectal wall passively distends so that the intraluminal pressure remains low.[48] In disease processes such as colitis[49] and in diseases conducive to constipation,[50, 51] in which the viscoelastic properties of the rectum are disturbed, the receptive capacity of the rectum is diminished or lost.

The rectoanal angle is maintained by the puborectal muscle and the deep portion of the external sphincter, which pulls the rectum anteriorly toward the pubis.[52] During rectal distention, the rectoanal reflex is elicited, which results in contraction of the internal sphincter. This event requires a spinal mechanism that is dependent on extrarectal structures. As the level of tension increases in the rectal wall, the urge to defecate is triggered, which involves a parasympathetic pathway.

The rectoanal inhibitory reflex is described as relaxation of the proximal portion of the anal canal and simultaneous contraction of the distal portion in response to acute rectal distention.[53–56] The role of the rectoanal inhibitory response is not fully understood. It has been hypothesized that following movement of intraluminal contents into the distal rectum, the character of the contents is recognized via contact with the sensitive mucosa of the proximal anal canal.[57] This process of sampling distinguishes among the three states of matter in the rectum—solid, liquid, and gas—and initiates appropriate reflex and voluntary muscle responses.

During defecation, the voluntary increase of intraabdominal pressure by straining changes the configuration of the rectum and anal canal by decreasing the rectoanal angle, changing the rectum to a funnel shape and shortening the anal canal.[58, 59] Defecation may result in massive emptying of the entire left colon or, more usually, only the stored contents in the sigmoid colon and rectum.[60] Following emptying, the closing reflex occurs,[61] which involves a brief contraction of the external anal sphincter and puborectal muscles. It is believed that this reflex facilitates the recovery of tonic activity of the internal anal sphincter and final closure of the anal canal.

CLINICAL MOTILITY DISORDERS

A number of clinical colonic disorders are thought to involve motility dysfunction, including irritable bowel syndrome, diverticular disease, aganglionosis of the colon, diarrhea, constipation, and postoperative ileus.

Irritable Bowel Syndrome

Irritable bowel syndrome (IBS) is characterized clinically by abdominal pain and altered bowel habits for which no organic cause can be found. In patients with IBS, the colon exhibits physiologically abnormal motor function and demonstrates abnormal responses to specific pharmacologic and physiologic stimuli. These factors include emotional stress, feeding, cholinergic drugs, gastrointestinal hormones, and rectal distention.[62–66] In patients with IBS, compared with healthy individuals, there may be a difference in colonic slow wave frequency.[21, 67] In a clinical study, a predominance of slower (3 cycles/min) activity was found in patients with IBS.[68]

Manometric studies of the sigmoid colon have shown that IBS patients with painless diarrhea have decreased motility. On the other hand, patients with the spastic colon or constipation variant of IBS exhibit hypermotility. Hypermotility also is observed in patients with constipation and diverticulosis. Because of the similarity of motility patterns in patients with IBS and those with diverticulosis, it has been suggested that the pathophysiologic mechanisms are the same.[69] The putative relationship between psychosomatic mechanisms in IBS and altered colonic motility is less clear.

Diverticulosis of the Colon

Diverticulosis is a common disease among both men and women in Western societies and is closely associated with disordered colonic motility.[70–72] Epidemiologic evidence suggests that the disease is most prevalent in countries in which a diet low in roughage is consumed. However, this hypothesis is difficult to validate, because there are no adequate animal models that mimic this disease condition.

Thickening of the intestinal wall due to hyperplasia of the circular muscle and shortening of the longitudinal axis of the colon secondary to retraction of the longitudinal muscle are regularly seen.[73] The thickening of the muscle wall is unexplained. Histologic studies, however, demonstrate an increase in the number of ganglion cells in the regions of the colon that contain diverticula.[74] Some studies have suggested that uncoordinated smooth muscle contractions coupled with increased intraluminal pressure may play a causative role. Following injection of morphine or neostigmine, high segmental pressures can be induced in the sigmoid colon of most patients with diverticular disease.

Aganglionosis of the Colon

Hirschsprung's disease results from the congenital absence of ganglia in the rectum and distal segments of colon and is characterized by spasticity of the involved segment. This is a disease of newborns and young children. Infrequently, symptoms have their onset later in life. Patients give a history of persistent and gradually worsening constipation. Usually, the aganglionic segment extends proximally from the anus for a variable distance upward in the rectum and the distal sigmoid colon. Because of the abnormal motility and spasticity of the aganglionic segment, propulsion does not occur and symptoms of obstruction and stasis become manifest.

Diarrhea and Constipation

It has been suggested that diarrhea is a manifestation of hypomotility, whereas constipation is a manifestation of hypermotility.[75] Idiopathic constipation may be caused by one of three disorders. First, the patient may experience rectoanal motility dysfunction due to Hirschsprung's disease or a constricted anus. Second, there may be pathologic stasis within the sigmoid colon. Finally, the entire colon may fail to propel stool.[76] These motility disorders can be demonstrated and differentiated by swallowed radiopaque markers.[77]

Psychogenic factors being the sole or primary cause of chronic constipation is a difficult hypothesis to validate; at present, there are no data to prove such a hypothesis. In the case of traumatic constipation (cauda equina syndrome or resection of the nervi erigentes), colonic motility is compromised and the internal sphincter becomes hypersensitive to rectal distention. The anus becomes hypertonic and the rectal wall atonic. In contrast, the rectoanal reflex is decreased.[78, 79]

Postoperative Ileus

In postoperative ileus there is temporary impairment of normal intestinal motility, characterized by abdominal distention, accumulation of gas and fluids in the bowel, obstipation, nausea, and vomiting on premature solid feeding. At present, the most reliable evidence suggests that the large bowel is the primary focus of the disordered motility in postoperative ileus.[16, 80, 81] Contrary to accepted dogma, experimental evidence suggests that the duration and type of operation do not greatly influence the severity of postoperative ileus.[16, 80–82]

Studies in monkeys[22, 81] and humans[15, 16, 26] have helped to characterize motility patterns during recovery from postoperative ileus. During the first 2 postoperative days, the colon exhibits spike bursts occurring at random. As recovery from ileus progresses, myoelectric activity becomes more organized, with the appearance of phasic short spike bursts followed by longer spike bursts that occur at a single site in the colon or show bidirectional migration. The resolution of post-

operative ileus is signaled by the appearance of long, aborally directed migrating spike bursts, which occur singly or in clusters. This type of electrical activity is associated clinically with the passage of flatus or defecation. Postoperative ileus has cleared when the patient is able to consume a solid diet and to defecate.

At present the physiologic mechanism inducing postoperative ileus is unknown. It has been suggested that it is mediated by stress-induced sympathetic hyperactivity, which inhibits bowel contraction. Peritoneal irritation by chemical or foreign materials, operative manipulation and dissection, electrolyte imbalance, and effects of analgesics and anesthetics may induce or prolong postoperative ileus. Peritoneal irritation or peritonitis may have a direct effect on the bowel, or the effect could be mediated by the adrenosympathetic system. Although sympathetic hyperactivity, as a response to surgical stress, may be involved in the cause of postoperative ileus, this possibility is still a matter of debate. Total blockage of the adrenergic system by guanethidine, or a combination of α-receptor blockade by phentolamine and parasympathetic stimulation by neostigmine, has been associated with resolution of postoperative ileus,[83, 84] but such pharmacologic manipulation failed when tested in a controlled clinical trial.[85]

Postoperative elevated circulating serum levels of epinephrine and norepinephrine support the hypothesis that there is a causal effect of sympathetic hyperactivity and ileus. The increase in epinephrine is most likely due to medullary secretion, whereas the norepinephrine increase is due to both sympathetic neural hyperactivity and adrenal medullary secretion. Furthermore, an increase in the synthesis of norepinephrine in the bowel has been demonstrated.[86] Patients with prolonged postoperative ileus have higher levels of epinephrine and norepinephrine, compared with patients with a more normal postoperative course.[86, 87] After 1 or 2 days, epinephrine levels return to baseline values, whereas norepinephrine may remain elevated for up to 5 days postoperatively. The return of normal colonic function coincides with normalization of circulating catecholamines in patients. Although current evidence suggests a link between postoperative ileus and catecholamine synthesis and release, there are other disease states in which elevation of catecholamines occurs without any associated ileus; examples are pheochromocytoma and severe burns.

Most postganglionic adrenergic sympathetic fibers innervating the colon appear to terminate in intramural ganglia or on blood vessels. The sympathetic nerves are believed to act primarily to modulate activity of intrinsic cholinergic nerves by inhibiting the release of acetylcholine. The action of norepinephrine on cholinergic nerves is mediated through α_1-receptors. Activation of α_1-receptors causes inhibition of gastrointestinal smooth muscle contractions. α_2-Receptors also are present in postganglionic sympathetic nerve terminals and act as a negative feedback mechanism to inhibit the release of norepinephrine. Very few sympathetic nerves terminate directly on smooth muscle cells. The few receptors located on smooth muscle are β-adrenergic and exert an inhibitory effect in response to circulating catecholamines such as isoproterenol and epinephrine. It appears that regional differences in adrenergic receptor concentration exist within each colonic segment. Studies in primates have shown that stimulation of α-receptors by low doses of adrenergic drugs is more effective in inhibiting left colon contractions.[88, 89] On the other hand, β stimulation inhibits contractions throughout the colon in a dose-related fashion. Although operative stress–induced sympathetic hyperactivity is an attractive mechanism to account for postoperative ileus, there is no conclusive evidence that this occurs.

Electrolyte imbalance has been suggested to play a causal role in the etiology of prolonged ileus. Patients may demonstrate low serum values of sodium, chloride, or magnesium; however, no direct linkage exists between these electrolyte alterations and the duration of ileus. At present, the only electrolyte-dependent etiology of ileus is severe hypokalemia. A study in primates suggests that severe hypokalemia significantly reduces fasting colon contractions and may thus play a role in the prolongation of postoperative ileus.[90] Furthermore, studies in patients with hypokalemia and protracted postoperative ileus showed reversal of ileus following potassium replacement.[91]

A role for general anesthesia in the genesis of postoperative ileus has been sought for over 8 decades. Studies in the early part of the twentieth century demonstrated slowing of transit time following the administration of diethyl ether.[92] It was observed in the 1920s that ether and chloroform delayed gastrointestinal transit during their administration, but the effect was transient with recovery within minutes to a few hours following termination of anesthesia.[93] A paradoxical increase in colonic activity, probably related to excitement, is seen following the administration of nitrous oxide. It has been reported that the administration of halothane and enflurane is associated with a significant depression of myoelectric and contractile activity in the colon intraoperatively. Recovery, however, occurs rapidly on cessation of anesthesia.[94] The mechanism of this inhibitory phenomenon is presently unknown. Because the effects of commonly used anesthetic agents on bowel motility are short-term and limited to the period of their administration, it is unlikely that these compounds play a major role in the etiology of postoperative ileus.

Studies of the effects of analgesics on bowel motility in primates[22] and humans[16] clearly demonstrate that morphine affects colonic motility. The effect is variable and dose-related. At low to moderate doses of morphine, there is an increase in the number of nonmigrating phasic random colonic contractions. In contrast, there is inhibition of colonic phasic myoelectric and contractile activity following higher doses. Morphine at all doses uniformly inhibits the aborally migrating contractions that are known to be the propulsive force in the large bowel and thus delays intestinal transit.

EDITORIAL COMMENT

It is universally accepted that a thorough and detailed knowledge of the anatomy of the hindgut is essential to the successful performance of operations involving the organs in it. An understanding of the physiology of the colon, rectum, and anus is no less essential for proper diagnosis, preoperative and intraoperative care, and postoperative management. Although our appreciation of the physiology and biochemistry of the large bowel is limited, the material set forth in this chapter has obvious clinical applications, ranging from operative planning through choice of anesthetic agents and postoperative care.

At the very least, students of surgery can appreciate what is known and what is not known regarding the physiology of the hindgut, enabling them to accept certain treatment modalities as founded on established knowledge, while rejecting others as having no adequate scientific basis.

REFERENCES

1. Hertz AF, Newton A. The normal movements of the colon in man. J Physiol (Lond) 1913;45–57.
2. Bockus HL. Gastroenterology. Philadelphia: WB Saunders, 1946.
3. Christensen J. Motility of the colon. In: Johnson LR, ed. Physiology of the Gastrointestinal Tract. New York: Raven Press, 1987.
4. Phillips SF. Absorption and secretion by the colon. Gastroenterology 1969;56:966–971.
5. Turnberg LS. Electrolyte absorption from the colon. Gut 1970;11:1049–1054.
6. Edmonds CJ. The gradient of electrical potential difference and of sodium and potassium of the gut contents along the caecum and colon of normal and sodium-depleted rats. J Physiol 1967;193:589–602.
7. Rask-Madsen J. Simultaneous measurement of electrical polarization and electrolyte transport by the entire normal and inflamed human colon during in vivo perfusion. Scand J Gastroenterol 1973;8:327–336.
8. Edmonds CJ, Marriott JC. The effect of aldosterone and adrenalectomy on the electrical potential difference of rat colon and on the transport of sodium, potassium, chloride and bicarbonate. J Endocrinol 1967;39:517–531.
9. Billich CO, Levitan R. Effects of sodium concentration and osmolarity on water and electrolyte absorption from the intact human colon. J Clin Invest 1969;48:1336–1347.
10. Binder HJ, Rawlins CL. Electrolyte transport across isolated large intestinal mucosa. Am J Physiol 1973;225:1232–1239.
11. Schultz SG. Ion transport by mammalian large intestine. In: Johnson LR, ed. Physiology of the Gastrointestinal Tract. New York: Raven Press, 1987.

12. Grady GF, Duhamel RC, Moore EW. Active transport of sodium by human colon in vitro. Gastroenterology 1970;59:583–588.

13. Hawker PC, Mashiter KE, Turnberg LA. Mechanisms of transport of Na, Cl, and K in the human colon. Gastroenterology 1978;74:1241–1247.

14. Brodribb AJM, Condon RE, Cowles V, DeCosse JJ. Effect of dietary fiber on intraluminal pressure and myoelectrical activity of left colon in monkeys. Gastroenterology 1979;77:70–74.

15. Frantzides CT, Condon RE, Cowles V. Early postoperative colon electrical response activity. Surg Forum 1985;38:163.

16. Condon RE, Frantzides CT, Cowles V, et al. Resolution of postoperation ileus in humans. Ann Surg 1986;203:574.

17. Taylor I, Duthie HL, Smallwood R, et al. Large bowel myoelectrical activity in man. Gut 1975;16:808.

18. Bueno L, Fioramonti J, Ruckebusch Y, et al. Evaluation of colonic myoelectric activity in health and functional disorders. Gut 1980;21:480.

19. Sarna SK, Waterfall WE, Bardakjian BL, Lind JF. Types of human colonic electrical activities recorded postoperatively. Gastroenterology 1981;81:61–70.

20. Sarna SK, Bardakjian BL, Waterfall WE, Lind JF. Human colonic electrical control activity (ECA). Gastroenterology 1980;78:1526–1536.

21. Snape WJ, Carlson GM, Cohen S. Colonic myoelectric activity in the irritable bowel syndrome. Gastroenterology 1976;70:326.

22. Frantzides CT, Condon RE, Schulte WJ, Cowles V. Effects of morphine on colonic myoelectric activity in subhuman primates. Am J Physiol 1990;21:247–252.

23. Flexino J, Bueno L, Fioramonti J. Diurnal changes in myoelectric spiking activity of the human colon. Gastroenterology 1985;88:1104.

24. Sarna SK, Latimer P, Campbell DM. Electrical and contractile activities of the human rectosigmoid. Gut 1982;23:698.

25. Taylor I, Duthie HL, Smallwood R. The effect of stimulation on the myoelectric activity of the rectosigmoid in man. Gut 1974;15:599.

26. Condon RE, Frantzides CT, Cowles V. Electrical activity of human colon. Poster presented to the XIIIth International Motility Symposium, Kobe, Japan, November 20, 1991.

27. Condon RE, Cowles VE, Schulte WJ, et al. The effect of whole gut lavage on colon motility and gastrocolic response in a subhuman primate. Surgery 1986;99:531.

28. Templeton RD, Lawson H. Studies in motor activity of large intestine. Am J Physiol 1931;96:667.

29. Adler HF, Atkinson AJ, Ivy AC. Supplementary and synergistic action of stimulating drugs on motility of human colon. Surg Gynecol Obstet 1942;74:809.

30. Ritchie JA. Colonic motor activity and bowel function. I. Normal movements of contents. Gut 1968;9:442.

31. Ritchie JA, Truelove SC, Ardan GM, et al. Propulsion and retropulsion of normal colonic contents. Am J Dig Dis 1971;16:697.

32. Hertz AF. The passage of food along the human alimentary canal. Guy's Hosp Rep 1907;61:389.

33. Holdstock DJ, Misiewicz JJ. Factors controlling colonic motility: Colonic pressures and transit after meals in patients with total gastrectomy, pernicious anemia and duodenal ulcer. Gut 1970;11:100.

34. Sarna SK. Physiology and pathophysiology of colonic motor activity. Dig Dis Sci 1991;36:827–862 and 998–1018.

35. Hagihara PF, Griffen WO Jr. Physiology of the colon and rectum. Surg Clin North Am 1972;52:797.

36. Pemberton JH. Anatomy and physiology of the anus and rectum. In: Condon RE, ed. Colon. Vol IV. Zuidema GD, ed. Shackelford's Surgery of the Alimentary Tract. 3rd ed. Philadelphia: WB Saunders, 1991.

37. Scharli AF, Kieswetter WB. Defecation and continence: Some new concepts. Dis Colon Rectum 1970;13:81–107.

38. Whitehead WE, Engel BT, Schuster MM. Irritable bowel syndrome: Physiological and psychological differences between diarrhea-predominant and constipation predominant patients. Dig Dis Sci 1980;25:404–413.

39. Kerremans R. Morphological and Physiological Aspects of Anal Continence and Defecation. Arscia, Ultgavin, Brussels, 1969.

40. Connell AM. The motility of the pelvic colon: Motility in normals and in patients with asymptomatic duodenal ulcers. Gut 1961;2:175–186.

41. Strom JA, Condon RE, Schulte WJ, et al. Glucagon, gastric inhibitory polypeptide and the gastrocolic response. Am J Surg 1982;143:155.

42. Connell AM, Logan CJH. The role of gastrin in gastroileocolic responses. Am J Dig Dis 1967;12:277.

43. Ruckebuch Y, Grivel ML, Fargeas MJ. Activité electique de l'intestin et prise de nouriture conditionelle chez le lapin. Physiol Behav 1971;6:359.

44. Snape WJ, Matarazzo SA, Cohen S. Effect of eating and gastrointestinal hormones on human colonic myoelectric and motor activity. Gastroenterology 1978;75:373.

45. Tansy MF, Kendall FM. Experimental and clinical aspects of gastrocolic reflexes. Am J Dig Dis 1973;18:521.

46. Tansy MF, Kendall FM, Mackowiak RC. The reflex nature of the gastrocolic propulsive response in the dog. Surg Gynecol Obstet 1972;135:404.

47. Collman PI, Grundy D, Scratcherd T, et al. Vago-vagal reflexes to the colon of the anesthetized ferret. J Physiol 1984;352:395.

48. Arhan P, Faverdin C, Persoz B, et al. Relationship between viscoeleastic properties of the rectum and anal pressure in man. J Appl Physiol 1976;41:677–682.

49. Colin DR, Galmiche JP, Geoffroy Y, et al. Elastic properties of the rectal wall in normal adults and in patients with ulcerative colitis. Gastroenterology 1979;77:45–48.

50. Arhan P, Devroede G, Danis K, et al. Viscoleastic properties of the rectal wall in Hirschsprung's disease. J Clin Invest 1978;62:83–87.

51. White JC, Verlot MG, Ehrentheil O. Neurogenic disturbances of the colon and their investigation by colonmetrogram. Ann Surg 1940;112:1042–1057.

52. Phillips SF, Edwards DAW. Some aspects of anal continence and defecation. Gut 1965;6:396–406.

53. Denny-Brown D, Robertson EG. Investigation of nervous control of defecation. Brain 1935;58:256–310.

54. Gowers WR. The automatic action of the sphincter ani. Proc Roy Med Soc (Lond) 1877;26:77–84.

55. Schuster MM, Hendrix TR, Mendeloff AI. The internal sphincter response: Manometric studies on its normal physiology, neural pathways, and alteration in bowel disorders. J Clin Invest 1963;42:196–207.

56. Schuster MM, Hookman P, Hendrix T, et al. Simultaneous manometric recording of internal and external anal spincteric reflexes. Bull Johns Hopkins Hosp 1965;116:79–88.

57. Duthie HL, Gairns FW. Sensory nerve-endings and sensation in the anal region of man. Br J Surg 1960;47:585–594.

58. Duthie HL, Bennett RC. The relation of sensation in the anal canal to the functional anal sphincter: A possible factor in anal continence. Gut 1963;4:179–182.

59. Tagart REB. The anal canal and rectum: Their varying relationship and its effect on anal incontinence. Dis Colon Rectum 1966;9:449–452.

60. Halls J. Bowel content shift during normal defecation. Proc Roy Soc Med 1965;58:859–860.

61. Bartolo DCC, Read NW, Jarratt JA, et al. Differences in anal sphincter function and clinical presentation in patients with pelvic floor descent. Gastroenterology 1983;85:68–75.

62. Almy TP, Hinckle LE, Berle B, et al. Alternation in colonic function in man under stress. III. Experimental production of sigmoid spasm in patients with spastic constipation. Gastroenterology 1949;12:437–449.

63. Connell AM, Jones FA, Rowlands EN. Motility of the pelvic colon. IV. Abdominal pain associated with colonic hypermotility after meals. Gut 1965;6:105–112.

64. Chaudhary NA, Truelove SC. Human colonic motility. A comparative study of normal subjects, patients with ulcerative colitis, and patients with the irritable colon syndrome. II. The effect of Prostigmin. Gastroenterology 1961;40:18–26.

65. Harvey RF, Read AE. Effect of cholecystokinin on colonic motility and symptoms in patients with the irritable bowel syndrome. Lancet 1973;1:1–3.
66. Mitra R, Chura C, Rajendra GR, et al. Abnormal responses to rectal distension in irritable bowel syndrome. Gastroenterology 1974;66:770.
67. Snape WJ, Carlson GM, Matarazzo SA, et al. Evidence that abnormal myoelectric activity produces colonic motor dysfunction in the irritable bowel syndrome. Gastroenterology 1977;72:383.
68. Taylor I, Darby C, Hammond P. Comparison of rectosigmoid myoelectrical activity in the irritable colon syndrome during relapses and remissions. Gut 1978;19:923.
69. Havia T. Diverticulosis of the colon. A clinical and histological study. Acta Chir Scand 1971;415:1.
70. Arfwidsson S. Pathogenesis of multiple diverticula of the sigmoid colon in diverticular disease. Acta Chir Scand 1964; 342 (suppl): 1–68.
71. Painter NS. Diverticulosis of the colon—fact and speculation. Am J Dig Dis 1967;12:222–227.
72. Williams I. Diverticular disease of the colon: A 1968 view. Gut 1968;9:498–501.
73. Slack WW. Bowel muscle in diverticular disease. Gut 1967; 7:668–670.
74. Macbeth WA, Hawthorne JH. Intramural ganglia in diverticular disease of the colon. J Clin Pathol (Lond) 1965;18:40–42.
75. Connell AM. The motility of the pelvic colon. II. Paradoxical motility in diarrhea and constipation. Gut 1962;3:342–348.
76. Martelli H, Devroede G, Arhan P, et al. Mechanisms of idiopathic constipation: Outlet obstruction. Gastroenterology 1978;75:623–631.
77. Pemberton JH, Ilstrup D. Evaluation and surgical treatment of severe chronic constipation. Presented to the American Surgical Association, Boca Raton, FL, April 12, 1991.
78. Devroede G, Lamarche J. Functional importance of extrinsic parasympathetic innervation to the distal colon and rectum in man. Gastroenterology 1974;66:273–280.
79. Devroede G, Arhan P, Duguay C, et al. Traumatic constipation. Gastroenterology 1979;77:1258–1267.
80. Woods JH, Erickson LW, Condon RE, et al. Postoperative ileus: A colonic problem? Surgery 1978;54:527.
81. Graber JN, Schulte WJ, Condon RE, et al. Relationship of duration of postoperative ileus to extent and size of operative dissection. Surgery 1982;92:87.
82. Wilson JP. Postoperative motility of the large intestine in man. Gut 1975;15:689.
83. Catchpole BN. Ileus: Use of sympathetic blocking agents in its treatment. Surgery 1969;66:811.
84. Neely J, Catchpole B. The restoration of alimentary tract motility by pharmacological means. Br J Surg 1971;58:21.
85. Heimbeck DM, Crout JR. Treatment of paralytic ileus with adrenergic neuronal blocking drugs. Surgery 1971;69:582.
86. Dubois A, Weise VK, Kopin IJ. Postoperative ileus in the rat: Physiopathology, etiology and treatment. Ann Surg 1973; 178: 781.
87. Smith J, Kelly KA, Weinshilbaum RM. Pathophysiology of postoperative ileus. Arch Surg 1977;112:203.
88. Esser MJ, Mahoney JL, Robinson JC, et al. Effects of adrenergic agents on colonic motility. Surgery 1987;102:416–423.
89. Salaymeh BM, Cowles VE, Tekin EO, et al. Selective adrenergic agonists and colon motility. Surgery 1992;111:694–698.
90. Schulte WJ, Cowles V, Condon RE. Hypokalemia and the gastrocolic response [Abstract]. Dig Dis Sci 1984;29:551.
91. Lowman RM. Potassium depletion states in postoperative ileus. The role of the potassium ion. Radiology 1977;98:691.
92. Cannon WB, Murphy FT. The movements of the stomach and intestines in some surgical conditions. Ann Surg 1906;43:512–536.
93. Miller GH. The effects of general anesthesia on the muscular activity of the gastrointestinal tract. J Pharmacol Exp Ther 1926;27:41–59.
94. Condon RE, Cowles V, Ekborn GA, et al. Effects of halothane, enflurane, and nitrous oxide on colon motility. Surgery 1987;101:81–85.

Diagnostic Approaches to Colorectal Disease

C H A P T E R   4

Ira M. Hanan

The clinical presentation of various colorectal disorders is variable. Often patients present with symptoms clearly referable to a disorder of the colon or rectum. On occasion, the presenting symptoms are a manifestation of a systemic disorder. In such circumstances, although a specific symptom prompts the patient to seek medical attention, the underlying cause, not the symptom alone, demands therapy. The physician must understand the potential underlying causes of various symptoms that may prompt a patient to see an internist, gastroenterologist, or colorectal surgeon. A systematic approach to various gastrointestinal symptoms can best uncover the etiology of the problem. Often a detailed history narrows the list of possible diagnoses. Not only does a thorough history aid in establishing a proper diagnosis, but it may limit unnecessary diagnostic evaluations.

DIARRHEA

A complaint of "diarrhea" often brings a patient to the internist. Frequently, however, the patient's meaning of the term and the internist's definition are not the same. Patients often consider rectal urgency, frequency, flatus, or even tenesmus as true diarrhea. As defined by the internist, diarrhea refers to acute or chronic conditions characterized by abnormal daily stool weight and liquidity. In normal individuals a 24-hour stool collection weighs less than 200 g, and the percentage of water is less than 8%.[1] Nevertheless, when rectal frequency (more than three stools per day) becomes excessive, it is generally associated with true diarrhea.

History

The assessment of the patient with diarrhea begins with a careful, detailed history that focuses on the patient's characterization of the problem. Attention must be paid to acuteness or chronicity and to abruptness of onset of the complaint. Acute diarrhea, often associated with an abrupt onset, is defined as diarrhea of less than 2 weeks' duration. Acute diarrhea is frequently of infectious origin and self-limited. Diarrhea lasting more than 2 weeks is considered chronic and implies an alternative differential diagnosis. Blood or mucus with the diarrhea implies either infectious or inflammatory etiology, further narrowing the differential diagnosis. In chronic diarrhea a careful dietary history is paramount in order to exclude lactose intolerance or sorbitol intolerance, which accounts for "chewing gum" or "soda pop" diarrhea.[2] The patient with such an intolerance is generally unaware that the frequent, high consumption of these products may induce chronic diarrhea. Strict avoidance of products containing the suspected nonabsorbed sugar should give prompt relief of diarrhea.

Medication History

A careful medication history excludes surreptitious or inadvertent laxative use by patients, particularly women, who constitute the majority of those found to abuse laxatives.[1] Magnesium-containing antacids, taken for a variety of symptoms including heartburn, abdominal pain, and nausea, frequently cause diarrhea. Phenolphthalein laxatives may be used by patients who are morbidly obese or are suffering from anorexia nervosa. Although pseudomembranous colitis may occur without antecedent antibiotic use, it should be strongly considered when the onset of diarrhea follows within days of antibiotic therapy. Many antibiotics have been associated with pseudomembranous colitis. Although clindamycin is associated with a high potential for causing pseudomembranous colitis, ampicillin is considered the most common instigating antibiotic because of its prevalent use. Many antibiotics, including cephalosporins, metronidazole, tetracycline, and penicillin, have been associated with the development of pseudomembranous colitis. The route of antibiotic administration does not alter the potential for a patient to develop antibiotic-induced pseudomembranous colitis. It may be seen following a course of oral or intravenous antibiotic therapy.

Medical History

The past medical history may provide clues to the origin of some forms of diarrhea. Chronic "postprandial diarrhea" originating soon after a cholecystectomy suggests postcholecystectomy diarrhea due to bile acid malabsorption. Although the mechanism of this form of diarrhea is not well understood, it complicates cholecystectomy in 2% of patients. The diagnosis may be supported by prompt improvement of diarrhea with cholestyramine treatment.[3] Severe diarrhea may complicate 8% of truncal vagotomized patients.[4] The incidence of diarrhea appears to be lower when selective or superselective vagotomy is performed.[1]

Any abdominal surgery that allows intestinal stasis, including gastrectomy with Billroth II anastomosis or intestinal bypass procedures, may permit bacterial overgrowth. Bacterial deconjugation of bile salts that results in bile acid malabsorption and bile salt depletion will cause diarrhea. Such forms of diarrhea are readily suggested by history and may be confirmed by the glucose breath test and the response to antibiotic therapy.

Most patients recognize that rectal urgency, when present, occurs within the hour following a meal. True diarrhea occurs at times unrelated to meals as well as at night. Diarrhea that awakens the sleeping patient is generally true diarrhea of significant pathologic origin, regardless of whether it is acute or chronic.

Unsuspected hyperthyroidism may be manifested by diarrhea or bowel frequency. Affected patients may fail to associate other symptoms, including heat intolerance, weight loss, smooth skin, tremors, and anxiety, with the onset of diarrhea.

Examination

Although examination of the patient infrequently gives a clue to the etiology of diarrhea, the severity of the diarrhea may indirectly narrow the differential diagnosis. Orthostasis and other signs of dehydration often accompany acute diarrhea, implying an acute infectious or inflammatory process. The absence of dehydration does not exclude true diarrhea, as many patients maintain adequate hydration. Tachycardia in the well-hydrated patient is significant and suggests that hyperthyroidism or another etiology such as malignancy or protein-losing enteropathy may account for diarrhea. Other physical findings, such as abdominal fullness or a palpable mass, may suggest inflammatory bowel disease. Remote lymphadenopathy may rarely be present in cases of small bowel lymphoma but is more likely to appear in the setting of metastatic colorectal or pancreatic carcinoma presenting with diarrhea. Finally, fecal impaction, particularly in the elderly patient, must always be excluded in the patient with diarrhea.

Laboratory Studies

Simple laboratory studies should be performed in the office or hospital ward laboratory as part of the initial evaluation. First, a characteristic diarrheal stool should be examined for fecal leukocytes. These are easily seen when counterstained with methylene blue. Their presence suggests an inflammatory process, usually acute colitis, of infectious etiology (e.g., *Shigella, Salmonella, Campylobacter jejuni*) or chronic idiopathic colitis, (i.e., ulcerative colitis or Crohn's colitis). The chronicity of the diarrhea generally aids in distinguishing between an acute colitis and a chronic colitis in such a setting. Although patients with small intestine Crohn's disease often present with the complaint of diarrhea, fecal leukocytes are rarely seen, and their absence does not exclude the diagnosis.

Potassium hydroxide alkalinization of the stool sample should be performed in order to detect surreptitious phenolphthalein use. One drop of 1N. potassium hydroxide should be added to several milliliters of liquid stool. A pink-red discoloration of the sample signifies the presence of phenolphthalein.

A qualitative fecal fat analysis is easily performed and excludes most cases of steatorrhea. A drop of stool is mixed with acetic acid on a slide, heated, and stained with Sudan III. The presence of more than 100 fat droplets correlates well with a daily 15-g fat excretion. If the result is positive, attention to further quantification of fat malabsorption should ensue.

Several fresh stool samples should be submitted to a reputable microbiology laboratory to screen for bacterial pathogens. Stool specimens must be collected prior to further investigations that may entail the use of barium or oil-containing laxatives as part of the preparation. These compounds as well as kaolin-pectin

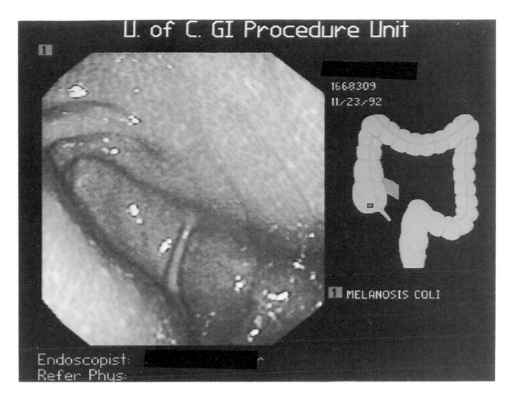

Figure 4–1. Melanosis coli. A flexible sigmoidoscopic examination of the lower colon and rectum may point to surreptitious laxative abuse in patients with diarrhea. Dark pigmentation of the colonic mucosa, as seen here, is typical of melanosis coli due to chronic ingestion of anthracene-containing laxatives.

(Kaopectate) interfere with proper identification of organisms in the stool. Commonly, bacterial infections account for acute, self-limited diarrhea. A variety of toxigenic *Escherichia coli* are among the most common pathogens to cause traveler's diarrhea. However, these organisms are rarely detected by routine laboratory cultures. *C. jejuni,* a large and small bowel pathogen, frequently causes a bloody, self-limited diarrhea that is often accompanied by fever. Although antibiotic therapy with erythromycin shortens the course of the illness, clearance of the organism generally occurs within 2 weeks. *Salmonella* and *Shigella* infections may account for acute or chronic diarrhea and often mimic idiopathic inflammatory bowel disease because of the chronicity of the illness.

Endoscopic and pathologic differentiation between these infectious colitides and idiopathic colitides may be difficult to accomplish. Therefore stool culture often provides the only clue to the true diagnosis. Stool culture is essential in the evaluation of patients with known inflammatory bowel disease, because these patients are prone to infectious flare-ups. Recurrent symptoms of bloody diarrhea following a period of remission in a patient with known ulcerative colitis or Crohn's colitis should be evaluated with a stool culture.

Examination for ova and parasites should be done on a fresh stool sample. Amebic cysts and *Giardia* cysts are the more common abnormalities found in an abnormal specimen. However, a single specimen may fail to reveal these pathogens. If the history supports a possible parasitic etiology, additional fresh samples should be submitted. Recently an enzyme-linked immunosorbent assay (ELISA) to detect giardiasis has become commercially available. Reports of high sensitivity and specificity suggest that this is an easy reliable screening examination for all patients with diarrhea.

In the setting of antibiotic-associated diarrhea, a liquidy stool should be screened for the presence of *Clostridium difficile* toxin. The latex agglutination test for the presence of *C. difficile* toxin A (the active subunit) is a highly sensitive, inexpensive test.[5] Culturing stool for *C. difficile* may occasionally reveal the organism, despite a negative toxin assay.[6] In such instances a treatment directed against the *C. difficile* organism generally results in improvement.

Sigmoidoscopy

The early assessment of diarrhea should include a proctosigmoidoscopic examination. Most clinicians find 35-cm or 60-cm flexible sigmoidoscopy preferable, because it allows easier examination of the sigmoid colon. However, rigid proctosigmoidoscopy should be performed if flexible sigmoidoscopy is not available. A negative proctosigmoidoscopy result excludes most instances of acute and chronic inflammatory bowel disease of the colon, melanosis coli (identifying anthracene laxative use) (Fig. 4–1), and most high-grade obstructive carcinomas of the distal colon. Of patients with idiopathic ulcerative colitis, 95% have involve-

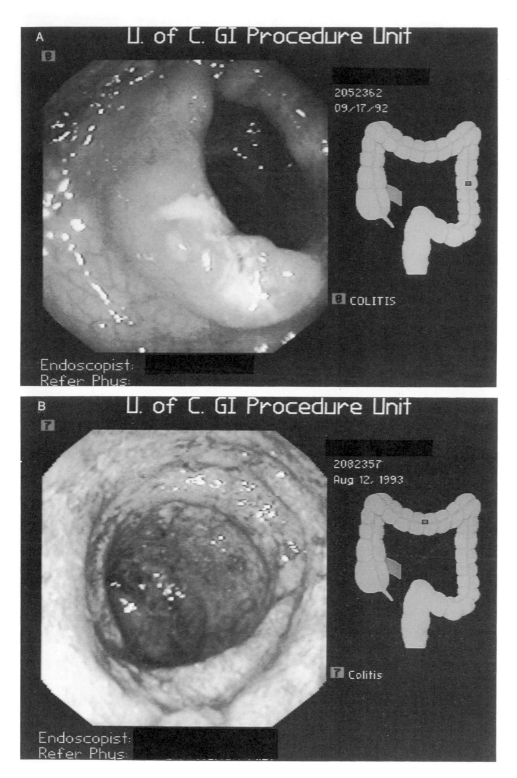

Figure 4–2. Crohn's colitis, ulcerative colitis. Longitudinal ulcers with normal-appearing surrounding mucosa are typical of Crohn's colitis (A), often allowing distinction from chronic ulcerative colitis in which diffuse involvement is present (B).

ment of the rectum and distal sigmoid colon,[7] whereas 67% of patients with Crohn's colitis may have involvement of these areas (Fig. 4–2).[8]

The sigmoidoscopic appearance of acute bacterial infections may mimic chronic inflammatory bowel disease, making differentiation difficult, even for an experienced endoscopist. *C. jejuni,* the most common

cause of acute bacterial diarrhea, may be endoscopically indistinguishable from ulcerative colitis. The colonic mucosa may appear diffusely involved with edema and ulceration. Alternatively, endoscopic features mimicking Crohn's colitis, segmental involvement and cobblestoning, may be observed.[9] Similarly, acute bacterial colitis induced by *Shigella* or *Salmonella* infections may resemble either left-sided ulcerative colitis or Crohn's colitis (Fig. 4–3). Although generally producing diffuse involvement, a predominantly right-sided colitis with skip lesions mimicking Crohn's disease may occur in *Salmonella* colitis.[10]

A pinch biopsy of the involved mucosa may aid in distinguishing acute bacterial colitis from chronic inflammatory bowel disease. Although biopsies of mucosa in acute bacterial colitis temporarily show acute inflammatory changes and occasionally crypt abscesses, they lack glandular distortion, a hallmark of chronic inflammatory bowel disease. When the inflammatory process is first discovered, a biopsy specimen should be taken to allow potential determination of etiology.

Pinch biopsy of normal colorectal mucosa is necessary to uncover some instances of melanosis coli as well as microscopic colitis. This unusual form of colitis may account for large-volume diarrhea in the patient with endoscopically normal colonic mucosa. Pronounced acute and chronic inflammation is seen microscopically.

Acute pseudomembranous colitis is quickly identified by characteristic pseudomembranes of the rectosigmoid in two thirds of cases; the remaining cases require total colonoscopy to detect these lesions in the right colon. The appearance of the colonic mucosa is important in such instances, because it estimates the severity of involvement, which in turn aids in approximating the length of therapy (Fig. 4–4).

An obstructing carcinoma of the rectosigmoid colon is rarely manifested as diarrhea alone. Failure to find such a lesion on flexible sigmoidoscopy does not exclude the diagnosis when other clinical features suggest colorectal cancer.

Any physician performing flexible sigmoidoscopy must be aware of the limitations of such an examination. The flexible sigmoidoscope creates a bow in the sigmoid colon, which leads to overestimating the length of region examined by the endoscope. An insertion to 60 cm in one instance may reach the splenic flexure, whereas in another may fail to reach the descending sigmoid colon junction. This variation has major ramifications for therapy when inflammatory bowel disease or colon carcinoma is encountered.

Further Diagnostic Assessment

The aforementioned initial assessment of the patient with diarrhea allows one to diagnose accurately many cases of diarrhea. Results of the early evaluation—positive or negative—guide further the diagnostic approach (Fig. 4–5). The finding of inflammatory bowel disease may necessitate additional radiographic or endoscopic evaluation of the right colon and small bowel. A stool specimen positive for fecal fat when stained

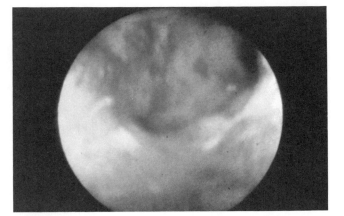

Figure 4–3. *Salmonella* colitis. Infectious colitis may mimic idiopathic ulcerative colitis or Crohn's colitis. The colonoscopic appearance of *Salmonella*-induced acute colitis may be indistinguishable from that of chronic ulcerative colitis. Biopsies may help distinguish between the two entities.

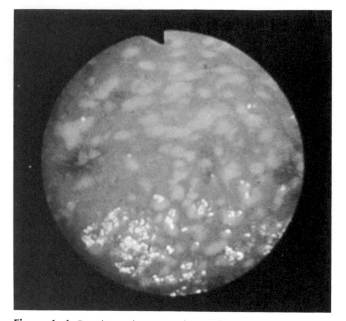

Figure 4–4. Pseudomembranous colitis. Yellowish-white pseudomembranes, typical of pseudomembranous colitis caused by *Clostridium difficile* infection. Although these characteristic pseudomembranes suggest antibiotic-associated colitis, their absence from the left colon does not exclude the diagnosis, as they are present in the rectosigmoid colon in only two thirds of cases.

with Sudan III suggests a diagnosis of malabsorption by the small bowel. This result necessitates small bowel radiography, assessment of carbohydrate absorption, possible small bowel biopsy, computed tomography, or endoscopic retrograde pancreatography. Confirmation of an infectious cause generally permits conclusion of the diagnostic assessment, initiation of therapy, and observation of response to therapy.

Further diagnostic assessment of diarrhea must continue in some patients. A 24-hour stool collection should be analyzed before one embarks on an additional workup. This analysis documents that the patient has true diarrhea, thereby heightening the likelihood that a pathologic process is responsible. Frequently the patient who complains of diarrhea may produce a small-volume 24-hour specimen with a low water content. Such a finding suggests either carbohydrate intolerance (lactose, sorbitol, or fructose intolerance) or irritable bowel syndrome. If more than 200 ml of a watery stool is collected, it should be analyzed for osmolality and sodium and magnesium concentration. The colon cannot produce a stool that is hypo-osmolar compared with the osmolality of serum, that is, less than 280 to 300. Osmolality of less than 240 mOsm suggests that water has been added to the collection, either by admixture of urine with the stool or by surreptitious means. Once stool osmolality has been measured, the stool osmolar gap should be calculated as follows: osmolar gap = total stool osmolality − stool [Na] × 2.

A stool osmolar gap greater than 50 mEq/l suggests the presence of an osmotic diarrhea. The causes of an osmotic diarrhea are limited and include disaccharidase (lactose) insufficiency, fructose malabsorption, sorbitol ingestion (chewing gum diarrhea), lactulose therapy, small bowel malabsorption disorders (e.g., celiac sprue), and excessive magnesium ingestion. The last can be diagnosed if the stool magnesium concentration is greater than 24 mEq/l.[11] The lactose breath test, which measures breath hydrogen following ingestion of lactose load, accurately identifies relative and absolute lactase deficiencies. However, the finding of a lactase deficiency in a patient may not account completely for an osmotic diarrhea, as this acquired abnormality is a common approach in 25% of healthy adults (Table 4–1).

Table 4–1. CAUSES OF OSMOTIC DIARRHEA

Lactose intolerance
Fructose intolerance
Sorbitol ingestion ("chewing gum" diarrhea)
Unmeasured cations: magnesium ingestion (e.g., magnesium citrate, magnesium-containing antacids)
Malabsorption (e.g., celiac sprue, tropical sprue)

1. Detailed history with particular attention to
   Patient's characterization of frequency, consistency of stool, duration of diarrhea (?acute or chronic)
   Nocturnal stooling present (suggests organic etiology)
   Detailed over-the-counter and prescription-drug history
   Detailed dietary history
   Surgical history to exclude postsurgical etiologies
   Sexual preference (see also discussion Gay Bowel Disease).

2. Physical examination with particular attention paid to
   Evidence of weight loss, wasting (suggests malabsorption, small bowel disease, or malignancy)
   Rectal examination to exclude fecal impaction, detect perirectal Crohn's disease.

3. Examination of stool specimen
   Is it really diarrhea?; formed specimen suggests functional etiology requiring limited evaluation
   Are fecal leukocytes present?
   Potassium hydroxide preparation: pink color indicates presence of phenolphthalein
   Sudan III stain: detects significant fat malabsorption.

4. Rigid or flexible sigmoidoscopy
   Useful in most cases of antibiotic-induced pseudomembranous colitis
   May detect inflammatory bowel disease
   May discover low-colon carcinoma.

5. Culture stool specimen for pathogens, including *Salmonella, Shigella,* and *Campylobacter*
   Ova and parasite examination by experienced technician
   Clostridium difficile toxin assay in cases of acute diarrhea following antibiotic use or
   when inflammatory bowel disease is present.

6. Small bowel radiography, air-contrast barium enema, or colonoscopy to rule out inflammatory bowel disease.

7. A 24-hour stool collection to quantitate diarrhea, measure osmolality.

Osmolality >350	Osmolality 240–350	Osmolality <240
Differential diagnosis of osmotic diarrhea (see Table 4–1)	Differential diagnosis of secretory diarrhea (see Table 4–2)	Unsatisfactory specimen (urine mixed with stool) or factitious diarrhea (water added to collection)

Steps 1 through 5 can be performed or initiated at first visit. Additional workup should proceed if diagnosis not made.

Figure 4–5. Evaluation of diarrhea.

The absence of a stool osmolar gap is evidence of a secretory component of the diarrhea. The differential diagnosis of secretory diarrhea is more expansive than that of osmotic diarrhea. Hormone or endotoxin-mediated as well as some laxative-induced diarrhea is a high-volume (more than 500 cc/day) secretory type. Diarrhea that continues despite fasting supports classifying it as secretory diarrhea. Chronic non–toxin-producing infections and inflammatory bowel disease may produce a largely secretory diarrhea.

If the stool collection analysis suggests a major secretory component of diarrhea, assessment should proceed with gastrointestinal roentgenography of the small bowel. The colon should be assessed by total colonoscopy and biopsy of colonic mucosa if a sigmoidoscopy has not been performed or by air-contrast barium enema if sigmoidoscopy has been unrevealing. If roentgenograms fail to reveal an etiology, the workup must move in a new direction.

If the evaluation has identified a chronic, high-volume secretory diarrhea (1 l/day), one must consider a hormonally mediated cause. Various benign and malignant tumors of amine precursor uptake and decarboxylase origin, arising in the pancreas or duodenum, produce intestinal secretagogues. A gastrinoma or vasoactive intestinal polypeptide–secreting tumor (VIPoma) can generally be excluded by history and stool quantitations, because these tumors produce profound, incapacitating diarrhea that often exceeds 1 l/day. In such instances, a fasting measurement of serum gastrin and vasoactive intestinal polypeptide (VIP) should be obtained. Table 4–2 lists causes of secretory diarrhea.

EVALUATING GASTROINTESTINAL SYMPTOMS IN HOMOSEXUAL MEN

The increasing prevalence of homosexual practices in urban and suburban populations has heightened awareness of sexually transmitted diseases, the "gay bowel" diseases and acquired immunodeficiency syndrome (AIDS)-related disorders affecting the gastrointestinal tract. Although homosexual or bisexual males may present with symptoms referable to anorectal infections, most are not associated with AIDS. Therefore the physician must consider any gastrointestinal disorder primarily affecting the colon and rectum of homosexual or bisexual individuals to be either a non–AIDS-related or AIDS-related disease (Fig. 4–6).

Non–AIDS-Related Diseases

Non–AIDS-related but sexually transmitted disease of the colon and rectum is not limited to only the homosexual and bisexual male population but may extend to the heterosexual female population practicing anal intercourse or anilingus. Anal sexual activity was reported by 25% of asymptomatic women surveyed in an urban gynecologic practice.[12] Therefore, the physician who sees any patient (male or female, homosexual, bisexual, or heterosexual) presenting with symptoms of anorectal pain, diarrhea, rectal bleeding, perianal discharge, and constipation must consider the diagnosis of sexually transmitted colorectal disease.

Whenever evaluating a patient with such symptoms, the physician must ask whether homosexual or anal sexual activity has been practiced. One can never assume that it has not, because most patients do not freely offer this information.

Perianal lesions and proctitis generally are accompanied by pain, discharge, bleeding, and possibly constipation. Generally these symptoms suggest local disease limited to the anus and rectum without extension to the rest of the colon. They may, however, be confused with idiopathic inflammatory bowel disease, such as ulcerative proctitis or Crohn's proctitis.

Following a detailed history and examination, proctoscopy should be performed to identify proctitis. Infectious proctitis can be caused by gonorrhea, syphilis, chlamydia, or herpes simplex. Proctoscopy may be very painful in a patient with infectious proctitis and should not be performed unless the physician is equipped to perform culture, biopsy, and dark-field microscopy on rectal tissue and exudate.

Gonorrhea Proctitis

Gonorrhea may be cultured in the rectum in as many as 45% of homosexual men,[13] although not all necessarily have symptoms. The appearance of gonorrhea proctitis is similar to that of idiopathic ulcerative proctitis. The mucosa is erythematous, friable, and edematous with exudate present. Inflammation is limited to the rectum and possibly the distal sigmoid colon. Inflammation extending beyond this region should raise the concern that *Shigella, Salmonella,* or amebic colitis is present.

A swab of exudate must be gram-stained and cul-

Table 4–2. CAUSES OF SECRETORY DIARRHEA

Certain laxatives (e.g., phenolphthalein, senna)
Tumors secreting hormones (e.g., gastrinoma, VIPoma)
Bile salt diarrhea (e.g., *Giardia,* AIDS-related infections)
Inflammatory bowel disease
Hyperthyroidism
Collagen vascular diseases (e.g., scleroderma)
Diabetic diarrhea

VIPoma = vasoactive intestinal polypeptide–secreting tumor;
AIDS = acquired immunodeficiency syndrome.

1. Assess for dehydration, may be profound.
2. Quantitate stool volume, fat.*
3. Culture stool for *Salmonella, Shigella, Campylobacter.*
4. Request direct stool examination for amebic cysts, trophozoites, *Giardia.*
5. Request acid-fast stain of stool for *Cryptosporidium, Isospora belli, Mycobacterium avium intracellulare* (MAI).

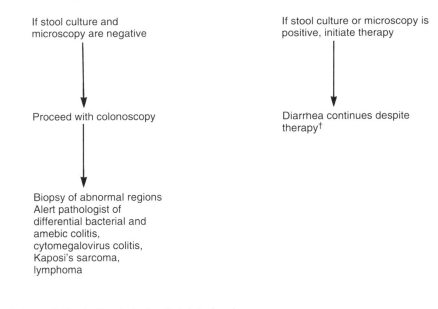

If stool culture and microscopy are negative

If stool culture or microscopy is positive, initiate therapy

Proceed with colonoscopy

Diarrhea continues despite therapy†

Biopsy of abnormal regions
Alert pathologist of
differential bacterial and
amebic colitis,
cytomegalovirus colitis,
Kaposi's sarcoma,
lymphoma

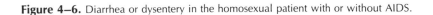

* A 24-hour fecal fat collection that exceeds 7 g signifies steatorrhea likely to be found.

† Isolated enteric pathogens may not account for symptoms in some patients since the carrier rate in this group of patients is high.

Figure 4–6. Diarrhea or dysentery in the homosexual patient with or without AIDS.

tured from *Neisseria gonorrhoeae.* In gonorrhea proctitis, Gram's stain of anorectal exudate reveals gram-negative diplococci within leukocytes. This factitious organism requires a special culture medium. A standard culture broth allows overgrowth of other organisms, which prevents isolation of *N. gonorrhoeae.* Thayer-Martin medium containing antibiotics to inhibit growth of other organisms may be used to culture *N. gonorrhoeae* from the rectum. Alternatively one can smear exudate onto chocolate agar. Incubation of either medium in a CO_2-rich environment for 48 hours is essential in order to isolate the organism.

Improper handling of the anal swab results in failure to isolate the organism, thereby potentiating misdiagnosis and improper treatment of gonorrhea proctitis. Growth of the gonorrhea organism in culture may be impaired if the rectal exudate is mixed with stool. Care must be taken to obtain a swab of the exudate alone and to discard any obviously contaminated swab. A stool specimen should never be used to diagnose rectal gonorrhea.

A biopsy of inflamed rectal mucosa should be obtained. Although nonspecific inflammatory changes indistinguishable from ulcerative proctitis may be observed, gonococci in the mucosa may be seen, confirming the diagnosis. The absence of gonococci in a rectal biopsy specimen does not exclude gonococcal proctitis.

Penicillin-resistant strains of *N. gonorrhoeae* have emerged over the past 2 decades, making treatment of infections difficult in some areas. Furthermore, gonococci isolated from homosexual males are more likely to be penicillin-resistant than those isolated from heterosexual patients.[14] Antimicrobial susceptibility should be requested if standard therapy fails to treat gonorrhea proctitis adequately.

Chlamydia trachomatis Proctitis

Chlamydia trachomatis infection of the rectum is common in homosexual men, carrier rates being as high as 15%. Both the lymphogranuloma venereum (LGV) strains and the non–lymphogranuloma venereum (non-LGV) strains may cause proctitis with features similar to those caused by *N. gonorrhoeae.* However, the extent of involvement may be greater, with inflammation extending through the sigmoid and descending colons. The LGV strains may be manifested as acute proctocolitis with fever and bloody diarrhea in addition to complaints of rectal pain and tenesmus. Inguinal lymphadenopathy may be present. Proctosigmoidoscopy shows discrete ulcerations, not unlike those seen with Crohn's colitis. LGV infection may form fibrosing strictures of the sigmoid colon, mimicking Crohn's stricture. Rectal biopsy, displaying crypt abscesses with granulomas and giant cells may be misinterpreted as indicating Crohn's disease. The non-LGV strains produce more local inflammation confined to the rectum. Proctoscopy reveals a more diffuse, less ulcerated process with nonspecific inflammation or rectal biopsy.

Because the proctoscopic and histologic appearances are nonspecific, the diagnosis of *C. trachomatis* proctitis rests heavily on the isolation of *Chlamydia* from the rectum. The organism can be cultured from a rectal swab, which should be part of any evaluation of proctitis in the homosexual patient. The culture technique is approximately 55% sensitive. Therefore, serologic evaluation should be included in suspected cases. The complement-fixation method lacks sensitivity and may not distinguish LGV from non-LGV strains. The preferred microimmunofluorescent antibody titer assay detects acute and chronic infections of both LGV and non-LGV strains. The LGV and non-LGV strains should be differentiated, because the former requires longer therapy with tetracycline in order to eradicate the organism.

Syphilis Proctitis

Anorectal syphilis may be confused with hemorrhoids, fissures, or anorectal abscesses. These painful anorectal chancres may develop several weeks after exposure. Alternatively, syphilis proctitis, with features indistinguishable from other infectious forms of proctitis, may be present. Dark-field examination of either the anal chancres or rectal exudate may reveal spirochetes, thereby confirming the diagnosis. However, the specimens must be examined within minutes of collection to ensure adequate motility of the organism. Rectal biopsy may reveal the *Treponema pallidum* organism when silver stained. Because many patients may present with symptoms before serologic tests (Venereal Disease Research Laboratory [VDRL], fluorescent treponemal antibody absorption [FTA-ABS]) are positive, they may fail to identify properly *Treponema* infection. If the VDRL is negative at the initial visit, it should be performed at a follow-up visit in 4 weeks in suspected but unconfirmed cases.

Herpetic Proctitis

Herpetic proctitis must be suspected in differential diagnosis of proctitis of both heterosexual and homo-sexual patients practicing anal sex. In addition to complaints of rectal pain and tenesmus, symptoms may include fever and malaise, sacral paresthesia, thigh pain, and inguinal lymphadenopathy. Sigmoidoscopy and mucosal biopsy are nonspecific, generally showing diffuse, inflammatory changes. Only occasionally, intranuclear inclusions or multinucleated giant cells may be present to support the diagnosis. Therefore rectal swabs or biopsy specimens should be sent for herpetic culture.

Genital Warts

Genital warts, caused by human papillomavirus, may be asymptomatic and discovered only during routine examination or when the patient presents with symptoms of coexisting sexually transmitted disease. The warts appear as a velvety or villous growth, often resembling a sessile polyp, in the perianal region or intra-anal canal. Most patients with intra-anal lesions have concomitant perianal disease, which facilitates detection of the warts. However, 10% of homosexual patients may have lesions intra-anally without perianal involvement, thereby making detection difficult. The intra-anal lesions are missed during proctoscopy; therefore anoscopy is essential during any anorectal evaluation in the homosexual male. Because condylomata acuminata has been associated with squamous cell carcinoma of the rectum, treatment should be instituted whenever the lesions are detected. There is a strong association between condylomata acuminata and anal squamous cell carcinoma. Previous gonococcal, chlamydial, or herpetic proctitis may also predispose the homosexual male to anal carcinoma.[15] For any atypical anal lesion, regardless of coexisting anorectal pathology, a biopsy should be done to exclude squamous cell carcinoma or its precursor, anal intraepithelial neoplasia.

Rectal Trauma

Usually anal intercourse is not associated with significant rectal trauma. Rectal incontinence is rarely noted, except when infectious proctitis is found. Anal sphincter tone may not be appreciably diminished in the homosexual male, unless there has been a previous tear of the anorectal sphincters. This latter finding is more apt to occur when foreign bodies are used in the practice of anorectal stimulation. Most rectal foreign bodies are expelled spontaneously. However, the patient may present with an inability to pass the object spontaneously without complaints of pain or bleeding.

Following assessment to ascertain that there is no intraperitoneal perforation, either by physical examination or radiography, digital examination of the rectum is performed. If the retained object is palpated, it can generally be removed transanally after local anesthesia is injected around the anus. Thereafter, proctosigmoidoscopy should be performed to ensure that there is no significant rectal tear. If the object cannot be palpated on digital examination, the patient should be hospitalized and observed until peristalsis propagates the foreign body to distal rectum, at which point the transanal removal can be done. This approach allows easy, safe removal of most foreign bodies without the need for laparotomy.[16] Fist penetration of the rectum is also apt to be associated with an anorectal trauma causing bleeding and pain.

Homosexuals often use lubricants and soaps prior to anal intercourse. These agents may cause a nonspecific, noninfectious proctitis that appear to be indistinguishable from several infectious forms (Fig. 4–7). Discontinuation of these irritants allows healing and resolving of symptoms.

Colonic Infections in Homosexuals

The homosexual male presenting with diarrhea, rectal bleeding, and abdominal cramps must be considered to have infectious colitis until it is proved otherwise. The clinical features of infectious colitis in the homosexual patient are similar to those of the heterosexual patient with either infectious or idiopathic colitis. The pathogenic organisms encountered usually are the same ones that cause infectious colitis in the heterosexual population, that is, *Shigella, Salmonella,* and *C. jejuni.* However, the frequency with which these infections are the cause of colitis is much greater among homosexuals. It is now well-recognized that these pathogens can be transmitted venereally.

The evaluation of the homosexual patient with suspected colitis should be like that of the heterosexual patient presenting with similar symptoms. The absence of rectal bleeding and physical findings of severe dehydration may not distinguish between colitis and infectious enteritis. A methylene blue–stained specimen should be examined for fecal leukocytes. Their presence strongly supports the diagnosis of infectious colitis. Sigmoidoscopy reveals the same nonspecific inflammatory changes, including inflammatory exudate, erythema, and granular and friable mucosa. The involvement may resemble Crohn's disease in some cases of *Salmonella* or *Campylobacter* infection, but rarely in cases of shigellosis. Therefore stool culture is essential to proper diagnosis of an infectious colitis and distinction among these three pathogenic causes. The therapy of choice is different for each of the three organisms.

Entamoeba histolytica infections are common in homosexual males, although most are asymptomatic carriers. Bowel symptoms may be rather mild, mimicking irritable bowel syndrome. Rarely, fulminant colitis that is clinically indistinguishable from other infectious colitides may ensue. Because symptoms vary widely, amebiasis should be considered in any homosexual male presenting with gastrointestinal complaints. Sigmoidoscopic findings are variable. The rectal mucosa may be normal or minimally inflamed. Erythema, mucosa friability, and ulcerations indistinguishable from ulcerative or Crohn's colitis may be seen.[9] Biopsies should be taken from regions where exudate is adherent to the mucosa, because these regions are most likely to contain the amebae. Nevertheless, rectal biopsy may fail to reveal amebae in nearly half the cases of amebiasis. Fresh, warm stool must carefully be examined for trophozoites or cysts. Formed stools are more apt to contain the cyst form, whereas diarrheal stools may allow identification of the mobile trophozoites. Serologic tests for amebiasis are both sensitive and specific, yet they do not readily identify asymptomatic carriers; nor do they infer active infection, as serologic tests remain positive for years after treatment.

AIDS-Related Infections

AIDS has not only increased the incidence of enteric infections in homosexual males but broadened the spectrum of pathogenic organisms identified in the gut.

Although cytomegalovirus (CMV) infection is common in the homosexual male population with and without AIDS, it is apt to be manifested as a serious infection in the patient with AIDS while being subclinical in most without AIDS. In the patient with AIDS, CMV may present with abdominal pain, diarrhea, and occasionally bleeding, which suggests an infectious colitis. The symptoms are nonspecific, thereby heightening the need for the physician to consider the diagnosis CMV colitis. The infection typically involves the right colon and terminal ileum and so resembles Crohn's disease (Figs. 4–8 and 4–9). Colonoscopic biopsies are thus paramount for proper diagnosis. Intranuclear inclusion suggests the diagnosis, but it should be confirmed by culture. A sample of the colonic mucosa, obtained by pinch biopsy at the time of colonoscopy, should be specifically cultured in viral culture media. Because CMV colitis may become fulminant and possibly cause colonic perforation, and in view of effective therapy provided by ganciclovir, an acyclovir analogue, earlier recognition of this colitis is essential.[17]

Large-volume, watery, nonbloody diarrhea in the patient with AIDS suggests an enteric infection. The incapacitating diarrhea has the hallmark of a secretory diarrhea, namely volumes exceeding 1 l/day, even when the patient is fasting. One of three pathogens is often

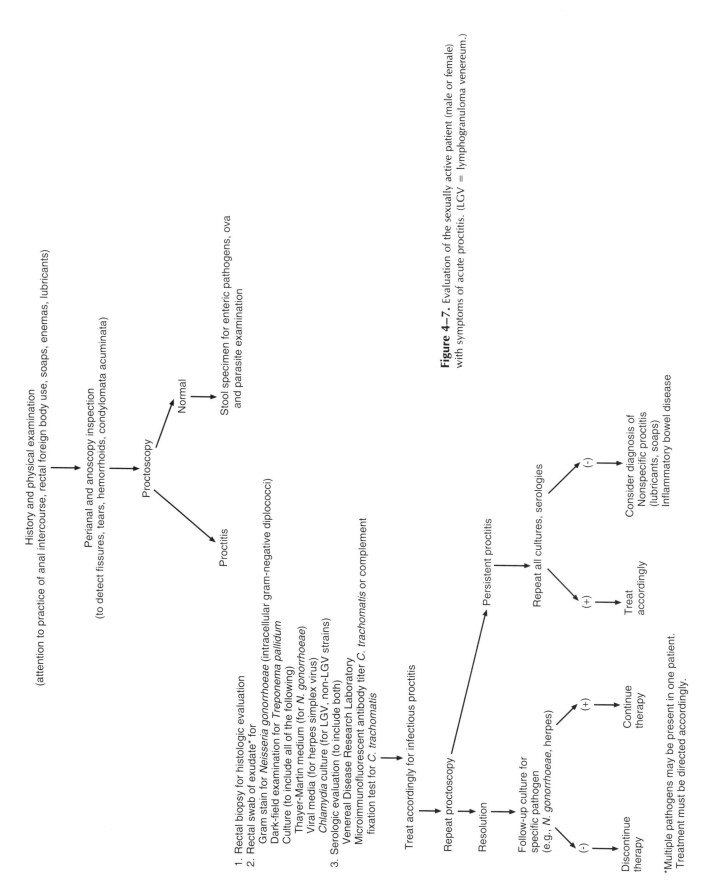

History and physical examination
(attention to practice of anal intercourse, rectal foreign body use, soaps, enemas, lubricants)

Perianal and anoscopy inspection
(to detect fissures, tears, hemorrhoids, condylomata acuminata)

Proctoscopy

Normal

Stool specimen for enteric pathogens, ova and parasite examination

Proctitis

1. Rectal biopsy for histologic evaluation
2. Rectal swab of exudate* for
   Gram stain for *Neisseria gonorrhoeae* (intracellular gram-negative diplococci)
   Dark-field examination for *Treponema pallidum*
   Culture (to include all of the following)
   Thayer-Martin medium (for *N. gonorrhoeae*)
   Viral media (for herpes simplex virus)
   Chlamydia culture (for LGV, non-LGV strains)
3. Serologic evaluation (to include both)
   Venereal Disease Research Laboratory
   Microimmunofluorescent antibody titer *C. trachomatis* or complement fixation test for *C. trachomatis*

Treat accordingly for infectious proctitis

Repeat proctoscopy

Resolution

Follow-up culture for specific pathogen
(e.g., *N. gonorrhoeae*, herpes)

(+)

Continue therapy

(-)

Discontinue therapy

Persistent proctitis

Repeat all cultures, serologies

(+)

Treat accordingly

(-)

Consider diagnosis of
Nonspecific proctitis
(lubricants, soaps)
Inflammatory bowel disease

*Multiple pathogens may be present in one patient. Treatment must be directed accordingly.

Figure 4–7. Evaluation of the sexually active patient (male or female) with symptoms of acute proctitis. (LGV = lymphogranuloma venereum.)

identified. *Cryptosporidium,* an opportunistic parasite that adheres to the small bowel brush border, can be diagnosed when stool is examined by using acid-fast stain. *Isospora belli,* which resembles *Cryptosporidium,* may be identified by using the same technique.

Alternatively, if clinical suspicion is high and stool samples fail to identify either organism, small bowel biopsy may be performed. With acid-fast stain, the organisms can be seen adhering to the brush border of the jejunum. *Mycobacterium avium intracellulare* can be diagnosed by acid-fast staining of either stool or small bowel mucosa; unlike the other two pathogens, blood culture may allow detection because the infection may disseminate. Whipple's disease, a small bowel infiltrative disorder manifested by malabsorption and diarrhea, may be indistinguishable from *M. avium intracellulare* on a biopsy of small bowel mucosa. Both entities reveal characteristic period acid–Schiff (PAS)-laden macrophages within the lamina propria of the jejunal mucosa, but only *M. avium intracellulare* reveals acid-fast organisms.

Unfortunately, despite easy detection of all three pathogenic organisms, therapy for *Cryptosporidium, I. belli,* and *M. avium intracellulare* infections has limited effectiveness. Anecdotal reports of successful antibiotic therapies for these organisms have spawned recent clinical trials.[18, 19]

Kaposi's sarcoma may be discovered coincidentally in any patient with AIDS who is undergoing sigmoidoscopy or colonoscopy as part of the evaluation of diarrhea, rectal bleeding, or rectal pain (Fig. 4–10). Although the incidence of Kaposi's sarcoma involving the gastrointestinal tract is not known, it is as high as 40% in those with known skin or nodal involvement by this tumor. Because most patients are asymptomatic, the lesion is often undetected unless coexisting infections prompt gastrointestinal evaluation. The lesions appear either macular with submucosal erythema or nodular. A reticulated pattern is common. Uncommon appearances, such as colonic ulceration with surrounding edema mimicking ulcerative or infectious colitis, have been noted.[20] Unfortunately, biopsy specimens from characteristic Kaposi's lesions usually do not provide a definitive diagnosis, because the lesions originate within the submucosa.

As with the unusual infectious complications of the gastrointestinal tract in patients with AIDS, malignant lymphoma may mimic inflammatory bowel disease. The terminal ileum appears to be a preferred site, as it is in Crohn's disease. When a diagnosis of malignant lymphoma is considered, endoscopic biopsy of the terminal ileum should be performed. It is important to obtain unfixed tissue for tumor-marker immunohistochemical staining.

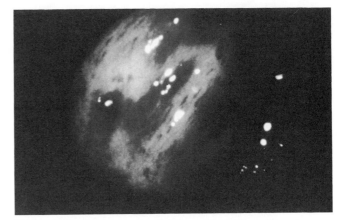

Figure 4–8. Cytomegalovirus (CMV) colitis. Inflammatory changes mimicking Crohn's disease or ulcerative colitis may be seen in the patient with AIDS. CMV infection may have a variety of endoscopic appearances. Biopsies and cultures help distinguish the disease from idiopathic ulcerative colitis or Crohn's colitis.

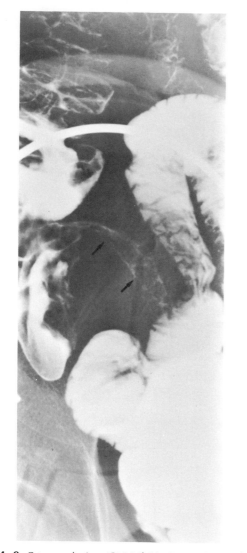

Figure 4–9. Cytomegalovirus (CMV) ileitis. Just as CMV colitis may mimic inflammatory bowel disease, so CMV ileitis may mimic small bowel Crohn's disease. The stricture and nodular appearance of CMV ileitis of terminal ileum was erroneously interpreted as Crohn's disease in this patient with AIDS.

LOWER GASTROINTESTINAL BLEEDING

Acute Lower Gastrointestinal Bleeding

Acute lower gastrointestinal bleeding is defined as bleeding from a site below the ligament of Treitz; this definition includes small intestinal as well as colonic etiologies. Occasionally, an upper gastrointestinal hemorrhage, usually from the duodenum, appears as rectal bleeding without hematemesis. The physician must use clinical judgment to try to determine the anatomic location and etiology of bleeding before embarking on a diagnostic evaluation. Because most patients who present with lower gastrointestinal bleeding are elderly, the average age being 65 years, invasive diagnostic procedures should be limited.

The history and physical examination are paramount in the evaluation of a bleeding patient. The patient's age must be considered when one investigates the differential diagnosis of bleeding. Brisk bleeding from an arteriovenous malformation is rarely congenital and is unlikely in a young patient. Although diverticular disease of the colon is reported in patients 40 years old or younger, the presentation is rarely one of bleeding. Massive bleeding in a previously well, young patient suggests bleeding from a Meckel's diverticulum or duodenal ulcer. Non–life-threatening bleeding in the younger patient suggests either benign anorectal conditions (hemorrhoids, fissures) or inflammatory bowel disease. Similar bleeding in the middle-aged or elderly patient requires exclusion of colorectal neoplasia.

The color of the blood passed may be misleading as to the site of bleeding. Bright red blood passed per rectum may arise from hemorrhoids, colonic diverticula, or duodenal ulcers. Associated symptoms, including syncope and lightheadedness, suggest hypotension and imply a brisk vascular bleed from the colon or higher sites. Vascular bleeding refers to larger arterial or arteriolar sites of bleeding. In the colon these include bleeding from arteriovenous malformations and diverticula. A duodenal ulcer eroding into a branch of the gastroduodenal artery may produce a similar clinical posture with massive rectal bleeding and hypotension without hematemesis. Hemorrhoids or other causes of anorectal bleeding rarely produce hypotension, except in the cirrhotic patient.

The passage of blood only, without stool, is also significant and implies a lesion above the rectum, often of a vascular etiology. Patients who report bleeding with a bowel movement and have no other symptoms are more inclined to have polyps, carcinoma, ulcerative proctitis, or other anorectal causes of bleeding.

Although melena generally implies duodenal or gastric bleeding, it may originate from bleeding in the right colon or small intestine. The rate of bleeding and colonic transit of the blood may allow its darkening to maroon or black, despite the relatively low site of origin.

A careful medication history is essential if upper gastrointestinal tract bleeding is contemplated in the differential diagnosis. The use of aspirin, aspirin-containing products (Anacin, Bufferin, Excedrin), or nonsteroidal anti-inflammatory drugs (NSAID) heightens the likelihood that a gastric or duodenal ulcer is present, which often prompts upper gastrointestinal evaluation first. The physical examination is important not only in identifying the type of bleeding but also in managing it. Orthostasis, hypotension, or tachycardia suggests significant blood loss from a vascular lesion. These signs necessitate prompt intravascular, as well as blood volume, replacement before diagnostic evaluations can proceed. Although volume restoration with crystalline fluid (e.g., normal saline or lactated Ringer's solution) normalizes blood pressure, the oxygen-carrying capacity may remain low, possibly resulting in myocardial or intestinal ischemia. Before the briskly bleeding patient is evaluated, efforts should be made to maintain the hematocrit at above 30%, systolic blood pressure above 100 mm Hg, and pulse rate under 120 beats/min.

Any gastrointestinal tract bleeding that occurs with signs of orthostasis, hypotension, or profound tachycardia should first be evaluated by excluding an upper gastrointestinal tract site. The physician must not make the erroneous assumption that the bleeding originates from below the ligament of Trietz if a nasogastric lavage is clear. Nearly 15% of patients with an upper gastrointestinal site of bleeding are found to have a clear nasogastric lavage on presentation.[21] Because esophagogastroduodenoscopy (EGD) is easily performed and promptly excludes bleeding from sites down to the third portion of the duodenum, it should be the first diagnostic evaluation performed following resuscitation in the hemodynamically unstable patient with gastrointestinal bleeding.

Once EGD has excluded an upper gastrointestinal site of bleeding, the physician has several options to pursue in identifying the site and cause of the bleeding. Consideration of the likely differential diagnoses for various age groups, as well as the presence of ongoing bleeding, helps direct further evaluation.

Emergent colonoscopy during severe bleeding has usually been avoided, because generally it is nondiagnostic and impractical. Visualization of the colonic mucosa is impaired in the unprepared bleeding patient. When the precise site is not seen, regional localization of bleeding may help limit surgical resection. However, retrograde flow of blood throughout long segments of

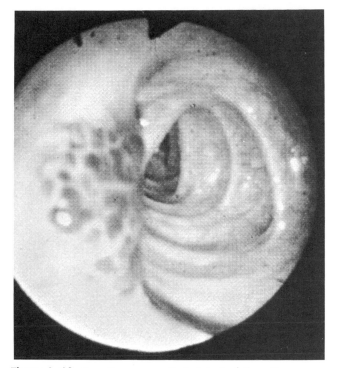

Figure 4–10. Kaposi's sarcoma. Gastrointestinal Kaposi's sarcomas are generally found coincidentally during a workup for rectal bleeding or diarrhea in a patient with AIDS. The reticulated, nodular appearance seen here is typical of Kaposi's sarcoma.

colon, and even into the terminal ileum, may falsely indicate the region of bleeding. Most endoscopists urge conservative support until bleeding has subsided or stopped before preparing the patient and proceeding with colonoscopy. Flexible sigmoidoscopy is of limited value in the bleeding patient and should generally be avoided in favor of complete colonoscopy. Colonoscopy may be used to establish the diagnosis of ischemic injury to the colon. Patients in whom the diagnosis is suspected should undergo "gentle" colonoscopic examination, because distention of the bowel with insufflating gas may result in perforation. If ischemic changes are noted in the left colon, complete examination of the entire colon is not necessary, except to limit the extent of surgical resection.

Endoscopic therapy exists for lower gastrointestinal bleeding. Lesions amenable to endoscopic therapy include angiodysplasia and bleeding from polypectomy sites. Endoscopic coagulation should be attempted by an experienced endoscopist, because it may prevent surgical intervention. Portable, easy-to-use bipolar electrocoagulation units can be used to control active bleeding or prevent recurrent bleeding from angiodysplasia of the colon. Because a transmural "burn" or perforation may result, especially during treatment for angiodysplasia of the cecum, low-current settings should be used. Higher-energy devices, such as lasers and monopolar coagulation devices, carry a greater perforation rate when used to treat lesions in the colon. Lavage of a bleeding diverticulum with epinephrine to control bleeding has been reported but is generally not feasible.[22]

Unfortunately, angiography requires active bleeding at the rate of at least 1 ml/min in order to allow detection. Bleeding must have a vascular origin, such as an artery within a diverticulum or arteriovenous malformation. Such bleeding is intermittent, which is likely to account for some reports that angiography is not sensitive for evaluating lower gastrointestinal bleeding. Therefore, prompt examination is essential when active bleeding is suspected by ongoing hypotension, orthostasis, or tachycardia. When instituted promptly in patients with massive lower gastrointestinal bleeding, superior and inferior mesenteric angiography may localize bleeding in over 70% of patients.[23] Localizing the site of bleeding may limit surgical resection or permit the use of angiographic therapy. Following identification of a bleeding site, selective infra-arterial infusion of vasopressin will halt bleeding in most patients. Operative mortality may be lower when angiographic therapy is initiated to stabilize the actively bleeding patient. Its use should be encouraged if an experienced angiographer is available.

Radionuclide bleeding scans are frequently used to localize bleeding sites in patients with lower gastrointestinal bleeding. Although the sensitivity may be greater than for angiography, its specificity may impair accurate diagnosis. Caution should be exercised against surgical intervention based on the results of a bleeding scan alone. Rather, the scan should redirect one's attention to specific sites of the gastrointestinal tract when one performs repeat angiography or endoscopy.

In the pediatric or young adult patient presenting with lower gastrointestinal bleeding, a nuclear isotope scan for Meckel's diverticula should be employed after endoscopy has ruled out an upper gastrointestinal source. The presence of ectopic gastric mucosa and its increased uptake of ^{99m}Tc pertechnetate permit the visualization of many Meckel's diverticula by scintigraphy. However, because the sensitivity is only 75%, a negative scan result does not exclude the diagnosis. If bleeding has stopped, small bowel radiography can be performed, occasionally revealing an erected Meckel's diverticulum.

Intraoperative endoscopy may be indicated in selected circumstances in which gastrointestinal bleeding is believed to arise from the small bowel. Intraoperative endoscopy should be considered only after attempts at conventional colonoscopy and EGD have failed to identify a definitive or suspected bleeding source. Furthermore, angiography should be performed before intraoperative endoscopy is considered. It may be useful to identify suspected angiodysplasia of the ileum, which may coexist in patients in whom cecal angiodysplasia is present. By identifying the uppermost extent of small bowel angiodysplasia, one can limit the length of resected small bowel.

Intraoperative endoscopy can be performed via the oral, rectal, or enterotomal route. After the abdomen is opened, a pediatric colonoscope can be introduced into the mouth. It can then be advanced easily to the ligament of Treitz. Thereafter, examination of the entire small bowel is facilitated by pleating the small bowel over the colonoscope. The endoscopist must take care to limit the amount of air insufflation, because excessive distention of the bowel will result in prolonged postoperative ileus. Complications of intraoperative endoscopy also include serosal lacerations and perforation. When the colonoscope is placed through an enterotomy site, contamination of the exposed peritoneum may occur, even if the colonoscope has been sterilized.

EDITORIAL COMMENT
The responsible surgeon must not allow the patient with major lower intestinal bleeding to be endlessly manipulated for the evanescent goals of "localization" or "therapy." If significant bleeding continues or if the patient becomes hemodynamically unstable, further nonoperative manipulations should be abandoned and the patient promptly resuscitated and operated on.

Chronic Lower Gastrointestinal Bleeding

The differential diagnosis of slower chronic forms of lower gastrointestinal bleeding is limited and more easily evaluated. The patient over the age of 30 years must be considered to have a colonic neoplasm until it is proved otherwise. Hemorrhoids or anorectal fissures found on anoscopic examination should not dissuade the physician from further evaluation by means of colonoscopy. The history alone is often misleading when one is trying to determine the cause of intermittent, non–life-threatening rectal bleeding. Typical symptoms of bright red blood streaking on the stool or passage of bright red blood with a bowel movement suggest anorectal or higher left colon sources of bleeding. However, a distinction between these two locations is important and often difficult to make on the basis of history alone. In one series, 16% of cases of rectal bleeding from colonic neoplasms (polyps and carcinomas) would have been misdiagnosed as benign anorectal disease (hemorrhoids and fissures). Flexible sigmoidoscopy frequently fails to reach the descending colon because the scope bows the sigmoid colon; therefore colonoscopy is essential in this clinical setting.

In the younger patient presenting with non–life-threatening lower rectal bleeding, anorectal lesions, inflammatory bowel disease, and juvenile polyps are frequently encountered. Anoscopy and flexible sigmoidoscopy may be employed, but further evaluation by total colonoscopy should not be withheld if the limited examination fails to identify a definitive source of bleeding or if iron-deficiency anemia is present.

Occult gastrointestinal bleeding is frequently discovered as part of a routine physical examination. Frequently, a physician tests a random stool specimen (obtained on a screening rectal examination) for the presence of blood. However, the predictive value of a positive test for fecal occult blood is not known, because several factors may influence the outcome of the assay. The standard fecal occult blood tests are employed to screen for colorectal carcinomas or large (wider than 1 cm) polyps. A fecal occult blood test (FOBT) should be performed annually as part of a program of screening for colorectal neoplasia in the patient 50 years of age or older. Properly performed, the FOBT may detect as many as 50% of these lesions.

The patient should be instructed to be on a low red meat, high-fiber diet for 2 days before and during stool sampling for FOBT. Red meat as well as foods high in peroxidase content (e.g., beets) may cause a false-positive result. A high-fiber diet may augment sensitivity by abrading a polyp or carcinoma, thereby promoting bleeding. Additionally, aspirin, NSAIDs, and iron can cause a false-positive reaction and should be avoided before and during testing. Vitamin C may cause a false-positive result and should be avoided.

If the test result of any of the three stool samples collected is positive, further colorectal evaluation by means of colonoscopy or flexible sigmoidoscopy and air-contrast barium enema should ensue without delay. Repeating FOBT, in the hope of obtaining a negative result, should not be done. Furthermore, FOBT should not be used in the evaluation of patients with symptoms that suggest colorectal neoplasia (e.g., thinning stool, gross rectal bleeding). Instead, these patients should immediately be evaluated with colonoscopy or barium enema.

Fecal occult blood loss may also be discovered during the evaluation of anemia. Commonly, occult blood loss results in iron-deficiency anemia. A serum iron–to–iron-binding capacity ratio of less than 10% or a serum ferritin of less than 20 in the patient with anemia should alert the physician to a diagnosis of iron deficiency. Regardless of the outcome of FOBT, colorectal evaluation should ensue, except in young female patients with menorrhagia.

Two strategies may be employed in the assessment of fecal occult blood loss. Colonoscopy is becoming a frequently used tool to assess for colorectal neoplasia in this setting. Proponents argue that it has greater efficacy in detecting polyps and carcinomas of significant size and permits polypectomy at the same time.[24] Alternatively, flexible sigmoidoscopy in conjunction with an air-contrast barium enema may be used. This approach is safer and often better-tolerated by elderly patients. Performing flexible sigmoidoscopy or air-contrast barium enema alone is not an acceptable alternative. Flexible sigmoidoscopy alone does not identify pathologic lesions above the left colon, whereas an air-contrast barium enema may fail to identify such lesions in a tortuous, redundant sigmoid colon. Single-contrast barium enema should not be used, because it lacks sensitivity in detecting mucosal lesions.

Opinions vary concerning which approach should be used in the evaluation of a positive FOBT result. Many physicians prefer colonoscopy, because its sensitivity for detecting polyps is greater than that of flexible sigmoidoscopy and air-contrast barium enema. Opponents of colonoscopy as the diagnostic procedure of choice argue that the cost of evaluation is lower when flexible sigmoidoscopy and air-contrast barium enema are employed. Obviously, cost analysis depends on individual charges by each physician and hospital as well as the age of patients included in the analysis. In older patients, there is a greater likelihood that a polyp of significant size will be discovered and that colonoscopy for removal will be necessary. This case would favor colonoscopy as the initial procedure of choice.

SCREENING FOR COLORECTAL NEOPLASIA

In addition to an annual FOBT, the American Cancer Society (ACS) recommends that patients 50 years of age or older have a flexible sigmoidoscopy performed annually for 2 consecutive years. If neither examination discovers a polyp, follow-up examination by flexible sigmoidoscopy is necessary every 3 years. However, FOBT should continue annually (Fig. 4–11).

Certain individuals may require alternative screening approaches. Patients who have had polypectomy for a benign adenomatous polyp should have colonoscopy repeated in 1 year. If no other polyps are identified, colonoscopic surveillance should continue every 3 years. If additional polyps are found, surveillance should be performed annually until a "clear" colonoscopy is identified, at which point colonoscopy may be performed every 3 years. Patients in whom a colon carcinoma has been resected should have follow-up colonoscopy performed in a similar manner.

Patients with a known history of colon cancer require additional surveillance utilizing serum carcinoembryonic antigen (CEA). The serum level of CEA should be established before a known or suspected colorectal carcinoma is resected. Serum CEA is less than 2.5 ng/ml in healthy individuals without colorectal carcinoma; it suggests that widespread metastatic disease is not likely. Furthermore, a normal preoperative CEA has been associated with a lower rate of occurrence.[25] A high preoperative serum CEA (greater than 10 ng/ml) is usually associated with metastatic disease. If an elevated preoperative CEA does not fall after resection, there is usually residual malignant disease.

The greatest usefulness of serum CEA determination is in screening asymptomatic patients who have undergone a resection for colorectal carcinoma.

A positive or rising serum CEA following cancer resection correlates well with the presence of recurrent or metastatic disease. CEA should be followed every 3 months for 3 years after resection. If it is found to be abnormal on two consecutive determinations drawn 3 months apart, reevaluation for recurrent or metastatic disease should ensue. This should entail colonoscopy to exclude a colonic recurrence, a computed tomographic scan of the abdomen and pelvis, and a chest radiograph.

Although the determination of serum CEA is valuable in the patient with a known history of colorectal carcinoma, it is rarely helpful as a screening examination for colorectal neoplasm in patients without an established diagnosis. Because as many as 40% of patients with early colorectal cancer may have a normal serum CEA, its sensitivity is low.[25] Conversely, smoking may elevate serum CEA,[25] erroneously suggesting

colorectal neoplasia. Furthermore, an elevated serum CEA is nonspecific. An elevated serum CEA may be associated with other forms of cancer, including pancreatic and breast cancer. However, these diseases generally are widely spread by the time the serum CEA is elevated.

The individual risk for colonic neoplasm if one first-degree relative is affected is two or three times that of the general population. The risk if two first-degree relatives are affected is substantially higher, approaching 30%. If a single first-degree relative is affected, standard screening employing yearly digital examination of the rectum, annual hemoccult testing, and flexible sigmoidoscopy every 3 years may be used. However, screening should begin at a younger age than for the general population. Screening should begin at 35 years of age. If two or more first-degree relatives have a history of colon cancer, full colon evaluation by means of colonoscopy should be performed every 3 years, beginning at age 35 (Fig. 4–12).

Familial adenomatous polyposis syndrome and Gardener's syndrome inevitably cause colon cancer if the colon is not removed. The average age of colon cancer diagnosis is 39 years. The polyps usually begin to appear in the second decade, although symptoms may not appear for 10 to 20 years thereafter. Because both syndromes are autosomal dominant with incomplete penetrance, screening of first-degree relatives is imperative. Annual flexible sigmoidoscopy should be performed in all first-degree relatives, beginning at the age of 12 years. Because both syndromes invariably involve the rectosigmoid colon early in life, full colonoscopy is not necessary for screening family members (Fig. 4–13).

For patients in whom a subtotal colectomy with ileorectal anastomosis has been performed for polyposis, yearly proctoscopic examination and fulguration of polyps are essential. Nonetheless, the cumulative incidence of cancer in such patients is 30% over 10 years, despite frequent endoscopic follow-up and fulguration.[26] Duodenal adenomas are common in Gardener's syndrome and familial adenomatous polyposis. Once either syndrome is identified, patients should undergo periodic screening for duodenal polyps. Screening by means of upper gastrointestinal endoscopy should continue every 3 to 5 years, even after colectomy has been performed.

There are no reliable data on the early detection of carcinoma in patients with chronic ulcerative colitis. Therefore, screening programs are not uniform and are often individualized by many physicians. Clearly, certain factors affect the risk of developing colon cancer in the patient with ulcerative colitis. These factors, including duration and extent of disease, determine the screening schedules for various individuals.

Total colonoscopy with random biopsies should be

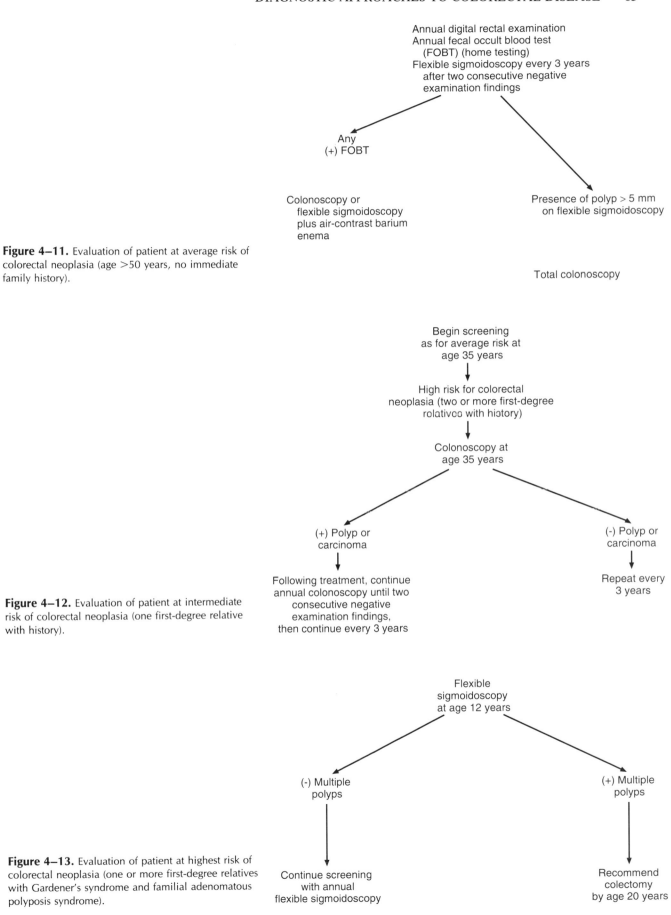

Annual digital rectal examination
Annual fecal occult blood test
(FOBT) (home testing)
Flexible sigmoidoscopy every 3 years
after two consecutive negative
examination findings

Any
(+) FOBT

Colonoscopy or
flexible sigmoidoscopy
plus air-contrast barium
enema

Presence of polyp > 5 mm
on flexible sigmoidoscopy

Total colonoscopy

Figure 4–11. Evaluation of patient at average risk of colorectal neoplasia (age >50 years, no immediate family history).

Begin screening
as for average risk at
age 35 years

High risk for colorectal
neoplasia (two or more first-degree
relatives with history)

Colonoscopy at
age 35 years

(+) Polyp or
carcinoma

(-) Polyp or
carcinoma

Following treatment, continue
annual colonoscopy until two
consecutive negative
examination findings,
then continue every 3 years

Repeat every
3 years

Figure 4–12. Evaluation of patient at intermediate risk of colorectal neoplasia (one first-degree relative with history).

Flexible
sigmoidoscopy
at age 12 years

(-) Multiple
polyps

(+) Multiple
polyps

Continue screening
with annual
flexible sigmoidoscopy

Recommend
colectomy
by age 20 years

Figure 4–13. Evaluation of patient at highest risk of colorectal neoplasia (one or more first-degree relatives with Gardener's syndrome and familial adenomatous polyposis syndrome).

used to screen for the development of dysplasia or cancer. The exact number and frequency of screening colonoscopies depend on the patient and physician. For the patient with a history of panulcerative colitis, colonoscopy and biopsy should begin 8 years after the onset of symptoms. If no dysplasia is identified, screening may continue to be done every 3 years for the next two examinations, at which time they should be performed every 2 years. Yearly colonoscopy and biopsy should be performed annually in patients with a disease duration exceeding 20 years. In these individuals with only left-sided disease, screening need not begin until symptoms have existed for 15 years. Ulcerative proctitis does not appear to place the patient at risk of developing rectal carcinoma, and therefore such patients do not require screening for dysplasia.

Despite recognition of the dysplasia cancer sequence in patients with long-standing ulcerative colitis, screening programs have not affected survival.[27] Comparison of large screened versus unscreened populations may provide information about the utility of dysplasia screening in ulcerative colitis.

CONSTIPATION

Constipation has different meanings for different patients, just as diarrhea has various meanings for patients and the physician. Because constipation is difficult to define, the physician must seek a clear, descriptive definition from the patient to allow a clearer understanding of the individual's symptoms. Some patients consider themselves constipated if they have hard, small bowel movements. Others use the term to describe infrequent bowel movements, whereas some may have complaints of incomplete evacuation. Although all forms of constipation may represent a benign symptom, generally without serious underlying colorectal disease, understanding of the patient's meaning of the term affects evaluation and therapy.

Most people on a Western diet have at least three bowel movements per week. Because some individuals may consider any less than one bowel movement per day to be constipation, this lower frequency must be understood to be normal. Nevertheless, 5% of Americans have fewer than three bowel movements per week and thus are considered to have constipation.[28] Because of the attention focused on primary prevention of colorectal cancer by consumption of a high-fiber diet, many individuals are concerned with the need to have large bowel movements daily, even though they may not have had such habits previously. Less-than-daily bowel movements may falsely be interpreted as constipation by the patient. Understanding what the patient means by "constipation" can thus prevent unnecessary and costly evaluation.

Significant constipation may be manifested as a sudden change of bowel frequency, along with dryness and hardness of stools that are difficult to pass. This acute form of constipation may result from several benign causes. A careful medication history is essential in the evaluation of the constipated patient. Narcotic analgesics (e.g., acetaminophen with codeine, oxycodone, meperidine), calcium channel blocking agents (e.g., nifedipine, verapamil), aluminum-containing antacids, tricyclic antidepressants, and sucralfate each may result in significant constipation (Table 4–3). Recent travel or recent illness with incapacitation may diminish colonic transit and result in constipation.

Constipation may produce rectal bleeding from anorectal trauma. However, carcinoma may cause constipation and bleeding, and the latter may mistakenly be attributed to fissures or hemorrhoids. The physician must be cautious in attributing bleeding to benign anorectal disease in the setting of constipation.

A history of constipation of years' duration, often with long-term laxative use, does not have an identifiable origin. One must ascertain whether laxatives or enemas are used chronically, because they may contribute to worsening of the complaint. Long-term laxative or enema use may damage the colon. Animal studies have shown that excessive ingestion of laxatives may cause megacolon with damage to the myenteric plexus.

Constipation may represent a symptom attributable to a systemic metabolic disorder. Hypothyroidism may present with constipation as the primary complaint. Hypercalcemia resulting from hypoparathyroidism or metastatic carcinoma may produce diminished colonic motility, leading to constipation. Progressive systemic scleroderma may cause either diarrhea (secondary to bacterial overgrowth) or profound constipation (due to fibrosis of intestinal muscle layers).

Physical examination of the constipated patient may occasionally uncover an underlying cause, such as in the case of hypothyroidism (presence of goiter, diminished deep tendon reflexes, bradycardia) or fecal impaction. Sclerodactyly suggests scleroderma as an underlying disorder.

The initial assessment of constipation should include

Table 4–3. DRUGS THAT MAY CAUSE OR EXACERBATE CONSTIPATION

Aluminum-containing antacids
Anticholinergic agents (e.g., bethanechol, urecholine)
Antidepressants (e.g., imipramine, amitriptyline)
Anti-Parkinson's agents
Calcium channel blocking agents (e.g., nifedipine, verapamil)
Iron supplements
Laxatives, enemas (long-term frequent use)
Narcotic analgesics (e.g., codeine, meperidine, oxycodone)
Sucralfate

screening of serum electrolytes, including calcium. Thyroid function tests should be performed routinely, because hypothyroidism may be difficult to detect clinically. Flexible sigmoidoscopy or rigid proctosigmoidoscopy should exclude a low sigmoid or rectal lesion. Flexible sigmoidoscopy may uncover melanosis coli that appears as dark pigmentation of the colonic mucosa. Melanosis coli in the constipated patient suggests long-term laxative use that may be significant enough to contribute to constipation.

An air-contrast barium enema should be performed in patients with recent onset of constipation, unless an obvious underlying cause, such as drug-related constipation, is apparent. In the patient who has a long history of constipation and in whom a barium enema has previously revealed no significant abnormality, additional barium enema examinations are generally not necessary.

The air-contrast barium enema uncovers anatomic abnormalities such as tumors or benign strictures of the left colon. However, the vast majority of patients have a "normal" examination that fails to identify a significant anatomic abnormality. In such patients the symptom of constipation is attributable to functional abnormality of colonic motility.

The evaluation of constipation ends here for most patients. Therapeutic trials of bulk laxatives, high-fiber diets, and exercise often aid in relief of the symptom. However, the physician may occasionally wish to carry the evaluation further. Measurement of colonic transit time can be assessed by sequential daily abdominal radiographs after the patient has ingested radiopaque markers. Films are taken until all markers are expelled, usually within 7 days of ingestion. This technique adds objectivity by quantitating the severity of constipation while it allows the physician to detect instances in which individuals overestimate or lie about the severity of constipation. Normal values of colonic transit have been established by means of this technique.[29]

Infrequently, the ultrashort form of Hirschsprung's disease may be manifested as adult-onset constipation. When constipation is profound and associated with marked rectal pressure, anorectal manometry should be performed to exclude this form of Hirschsprung's disease. Failure of internal sphincter relaxation suggests the diagnosis of the ultrashort form of the disease. Other abnormal tracings may be seen in the adult. The presence of the inhibiting reflex with a high threshold suggests high compliance of the rectum or loss of sensory perception, as in the case of spinal cord injury. Anorectal manometry is a prerequisite to considering connective anorectal sphincter surgery for constipation. Obviously a constipated patient with a low resting internal sphincter pressure would not be well-served by sphincterotomy. Other causes of constipation must be sought.

When a child presents with constipation, it is important to exclude Hirschsprung's disease as the cause. Diagnosis of the disorder is often reached within the first few days of life; the infant presents with signs of colonic obstruction, having failed to pass meconium within the first 48 hours. The disease may present as constipation in the older child. The diagnosis is easily made in children by barium enema and rectal biopsy. In most cases the barium enema reveals a transition zone from distended to nondistended colon. A partial-thickness rectal biopsy specimen obtained by using a pediatric suction biopsy technique is preferred, because it is easily performed without the need for general anesthesia. However, only mucosal and Meissner's submucosal complex tissue is obtained. The biopsy should be taken at least 2 cm above the anal verge, because ganglion cells are sparse in the anus. The absence of ganglion cells and replacement by fibrous tissue is pathognomonic. Because necrons in both Meissner's and Auerbach's plexi are simultaneously absent, the submucosal partial-thickness biopsy is generally sufficient. The specimen should be reviewed by an experienced pathologist, as the pathologic diagnosis is not always apparent. Various histochemical techniques may enhance diagnostic accuracy.

In some instances Hirschsprung's disease may involve only a short segment of the distal rectum. A suction biopsy may be falsely negative if the biopsy is taken above the short aganglionic segment. Furthermore, the distal rectum, near the anus, generally contains fewer ganglion cells. Therefore, biopsies taken from this region may be difficult to interpret. In such instances anorectal manometry may be the only reasonable means of establishing the diagnosis. The absence of the rectoanal inhibiting reflex uncovers the diagnosis. The normal premature neonate, who has no Hirschsprung's disease, lacks the normal anorectal inhibiting reflex for up to the first several weeks of life. Anorectal manometry may mislead the physician to make a diagnosis of Hirschsprung's disease in such infants. Anorectal manometry should be included as part of the evaluation of the child in whom Hirschsprung's disease is suspected but not confirmed by suction biopsy. Despite concern about the diagnosis of Hirschsprung's disease, most children referred for constipation have neither that disease nor other abnormalities accounting for constipation.

REFERENCES

1. Fine KD Krejs GJ, Fordtran JS. Diarrhea. In: Sleisenger MH, Fordtran JS, eds: Gastrointestinal Disease. Philadelphia: WB Saunders, 1989.
2. Goldberg LD, Ditchek NT. Chewing gum diarrhea. Dig Dis Sci 1978;23:568.

3. Hutcheon DF, Bayless TM, Gadacz TR. Postcholecystectomy diarrhea. JAMA 1979;241:823.
4. Raimes SA, Wheldon EJ, Smirniotis V, et al. Postvagotomy diarrhea put into perspective. Lancet 1986;2:851.
5. Shahrabadi MS, Bryan LE, Gaffney D, et al. Latex agglutination test for detection of *Clostridium difficile* toxin in stool samples. J Clin Microbiol 1984;20:339–341.
6. Lashner BA, Todorczuk J, Sahm DF, Hanauer SB. *Clostridium difficile* culture-toxin–negative diarrhea. Am J Gastroenterol 1986;81:940–943.
7. Burnham WR, Ansell ID, Langman MJS. Normal sigmoidoscopic findings in severe ulcerative colitis: An important and common occurrence. Gut 1980;21:A460.
8. Mekhjian HS, Switz DM, Melnyk CS, et al. Clinical features and natural history of Crohn's disease. Gastroenterology 1979;77:898–906.
9. Blackstone MO. Endoscopic Interpretations. New York: Raven Press, 1984.
10. Saffouri B, Bartolomeo RS, Fuchs B. Colonic involvement in salmonellosis. Dig Dis Sci 1979;24:203–208
11. Ewe K, Karbach U. Factitious diarrhoea. Clin Gastroenterol 1986;15:723–740.
12. Bolling DR Jr. Prevalence, goals and complications of heterosexual anal intercourse in a gynecologic population. J Reprod Med 1977;19:120–124.
13. Klein EJ, Fisher LS, Chow AW, et al. Anorectal gonococcal infection. Ann Intern Med 1977;86:340–346.
14. Morse SA, Johnson SR, Biddle JW, et al. High-level tetracycline resistance in *Neisseria gonorrhoeae* is result of acquisition of streptococcal tetM determinant. Antimicrob Agents Chemother 1986;30:664–670.
15. Daling JR, Weiss NS, Hislop G, et al. Sexual practices, sexually transmitted diseases, and the incidence of anal cancer. N Engl J Med 1987;317:973–977.
16. Sohn N. Surgical conditions of the anus and rectum in male homosexuals. Pract Gastroenterol 1985;9:46–49.
17. Peppercorn MA. Enteric infections in homosexual men with and without AIDS. Contemp Gastroenterol 1989;2:23–32.
18. Portnoy D, Whiteside ME, Buckley E III, Macleod CL. Treatment of intestinal cryptosporidiosis with spiramycin. Ann Intern Med 1984;101:202–204.
19. DeHovitz JA, Pape JW, Boncy M, Johnson WD Jr. Clinical manifestations and therapy of *Isospora belli* infection in patients with the acquired immunodeficiency syndrome. N Engl J Med 1986;315:87–90.
20. Weber JN, Carmichael DJ, Boylston A, et al. Kaposi's sarcoma of the bowel—presenting as apparent ulcerative colitis. Gut 1985;26:295–300.
21. Silverstein FE, Gilbert DA, Tedesco FJ, et al. The national ASGE survey on upper gastrointestinal bleeding. Gastrointest Endosc 1981;27:80–93.
22. Mauldin JL. Therapeutic use of colonoscopy in active diverticular bleeding. Gastrointest Endosc 1985;31:290.
23. Browder W, Cerise EJ, Litwin MS. Impact of emergency angiography in massive lower gastrointestinal bleeding. Ann Surg 1986;204:530–536.
24. Lashner BA, Silverstein MD. Evaluation and therapy of the patient with fecal occult blood loss: A decision analysis. Am J Gastroenterol 1990;85:1088–1095.
25. Fletcher RH. Carcinoembryonic antigen. Ann Intern Med 1986;104:66–73.
26. Bess MA, Adson MA, Elveback LR, Moertel CG. Rectal cancer following colectomy for polyposis. Arch Surg 1980;115:460–467.
27. Lashner BA, Silverstein MD, Hanauer SB. Hazard rates for dysplasia and cancer in ulcerative colitis: Results from a surveillance program. Dig Dis Sci 1989;34:1536–1541.
28. Drossman DA, Sandler, RS, McKee DC, Lovitz AJ. Bowel patterns among subjects not seeking health care. Use of a questionnaire to identify a population with bowel dysfunction. Gastroenterology 1982;83:529–534.
29. Arhan P, Devroede G, Jehannin B, et al. Segmental colonic transit time. Dis Colon Rectum 1981;24:625.

Principles of Resection and Anastomosis

C H A P T E R   5

George E. Block
A. R. Moossa

Implicit in the successful execution of operations on the gastrointestinal tract is the ability to properly excise various segments of intestine and their adnexae and to re-establish intestinal continuity by means of a perfect anastomosis. An improperly performed excision or a faulty anastomosis results in leakage of intestinal contents with catastrophic consequences.

Various bowel resections and repair have occupied the imagination of surgeons for centuries, but it was not until Halsted published his experiments on anastomosis of the small intestine that the principles of surgical anastomosis were established.[1] A review of the hundreds of methods of resection and anastomosis will not be attempted here.[2] Rather, we present certain principles essential to proper intestinal resection and anastomosis and our preferred techniques.

INTESTINAL RESECTION

Resection of the intestine is termed *enterectomy* when the excised bowel is the jejunum and/or the ileum; *colectomy* is the term reserved for resections of the large bowel. In practice the small or large bowel may be removed separately or in various combinations, so that the techniques merge together. Therefore, they will be considered as one, with minor variations in technique depending on the segment of bowel to be resected.

It is obvious that the site or sites of bowel to undergo resection depend on the disease entity and its extent. In addition to this basic consideration, other fundamental factors are of prime importance in the excision of bowel: adequate exposure; exploration and visualization of the entire abdomen, so that the extent of disease or coexisting disease is not overlooked and the outcome of the resection not prejudiced; and following resection of the bowel and its related mesentery, the portions to be anastomosed must be healthy, be supple, have an adequate blood supply, and be tension free. The surgeon must determine the length of bowel to be resected, the amount of any surrounding tissue to be excised, and the extent of mesenteric resection required.

With the exception of certain portions of the esophagus, duodenum, and rectum, it is appropriate to mobilize the bowel to be resected and anastomosed into the surgical wound for adequate exposure, visualization, and convenience of manipulation. Anastomoses of the esophagus, biliary tract, duodenum, and rectum perforce are done within the recesses of the abdominal cavity because of the inability to mobilize these organs from the abdomen.

Resections of the small and large gut vary somewhat because of the differences in their blood supply and the attachment of the omentum to the midcolon.

Techniques of Resection

The blood supply of the small bowel is configured as connecting primary and secondary arcades, the arcades being more complex in the ileum than in the jejunum. From the convexities of the terminal arcades, small parallel vessels (vasa recta) extend to the mesenteric border of the bowel, where they bifurcate to nourish the bowel. The jejunum has one or two arterial arcades

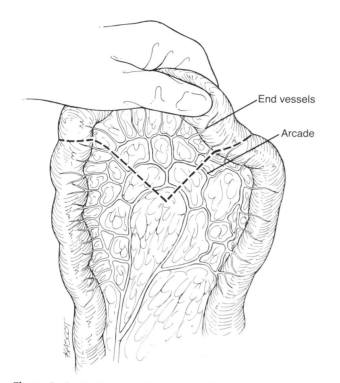

Figure 5–1. The blood supply of the small bowel showing the arcades and parallel end vessels. Resection of the small bowel is based on the anatomy of the arcades and preservation of the end vessels.

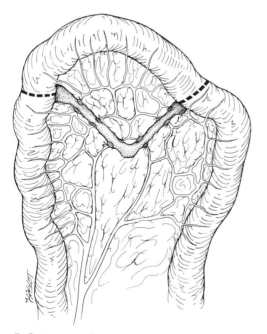

Figure 5–2. Division of the mesentery. The arcade vessels are suture-ligated, and hemostats are not allowed to accumulate in the operative field.

with long parallel end vessels, whereas the ileum has two to three arterial arcades with short terminal vessels (Fig. 5–1).

After the site and limits of the resection have been determined, the thin peritoneum on the anterior and posterior surfaces of the mesentery is lightly incised with a scalpel along the lines of proposed resection. The mesentery with its contained blood vessels is then serially clamped and divided between hemostats, and secure hemostasis is obtained by means of suture ligatures of fine (3-0 or 4-0) nonabsorbable sutures such as silk. In the application of the hemostats, small bites should be taken and an accumulation of hemostats should be avoided. After one or two pairs of hemostats have been applied to the mesentery, the vessels within these clamps are suture-ligated to prevent tearing of the mesentery by the mere weight of the hemostats.

In thick mesenteries the subperitoneal fatty tissue may be serially clamped and ligated so that the mesenteric vessels can be clamped and ligated individually to avoid large bites of tissue within the hemostats. Similarly, in fatty mesenteries the suture ligation should be in the form of a U-stitch encompassing at least one layer of peritoneum to ensure that the vascular-mesenteric complex does not slip from the ligature (Fig. 5–2).

The blood vessels are divided in continuity and ligated. The points selected for division of bowel are cleared of mesentery for a length of 4 to 8 mm, so that 360 degrees of bowel wall is visible to the surgeon for precise placement of sutures at the time of the anastomosis. In the division of the mesentery, care must be taken that an excessive vascular pedicle is not removed, which would lead to ischemia of the bowel (Fig. 5–3).

The operative field is then isolated with large packs, the margins of the abdominal incision having been previously covered with protective sheeting. Noncrushing bowel clamps are preferred (Block-Potts clamps, Edward Weck & Company). These clamps are placed with their points at the mesenteric portion of the bowel and with a slight angulation away from the excised segment. This angulation increases the diameter of the lumen and allows for an adequate mesentery and its accompanying blood supply.

The principles of resection of the colon are similar to those for resection of the small bowel, but the technique differs somewhat because of the difference of blood supply and the attachments of the omentum. The colon derives its blood supply on the right from the ileocolic, right colic, and middle colic vessels. The left side of the bowel is nourished by branches of the inferior mesenteric vessel. In cancer operations in which a wide lymphadenectomy is essential, the mesenteric division is at the site of origin of these vessels or at least their primary branches. These vessels eventuate to an anastomosing marginal artery that extends from the ileocecal valve to the rectosigmoid junction. The marginal colic artery, which forms an anastomosis between the right colic and middle arteries and the middle colic and left colic arteries, is the critical point in colonic resections.

Depending on the nature of the operation, either the main branches of the superior mesenteric artery or the branches of the inferior mesenteric artery or the inferior mesenteric artery itself may be chosen for ligation and division. In lesser resections the branches of these arteries are chosen for division after the intra-abdominal colon is adequately mobilized. Nevertheless, in all of these operations the marginal artery must be divided and suture-ligated with preservation of the arteriae rectae, which are the arteries nourishing the colon segments (Fig. 5–4). The pelvic colon is supplied by the superior rectal artery which anastomoses below with branches of the middle and inferior rectal arteries.

In the past the blood supply to the terminal sigmoid and upper rectum was considered to be precarious and termed *Sudeck's critical point*, but modern experience does not bear out this conception.[3] In fact, there is a rich collateral circulation in the distal arches. In resections of the rectum, the mesorectum must be mobilized and divided between hemostats at right angles to the point of resection of the rectum. Excision of an inadequate amount of mesorectum compromises an adequate lymphadenectomy, and an overly vigorous resection results in an ischemic upper rectal segment.

For resection of the intra-abdominal colon, the earlier-named branches of the arterial supply to the colon are exposed in the mesentery, clamped, divided, and suture-ligated. For large vessels, such as the inferior mesenteric or middle colic arteries, it is recommended to doubly ligate these stumps with fine silk. After transection and ligation of the marginal artery, the *arteriae rectae* are spared and division is made between a pair of these straight arteries. The mesentery is cleared from the proposed site of transection for a distance of approximately 3 to 7 mm, in order to visualize the bowel wall at the mesenteric edge.

In addition to dividing the colonic mesentery, it is necessary to divide and remove the attachment of the greater omentum from the superoanterior surface of the midcolon. Obviously, the omental apron must be divided between hemostats and suture-ligated. Following division of the mesentery and omentum, all subserosal fat and epiploic appendages immediately adjacent to the proposed area of anastomosis are cleared of fat. This gives a direct view of the muscular coat of the colon for a proper anastomosis.

Removal of fat is best accomplished by using a sharp scalpel in a "cutting and combing" technique. In this maneuver the peritoneum overlying the fatty deposit is incised, and the fat deposits and/or epiploic append-

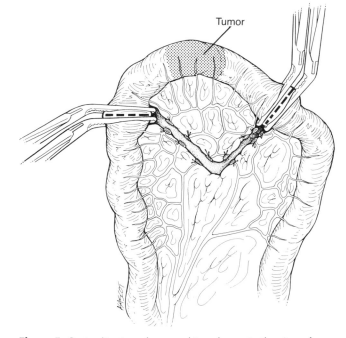

Figure 5–3. Application of noncrushing clamps to the sites of resection. The points of the bowel clamps are at the mesenteric surface and are angled to preserve mesentery and to enlarge the lumen. There is clearance of mesentery and fatty areolar tissue from the bowel wall for a length of 3 to 4 mm.

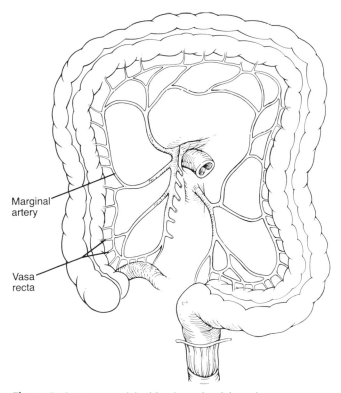

Figure 5–4. Diagram of the blood supply of the colon, emphasizing the anastomotic pattern of the marginal artery and vasa recta, which must be preserved.

ages are pushed away from the line of anastomosis. Small vessels encountered during this maneuver can be controlled by electrocoagulation, but one must spare as many vessels as possible. On completion of these maneuvers, the ends of the colon are free of mesenteric and omental attachments as well as subserosal fat, and the colon is ready to be divided.

Noncrushing bowel clamps are applied in an angled fashion, so that there is a greater length of mesenteric surface than antimesenteric surface, and intestinal contents are milked into the segment to be resected. If the proposed anastomosis is to be an end-to-side or a side-to-end anastomosis, the blind end of the colon may be transected by using a stapler-cutter that is convenient and allows the specimen to be free of cumbersome clamps.

Following application of noncrushing clamps at the proximal and distal segments, the colon is divided between the clamps by the cutting phase of the electrocautery. The ends of the bowel to be anastomosed are approximated to ensure that there is no tension. If this trial of approximation indicates any tension, the two segments of bowel are further mobilized until a tension-free approximation results.

INTESTINAL ANASTOMOSIS: HANDSEWN METHOD

Numerous factors influence the outcome of an intestinal anastomosis. These include general and regional influences as well as the details of the anastomosis itself. A thorough mechanical preparation of the bowel improves the outcome of intestinal—particularly colonic—anastomosis, but anastomosis may be safely accomplished in nonprepared bowel in carefully selected instances. Antibiotic prophylaxis (oral, systemic, or a combination) further reduces the septic complications associated with intestinal anastomosis. To perform a perfect intestinal anastomosis, it is essential to have adequate exposure, access, mobilization, and assistance.

Halsted developed certain principles for intestinal anastomosis, which emphasized a circular end-to-end anastomosis, incorporation of the submucosa by the suture without penetration of the mucosa, inversion of the mucosa, adequate blood supply, and absence of tension.[1] He also advocated a single-layer anastomosis without closure of the mesentery for fear of compromise of the blood supply. Although Halsted's tenets are pertinent today, modern experience has de-emphasized the single-layer anastomosis in favor of the two-layer technique. Closure of the mesenteric defects and alignments other than an end-to-end configuration are commonplace.

The authors have for many years practiced a two-layer anastomosis by using noncrushing clamps, fine nonabsorbable suture material (4-0 silk), and fine intestinal needles (taper, RB-1, control release: Ethicon, a Johnson & Johnson Company). We prefer an interrupted technique, because continuous sutures, although excellent for hemostasis, tend to compromise the blood supply, constrict the anastomosis, and are at risk should breakage occur anywhere along the course of the continuous suture.

We illustrate our preferred technique as an end-to-end anastomosis, but the identical technique is easily adaptable to end-to-side, side-to-end, or even the rarely indicated side-to-side anastomosis. While emphasizing our preferred technique we acknowledge countless excellent methods of intestinal anastomosis in which innumerable combinations and permutations in technique are used.[4] Our method of anastomosis is most easily performed by using noncrushing intestinal clamps, but if staples or crushing clamps are utilized, the crushed or stapled ends of the bowel are merely excised after the outer, posterior row is placed.

Posterior Layers

The ends of the bowel are approximated by the assistant's manipulation of the intestinal clamps. Mesenteric and antimesenteric alignment is obtained, and the bowel is inspected to confirm that 360 degrees of bowel wall is visible. The bowel segments are oriented so that the antimesenteric borders are referred to as the twelve o'clock position and the mesenteric borders as six o'clock (Fig. 5–5, *left*).

The first suture is placed at the antimesenteric border and is a simple Lembert suture at the eleven-thirty and twelve-thirty positions of the proximal and distal segments. This suture, like all others in this layer, include serosa, muscle, *and* submucosa without penetrating the mucosa. This row of sutures is placed far enough away from the cut end of the bowel that there is room for a second layer without the formation of a large valve; in practice, this distance is about 4 to 5 mm from the ends of the bowel.

The seromuscular-submucosal suture is continued parallel to the bowel ends to the mesenteric edge, where a similar Lembert suture is introduced at the five-thirty and six-thirty positions. These outer-layer posterior sutures may be tied as they are applied or, as we prefer, tied after the entire row of sutures has been placed.

A variant of this technique is useful if there is a disparity between the diameters of the two segments of bowel being anastomosed. If this situation exists, the first sutures are placed at the twelve and six o'clock positions, and the next is placed at the midpoint of the

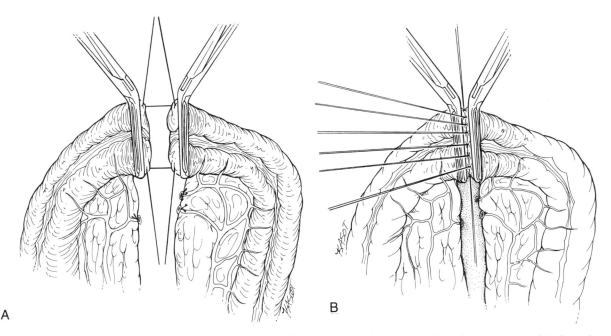

A B

Figure 5–5. Outer layer, posterior row. Traction sutures applied at the mesenteric and antimesenteric ends are maintained (*Left*), and Lembert sutures of 4-0 silk spaced 3 mm apart constitute the outer layer of the posterior row (*Right*).

wall of the two segments of bowel. The remaining sutures are placed halfway between the midpoint and end sutures, and midpoint placement continues until the row is complete. In this fashion one accommodates disparity in size. Obviously, great discrepancies in bowel size do not accommodate an end-to-end anastomosis, and another technique (e.g., end-to-side or antimesenteric slit) should be chosen (Fig. 5–6).

After the outer layer of the posterior sutures is placed, the sutures are cut on the knots at all but the extremity sutures to which hemostats are applied, so as to orient the suture line and give continuous visualization of the ends of the row of sutures.

Padded clamps are applied to the proximal and distal limbs 4 to 5 inches from the ends in order to occlude the lumens and prevent contamination of the proposed anastomosis by intestinal content. The bowel clamps are removed or, conversely, the crushed or stapled ends of the bowel are excised. Any intestinal contents are removed by suction, irrigation, and swabbing with cotton balls. The inner layer of the posterior row is now ready for joining. Any bleeding points are controlled by simple suture ligation or coagulation.

The inner layer is a through-and-through suture of all layers. Mucosa and serosa are visualized for each suture so that if the mucosa and serosa are within the arc of the needle, the submucosa is obviously included. The sutures of the inner row are placed at each end and continue to be placed 3 to 4 mm apart. The sutures are tied after each placement and cut at the knot. It is

helpful to alternate sutures, first at the mesenteric side, then at the antimesenteric side, so that any disparity is in the middle and not at the ends of this row (Fig. 5–7).

Anterior Layers

After the inner layer of the posterior row is placed, attention is turned to the inner layer of the anterior portion of the anastomosis. This layer is all-important, because this is where inversion occurs, hence it is also the site of errors and leakage from improper inversion. For this layer we utilize interrupted fine silk sutures, although synthetic or absorbable sutures may be used, depending on the surgeon's preference. The inverting suture that we prefer is a Czerny suture, which is a simple U-stitch with the loop on the serosal side. A small bite of mucosa is taken with a slightly larger bite of bowel wall. By this means the suture goes through the bowel wall at an angle. After the suture is placed, the two ends of the suture are pulled back and forth (running), which inverts the bowel wall. The sutures are individually tied and are cut at the knot, which now rests within the lumen.

The first suture is placed at the antimesenteric surface at the eleven-thirty and twelve-thirty positions. Two or three similar sutures are placed 3 mm apart, so as to completely turn in the antimesenteric corner. A similar maneuver is accomplished at the mesenteric border with sutures placed first at the five-thirty and

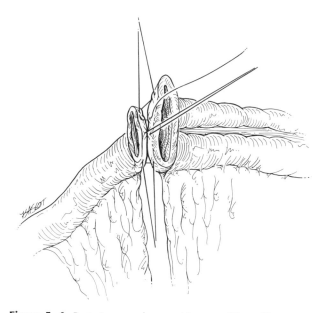

Figure 5–6. Posterior row placement in a condition of lumen disparity. The mesenteric and antimesenteric seromuscular sutures are first placed at each limb and the remaining spaces divided in "halves" to compensate for the disparity in size.

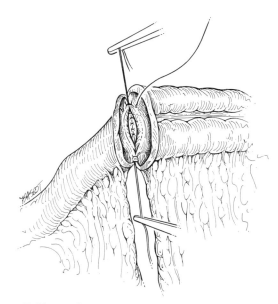

Figure 5–7. Inner layer, posterior row. Through-and-through seromuscular sutures piercing mucosa and serosa (to incorporate submucosa) are placed from the mesenteric to the antimesenteric borders.

six-thirty positions. This corner is turned in with two or three sutures again placed 3 mm apart until the corner is well inverted.

The remaining anterior defect is closed with interrupted inverting Czerny sutures placed 3 to 4 mm apart. When this layer is complete, a watertight closure has been accomplished. The occluding clamps are removed from the bowel, and the anastomotic integrity is tested by inspection and manipulation (Fig. 5–8).

The final layer is the outer layer of the anterior row. This layer achieves serosa-to-serosa approximation as well as hemostasis. Simple Lembert sutures of 4-0 silk are applied beyond the stay sutures of the outer layer of the posterior row. These so-called seromuscular (submucosal) sutures approximate the serosa outside of the stay sutures (which are now cut) to ensure complete serosal approximation. This row is continued along the suture line as interrupted seromuscular sutures, and serosa approximation is achieved without turning in a large valve.

After the outer layer of the anterior closure is completed, the mesentery defect is carefully closed, care being taken to avoid hematoma formation or devascularization. The lumen is tested between thumb and forefinger to ensure its adequacy. The anastomosis is now complete (Fig. 5–9).

A satisfactory bowel anastomosis requires a good blood supply. It must be tension-free, and there should be no stenosis of the lumen. Anastomosis should not be attempted in the case of gross contamination or distal obstruction. The anastomosis should be watertight; serosal apposition is desired; and mesenteric defects should be closed without tension.

The closed and the single-layer anastomoses, although acceptable, are techniques that have been supplanted in our practices by the two-layer, inverting anastomosis done via an open technique with modifications to avoid fecal contamination. This method of anastomosis can be applied from the pharynx to the anal canal.

The empiric use of drains is contraindicated, because drains in contact with the suture line are associated with anastomotic leaks. Fecal diversion or decompression proximal to an anastomosis is appropriate in certain selected situations, but generally implies that the surgeon is insecure about the fate of the anastomosis. A proximal colostomy does not reduce the incidence of anastomotic dehiscence or leak but substantially reduces the contamination and abdominal or pelvic peritonitis associated with such a leak. If the surgeon is dissatisfied with the anastomosis, primary anastomosis should be abandoned or the anastomosis redone until the surgeon is satisfied with the integrity of the anastomosis.

We have presented our preferred method of intestinal anastomosis. Although we have relied on this technique for many years, countless other anastomotic techniques are advocated by surgeons of skill and experience and are generally acceptable. The reader is referred to standard texts of operative surgery for details of various anastomotic techniques.[2, 4–7]

STAPLES FOR RESECTION AND ANASTOMOSIS

The introduction in the 1960s of commercially available stapling devices by Ravitch and Steichen was met with immediate acceptance by gastrointestinal surgeons and resulted in a revolution in operative technique.[8] Surgical staplers can reduce operating time and tissue manipulation, allow for anastomosis low in the pelvis and high in the thorax, and have proved to be effective and safe.

Surgical staplers are not a panacea. The same principles that control the fate of handsewn anastomoses apply to stapled anastomoses. The requirements of an adequate blood supply, freedom from tension, and adequacy of lumen apply to all types of anastomoses—stapled and sewn. Violation of these principles results in anastomotic failure, irrespective of the technique employed.

The ingenuity of surgeons has resulted in countless variations of technique and the application of suturing devices for resection and anastomosis from the cervical esophagus to the anal canal. In this presentation we describe the techniques we commonly employ. The reader is referred to several splendid texts, monographs, journals, and atlases for further exposition of this subject.[8–13]

Resection Utilizing Stapler-Cutter Devices

The enteric segment to be resected is freed from its mesenteric attachments, and the bowel wall is cleared in the usual fashion. The GIA instrument is placed across the bowel at the point of resection in a scissors-like fashion. The instrument is closed, care being taken to confirm that the tissue does not extend beyond the zero calibration of the instrument. The stapler is fired, and the bowel is divided between two parallel rows of staples. Any bleeding points are coagulated, and the row of sutures may be inverted by fine interrupted sutures, according to the surgeon's preference. This operation is repeated at the opposite end of the segment to be resected. The result is an excision of bowel and closure of both the proximal and distal lumens (Fig. 5–10).

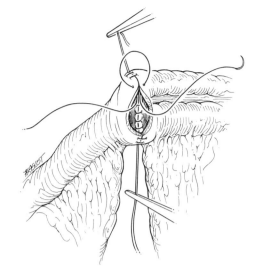

Figure 5–8. Placement of inverting Czerny sutures. The mesenteric and then the antimesenteric ends are inverted first, and the midpoint of the lumen is finally closed with the inverting suture. The inverting suture takes a small bite of mucosa and a larger bite of serosa, thus angling through the bowel wall.

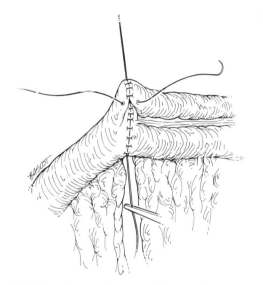

Figure 5–9. Serosal approximation of the outer layer, anterior row. Interrupted Lembert seromuscular sutures invert the inner layer.

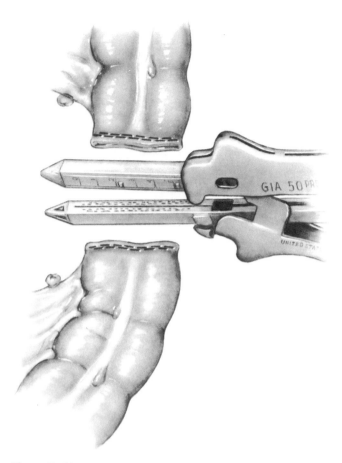

Figure 5–10. Transection of bowel with the GIA. A double-row staggered staple closure is placed both on the retained bowel and on the specimen side. (Copyright 1974, 1980, 1988, United States Surgical Corporation. All rights reserved. Reprinted with the permission of the United States Surgical Corporation.)

Anastomotic Techniques Utilizing Staplers

End-to-End Anastomoses

Method #1. For bowel that can be easily rotated (i.e., mid–small bowel), an end-to-end anastomosis may be fashioned by using a triangulation technique and staples. In this technique three everting traction sutures are placed equidistantly to approximate the bowel ends, mucosa to mucosa. The traction sutures are first placed at the mesenteric borders, and the two remaining sutures at one-third intervals.

The jaws of a TA-30 instrument are placed beneath the first two traction sutures. Approximation of the bowel ends between the traction sutures is facilitated by grasping the ends with an Allis clamp. The stapler is fired, and the tissue that protrudes above the staple line is excised, care being taken to preserve the traction sutures. The maneuver is repeated for the remaining two segments of the triangulated bowel. Each new staple line should overlap the prior staple line. As in all stapled anastomoses, the staple line is inspected for mechanical imperfections or for bleeding points (Figs. 5–11 and 5–12).

Method #2. A variant of the triangulation technique is an end-to-end anastomosis in which the posterior walls of the bowel are first approximated with inverting traction sutures in a serosa-to-serosa approximation. Again, an Allis clamp is placed at the midpoint to ensure approximation of tissue edges, and the posterior wall is joined with staples by utilizing a Roticulator-55. After the instrument is fired, the tissue protruding from the jaws of the instrument is excised.

The anterior walls of the bowel are bisected with everting traction sutures, and this now forms a triangle in which a stapled posterior row is the base. Each arm of the triangle is closed with the TA-55, care being taken to include each end of the posterior row in the staple line.

This technique is particularly adaptable to the left colon. The anastomosis consists of one inverted posterior row and two everted anterior rows, which may be inverted with seromuscular sutures if the surgeon so chooses (Figs. 5–13 to 5–15).

Method #3. This method is particularly useful for colocolonic anastomosis and involves the EEA instrument with its anvil and cartridge. The diameter of the colon is determined with sizers, and a corresponding EEA instrument is chosen. The instrument is introduced through a colotomy incision 3 to 4 cm from the proposed anastomotic site. The instrument is opened, the anvil advanced through the bowel end, and a pursestring suture of 2-0 monofilament material tied around the shaft. Any fatty tissue is removed from the pursestring-sutured end of the colon.

Text continued on page 79

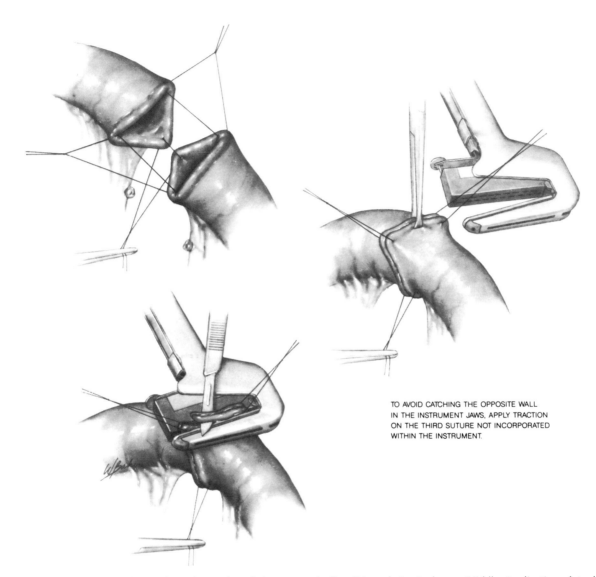

TO AVOID CATCHING THE OPPOSITE WALL
IN THE INSTRUMENT JAWS, APPLY TRACTION
ON THE THIRD SUTURE NOT INCORPORATED
WITHIN THE INSTRUMENT.

Figure 5–11. Triangulation technique for end-to-end stapled anastomosis. *Top,* Triangulation is shown. *Middle,* Application of staple device to one third of the everted bowel wall is illustrated. *Bottom,* Excision of redundant tissue after application of staple line is shown. (Copyright 1974, 1980, 1988, United States Surgical Corporation. All rights reserved. Reprinted with the permission of the United States Surgical Corporation.)

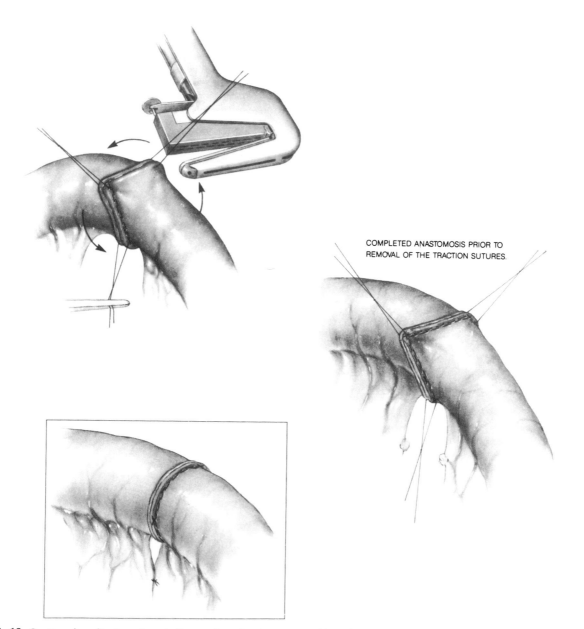

COMPLETED ANASTOMOSIS PRIOR TO
REMOVAL OF THE TRACTION SUTURES.

Figure 5–12. Continued application of staple line to triangulated segments of bowel. *Top,* Bowel is rotated in a counterclockwise manner, and a second segment is then stapled. *Middle,* Staples overlap at each end. *Bottom,* Completed end-to-end stapled anastomosis. (Copyright 1974, 1980, 1988, United States Surgical Corporation. All rights reserved. Reprinted with the permission of the United States Surgical Corporation.)

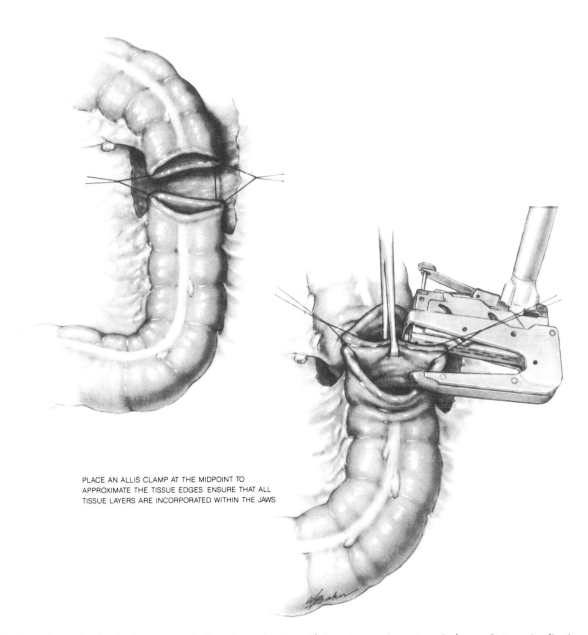

PLACE AN ALLIS CLAMP AT THE MIDPOINT TO
APPROXIMATE THE TISSUE EDGES. ENSURE THAT ALL
TISSUE LAYERS ARE INCORPORATED WITHIN THE JAWS.

Figure 5–13. End-to-end colocolonic anastomosis. *Top,* Approximation with inverting traction sutures is shown. *Bottom,* Application of Roticulator to posterior walls of approximated bowel is illustrated. (Copyright 1974, 1980, 1988, United States Surgical Corporation. All rights reserved. Reprinted with the permission of the United States Surgical Corporation.)

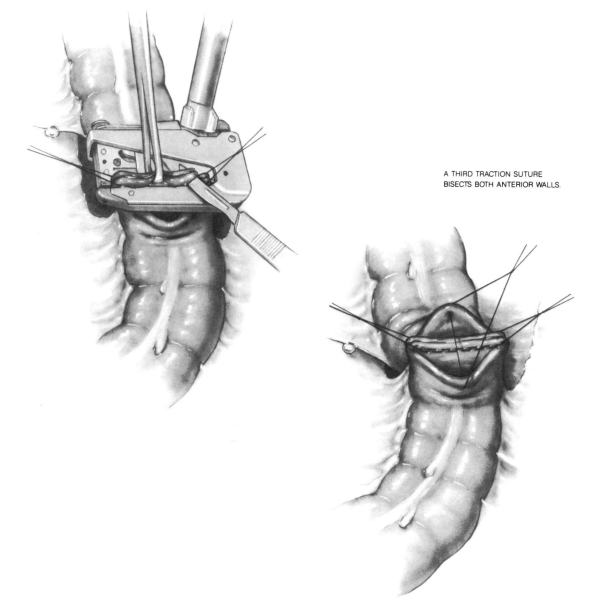

A THIRD TRACTION SUTURE
BISECTS BOTH ANTERIOR WALLS.

Figure 5–14. *Top,* Excision of redundant tissue from posterior wall. *Bottom,* Traction sutures are placed at the mesenteric and antimesenteric ends of the stapled posterior wall, and an everting traction suture is placed through the midportion of the anterior wall. (Copyright 1974, 1980, 1988, United States Surgical Corporation. All rights reserved. Reprinted with the permission of the United States Surgical Corporation.)

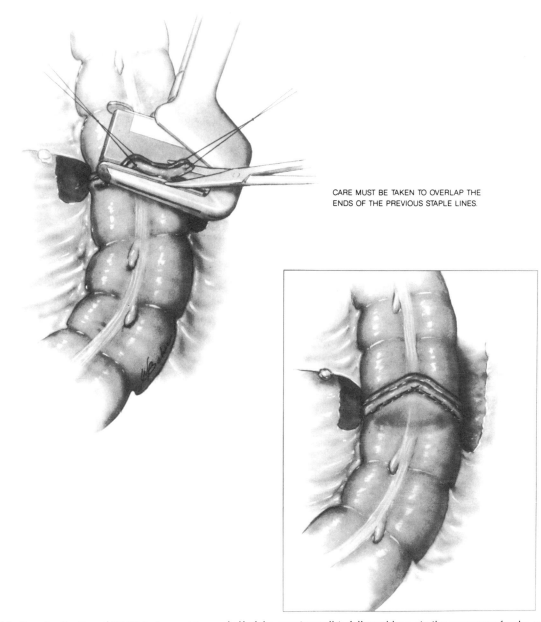

CARE MUST BE TAKEN TO OVERLAP THE
ENDS OF THE PREVIOUS STAPLE LINES.

Figure 5–15. *Top,* Application of TA-30 instrument to one half of the anterior wall is followed by a similar maneuver for the other half. Staples should overlap at the midportion of this anterior wall closure. *Bottom,* The completed anastomosis has one inverted and two everted staple lines. (Copyright 1974, 1980, 1988, United States Surgical Corporation. All rights reserved. Reprinted with the permission of the United States Surgical Corporation.)

The anvil is placed into the distal colonic segment with the aid of an Allis forceps. Another pursestring suture is placed around the shaft of the anvil, and fatty tissue is once again removed from this end. An automatic pursestring applier is a convenient modification of this technique.

The EEA instrument is closed snugly and fired. The instrument is opened slightly, the suture line is lifted over the anvil, and the instrument is removed. The suture line is inspected through the colotomy, which may then be closed with a TA-55 instrument. With each use of the EEA, the excised segments of bowel ("doughnuts") are inspected to ensure complete excision of the closed ends and circumferential staple placement (Figs. 5–16 to 5–18).

Method #4. This method is valuable for coloproctostomy in anterior resections of the rectum. It involves a double-staple technique, but the two-pursestring technique described under Method #3 may also be employed.

The segment of rectum and colon to be excised is mobilized, and the rectum is closed with the Roticulator-55. The rectum is transected on the edge of the Roticulator.

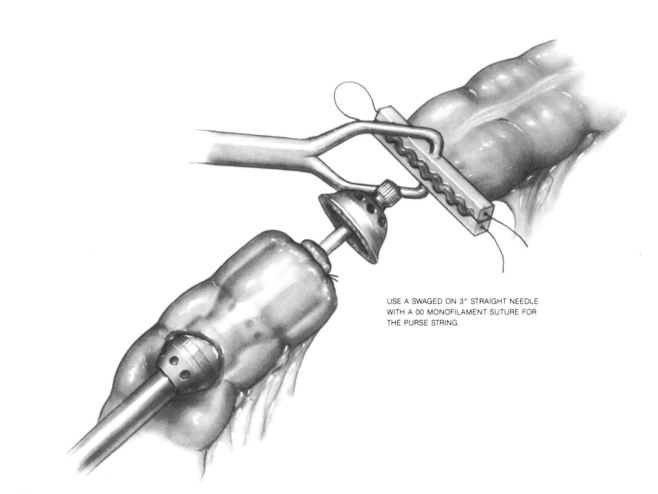

USE A SWAGED ON 3″ STRAIGHT NEEDLE
WITH A 00 MONOFILAMENT SUTURE FOR
THE PURSE STRING.

Figure 5–16. Introduction of the EEA through a colotomy 3 to 4 cm from the closed end of the proximal limb. The anvil is pushed through the open end of the colon, and a pursestring suture of 2-0 monofilament suture is applied snugly around the shaft. The distal limb has been divided across the automatic pursestring device. (Copyright 1974, 1980, 1988, United States Surgical Corporation. All rights reserved. Reprinted with the permission of the United States Surgical Corporation.)

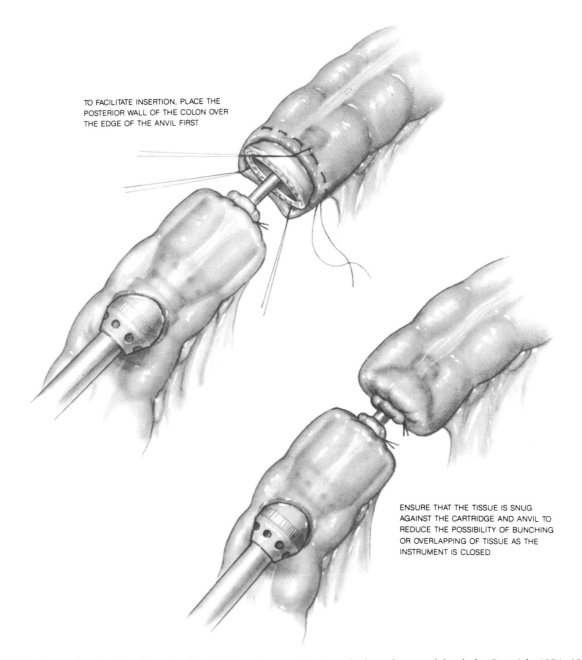

TO FACILITATE INSERTION, PLACE THE
POSTERIOR WALL OF THE COLON OVER
THE EDGE OF THE ANVIL FIRST.

ENSURE THAT THE TISSUE IS SNUG
AGAINST THE CARTRIDGE AND ANVIL TO
REDUCE THE POSSIBILITY OF BUNCHING
OR OVERLAPPING OF TISSUE AS THE
INSTRUMENT IS CLOSED.

Figure 5–17. The anvil is introduced into the distal limb, and a pursestring is applied snugly around the shaft. (Copyright 1974, 1980, 1988, United States Surgical Corporation. All rights reserved. Reprinted with the permission of the United States Surgical Corporation.)

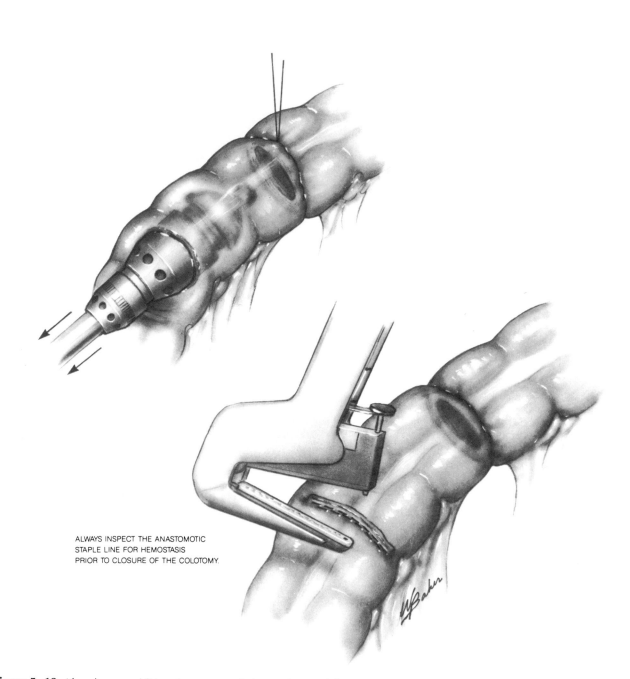

ALWAYS INSPECT THE ANASTOMOTIC
STAPLE LINE FOR HEMOSTASIS
PRIOR TO CLOSURE OF THE COLOTOMY.

Figure 5–18. After closure and firing, the anastomosis is complete, and the instrument is slightly opened and removed from the colotomy. The colotomy incision is closed with a TA-55 stapler. (Copyright 1974, 1980, 1988, United States Surgical Corporation. All rights reserved. Reprinted with the permission of the United States Surgical Corporation.)

The pursestring instrument is placed at the site of proximal division, and the colon is transected. The Premium CEEA stapler is employed in this method. After sizing, the anvil is placed into the proximal colon, and the pursestring is tied. The Premium CEEA without the anvil is introduced transanally and advanced to the stapled closure of the rectum. A small incision is made with scissors at the midpoint of the rectal closure, and the trocar of the Premium CEAA is advanced through this opening. The trocar is removed, and the anvil shaft is placed firmly into the opening vacated by the trocar. At this point care must be taken to ensure proper orientation of the colonic segment and its mesentery to avoid torsion.

The CEEA is closed snugly and fired. The instrument is opened slightly and withdrawn by lifting the staple line over the anvil while gently rotating the instrument.

Again, the proximal and distal doughnuts are inspected, and the anastomosis is tested by transanal instillation of saline and air to ensure that there are no leaks. If an air or water leak is found, it is closed by sutures. Testing is done until the anastomosis proves to be airtight and watertight (Figs. 5–19 to 5–22).

Side-to-Side Anastomoses

Method #1. This side-to-side anastomosis is adaptable to enteroenterostomies and enterocolostomies and is termed a *functional end-to-end anastomosis.* Despite this terminology the anastomosis has a side-to-side configuration and is subject to the sequelae of this configuration.

The antimesenteric borders of the two limbs of bowel are approximated, and one fork of a GIA stapler-cutter is inserted into each lumen. The bowel ends are aligned evenly on the forks, the instrument is closed and fired. Two double, staggered staple lines join the bowel; simultaneously the knife blade creates a stoma between the staple lines. The suture line is inspected for hemostasis. The ends of the bowel are everted with traction sutures at each end, Allis forceps or a third traction suture approximates all layers at the midpoint, and the open ends are closed with a TA-55 instrument. Tissue protruding beyond the jaw of the TA-55 is excised. If the surgeon so elects, the staple lines may be reinforced with inverting seromuscular sutures (Figs. 5–23 and 5–24).

Method #2. The bowel resection is performed with two applications of a GIA instrument, thus closing the proximal and distal ends. The antimesenteric corners of each limb with its closing staples are excised widely enough to accommodate one fork of the GIA. The antimesenteric borders of the bowel are approximated, and one fork of the GIA is inserted into the proximal and distal lumens. The bowel is aligned evenly on the

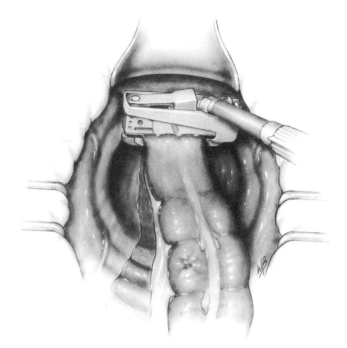

Figure 5–19. Application of the Roticulator at the chosen line of resection. The rectum is transected on the Roticulator. (Copyright 1974, 1980, 1988, United States Surgical Corporation. All rights reserved. Reprinted with the permission of the United States Surgical Corporation.)

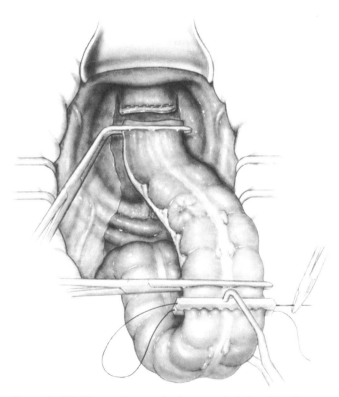

Figure 5–20. The rectal stump is shown stapled closed by the Roticulator and the proximal line of resection is at the application of the automatic pursestring device. (Copyright 1974, 1980, 1988, United States Surgical Corporation. All rights reserved. Reprinted with the permission of the United States Surgical Corporation.)

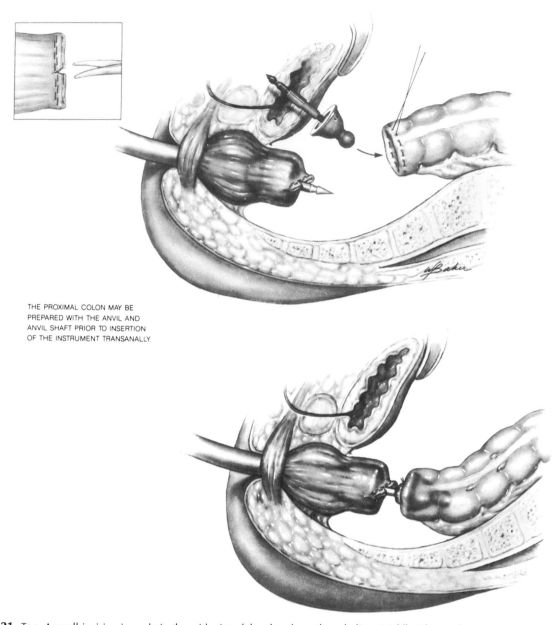

THE PROXIMAL COLON MAY BE
PREPARED WITH THE ANVIL AND
ANVIL SHAFT PRIOR TO INSERTION
OF THE INSTRUMENT TRANSANALLY.

Figure 5–21. *Top,* A small incision is made in the midpoint of the closed rectal staple line. *Middle,* The anvil is inserted into the descending colon, and the pursestring suture is tied snugly on the anvil. Simultaneously, the trocar is advanced through the rectal suture line. The trocar is removed, and the anvil shaft is inserted into the shaft of the CEEA. *Bottom,* The anvil is shown within the descending colon, and the CEEA abuts onto the staple closure of the rectum. (Copyright 1974, 1980, 1988, United States Surgical Corporation. All rights reserved. Reprinted with the permission of the United States Surgical Corporation.)

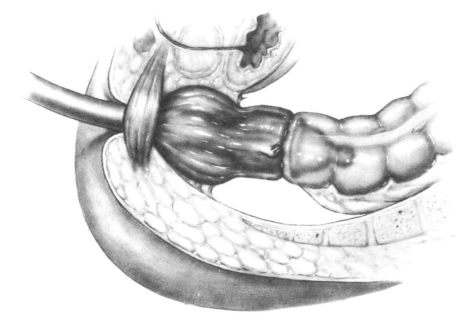

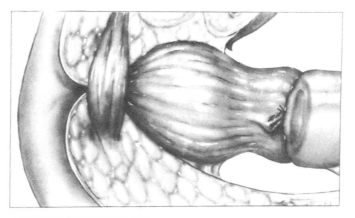

ALWAYS INSPECT THE ANASTOMOTIC
STAPLE LINE FOR HEMOSTASIS.

Figure 5–22. The stapler is closed snugly and fired, resulting in a circular end-to-end anastomosis. The instrument is opened slightly, manipulated past the suture line, and removed. The suture line is tested for integrity. (Copyright 1974, 1980, 1988, United States Surgical Corporation. All rights reserved. Reprinted with the permission of the United States Surgical Corporation.)

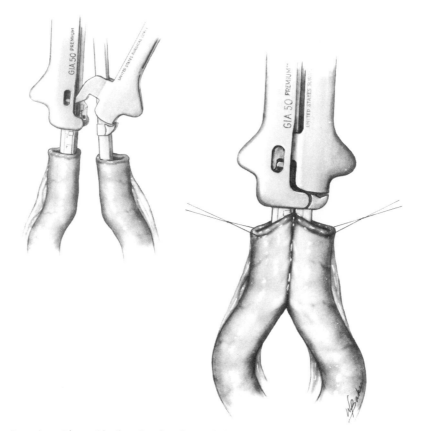

Figure 5–23. Enteroenterostomy in a side-to-side (functional end-to-end) fashion. *Top,* The antimesenteric borders of the bowel are approximated, and the GIA-50 is inserted with one limb of the fork in each lumen. *Bottom,* The forks are fully inserted to ensure the maximal stomal size. The forks are approximated and the instrument closed and fired, creating a side-to-side stoma. (Copyright 1974, 1980, 1988, United States Surgical Corporation. All rights reserved. Reprinted with the permission of the United States Surgical Corporation.)

instrument forks, and the instrument is closed and fired to create a side-to-side stoma. The TA-55 is employed to close the common end opening. The redundant tissue is excised and the anastomosis is complete. This technique is adaptable to colocolostomies and enterocolostomies (Figs. 5–25 to 5–27).

BIOFRAGMENTABLE ANASTOMOTIC RING

Another technique of achieving a bowel anastomosis has recently gained considerable attention. The biofragmentable anastomotic ring (BAR: Valtrac, Davis & Geck Medical Device Division, Wayne, NJ) (Fig. 5–28) was developed by Hardy et al,[14] but in fact it is a modification of the historic Murphy Button.[15] The device consists of two interlocking rings of polyglycolic acid rendered radiopaque by the addition of barium sulfate. After appropriate bowel resection is done, the technique is performed by inserting the two halves of the BAR inside the proximal and distal ends of the

transected bowel. Each half of the device is held in place by a pursestring suture. A variety of diameter and gap sizes are manufactured to suit the anatomic situation, which varies with the width of the bowel ends and the thickness of the bowel wall.

The anastomosis is accomplished by compressing together the two pieces of the BAR, which lock with a definite "click." The design of the BAR is such that it fragments as a result of hydrolysis; the subsequent loss of tensile strength leads to its expulsion from the body at about 18 days.[16]

In a recently completed randomized trial, the BAR was compared with sutured and stapled anastomoses. This trial revealed no significant differences in wound complications, abscess formation, bleeding, anastomotic leaks, ileus, mechanical obstruction, or death.[17]

The BAR is clearly not suitable as a low rectal or anal anastomosis in such situations. It is ideally suited for an intra-abdominal end-to-end anastomosis. Special attention must be paid to closing the mesenteric defect, not only to prevent internal herniation but also to provide additional support to the anastomotic line.

Text continued on page 91

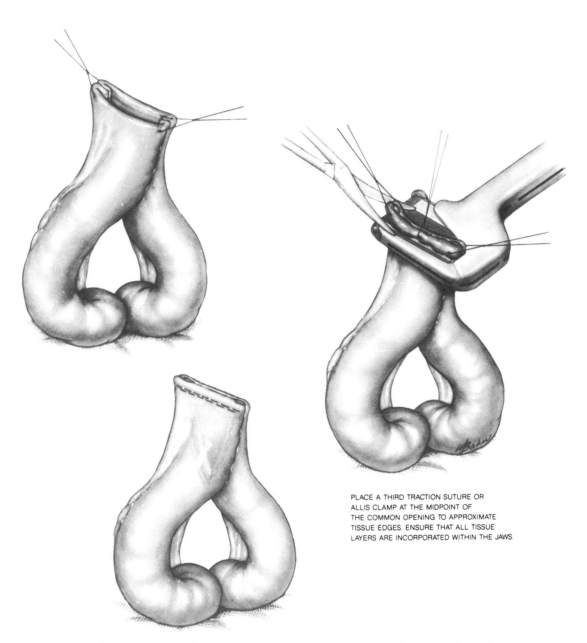

PLACE A THIRD TRACTION SUTURE OR
ALLIS CLAMP AT THE MIDPOINT OF
THE COMMON OPENING TO APPROXIMATE
TISSUE EDGES. ENSURE THAT ALL TISSUE
LAYERS ARE INCORPORATED WITHIN THE JAWS.

Figure 5–24. The open ends of the bowel are fixed with everting traction stay sutures, and the open ends are closed by a TA-55 instrument. The instrument is fired and the redundant tissue is excised. *Bottom,* The completed anastomosis. (Copyright 1974, 1980, 1988, United States Surgical Corporation. All rights reserved. Reprinted with the permission of the United States Surgical Corporation.)

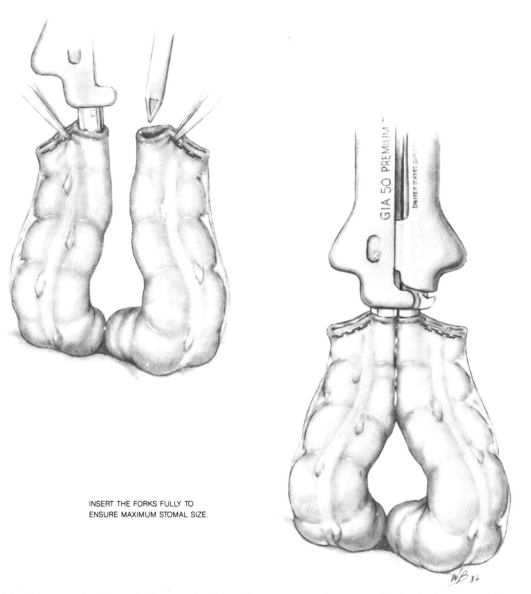

INSERT THE FORKS FULLY TO
ENSURE MAXIMUM STOMAL SIZE.

Figure 5–25. Colocolostomy with side-to-side (functional end-to-end) anastomosis. The section of colon has been excised by using the GIA-50, resulting in a complete suture closure of the proximal and distal ends of bowel. *Top,* The staples are excised at the antimesenteric border of each limb widely enough to allow insertion of one fork of the GIA-50. *Bottom,* The GIA-50 instrument is approximated after being inserted fully, is closed, and is fired. (Copyright 1974, 1980, 1988, United States Surgical Corporation. All rights reserved. Reprinted with the permission of the United States Surgical Corporation.)

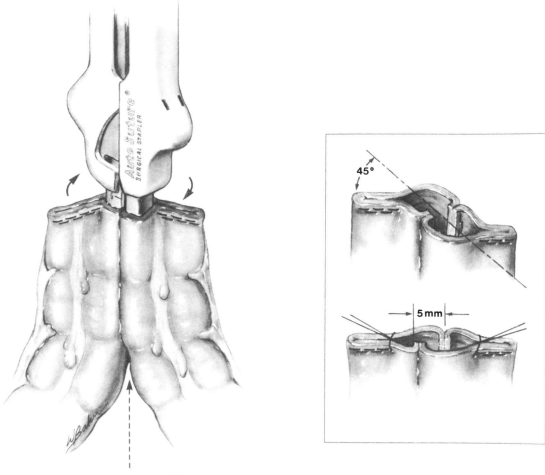

BOWEL WALLS
OVERLAP SLIGHTLY

Figure 5–26. A modification of the side-to-side anastomosis in which the instrument is rotated 45 degrees relative to the transection staple lines. This results in an offset method as shown on the right. (Copyright 1974, 1980, 1988, United States Surgical Corporation. All rights reserved. Reprinted with the permission of the United States Surgical Corporation.)

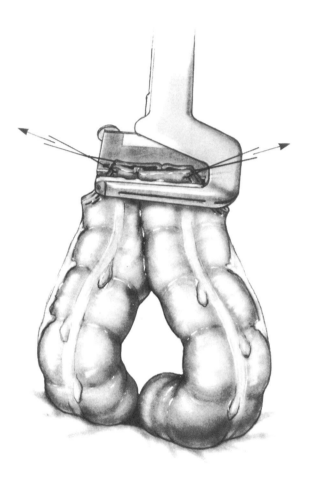

CARE MUST BE TAKEN TO OVERLAP THE
ENDS OF THE PREVIOUS STAPLE LINES.

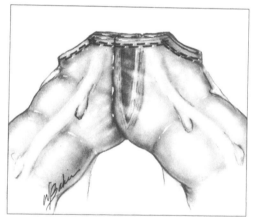

AN ANCHOR SUTURE MAY BE PLACED AT THE BASE
OF THE ANASTOMOSIS FOR ADDITIONAL SECURITY.

Figure 5–27. *Top,* The TA-55 is used to close the common opening while stay sutures evert the bowel wall. The ends of all staple lines and all tissue layers are included within the jaws of the TA-55 instrument. *Bottom,* The side-to-side (functional end-to-end) colocolostomy is depicted. (Copyright 1974, 1980, 1988, United States Surgical Corporation. All rights reserved. Reprinted with the permission of the United States Surgical Corporation.)

The exact role of the BAR in the armamentarium of anastomotic techniques remains to be evaluated. How it will compare with the time-honored suture and stapler techniques for practical issues such as cost and time savings remains an unanswered question.

We have chosen to present stapled anastomotic techniques we commonly employ in operations on the hindgut. There are, of course, numerous other modifications and techniques adaptable to all portions of the gastrointestinal tract. We have also described our techniques by citing instruments produced by the Auto Suture Company, a Division of the United States Surgical Corporation. We have done so because we are most familiar with these instruments. However, a number of other manufacturers produce similar high-quality instruments that may be chosen for all of the techniques illustrated in this chapter.

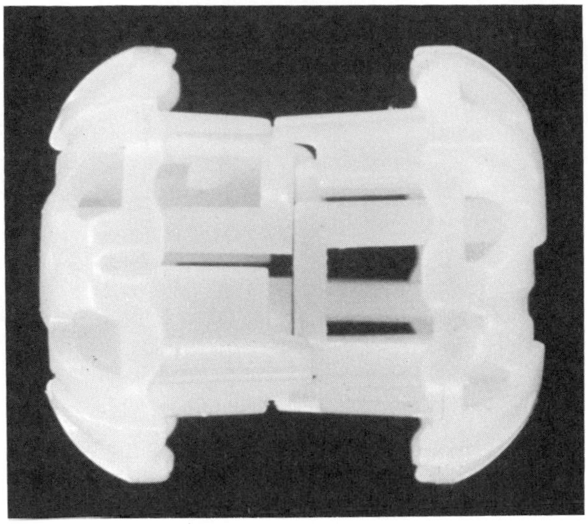

Figure 5–28. The Biofragmentable Anastomotic Ring, BAR (Voltrac®).

REFERENCES

1. Halsted WH. Circular suture of the intestine: An experimental study. Am J Med Sci 1887;94:436.
2. Nelson RL. Surgical techniques and care of obstruction of the small intestine. In: Nyhus LM, Baker RJ, eds. Mastery of Surgery. Vol II. Boston: Little, Brown & Company, 1984, p 887.
3. Anson BJ, McVay CB. Abdominal Cavity and Contents in Surgical Anatomy. 5th ed. Vol. 1. Philadelphia: WB Saunders, 1971, pp 643–681.
4. Maingot R. Abdominal Operations. 7th ed. New York: Appleton-Century-Croft, 1980.
5. Maingot R. Abdominal Operations. 9th ed. In: Schwartz SL, Ellis H, eds. Norwalk, CT: Appleton & Lange, 1989.
6. Nora PF, ed. Operative Surgery—Principles and Technique. Philadelphia, WB Saunders, 1990.
7. Goligher JC. Surgery of the Anus, Rectum and Colon. 4th ed. London: Bailliere Tindall, 1980.
8. Ravitch MM, Steichen FM. Atlas of General Thoracic Surgery. Philadelphia: WB Saunders, 1988.
9. Ravitch MM, Steichen FM. Principles and Practice of Surgical Stapling. Chicago: Year Book, 1987.
10. Steichen FM, Ravitch MM. Stapling in Surgery. Chicago: Year Book, 1984.
11. Shires GT, et al, eds. Advances in Surgery. Vol 17. Chicago: Year Book, 1984.
12. Nelson RL, Nyhus LM. Surgery of the Small Intestine. Norwalk, CT: Appleton-Century-Croft, 1987.
13. Chassin JL. Operative Strategy in General Surgery—An Expositive Atlas. New York: Springer-Verlag, 1980.
14. Hardy TG, Pace WG, Meheny JW, et al. A biofragmentable ring for sutureless bowel anastomosis—an experimental study. Dis Colon Rectum 1985;28:484.
15. Hamilton B, Bishop WJ. In: Notable Names in Medicine and Surgery. 2nd ed. London: HK Lewis Publishers, 1946, p 152.
16. Hardy TG, Aguilar PS, Steward WRC, et al. Initial clinical experience with a biofragmentable ring for sutureless bowel anastomosis. Dis Colon Rectum 1987;30:55.
17. Bubick NP, Corman ML, Cahill CJ, et al. Prospective randomized trial of the biofragmentable anastomotic ring. Am J Surg 1991;161:136.

Perioperative Management of Disorders of the Colon, Rectum, and Anus

C H A P T E R 6

Charles D. Dietzen
Isidore Cohn, Jr.

Attention to precise surgical technique is essential for the safe and successful outcome of any operation. Of equal importance, however, are the correct choice and optimum timing of the procedure and proper perioperative management. Perioperative care—preoperative planning, intraoperative decision-making (excluding technique), and postoperative management—is the subject of this chapter.

All aspects of perioperative care are discussed, with the arbitrary division into preoperative, intraoperative, and postoperative phases. This separation is made with the full realization that certain aspects of patient care often involve more than one phase of the clinical course. Additionally, the possibility of duplication of information from other chapters (such as those describing colorectal emergencies and complications) is inevitable.

Perioperative care for elective abdominal colorectal operations differs in some aspects from that for emergency colorectal procedures and anorectal operations, both elective and emergency. For simplification, the discussion refers to elective abdominal colorectal cases, unless otherwise stated.

PREOPERATIVE CARE

Careful preparation and planning are the mainstays of effective preoperative care. Thorough knowledge of the patient's general medical status, the disease process requiring operative management, and the intended surgical procedure prevents omissions in patient preparation and minimizes the chance of complications.

Cardiovascular Status

A comprehensive discussion of cardiovascular management exceeds the purpose and scope of the chapter. It is incumbent on the surgeon to seek medical consultation judiciously when assistance is indicated. This requires recognition by the surgeon of patients with cardiovascular risk factors. Recent myocardial infarction, cardiac arrhythmias, and congestive heart failure, and the presence of cardiac valvular disease (especially aortic stenosis) are major cardiovascular risk factors.[1, 2] Sophisticated evaluation and management, including stress testing, arteriographic studies, pharmacologic management, and perioperative use of the pulmonary artery catheter are warranted in selected cases.

Patients with a recent myocardial infarction who undergo a major procedure are at a significantly increased risk of reinfarction for up to 6 months; they should not undergo operative therapy during that interval unless the surgical indications and urgency of the situation make delay a greater threat to life.[2] Medical or surgical treatment of coronary artery disease with appropriate indications for such should take precedence over treatment of the colorectal problem, except in the case of a colorectal emergency that cannot be postponed.

Although stable hypertension is not a major independent risk factor for noncardiac surgery, studies suggest the safety and efficacy of maintaining control of hypertension by continuing antihypertensive medications up to the time of operation.[2] For patients taking cardiac or antihypertensive medications, the possibility of toxic or withdrawal reactions, such as with digoxin and β-blockers, as well as untoward reactions to drug combinations (e.g., β-blockers and calcium channel blockers) must be kept in mind.

A history of congenital heart disease, cardiac valve replacement, or acquired valvular heart disease mandates bacterial endocarditis prophylaxis in patients undergoing colorectal procedures more extensive than proctoscopy without biopsy.[3] The recommended regimen requires ampicillin (or vancomycin in the case of penicillin allergy) and gentamicin (Table 6–1).

Cerebrovascular symptoms or known disease may warrant noninvasive and, possibly, angiographic evaluation. A similar situation exists for an asymptomatic abdominal aortic aneurysm. The approach to treatment of coexistent colorectal and vascular disease parallels the situation with colorectal and coronary artery disease. The relative urgency of each disease process and risk of delayed treatment should dictate the order of treatment. Combined procedures generally are not recommended.

Pulmonary Status

Patients undergoing general anesthesia are always at risk of postoperative pulmonary complications, especially when there is pre-existing pulmonary disease and when an upper abdominal incision is required. If the anticipated risk of postoperative pulmonary complications is great, preoperative pulmonary function testing may be helpful. Improvement in pulmonary function after bronchodilator therapy indicates that short postponement of operation, time permitting, and aggressive preoperative pulmonary therapy can lessen the pulmonary risk. As with high-risk cardiovascular patients, judicious consideration of medical consultation is recommended.

Hematologic Status

Anemia is often encountered in patients with colorectal disease. The generally accepted minimal preoperative hemoglobin level is 10 g/dl (corresponding to a hematocrit of 30%). Using this guideline, one must bear in mind ongoing blood loss in selected patients and transfuse accordingly. Furthermore, although young, healthy patients may tolerate a perioperative hemoglobin level considerably less than 10 g/dl, selected patients, specifically those with angina or chronic obstructive pulmonary disease, may best respond to an operative procedure with a hemoglobin level greater than 10 g/dl, providing greater oxygen-carrying capacity.[4] Patients with cardiac disease should have a hemoglobin level of 12 to 13 g/dl. Patients with chronic pulmonary disease and secondary polycythemia should also be maintained at a higher hemoglobin level.

Preoperative coagulation function can be screened with a prothrombin time, checking the extrinsic pathway, and a partial thromboplastin time, checking the intrinsic coagulation pathway. Depending on the clinical situation, vitamin K, fresh frozen plasma, or other blood products may be given to correct clotting factor deficits.

Platelet quantity and function can be checked with a platelet count and bleeding time (obviously a preoperative bleeding time is not necessary in every case). Although spontaneous bleeding does not occur below platelet counts of 10,000 to 20,000/μl, pre-existing bleeding usually does not stop with a platelet count of less than approximately 100,000/μl.[4] One unit of platelets will increase the platelet count by approximately 10,000. The influence of aspirin to produce diminished platelet function for 7 to 10 days following ingestion is well described. In the case of recent aspirin use, depending on the urgency of the disease, consideration should be given to delay of selected colorectal procedures (particularly colonoscopy with electrosnare polypectomy) for 7 days or until the patient's bleeding time reverts to normal.

Table 6–1. SUBACUTE BACTERIAL ENDOCARDITIS PROPHYLAXIS IN COLORECTAL SURGERY

Standard			
Ampicillin	2.0 g	(50 mg/kg for children)	IM or IV
Plus			
Gentamicin	1.5 mg/kg	(2.0 mg/kg for children)	IM or IV
Penicillin Allergic			
Vancomycin	1.0 g	(20 mg/kg up to 1.0 g for children)	IV
Plus			
Gentamicin	1.5 mg/kg	(2.0 mg/kg for children)	IM or IV

The standard regimen should be given 30 minutes prior to procedure. The penicillin-allergic regimen is designed for slow infusion of vancomycin over 1 hour and with the vancomycin and gentamicin infusions completed 1 hour prior to the procedure. With both regimens the dose can be repeated once after 8 hours.

From Shulman ST, Amren DP, Bisno AL, et al. Circulation 1984; 70:1123A–1127A.
IM = intramuscular; IV = intravenous.

Fluid and Electrolyte Status

The majority of patients in need of a colorectal procedure have normal fluid and electrolyte balance. However, there are specific situations in which deficiencies requiring preoperative correction exist. Patients taking diuretics, particularly kaliuretics, and patients undergoing prolonged mechanical bowel preparation are prone to volume and potassium deficits, sometimes quite severe ones. Replenishment prior to the autonomic inhibition associated with general anesthesia is critical to maintenance of maximum tissue perfusion during the operative procedure.

Patients with urgent colorectal problems, such as diverticulitis or colon obstruction, and chronic colorectal disease, such as inflammatory bowel disease, may also need correction of fluid and electrolyte deficiencies preoperatively. Careful scrutiny of serum electrolyte concentrations and maintenance of normal urinary volume are essential to satisfactory preoperative preparation.

The phenomenon of dehydration, hypokalemia, and mucous diarrhea associated with colorectal villous adenoma merits mention. In some cases, sodium and chloride losses can be severe and may be related to the variable metabolic acidosis or alkalosis noted.[5, 6] When present, these abnormalities should be repaired prior to surgical intervention.

Endocrine, Immunologic, and Nutritional Status

Colorectal problems are not generally associated with endocrine disease. However, inflammatory bowel disease is often treated with corticosteroids, resulting in suppression of the hypothalamic-pituitary-adrenal axis and altering the patient's ability to mount an endocrine response to stress. Adrenal suppression is dependent on the steroid dose, duration, frequency, and time and route of administration. Suppression for 1 week or longer can occur after as little as 5 to 7 days of daily treatment with large doses (greater than 40 mg/m² prednisone or its equivalent).[7] Length of time for full recovery of adrenal function is variable and has been reported to be greater than 1 year in some cases.[8]

When patients have had glucocorticoid treatment capable of adrenal suppression within 1 to 2 years of a proposed operation, it is recommended to anticipate the necessary endocrine response to operative stress and administer exogenous steroids perioperatively.[9, 10] A number of regimens have been suggested. Most involve giving approximately 300 mg per day of hydrocortisone, or its equivalent, in divided doses (Table 6–2). This amount represents the response of the normal adrenal gland to major stress.[9]

After 1 to 2 postoperative days, the steroid dose can usually be safely reduced to maintenance level over 5 days, after which further reduction should be carried out more slowly. Unexpected postoperative stress from

Table 6–2. PERIOPERATIVE STEROIDS IN THE ADRENAL-SUPPRESSED PATIENT

Day of operation, preoperative hydrocortisone	100 mg	IM on call
Day of operation, postoperative hydrocortisone	50 mg	IM or IV q6h
		(Start in recovery room)

On postoperative day 2, begin gradual taper over 3 to 5 days to maintenance therapy. Revert to original dosage for complications and added stress.

Modified from Bergland RM, Gann DS, DeMaria EJ. Pituitary and adrenal. In: Schwartz SI, Shires GT, Spencer FC, eds. Principles of Surgery. 5th ed. New York: McGraw-Hill, 1989.

IM = intramuscular; IV = intravenous.

complications or signs of steroid withdrawal warrant resumption of the original high dose until the problem is rectified. It has been suggested that the frequency of steroid withdrawal after too-rapid tapering may be underappreciated and often misdiagnosed as intestinal obstruction.[11]

To date, no scientifically valid data have proved that preoperative nutritional supplementation, enteral or parenteral, significantly alters the outcome of major colorectal operations. The literature contains numerous reports of preoperative nutritional repletion in surgical patients. Most of these studies are flawed by nonuniformity of a number of variables: randomization (lack of it); definition of nutritional status; content and quantity of solutions administered; end point of administration; definition of complications. Nevertheless, there is a suggestion that in patients who are severely malnourished, in whom immunologic and nutritional deficits are reversed with preoperative nutritional repletion, a decreased postoperative complication rate accrues following major abdominal surgery. This suggestion probably can be extrapolated to colorectal operations, including those for inflammatory bowel disease.[12–14] Until there are more reliable data to clarify this issue, the surgeon managing a malnourished pa-

EDITORIAL COMMENT

Although convincing data may be lacking to endorse the use of nutritional repletion in the patient undergoing major colonic or rectal operations, there are practical considerations that favor the concept. Total parenteral nutrition (TPN) allows for a leisurely mechanical preparation of the bowel in patients with partial obstruction, severe inflammatory bowel disease, and perineal sepsis, while allowing adequate caloric and protein intake. Starvation can be avoided in the postoperative period pending return of gastrointestinal function and ensured venous access. TPN is now part and parcel of the gastrointestinal surgeon's armamentarium, and its widespread use and acceptance are warranted.

tient requiring a colorectal operation has two reasonable choices: either administer 7 to 10 days or more of alimentation prior to the procedure, or perform the necessary operation without further delay and begin parenteral alimentation in the immediate postoperative period.

Gastrointestinal Status

Occasionally patients with a history of peptic ulcer disease or another upper gastrointestinal condition who are under medical management require a colorectal operation (for unrelated disease). In this situation, the surgeon should be satisfied that the upper gastrointestinal process is controlled by utilizing endoscopy or radiologic contrast studies, if indicated. Specifically, patients with a history of peptic ulcer should be treated with H$_2$ receptor antagonists during the perioperative period to prevent reactivation of disease.

Likewise, in a patient with known cholelithiasis, a history of appropriate symptoms should be sought and the propriety of removal of the gallbladder in combination with the colorectal operation should be discussed with the patient. We recommend selective performance of cholecystectomy in this situation, depending on the preoperative symptoms, intraoperative findings, and intraoperative condition of the patient.

It has been generally accepted that steroid use is associated with an increased incidence of peptic ulcer disease. However, there are no confirmed data to substantiate such an association.[15] Therefore, surgeons who, based on experience, think that H$_2$ blockers should be used as "prophylaxis" in these cases should be aware of all possible side effects to avoid iatrogenic complications. The routine use of H$_2$ blockers perioperatively for patients on steroids who have no history of ulcer disease cannot be recommended at present.

The use of H$_2$ blockers for "prophylaxis" against stress ulceration in the critically ill patient is also controversial. Although their use is a common practice, scientific evidence to justify it is not available. These agents have not been approved by the Food and Drug Administration for prevention of stress ulceration. If the surgeon gives H$_2$ blockers for this indication, it is necessary to be aware of the possible complications of the drug.[16, 17]

Prophylaxis: Deep Vein Thrombosis and Pulmonary Embolism

Very few studies have addressed prophylaxis against deep vein thrombosis (DVT) and pulmonary embolism (PE) in colorectal operations alone. The most recent study of this type, comparing low-dose heparin to no treatment in colorectal resection, found no significant difference for thromboembolic complications.[18] A number of trials limited to general surgical operations (including colonic surgery) have indicated a significant reduction in DVT, PE, or both with a variety of methods. A review by Clagett and Reisch[19] summarizes these studies. Briefly, only low-dose heparin and dextran have been shown to be efficacious in preventing DVT *and* PE. Dihydroergotamine-heparin, intermittent pneumatic compression devices, and graded elastic stockings offer effective prophylaxis against DVT, but there are insufficient data to evaluate their worth in preventing PE.[19] Kakkar et al[20] found that a daily dose of 0.5 mg dihydroergotamine mesylate in combination with 1,500 IU of low-molecular-weight heparin by subcutaneous injection provided prophylaxis against DVT equal to low-dose heparin (5,000 IU unfractionated heparin plus 0.5 mg dihydroergotamine mesylate twice daily). Dihydroergotamine has subsequently been banned owing to concern over vasospastic side effects. Prophylaxis was started preoperatively and continued at least 7 days postoperatively.

Many patients undergoing major colorectal operations fall into a moderate- to high-risk category for DVT or PE (past history of thromboembolic disease, obesity, age greater than 40 years, malignant disease). Until further trials can disprove the benefit of DVT and PE prophylaxis for colorectal operations, it seems prudent to use one of the aforementioned methods when a colorectal operation is planned with general anesthesia for patients at increased risk. Our recommendation would be the intermittent pneumatic compression devices or low-dose subcutaneous heparin, according to the preference of the surgeon. Postoperatively, patients should be walking actively before discontinuance of prophylaxis.

EDITORIAL COMMENT
The use of heparin as a prophylaxis against DVT and PE is appealing but not without danger. The colitic patient (with ulcerative colitis or extensive Crohn's colitis) may suffer devastating hemorrhage as a result of anticoagulation. For the high-risk patient with colitis, mechanical measures to prevent PE (caval filter or clip) offer protection without the risk of hemorrhagic complications.

Bowel Preparation

Mechanical Preparation

It is well established that infectious complications with colorectal resection are reduced when satisfactory bowel preparation is carried out.[21, 22] Adequate preparation is accomplished by mechanical purgation of solid fecal matter (which contains as much as 30% bacteria by wet weight), to reduce the gross *quantity* of bacteria within the large bowel, and antimicrobial preparation to reduce the *concentration* of bacteria in the colon residue.[23, 24]

Two methods of mechanical bowel cleansing are available. The older, traditional method consists of a low-residue or liquid diet in combination with cathartics and enemas beginning 2 to 5 days prior to the procedure. The second method involves prograde intestinal lavage 1 day prior to operation. Peroral lavage was initially described with mannitol or saline, but a polyethylene glycol (PEG)–electrolyte solution has been developed. Studies indicate that the PEG–electrolyte oral lavage is as effective as the traditional bowel preparation and reduces the number of preoperative hospital patient days.[25, 26] The PEG–electrolyte solution does not cause the significant fluid or electrolyte alteration sometimes associated with several days of cathartics and enemas or antegrade saline or mannitol lavage.[27] Although a survey indicates that more than 50% of surgeons continue to favor the traditional method,[28] we recommend the oral lavage with PEG–electrolyte solution, reserving cathartics and enemas for those patients unable to satisfactorily carry out oral lavage. In selected patients receiving cathartics and enemas, intravenous fluids should be given during the preparation period to avoid dehydration.

Obviously preoperative mechanical bowel preparation in the presence of complete large bowel obstruction is not possible; however, there are reports of *intraoperative* colonic cleansing under such circumstances. This technique has not gained wide acceptance, but more reports are anticipated in the future.[29]

Antibiotic Preparation

Although it is clear that antibiotic colon preparation, in combination with mechanical purgation, significantly lowers infectious complications, the optimum agents and routes of antibiotic administration are yet to be determined. Perhaps a definitive regimen has not been forthcoming because of flaws in many of the previous investigations.[30] However, a review of the literature allows some general statements. There is a significantly greater infection rate with mechanical preparation alone compared with mechanical *plus* antibiotic preparation. This finding is almost universally accepted.

The most effective antibiotic regimens utilize agents to which the major colon pathogens, anaerobes (predominantly *Bacteroides* species) and gram-negative aerobes (predominantly *Escherichia coli*), are sensitive. This holds for both oral and parenteral agents.

"Coverage" by agents, either by intraluminal suppression with oral antibiotics or by serum levels of parenteral antibiotics, needs to be achieved only in the perioperative period, that is, just prior to the procedure, during the procedure, and for a short time (6 to 48 hours) postoperatively. Failure of *preoperative* initiation of antibiotics negates the beneficial effect. Prolonged antibiotic use for longer than 48 hours postoperatively offers no greater protection from infection than perioperative use alone.

In reviewing studies comparing oral antibiotic preparation with parenteral antibiotic coverage, preparation by the oral route *tends* to be equal to or better than the parenteral method in preventing infection. However, enough studies show equivalence of the two methods to create uncertainty about one being superior.

In evaluating studies comparing oral preparation with the combination of oral and parenteral preparation, it is suggested, but not substantiated, that the combination method may offer added protection.[24] A survey of colorectal surgeons shows that the majority use both oral antibiotics and parenteral antibiotics for elective colorectal resection.[28]

The most frequently employed oral agents are neomycin or kanamycin and erythromycin or metronidazole, covering gram-negative aerobes and anaerobes, respectively. These are usually given during the day prior to operation. A number of agents, singly or in combination, have been used for parenteral coverage: cephalosporins, aminoglycosides in combination with metronidazole or clindamycin, "broad-spectrum" penicillins (e.g., ticarcillin), and others.[24] In light of the data available, one method (oral or parenteral, or both) cannot be recommended as superior. Patients for elective colorectal resection should receive antibiotics perioperatively, surgeons using the routes and agents of their choice.

Unusual Circumstances

Urgent colorectal problems, marked by complete obstruction or possible perforation, do not allow the luxury of mechanical and antimicrobial preparation. In this situation, broad-spectrum parenteral coverage of colonic pathogens extending 5 to 10 days postoperatively may be needed.

Although patients who are immunocompromised or ascitic, or who have undergone pelvic radiotherapy may be at increased risk of postoperative infectious complications, there is no evidence that prolonged postoperative antibiotics or preoperative maneuvers (save reversal of immunosuppression or ascites) in addition to preparation as outlined previously are helpful in preventing infection in the "clean contaminated" situation. Obviously the severely neutropenic patient is an exception. These individuals require broad-spectrum antibiotic protection regardless of need of operation.

Anorectal Procedures

Previous clinical experience has shown that many ano-rectal procedures require neither mechanical nor anti-biotic preparation of the large bowel preoperatively. Examples include hemorrhoidectomy, anal fistulotomy, and lateral internal anal sphincterotomy. These procedures require, at most, an enema shortly before the procedure to evacuate the lower colorectum, and no antibiotics unless an immune deficit or systemic sepsis is present.

Anorectal procedures of a higher order of magnitude, for example, repair of rectovaginal fistula, per-anal excision of low rectal lesions, and perineal recto-sigmoidectomy usually involve more extensive dissection, with greater hazard from postoperative wound sepsis. For these types of procedures, therefore, preparation of the large bowel should be similar to that for elective transabdominal colorectal resection.

Urologic Considerations

The proximity of the components of the urinary system to the colon and rectum, along with its blood and nerve supply, necessitates consideration for urologic evaluation preoperatively. Some surgeons recommend that an intravenous pyelogram (IVP) be performed prior to all colonic and rectal resections. Advocates of the routine IVP cite a high incidence of unexpected abnormalities discovered with this practice.[31] However, some literature suggests that the urologic injury rate is not significantly different for patients who do *not* routinely have a preoperative IVP.[32]

Until a randomized trial clarifies the value of a mandatory IVP versus a selective IVP prior to colo-rectal resection, this should be the surgeon's choice. In patients with potential urologic disease suggested by history or examination or with involvement from contiguous large bowel disease (e.g., complicated di-verticulitis, extensive rectal cancer), and in instances of planned pelvic surgery, there is great advantage in the preoperative knowledge of the function and location of the kidneys and ureters.

As with the IVP, preoperative placement of ureteral catheters is a practice based solely on the preference of the surgeon, and most probably is done on a selective basis. The disadvantages of stent placement include added time needed for the procedure, bladder or ureteral injury during placement, urinary infection, and a false sense of security from over-reliance on the ability to palpate stents to avoid injury. The advantages include added help with identification of the ureter in difficult cases and a greater likelihood of identification and repair of an unintended ureteral injury at the primary procedure. All things considered, it would seem prudent to obtain an IVP and place ureteral catheters in selected cases, at the very least, if difficulty is anticipated. The most important factors in avoidance of ureteral injury are knowledge of normal and variant ureteral anatomy, knowledge of the possible alterations in ureteral anatomy with complicated colorectal dis-ease, and surgical experience.

EDITORIAL COMMENT

Ureteral injury most often occurs during rectosigmoid re-section at two locations: the left ureter may be injured during isolation and division of the inferior mesenteric ar-tery and vein; the left ureter may also be damaged at the level of the origin of the hypogastric artery during re-resection of the rectum. At the higher level, ureteral cath-eters should not be necessary; identification of the ureter prior to mesenteric division should suffice. In re-resec-tions, the ureter is often medial from its normal position and adherent to the rectal mesentery. In this situation there is often dense scar tissue through which only an extremely large ureteral catheter can be palpated. These large catheters themselves may cause ureteral injury. The editors prefer careful dissection and repeated identifica-tion of the ureter rather than the employment of cathe-ters.

During pelvic dissection for rectal cancer, the pelvic autonomic nervous system may be damaged or sacrificed, resulting in bladder atony. Following these dissections, cystometrograms should be performed prior to the dis-continuance of the bladder catheter.

A last urologic consideration concerns the elderly male with pre-existing subclinical prostatic hypertrophy and development of urinary retention after abdomi-noperineal resection or low anterior resection. This patient can benefit from preoperative urologic evalua-tion with urodynamics to plan more effectively the intra- and postoperative management of the prostate and bladder. In this patient, liberal urologic consulta-tion prior to the operation is recommended.

Ostomy Considerations

The possible need for a stoma should be assessed by the surgeon preoperatively, and if ostomy is certain, possible, or even remote, the subject should be dis-cussed in an appropriate context with the patient.

Of equal importance is consultation with an enter-ostomal therapist when the possibility of an ostomy is envisioned. These nurse specialists are invaluable in the psychological preparation and education of the patient as well as in the determination of the most suitable abdominal skin sites for a stoma.

Emergency Situations

Depending on the severity and subsequent urgency of the situation, some colorectal problems are inappropriate for elective preparation and operation. These problems usually fall into one or more of the following categories: complete obstruction, massive hemorrhage, infection (with or without perforation), and ischemia (Table 6–3). In contrast to the elective situation, these processes usually preclude mechanical and oral antibiotic colon preparation before the operation. As with other abdominal emergencies, the tenets of preoperative preparation are more critical illness–directed than colon-directed: nasogastric decompression (almost all of these patients have a paralytic ileus); fluid, electrolyte, and acid-base repair; urinary catheterization and critical care monitoring (in many cases); repair of blood product deficits; and systemic, broad-spectrum antibiotics effective against gram-negative coliforms and anaerobes (Table 6–4). Further discussion of the management of gram-negative sepsis, septic shock, or hemorrhagic shock is beyond the scope of this chapter. These patients should be converted to the highest-possible hemodynamic status, for the particular situation encountered, before operative treatment is initiated.

Patient Hospitalization

In the past decade there has been a trend toward reduced hospitalization stays and greater use of outpatient facilities ("one-day-stay surgery," "same-day surgery") for many surgical disciplines, including colonic and rectal surgery. This trend was probably engendered, in part, by increasing medical costs and has been embraced by third-party carriers. Regardless of physician reluctance, patients have apparently not suffered from the shift of surgical services from the hospital to the office or outpatient facility. A number of anorectal procedures have been conducted successfully on an outpatient basis.[33] It is probable that same-day admission for major colorectal resection, at least for selective patients, will be practiced in the future.

Table 6–3. COLORECTAL EMERGENCIES
PRECLUDING BOWEL PREPARATION

Complete obstruction
Massive hemorrhage
Infection
Acute diverticulitis
Active inflammatory bowel disease
Trauma
Ischemia

Table 6–4. PREOPERATIVE MANAGEMENT OF
COLORECTAL EMERGENCIES

Nasogastric decompression
Fluid, electrolyte, and acid-base repair
Urinary catheterization
Correction of blood product deficits
Broad-spectrum antibiotics (parenteral)
Critical care monitoring
(Arterial catheterization, central venous or Swan-Ganz catheterization), as needed

No medical organization exists to give its imprimatur to the safety and propriety of these practices. Therefore, the utilization of the office or outpatient facility and of same-day admission for colorectal procedures should be the surgeon's choice based on the intended procedure, the health of the patient, and the surgeon's previous experience.

INTRAOPERATIVE CARE

The general conduct of a colorectal operation involves much more than the technical act of dissection, excision, suture, and repair. Although the cases may have similarities to one another, each likewise has differences necessitating intraoperative decision-making and, occasionally, change in plan. Anticipation of all possible situations leads to forethought, planning, and smoother operations.

Unexpected Findings

Gallstones

When cholelithiasis is discovered during a colorectal procedure, several factors come into play in deciding whether to perform cholecystectomy in addition to the colorectal operation. The appearance of the gallbladder is one determinant. If there are signs of subacute or recent inflammation, it is probably best to remove the gallbladder, regardless of the presence or absence of preoperative symptoms.

When symptoms consistent with gallbladder disease have been elicited prior to operation and gallstones are found, cholecystectomy should be done if the intraoperative condition is stable.

If unforeseen events during the procedure lead to an unstable patient, any plan for additional cholecystectomy should be abandoned. In a patient undergoing an emergency colorectal operation, it is probably unwise to add cholecystectomy unless the surgeon is convinced from the intraoperative findings that acute cholecystitis is likely to complicate the postoperative course.

The subset of patients with asymptomatic stones and no inflammation in the gallbladder poses an interesting problem. Truly asymptomatic patients with stones have approximately a 2% per year rate of developing symptoms with subsequent mortality and morbidity similar to those in patients having cholecystectomy. Therefore, incidental cholecystectomy should not be performed in these patients unless the surgeon is confident that it can be done safely.[34] In addition, the incidental procedure should be performed safely *without* excessive extension of the abdominal incision.

Abdominal Aortic Aneurysm

The best management of coexistent colonic disease and abdominal aortic aneurysm (AAA) is controversial. Surgical department chairmen and section directors of vascular surgery of 46 medical schools were surveyed on the proper management of synchronous colon cancer and AAA.[35] Except for two surgeons who expressed a preference for resection of the colon and aneurysm at the same operation, there was agreement on staged procedures. Their opinions were approximately equally divided on initial resection of the colon cancer or the aneurysm, or on basing the decision on intraoperative findings. Thomas' review[36] summarizes the literature and offers the same conclusions and recommendations, with minimal modification, as in the classic paper of Szilagyi et al (Table 6–5).[37] Thomas' recommendations, with which we agree, hold for patients with benign colonic disease as well. He states that symptoms of expansion or rupture mandate aneurysm repair and that signs of emergency colon disease (hemorrhage, perforation, obstruction) mandate colon resection. If a patient is seen with these "absolute indications," such as aneurysm rupture and colonic obstruction, treatment of both problems at the same procedure is indicated. If only one organ has so-called absolute indications for treatment, it should be appropriately managed and the other organ managed at a secondary procedure. In the absence of absolute indications, the preference is resection of the more extensive disease (aneurysm, if large; colon, if aneurysm is small) with treatment of the less advanced process at a secondary procedure. If "controlled" metastatic malignant disease is present, AAA resection is indicated with a rupture, symptoms of expansion or leak, or an asymptomatic aneurysm that is greater than 6 cm in diameter.

Thomas also draws attention to a subset of small-diameter aneurysms that are thin-walled or have formed blebs. He ascribes an increased risk of rupture to aneurysms in this category, similar to the risk for those greater than 6 cm.

Colorectal Cancer: Contiguous or Distant Tumor Involvement

Spread of a colorectal tumor into adjacent organs necessitates a decision regarding the extent of resection. Because of difficulty distinguishing inflammatory reaction from actual tumor growth into adjacent organs, the surgeon should always assume the latter. This finding does not necessarily worsen the prognosis.[38] If the tumor can be removed en bloc with negative margins, the patient is potentially curable. The particular organ and extent of involvement determine the potentially considerable morbidity and mortality associated with extended resection.[38] Few surgeons would hesitate to add limited small bowel or abdominal wall resection to a colorectal resection; however, additional cystectomy with ileal conduit or pancreatic resection is a complicated undertaking that is best anticipated, evaluated, and discussed preoperatively. When this type of situation exists, the surgeon must use clinical judgment to choose the best procedure for the particular patient and particular organ involved.

The same strategy holds for unexpected distant metastasis to the liver or other organs. The intended colon resection *and* resection of metastases may be performed, depending on the extent and location of disease. For extensive distant metastasis limited colon resection, bypass, or diversion probably is preferred. Patients with extensive liver metastasis that is resectable should undergo conventional excision of the primary tumor, biopsy of the liver lesion for histologic

Table 6–5. AORTIC ANEURYSM ENCOUNTERED AT COLORECTAL OPERATION

	Colon	Aortic Aneurysm
Absolute indications for resection or repair at initial operation:	Obstruction Hemorrhage Perforation	Rupture Symptoms

Staged procedures are the rule. The *only* exception is absolute indications in *both* organs, warranting resection of aneurysm *and* colon at the same procedure.

Absolute indications in one organ warrant treatment of that organ as the first stage.

Absolute indications in neither organ warrant treatment of the more extensive disease (aneurysm, if diameter > 6 cm; otherwise, the colon) as the first stage.

Symptoms or rupture warrants treatment of aneurysm in the face of metastatic disease. Diameter > 6 cm, thin wall, or bleb formation in a small aneurysm warrants treatment of the aneurysm in the face of metastatic disease *effectively controlled.*

Modified from Thomas JH. Abdominal aortic aneurysmorrhaphy combined with biliary or gastrointestinal surgery. Surg Clin North Am 1984; 69:807–815.

confirmation, and re-evaluation for hepatic resection after recovery.[39]

Intraoperative Contamination

Unanticipated contamination during elective colorectal resection is an infrequent occurrence. It usually results from unrecognized, inadequate mechanical preparation in combination with a technical mishap allowing spillage of stool, or from disruption of an unsuspected, contained subacute or chronic perforation. When this happens the surgeon is faced with the decision to carry out the procedure as intended or to alter the plan. If an abdominoperineal resection or proctocolectomy with ileostomy was elected, most would continue the procedure without change. The major question arises when a large bowel anastomosis is planned. Strength and integrity of the anastomotic suture line are compromised, probably from increased fibrin deposition in the presence of peritonitis or increased collagen breakdown in the presence of intraluminal stool.[40, 41]

Numerous reports address the merits of staged (diverting stoma with later stoma closure) versus primary (one-stage) anastomosis for conditions such as complicated diverticulitis or perforative colon injury, where there is less-than-satisfactory mechanical preparation of the colon.[42–44] Unfortunately, each case has its unique characteristics, making blanket recommendations impossible. This issue is further complicated by technical innovations such as intraoperative colon lavage and intracolonic bypass tube, as well as scientific discoveries such as the use of tissue plasminogen activator in the presence of peritonitis.[29, 41, 45] The place of these breakthroughs in present-day clinical practice is yet to be defined.

With the controversy surrounding primary anastomosis in the presence of fecal loading, excessive fecal spillage, or diffuse peritonitis, it is probably wise to divert the fecal stream, accepting a second operation for stoma closure unless the surgeon has previous experience and confidence in a one-stage approach.

Although the usually recommended management of contaminated and dirty wounds is delayed primary closure or secondary closure,[46] many surgeons accept the increased risk of wound infection and perform primary closure. However, some patients in this category are critically ill and do not tolerate wound infection well. Because of the potential systemic and local complications associated with delayed detection of wound infection we recommend delayed primary closure or secondary closure for most contaminated or dirty wounds.

Use of Drains

Often the intra- and postoperative use of drains is based on the surgeon's previous training and past experience rather than scientifically proven principles. Despite uncertainty about the need for some types of drains, the surgeon should be acquainted with their proper use to avoid iatrogenic mishaps.

Bladder Drainage

The fluid shifts associated with most intraperitoneal colorectal operations ("third-space" loss, blood loss) necessitate bladder drainage to accurately quantitate urinary volumes and maintain hydration. Additionally, extensive pelvic dissection and complex anorectal cases are often accompanied by a short period of bladder dysfunction best managed with catheter placement. Less extensive anorectal cases (e.g., hemorrhoidectomy, sphincterotomy) do not warrant catheterization under most circumstances, unless postoperative urinary retention occurs. This is usually avoided by infusion of minimal necessary intravenous fluids perioperatively.

Discontinuance of the catheter at the earliest-possible time minimizes secondary urinary tract infection. The surgeon should be satisfied that there is recovery without hemorrhage or intraperitoneal infection before discontinuing bladder drainage. In addition, the patient should be able to empty the bladder successfully at the time of catheter removal. An elderly patient may experience retention if the catheter is discontinued during the phase of mobilization of third-space losses. Usually the catheter can safely be removed 3 to 5 days postoperatively. Extensive pelvic dissection with bladder trauma and autonomic disturbance responds more favorably with a longer period (6 to 7 days) of catheterization. This latter category would include low anterior resection, abdominoperineal resection, and colon resection with repair of a colovesical fistula.

Abdominal (Anastomotic) Drainage

Drainage of intra-abdominal colonic anastomoses is not done routinely in the United States, although it may be practiced frequently in other countries.[47] Clinical studies have shown no advantage to the use of drains, and animal studies indicate a possible deleterious effect on healing.[48, 49] We do not advocate this practice.

Large bowel anastomoses located below the pelvic peritoneum that may become sealed off from the peritoneal cavity soon after operation *may* be appropriate for drainage, although this is not substantiated by clinical studies. In this situation (e.g., low anterior resection, ileal pouch anal anastomosis), if drainage is selected we recommend a closed, Silastic drain, under low suction pressure, exiting via an independent, lower abdominal site. The drain should be placed near, but not in direct contact with, the suture line. Drain removal is usually safe when daily volume is less than 25 to 50 ml.

Abdominal drainage is indicated for infection with organized abscess cavities that have walled off from the peritoneal cavity. We advocate large, soft sump drains, placed through wounds separate from the operative incision. Suction pressures on these drains should be kept at the lowest setting, which allows sump function to reduce trauma to adjacent intestine and fistula formation. These drains should remain in place until the cavity has collapsed and drainage is negligible; graduated removal of the drain over several or more days, allowing the drain track to collapse, is recommended.

Anorectal Drainage

Infectious cases and clean contaminated cases of the anorectum are often appropriate for drainage. Depending on the disease process, consistency of drainage fluid, and preference of the surgeon, open, dependent capillary drainage with latex (Penrose drain) or closed, suction drainage with a Silastic device is effective.

Nasogastric and Intestinal Tubes

As with intraperitoneal drainage, the past use of nasogastric tubes in colorectal operations more often has been based on previous training and experience than on sound clinical research. It is now evident that nasogastric drainage for routine, elective colorectal resection offers no added benefit to most patients with respect to anastomotic or fascial healing or protection from aspiration. Statistically valid studies substantiate these findings; only 4% to 13% of patients treated initially without a tube subsequently needed gastric decompression for nausea or vomiting.[50–53]

Patients with emergent colorectal problems associated with ileus and bowel distention and patients at high risk of postoperative aspiration or gastric atony are most effectively managed with nasogastric or gastrostomy drainage.

Rectal tube decompression for left-sided colon anastomoses has been described.[54] A clinical advantage of decreased infectious complications has never been proven. We do not practice this technique.

POSTOPERATIVE CARE

The aspects of postoperative management related to preoperative and intraoperative care have been discussed: antibiotics, drains, intestinal and urinary catheters, and DVT prophylaxis. This section covers the features of patient care specific to the postoperative period.

Dietary Progression

Colonic function in the form of flatus or bowel motion usually returns 3 to 5 days after major colon resection. Although earlier institution of postoperative feedings may be well tolerated in some patients, forced oral feeding in the presence of an intestinal ileus usually does not shorten the period of postoperative bowel dysfunction. We advocate no oral intake until colon function returns. Progression from clear liquids to a solid diet over 1 to 3 days, depending on the oral intake and appetite, can then be carried out.

For most anorectal cases, dietary progression can begin when the patient recovers from the anesthesia and is experiencing no nausea.

Bowel Stimulants and Depressants

Laxatives, cathartics, and enemas in the postoperative period, especially in the presence of an anastomotic suture line, are unwise. Abnormal intracolonic pressures, exceeding the bursting strength of the anastomosis, may occur. If colonic function has not returned in a reasonable time after the operation, radiologic evaluation with computed tomography, ultrasonography, or water-soluble contrast enema under low pressure, may be indicated.

Metoclopramide has little pharmacologic effect on large bowel motility and cannot be recommended for postoperative augmentation of colonic function.[55] Cisapride is a relatively new agent, not approved by the Food and Drug Administration for use in the United States.[56] Cisapride has been shown to promote colonic peristalsis. Clinical utility after major colorectal surgery no doubt will be evaluated. However, it may prove more valuable in the management of chronic, severe constipation and colonic pseudo-obstruction (Ogilvie's syndrome).

After removal of most or all of the large intestine, patients often experience increased stool frequency and fluid loss. If this situation proves burdensome, agents such as diphenoxylate or loperamide may be used to counteract the diarrhea. In many patients the remaining bowel adapts, and these drugs are needed only temporarily. Some patients, however, require long-term antidiarrheal medication. The surgeon initiating this therapy in the postoperative course must be satisfied that the patient has truly resumed bowel function and that the diarrhea is a manifestation of large bowel loss rather than of partial intestinal obstruction from anastomotic narrowing or other causes.

In patients undergoing less extensive anorectal procedures without preoperative purgation of the entire colon, prevention of postoperative constipation is important. Pain in the anal region, narcotic usage for analgesia, and fear of bowel motion (with accentuation of pain) promote large bowel stasis. The patient should be warned of this possibility, and early resumption of ambulation and adequate hydration should be encouraged. Bulk agents such as psyllium are also recommended after most anorectal procedures. If these measures are unsuccessful in the initiation of defecation by 3 days postoperatively, an oral laxative should be taken, but enema tips near the operative site are unwise. A magnesium-based compound is usually effective. After the first bowel passage these agents usually are no longer needed.

Pain Control

Although narcotics continue as the mainstay for postoperative pain relief, several developments deserve discussion. Patient-controlled analgesia (PCA), the self-administration of intravenous narcotic by the patient via a mechanical pump, was described over 20 years ago.[57] It became more widely used only in the past few years. The pumps are constructed in such a way that the physician can place limits on the maximum dose. The narcotic is stored within a locked reservoir in the pump and not directly accessible by the patient. Advantages may include more rapid alleviation of postoperative pain and reduction of the nurse's workload, allowing attention to other aspects of patient care. There may be psychological benefits, such as the patient experiencing more control during the clinical course. This technique is successful and safe, although it is difficult to demonstrate its superiority over conventional intramuscular narcotics.[57]

Another increasingly popular technique is epidural analgesia.[58] Selective blockade of pain sensation is achieved in the absence of any change in remaining sensory or motor function. The advantages of epidural analgesia include less sedation, although as with intramuscular narcotics, respiratory depression is possible; improved pulmonary function; shorter time until walk-

ing begins after completion of the operation; and decreased morbidity. Besides respiratory depression, which may be prolonged, potential disadvantages include prolonged gastric emptying, urinary retention, nausea, and itching.[58] This method probably will be more common in the future in patients with pre-existing pulmonary disease.

A parenteral nonsteroidal anti-inflammatory agent, ketorolac, has become available.[59] The drug, designed for intramuscular administration only, has more analgesic than anti-inflammatory potency. A dose of 30 to 90 mg has an analgesic effect comparable to that of 6 to 12 mg morphine. Although respiratory depression and euphoria are not recognized adverse effects of ketorolac, it appears to inhibit platelet aggregation induced by arachidonic acid and collagen, and can prolong bleeding time. This drug, or similar ones, may be most useful as supplements to narcotics for postoperative pain control.[59]

Postoperative Pulmonary Care

Postoperative pulmonary complications after all types of operations occur 2% to 9% of the time.[60] In abdominal operations, especially in patients with pre-existing pulmonary disease, the risk is even greater. As with other complications, anticipation is the key to prevention or diminution of pulmonary morbidity. This can be accomplished by preoperative screening, treatment, and patient education (see Preoperative Care) and appropriate postoperative care.

Abdominal incisions inhibit primary muscles of respiration. This effect results in reduced tidal volume, reduced functional residual capacity, and interference with normal mucociliary clearance. If not corrected, atelectasis and pneumonia will eventuate. Preoperative patient education, early assumption of the upright position after operation, walking, coughing, and deep breathing are helpful. Adequate numbers of competent ancillary staff to assist patients with these maneuvers are critical to minimizing pulmonary complications.

Surgeons must individualize the care of each patient, based on knowledge of the patient and the pulmonary risk. They must choose a method of analgesia that allows optimal recovery of pulmonary parameters and specific respiratory techniques to ensure smooth recovery. The most common techniques in maintaining pulmonary function in the surgical patient probably include intermittent positive-pressure breathing (IPPB), chest physical therapy (CPT), and incentive spirometry (IS).

IPPB may be the most misused of these methods. Even though it has been shown to be very helpful in the intrabronchial delivery of medications (broncho-

---

EDITORIAL COMMENT

A variant of epidural analgesia is the continuance of epidural *anesthesia* postoperatively for pain control. Although this conductive anesthetic method is excellent, it poses particular problems for patients who have undergone operation in a modified lithotomy position. Sensory and motor function may be absent so that the usual symptoms of limb ischemia (pain, inability to extend or flex the feet) may be lacking. In this setting careful and continued examination of the lower extremities is mandatory until the anesthesia is discontinued.

dilators, mucolytics), IPPB is often inappropriately ordered solely for prevention of atelectasis.

A number of techniques fall under the description of CPT: postural drainage, percussion, vibration, and directed coughing.[61] CPT is most helpful in mucociliary clearance of excessive secretions and treatment of established lobar atelectasis. Postural drainage and coughing maneuvers seem to be the dominant components of CPT.

Although some controversy may exist over the benefit of IS in the prevention and treatment of atelectasis, it is relatively uncomplicated, well-received by surgeons, and employed extensively. Through sustained voluntary inspiration, alveolar collapse may be averted.

The least emphasized, and perhaps most important, ingredient in postoperative pulmonary care is informed, competent ancillary personnel to assist patients with early walking, frequent position change, and proper use of IPPB, CPT, and IS. Without therapists and other staff to apply these methods appropriately, they will rarely work.

REFERENCES

1. Brown DL, Kirby RR. Preoperative evaluation of high-risk elective surgical patients. In: Civetta JM, Taylor RW, Kirby RR, eds. Critical Care. Philadelphia: JB Lippincott, 1988, pp 137–144.
2. Goldman L. Cardiac risks and complications of noncardiac surgery. Ann Intern Med 1983; 98:504–513.
3. Shulman ST, Amren DP, Bisno AL, et al. Prevention of bacterial endocarditis. A statement for health professionals by the Committee on Rheumatic Fever and Infective Endocarditis of the Council on Cardiovascular Disease in the Young. Circulation 1984; 70:1123A–1127A.
4. Yeston NS, Niehoff JM, Dennis RC. Transfusion therapy. In: Civetta JM, Taylor RW, Kirby RR, eds. Critical Care. Philadelphia: JB Lippincott, 1988, pp 1481–1493.
5. Jeanneret-Grosjean AJ, Tse GN, Thompson WG. Villous adenoma with hyponatremia and syncope: Report of a case. Dis Colon Rectum 1978; 21:118–119.
6. Tannen RL. Potassium disorders. In: Kokko JP, Tannen RL, eds. Fluids and Electrolytes. 2nd ed. Philadelphia: WB Saunders, 1990, pp 195–300.
7. Spiegel RJ, Oliff AI, Bruton J, et al. Adrenal suppression after short-term corticosteroid therapy. Lancet 1979; 1:630–633.
8. Salassa RM, Bennett WA, Keating RF Jr, Sprague RG. Postoperative adrenal cortical insufficiency: Occurrence in patients previously treated with cortisone. JAMA 1953; 152:1509–1515.
9. Roizen MF. Anesthetic implications of concurrent diseases. In: Miller RD, ed. Anesthesia. 2nd ed. Vol 1. New York: Churchill Livingstone, 1986, pp 255–357.
10. Bergland RM, Gann DS, DeMaria EJ. Pituitary and adrenal. In: Schwartz SI, Shires GT, Spencer FC, eds. Principles of Surgery. 5th ed. New York: McGraw-Hill, 1989, pp 1545–1612.
11. Stelzner M, Phillips JD, Fonkalsrud EW. Acute ileus from steroid withdrawal simulating intestinal obstruction after surgery for ulcerative colitis. Arch Surg 1990; 125:914–917.
12. Albina JE, Koruda MJ, Rombeau JL. Perioperative total parenteral nutrition. In: Rombeau JL, Caldwell MD, eds. Clinical Nutrition. Vol 2. Parenteral Nutrition. Philadelphia: WB Saunders, 1986, pp 370–379.
13. Muller JM, Dienst C, Brenner U, Pichlmaier H. Preoperative parenteral feeding in patients with gastrointestinal carcinoma. Lancet 1982; 1:68–71.
14. MacLean LD. Host resistance in surgical patients. J Trauma 1979; 19:297–304.
15. McGuigan JE. Peptic ulcer. In: Braunwald E, Isselbacher KJ, Petersdorf RG, Wilson JD, Martin JB, Fauci AS, eds. Principles of Internal Medicine. 11th ed. New York: McGraw-Hill, 1987, pp 1239–1253.
16. Reines HD. Do we need stress ulcer prophylaxis? Crit Care Med 1990; 18:344.
17. Zuckerman GR, Shuman R. Therapeutic goals and treatment options for prevention of stress ulcer syndrome. Am J Med 1987; 83(6A):29–35.
18. Wille-Jorgensen P, Kjaergaard J, Jorgensen T, Larsen TK. Failure in prophylactic management of thromboembolic disease in colorectal surgery. Dis Colon Rectum 1988; 31:384–386.
19. Clagett GP, Reisch JS. Prevention of venous thromboembolism in general surgical patients. Ann Surg 1988; 208:227–240.
20. Kakkar VV, Stringer MD, Hedges AR, et al. Fixed combinations of low-molecular weight or unfractionated heparin plus dihydroergotamine in the prevention of postoperative deep vein thrombosis. Am J Surg 1989; 157:413–418.
21. Cohn I Jr. Intestinal antisepsis. Surg Gynecol Obstet 1970; 130:1006–1014.
22. Nichols RL, Broido P, Condon RE, et al. Effect of preoperative neomycin-erythromycin intestinal preparation on the incidence of infectious complications following colon surgery. Ann Surg 1973; 178:453–462.
23. Moore WEC, Holdeman LV. Human fecal flora: The normal flora of 20 Japanese-Hawaiians. Appl Microbiol 1974; 27:961–979.
24. Walker AP, Condon RE, Jones FE. Infections of the colon. In: Howard RJ, Simmons RL, eds. Surgical Infectious Diseases. 2nd ed. Norwalk, CT: Appleton & Lange, 1988, pp 713–755.
25. Fleites RA, Marshall JB, Eckhauser ML, et al. The efficacy of polyethylene glycol-electrolyte lavage solution versus traditional mechanical bowel preparation for elective colonic surgery: A randomized, prospective, blinded clinical trial. Surgery 1985; 98:708–716.
26. Wolff BG, Beart RW Jr, Dozois RR, et al. A new bowel preparation for elective colon and rectal surgery: A prospective, randomized clinical trial. Arch Surg 1988; 123:895–900.
27. Davis GR, Santa Ana CA, Morawski SG, Fordtran JS. Development of a lavage solution associated with minimal water and electrolyte absorption or secretion. Gastroenterology 1980; 78:991–995.
28. Beck DE, Fazio VW. Current preoperative bowel cleansing methods: Results of a survey. Dis Colon Rectum 1990; 33:12–15.
29. Saadia R, Schein M. The place of intraoperative antegrade colonic irrigation in emergency left-sided colonic surgery. Dis Colon Rectum 1989; 32:78–81.
30. Evans M, Pollock AV. The inadequacy of published random control trials of antibacterial prophylaxis in colorectal surgery. Dis Colon Rectum 1987; 30:743–746.
31. Prager E, Swinton NW, Corman ML, Veidenheimer MC. Intravenous pyelography in colorectal surgery. Dis Colon Rectum 1973; 16:479–481.
32. Tartter PI, Steinberg BM. The role of intravenous pyelogram in operations performed for carcinoma of the colon and rectum. Surg Gynecol Obstet 1986; 163:65–69.
33. Davis JE. Major ambulatory surgery of the general surgery patient: Management of anorectal conditions, peripheral vascular problems, and gastrointestinal endoscopy. Surg Clin North Am 1987; 67:761–790.
34. Nahrwold DL. Chronic cholecystitis and cholelithiasis. In: Sabiston DC Jr, ed. Textbook of Surgery: The Biologic Basis of Modern Surgical Practice. 13th ed. Philadelphia: WB Saunders, 1986, pp 1147–1153.
35. Lobbato VJ, Rothenberg RE, LaRaja RD, Georgiou J. Coexistence of abdominal aortic aneurysm and carcinoma of the colon: A dilemma. J Vasc Surg 1985; 2:724–726.
36. Thomas JH. Abdominal aortic aneurysmorrhaphy combined with biliary or gastrointestinal surgery. Surg Clin North Am 1989; 69:807–815.

37. Szilagyi DE, Elliot JP, Berguer R. Coincidental malignancy and abdominal aortic aneurysm: Problems of management. Arch Surg 1967; 95:402–412.
38. Sugarbaker PH. Carcinoma of the colon—prognosis and operative choice. Curr Prob Surg 1981; 18:753–802.
39. Foster JH, Lundy J. Liver metastases. Curr Prob Surg 1981; 18:157–202.
40. Cronin K, Jackson DS, Dunphy JE. Specific activity of hydroxyproline-tritium in the healing colon. Surg Gynecol Obstet 1968; 126:1061–1065.
41. Houston KA, McRitchie DI, Rotstein OD. Tissue plasminogen activator reverses the deleterious effect of infection on colonic wound healing. Ann Surg 1990; 211:130–135.
42. Hinchey EJ, Schaal PGH, Richards GK. Treatment of perforated diverticular disease of the colon. Adv Surg 1978; 12:85–109.
43. Madden JL. Primary resection in the treatment of acute perforations of the colon with abscess or diffuse peritonitis. In: Delaney JP, Varco RL, eds. Controversies in Surgery II. Philadelphia: WB Saunders, 1983, pp 349–354.
44. Stone HH, Fabian TC. Management of perforating colon trauma: Randomization between primary closure and exteriorization. Ann Surg 1979; 190:430–436.
45. Keane PF, Ohri SK, Wood CB, Sackier JM. Management of the obstructed left colon by the one-stage intracolonic bypass procedure. Dis Colon Rectum 1988; 31:948–951.
46. Alexander JW. Surgical infections and choice of antibiotics. In: Sabiston DC Jr, ed. Textbook of Surgery: The Biologic Basis of Modern Surgical Practice. 13th ed. Philadelphia: WB Saunders, 1986, pp 259–283.
47. Goligher J. Surgery of the anus, rectum, and colon. 5th ed. London: Bailliére Tindall, 1984.
48. Hoffman J, Shokouh-Amiri MH, Damm P, Jensen R. A prospective, controlled study of prophylactic drainage after colonic anastomoses. Dis Colon Rectum 1987; 30:449–452.
49. Khoury GA, Waxman BP. Large bowel anastomoses. I. The healing process and sutured anastomoses: A review. Br J Surg 1983; 70:61–63.
50. Burg R, Geigle CF, Faso JM, Theuerkauf FJ Jr. Omission of routine gastric decompression. Dis Colon Rectum 1978; 21:98–100.
51. Bauer JJ, Gelernt IM, Salky BA, Kreel I. Is routine postoperative nasogastgric decompression really necessary? Ann Surg 1985; 201:233–236.
52. Cheadle WG, Vitale GC, Mackie CR, Cuschieri A. Prophylactic postoperative nasogastric decompression: A prospective study of its requirement and the influence of cimetidine in 200 patients. Ann Surg 1985; 202:361–366.
53. Wolff BG, Pemberton JH, van Heerden JA, et al. Elective colon and rectal surgery without nasogastric decompression: A prospective, randomized trial. Ann Surg 1989; 209:670–675.
54. Balz J, Samson RB, Stewart WRC. Rectal-tube decompression in left colectomy. Dis Colon Rectum 1978; 21:94–97.
55. Pinder RM, Brogden RN, Sawyer PR, Speight TM, Avery GS. Metoclopramide: A review of its pharmacologic properties and clinical use. Drugs 1976; 12:81–131.
56. McCallum RW, Prakash C, Campoli-Richards DM, Goa KL. Cisapride: A preliminary review of its pharmacodynamic and pharmacokinetic properties, and therapeutic use as a prokinetic agent in gastrointestinal motility disorders. Drugs 1988; 36:652–681.
57. Veselis RA. Intravenous narcotics in the I.C.U. Crit Care Clin 1990; 6:295–313.
58. Crews JC. Epidural opioid analgesia. Crit Care Clin 1990; 6:315–342.
59. Buckley MM-T, Brogden RN. Ketorolac: A review of its pharmacodynamic and pharmacokinetic properties, and therapeutic potential. Drugs 1990; 39:86–109.
60. Pontoppidan H. Mechanical aids to lung expansion in nonintubated surgical patients. Am Rev Respir Dis 1980; 122:109–119.
61. Kirilloff LH, Owens GR, Rogers RM, Mazzocco MC. Does chest physical therapy work? Chest 1985; 88:436–444.

Anesthesia for Colorectal Operations

CHAPTER 7

William C. Wilson
Harvey M. Shapiro

Anesthetic considerations for colorectal operations are numerous, and procedures on the colon, rectum, and anus constitute a large fraction of those performed by the general surgeon. Despite this fact, few reports have focused on this subject.[1]

High-quality anesthetic care for patients undergoing colorectal operations depends on clear communication between the surgeon and anesthesiologist. Detailed surgical issues are covered elsewhere in this text. This chapter elucidates the main issues pertinent to anesthetic care in a format relevant to surgeons.

Anesthetic considerations begin with preoperative evaluation (including history, physical examination, and analysis of laboratory data) and risk assessment. Preoperative preparation is conceptually different from evaluation; however, the two may proceed concomitantly in acute situations, and preparation is dictated by the patient's physical status, the resuscitative requirements, and the operation planned. Monitoring needs vary with patient condition and operative procedure. The choice of anesthetic technique is based on the preceding considerations and can include general, regional, or local infiltration anesthesia in various situations. Positioning is an important factor in all operations, and especially so in colorectal procedures. The aforementioned factors all impinge on the likelihood of intraoperative and postoperative complications. Postoperative analgesia following colorectal procedures has developed to the point of providing a number of effective methods for alleviating pain.

Pediatric patients have several unique anesthetic requirements, and these issues are discussed with emphasis on colorectal operations. Additionally, unique anesthetic implications for certain special elective colorectal procedures are described.

PREOPERATIVE EVALUATION

Anesthesiologists conduct the preoperative evaluation of patients undergoing colorectal procedures in order to assess their overall readiness for surgery, paying particular attention to volume status and significant cardiovascular, pulmonary, and other medical conditions. The increasing trend toward ambulatory evaluation and preparation of surgical patients places additional burdens of communication and planning upon the surgical-anesthesia team to ensure smooth patient flow and efficient resource utilization. It is essential that adequate patient information (i.e., chart with pertinent consultation notes and preoperative workup) be available in a timely fashion and that additional data and changes in patient status are effectively transmitted to all participating medical teams. Although a complete physical examination is required for the most severely ill patients, the following systems approach is most relevant to anesthesia for colorectal procedures.

Airway Assessment

Preoperative evaluation for colorectal surgical procedures, as for all operations, begins with assessment of the airway. Physical characteristics that impair direct laryngoscopy are listed in Table 7–1 and include obesity (>110 kg), "buck teeth," large tongue, decreased jaw movement, decreased head and neck movement, and receding mandible (in the fully extended adult neck, if the distance between the mandible and the upper border of thyroid cartilage is <6.5 cm, visualization of the vocal cords is predictably difficult).

Table 7–1. PREDICTORS OF DIFFICULT INTUBATION

Obesity (>110 kg)
Buck teeth
Small mouth
Large tongue
Decreased jaw movement
Decreased head extension or neck flexion
Receding mandible or anterior larynx

Intravascular Volume Assessment

Fluid balance abnormalities are frequently encountered in patients awaiting colorectal surgery, the typical situation being depletion of intravascular volume. Fluid loss can occur by means of a number of mechanisms. Fasting and vigorous bowel preparation can deplete intravascular volume, whereas bowel obstruction, necrosis, or abscess can sequester fluids into the bowel lumen, bowel wall, adjacent soft tissues, and peritoneum. Additionally, patients may have significant extrinsic losses from fistulas, nasogastric tubes, or episodes of emesis or diarrhea. One begins assessment of intravascular volume with the clinical evaluation of mental status, skin color, warmth, turgor, capillary refill, jugular venous pulse height, blood pressure, heart rate, and postural effects, as well as with an assessment of urine output. If the volume status remains unclear, then central venous or pulmonary artery catheters should be employed preoperatively. Although a complete review of blood volume and fluid requirements is beyond the scope of this text, Tables 7–2 and 7–3 provide estimates of circulating blood volume, maintenance fluid requirements, and insensible losses due to fever. Requirements for third-spacing losses and blood losses are additions to these baseline requirements.

Cardiovascular Assessment

In the preoperative evaluation, it is essential to detect any limitation in cardiovascular reserves. Critical information includes exercise tolerance and history and timing of previous myocardial infarction, congestive heart failure, arrhythmia, angina, or hypertension. Cardiac medications are noted. A recent electrocardiogram (ECG) is mandatory for all patients with a known history of coronary artery disease, arrhythmia, or hypertension. The ECG is unnecessary for elective surgery in patients who are asymptomatic, have no significant risk factors for coronary artery disease (CAD), and are under age 45 years (men) or 55 years (women).[2] Patients with evidence of CAD (by history

Table 7–2. ESTIMATING CIRCULATING BLOOD VOLUME AND FLUID REQUIREMENTS

Estimating circulating blood volume
    Adult 7% body weight: i.e., 70 ml/kg (5 liters in 70-kg adult)
    Child 8% body weight
    Newborn 9–10% body weight

Maintenance fluid requirements
    4 ml $\cdot$ kg^{-1} $\cdot$ hr^{-1} for the first 10 kg
    2 ml $\cdot$ kg^{-1} $\cdot$ hr^{-1} for the second 10 kg
    1 ml $\cdot$ kg^{-1} $\cdot$ hr^{-1} for subsequent kg

Insensible fluid loss
    Fever 10 ml $\cdot$ kg^{-1} $\cdot$ day^{-1} 1°C temperature rise
    0.5 ml $\cdot$ kg^{-1} $\cdot$ hr^{-1} 1°C temperature rise

or physical examination) or patients with risk factors and an ECG consistent with ischemia should have an exercise (treadmill) thallium test. Those unable to exercise should receive a thallium dipyridamole (Persantine) scan and receive an evaluation by a cardiologist to determine the need for additional diagnostic tests (i.e., cardiac catheterization or echocardiogram). Cardiac catheterization is generally reserved for patients with reversible defects identified on a thallium dipyridamole scan. An echocardiogram is helpful in evaluating patients with valvular heart disease and as an assessment of left ventricular function (i.e., ejection fraction), chamber size, and wall motion.

Pulmonary Assessment

A significant history of pulmonary disease should be sought, with focus on tobacco use, reactive airway disease, and emphysema. Patients requiring bronchodilators should be encouraged to use their nebulizers the night before and immediately prior to surgery. A recent chest film is mandatory for the patient with known active lung disease (acute respiratory distress syndrome, pneumonia, pleural effusions, or prolonged mechanical ventilation for any reason). However, in the asymptomatic patient under 60 years of age who is being considered for elective colorectal surgery, the

Table 7–3. CLINICAL ASSESSMENT OF FLUID STATUS

Mental status
Skin color, warmth, and turgor
Capillary refill
Mucosa and auxiliary moisture
Jugular venous pressure
Vital signs (and postural effects)
Urine output
Fontanelles (in pediatrics)

risks of radiation exposure from chest radiography probably exceed the benefits.[3]

Preoperative pulmonary function testing has been shown to improve outcome prediction measurably in lung resection candidates. Preoperative forced expiratory volume in 1 second that is less than 1,000 ml is a high-risk indicator. However, in contrast, pulmonary function tests in healthy patients are seldom helpful, and in patients with pulmonary disease who are undergoing a noncardiothoracic operation, are not predictive. Similarly, preoperative arterial blood tests are not indicated in otherwise healthy patients undergoing colorectal surgical procedures. Yet baseline arterial blood gas measurements are helpful for patients with chronic lung disease.

Other Organ System Evaluation

Evidence of renal or hepatic dysfunction is sought, as anesthetic drug clearance, metabolism, and intravascular fluid status may be affected by the presence of severe renal or hepatic insufficiency. Currently available anesthetics and anesthetic adjuvants offer choices of preferential metabolic degradation pathways, and thus they can be matched appropriately to individual patient needs.

Central nervous system disorders are not particularly relevant to the colorectal evaluation. Deficits in mental acuity and gross central nervous system lesions are generally discovered during the basic history and physical examination; however, patients with histories of central nervous system injury or disease require a more focused and rigorous examination.

Potential vascular access and sites for establishing regional anesthesia are also evaluated preoperatively.

Evaluation of Preoperative Laboratory Data

Other than a baseline hematocrit, no specific laboratory tests are considered routine for colorectal procedures. Guidelines for rational use of electrocardiography, chest radiography, pulmonary function tests, and arterial blood gas evaluations are offered in previous discussions under Cardiovascular Assessment and Pulmonary Assessment. All additional laboratory testing decisions should be based on the specific procedure planned and the findings discovered during the history and physical examination.

Hematocrit

Although it is difficult to justify proceeding with a major colorectal operation in a patient with an unex-plained anemia (hematocrit <30), there is no rigid cutoff, especially in the chronically stable anemic patient. Christopherson et al[4] demonstrated a significantly increased risk of cardiac ischemia on postoperative Day 2 in high-risk patients who had postoperative hematocrit values of less than 29 (55%) compared with those who had hematocrit values greater than 29 (16%). However, patients with hematocrit values below 30 occurring relatively acutely should probably be transfused preoperatively when major blood loss is anticipated. The level to which one allows the hematocrit to drop during a procedure is most accurately decided by monitoring the mixed venous saturation and base deficit. The starting hematocrit level should be known for all elective surgeries.

Platelets

Platelet count and bleeding time should be sought preoperatively only (1) if indicated by the history or physical examination (chemotherapy, renal failure, aspirin or nonsteroidal anti-inflammatory drug use, bleeding gums, nosebleeds, bruising easily); (2) if the procedure is likely to involve platelet destruction (use of cell saver); or (3) if great blood loss is likely (major re-operations). They should also be sought when regional anesthesia is planned.

Coagulation Studies

As with platelets, coagulation studies (prothrombin time, partial thromboplastin time) are indicated only if the history or physical examination suggests need (i.e., one should check the prothrombin time if the patient is receiving sodium warfarin (Coumadin) or has known liver disease, and the partial thromboplastin time if the patient has received heparin).

Electrolytes, Blood Urea Nitrogen, Creatinine, and Glucose

Electrolytes, blood urea nitrogen, creatinine, and glucose determinations are helpful only when the history or physical examination reveals risk factors. Examples of risk factors include use of diuretics (K^+), diabetes (lytes, glucose), renal insufficiency, and suspected intravascular volume deficit (blood urea nitrogen and creatinine). Unexpected abnormalities in sequential multiple analysis–12 occur in only 2.5% of patients under 40 years old and in 7.5% of patients more than 60 years old (70% of the unexpected findings are in blood urea nitrogen and creatinine, or glucose). However, patients with advanced colorectal cancers may have significant electrolyte and nutritional imbalances.

Liver Function Tests

Liver function tests are useful in evaluating hepatic involvement of colorectal cancers, and the presence of jaundice or a history of heavy alcohol use is an indication for testing. In contrast, only 1 in 750 otherwise healthy patients will demonstrate an unexpected abnormal liver function test, and only 1 in 3 of these will subsequently become jaundiced.

Assessment of Risk

No large-scale studies of anesthetic morbidity and mortality for colorectal procedures have been conducted, and the hazards of anesthesia are frequently difficult to distinguish from those due to surgery. The risk of death attributed solely to an anesthetic varies from between 1 in 10,000 and 1 in 20,000 anesthetics.[5]

In an attempt to quantify the risk of cardiac arrest during anesthesia, Keenan and Boyan presented statistics for the 15-year epoch prior to 1985 at the Medical College of Virginia.[6] Cardiac arrest solely due to anesthesia occurred 1.7 times per 10,000 anesthetic administrations; 50% of the patients died. Inability or failure to ventilate was responsible for one half of the cardiac arrests. One third of these cardiac arrests resulted from an absolute overdose of inhalational anesthetic. Pediatric patients were three times more likely than adults to have cardiac arrests.

We cannot, with certainty, assign a numeric anesthetic risk for any given patient. However, as part of the preoperative evaluation, the anesthesiologist assigns a standardized American Society of Anesthesiology (ASA) physical status score for each patient (Table 7–4).

Although this score does correlate with overall perioperative mortality and morbidity, it was never intended to define operative risk (as it does not consider hazards inherent in specific surgical procedures or operator skill), but rather to define preoperative physical status.

After the ASA physical status is determined, preoperative preparation, intraoperative monitoring needs, and anesthetic technique are planned.

PREOPERATIVE PREPARATION

The goal of preoperative preparation is to deliver the patient to the operating room in optimal medical condition. "Optimal" remains a relative term that should be defined within the context of what is feasible for a particular patient and the urgency of the planned surgical procedure. Therefore, the preoperative anesthetic evaluation may lead to additional laboratory studies or even a request for consultation regarding medical conditions not previously recognized or apparently not under adequate control. When conflict emerges between the need for optimal medical preparation and urgency, a coordinated anesthesia-surgical decision is required. For instance, the risk of perioperative myocardial ischemia and/or infarction is increased when procedures are performed emergently in older patients. This finding probably reflects the seriousness of the problem as well as the lack of time to optimize potentially complex medical conditions.

Bowel Preparation

Bowel preparation protocols can result in dehydration, and the anesthesiologist may suggest intravenous (IV) hydration prior to the patient's arrival in the operating room. Induction of anesthesia is often associated with reduction in cardiac function and/or sympathetic nervous system tone, and a resultant fall in arterial pressure is exacerbated by intravascular depletion. Not infrequently, patients undergoing major colorectal surgical procedures are emaciated, anemic, and hypoalbuminemic, and have fluid and electrolyte abnormalities, all of which further complicate the preoperative preparation.

Fasting

Gastric emptying prior to surgery for nonabdominal procedures is typically normal.[7] However, trauma,

Table 7–4. AMERICAN SOCIETY OF ANESTHESIOLOGISTS (ASA) PHYSICAL STATUS CLASSIFICATION

ASA-1	No organic, physiologic, biochemical, or psychiatric disturbance
ASA-2	Mild to moderate systemic disease (Mild DM, controlled HTN, extremes of age, morbid obesity, anemia)
ASA-3	Severe systemic disease that limits activity (Stable CRF, poorly controlled HTN, DM with vascular complications, exercise-limited COPD, angina, history of prior MI)
ASA-4	Severe systemic disease that constantly threatens life (Persistent angina; CHF; rapidly advancing renal, pulmonary, or liver failure)
ASA-5	Moribund patient not expected to live longer than 24 hr (Ruptured AAA, cerebral trauma with increased ICP)

DM = diabetes mellitus; HTN = hypertension; CRF = chronic renal failure; COPD = chronic obstructive pulmonary disease; MI = myocardial infarction; CHF = congestive heart failure; AAA = abdominal aortic aneurysm; ICP = intracranial pressure.

apprehension, narcotics, and gastrointestinal disorders are associated with an increased volume of gastric contents.[3] Pain, trauma, burns, and apprehension decrease the gastric pH,[8] further increasing the risk that passive regurgitation would progress to aspiration syndrome. Therefore, all acute abdomen or trauma patients are considered to have full stomachs, and a rapid-sequence induction with endotracheal intubation to protect the airway is indicated. Elective surgical operations have less risk of aspiration; however, the correct time for preoperative fasting has yet to be established. In 1826 Beaumont observed that gastric fluids empty rapidly (within 1 hour), whereas solids require longer periods to empty.[9] There is growing evidence that small amounts of clear liquids may enhance gastric emptying. Indeed, patients given 150 ml of water $2\frac{1}{2}$ hours preoperatively have significantly lower gastric volumes than patients who have fasted.[10] Additionally, gastric pH increases significantly higher than with placebo following the administration of ranitidine, 150 mg $2\frac{1}{2}$ hours preoperatively (pH >5 versus <2).[10] Thus, our present state of knowledge indicates that an 8-hour fast for solid food is indicated, whereas clear liquids up to a volume of 250 ml are safely taken as late as $2\frac{1}{2}$ hours preoperatively. Ranitidine 150 mg (or another H_2 blocker) is indicated for patients deemed at increased risk of regurgitation and aspiration.

Preoperative Medication

There is no single recipe for preoperative medication, and an adequate preoperative explanation often obviates or reduces the need for preoperative anxiolytic medications. The goal in preoperative medication is to diminish the anxiety and stress of the operative experience (e.g., with sedatives and analgesics), and maximize safety of the procedure (e.g., with H_2 blockers, reducing gastric volume and acidity).

Premedication protocols may also be directed at modifying autonomic nervous system influences. For instance, premedicant sympatholysis can be designed to attenuate perioperative hypertension and tachycardia in patients with coronary artery disease as well as reduce the subsequent dose of potent inhalational anesthetics. Adverse effects of premedication may include opiate-induced decreased gastric emptying and nausea in some patients. Most importantly, excessive sedative-analgesic premedication in frail and/or nonmonitored patients can lead to a cardiopulmonary arrest.

Bronchodilators, such as albuterol, are indicated for patients with a history of reactive airway disease. Albuterol delivery via a metered-dose inhaler should be administered the night before as well as on the morning of the operation.

Anticholinergics such as atropine and glycopyrrolate as routine premedications are now relegated solely to pediatric patients, because most modern anesthetics, other than ketamine, do not increase salivation, and, moreover, anticholinergics decrease gastric emptying. Patients with increased risk of regurgitation (those with obesity, pregnancy, diabetes, history of a hiatal hernia, or gastric reflux) generally receive metoclopramide (to increase gastric emptying and decrease nausea) as well as either an H_2 blocker (to decrease gastric acidity and volume) or a nonparticulate antacid, such as sodium citrate rather than a particulate antacid, which increases pulmonary inflammation if aspirated.

Sedatives

Benzodiazepines are the sedative-anxiolytics most often used in today's practice because of their wide margin of safety compared with barbiturates or narcotics. Also, benzodiazepines rarely cause allergic reactions and are safely reversible, even in patients with coronary artery disease, by the specific benzodiazepine antagonist flumazenil.[11] Benzodiazepines have excellent amnestic properties and produce mild skeletal muscle relaxation. Benzodiazepines exert their antianxiety and skeletal muscle relaxing effects by increasing the availability of the inhibitory neurotransmitter glycine. Their sedative effects result from the facilitation of the inhibitory neurotransmitter γ-aminobutyric acid (GABA). Diazepam is the standard with which most benzodiazepines are compared. However, some of the newer benzodiazepines have significant clinical advantages over diazepam.

Midazolam has several advantages over diazepam. Water solubility, immediate onset with rapid metabolism, and elimination all contribute to a speedy recovery after the operation. Midazolam can be given orally (0.1 to 0.5 mg/kg), injected intramuscularly (0.1 to 0.5 mg/kg), or given intravenously (0.05 to 0.1 mg/kg).[12] Flumazenil, the specific benzodiazepine antagonist, administered in a dose of 0.1 mg/kg will reverse benzodiazepine-induced respiratory depression, yet it has relatively few respiratory or cardiovascular effects when given alone.[13]

Analgesics

Opioid agonists are the best-known and most potent analgesics available. Opioids act at specific receptor sites throughout the central nervous system. There are many opioid receptor subtypes: the μ_1-receptors are responsible for supraspinal analgesia; μ_2-receptors depress ventilation, decrease heart rate, and produce euphoria; and κ-receptors are responsible for analgesia (particularly in the spinal cord) and sedation. Morphine given intramuscularly has been the most popularly applied preoperative analgesic. Narcotics allow for a reduction of the total dose of inhalational anesthetic required to maintain anesthesia, and they serve to minimize hemodynamic fluctuations associated with variations in surgical stimuli.

Small doses of fentanyl or sufentanil IV given just prior to induction of general anesthesia have become popular, as they permit immediate observation and titration for narcotic effects and avoid the possibility of unobserved respiratory depression following opioid administration outside the surgical suite.

Antibiotics

When blood culture results are known, specific drug therapy can be instituted; however, presumptive therapy is often employed. The most common organisms encountered in colorectal surgery are *Escherichia coli*, enterococci, and the anaerobes *Bacteroides fragilis* and *Clostridium* spp. If biliary sepsis is involved, *Klebsiella*, *Pseudomonas*, and *Proteus* should be covered as well.[14] In most cases ampicillin, gentamicin, and metronidazole (or clindamycin), given preoperatively or at the induction of anesthesia, provide suitable coverage of the probable pathogens until culture results are available.

Several types of antibiotics enhance the neuromuscular blockade produced by nondepolarizing neuromuscular blocking drugs; chief among these are the aminoglycosides. The reversal of antibiotic-exacerbated neuromuscular blockade is unpredictable, and thus caution should be employed in assessing extubation parameters for patients in this category. The penicillins and cephalosporins are devoid of neuromuscular blocking effects.

MONITORING

There are no monitoring techniques specifically required for routine colorectal surgery because continuous pulse oximetry, noninvasive blood pressure monitoring, end-tidal CO_2 (PET_{CO_2}), ECG, and peak inspiratory pressure (PIP) monitoring are all considered standard care. The decision to use additional, often invasive, monitoring is based on the severity of the patient's medical condition and the extensiveness of the operation.

PATIENT POSITIONING

Clear cooperative preoperative planning for positioning requirements in colorectal surgery greatly promotes trouble-free anesthetic preparation and the subsequent positioning sequence. In certain instances the anesthesiologist may suggest exploration of alternative positions because of nuances in individual patients. If the following guidelines for patient positioning are observed, complications can be minimized.

Supine

The supine position is used primarily for abdominal approaches to the colon and upper rectum. The supine position is considered by some to be a natural position; however, several complications can occur. For example, when the arms are extended in the spread-eagle or crucifix position, traction can be placed on the brachial plexus, especially if the arms are brought cephalad greater than 90 degrees relative to the spinal axis. Furthermore, pressure necrosis can occur at bony contact points including the occiput, elbows, sacrum, and heels; thus, these areas should be padded. Additionally, hemodynamic compromise can be provoked by the placement of deep abdominal packs and retraction against the major vessels. Finally, postoperative leg and back pain occurs frequently after prolonged procedures in the supine position, owing to stretch upon the nerves and tendons on the flexor side of the extremity. Thus, when possible, a contoured supine or "lawn chair" position (Fig. 7-1) is used in order to relieve the tension on these flexor tendons and muscles.[15]

Lithotomy

The basic lithotomy position (Fig. 7-2) is frequently chosen in anorectal procedures such as anoscopy, colonoscopy, incision and drainage of perirectal abscess, lateral internal sphincterotomy, and hemorrhoidectomy. Nivatvongs et al have categorized buttock shape as a guide for selecting patient positioning for anorectal surgery.[16]

Typically the patient is anesthetized first, by a regional technique or by general anesthesia. Alternatively the patient may be positioned first, and then a local infiltrative anesthetic technique may be employed. In either case, the legs should be wrapped or a sequential calf-squeezing apparatus should be used to prevent venous stasis injury. In the anesthetized patient, it is essential that a particular positioning sequence be followed in order to minimize the chance of injury, especially hip dislocation. The legs are elevated and flexed in the midline simultaneously initially without abduction or rotation of the thighs. Next the legs are simultaneously and gently placed within the stirrups with moderate external rotation and abduction.

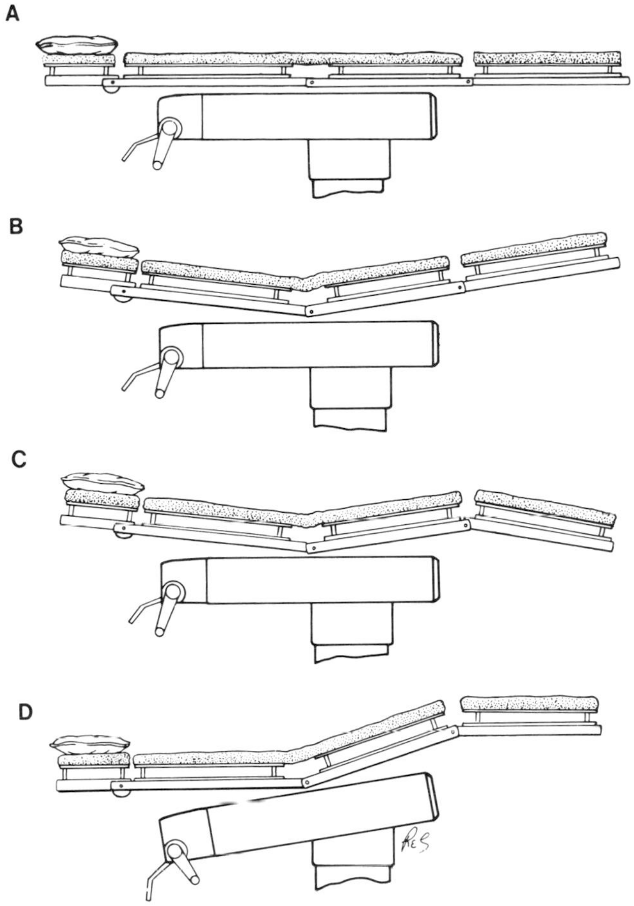

A

B

C

D

Figure 7–1. Establishment of the lawn chair (contoured supine) position: A, flat table top; B, forward flexion at the hips; C, flexion at the knees; D, trunk section leveled to allow attachment of floor standing arm board when desired. (From Martin JT. Positioning in Anesthesia and Surgery. Philadelphia: WB Saunders, 1987.)

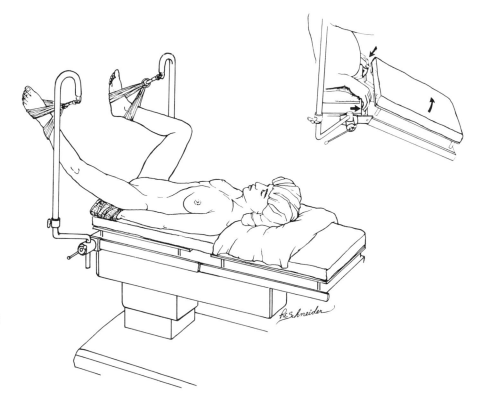

Figure 7–2. Basic lithotomy position. Note that the legs are flexed, abducted, and externally rotated to minimize joint stress. The hands can be gently wrapped to protect them from a pinching or shearing type injury as the leg portion of the table is elevated to the level position. The padding between the support bar and the leg, as well as the leg wrappings, are not shown for the sake of clarity. (From Martin JT. Positioning in Anesthesia and Surgery. Philadelphia: WB Saunders, 1987.)

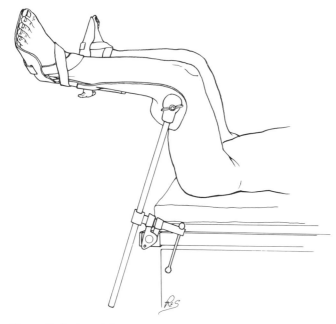

Figure 7–3. Basic lithotomy position using supportive leg/foot brace. The sacral pad and padding between the supportive braces and the leg/foot, as well as the leg wrappings, are not shown for the sake of clarity. (From Martin JT. Positioning in Anesthesia and Surgery. Philadelphia, WB Saunders, 1987.)

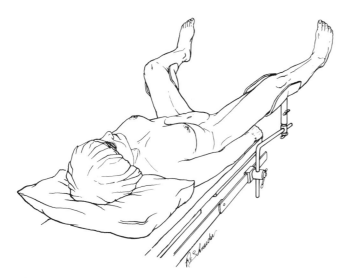

Figure 7–4. Modified lithotomy for abdominal perineal resection (APR). Note that the legs are flexed at the thighs, abducted, and externally rotated; however, the leg elevation is less than in the standard lithotomy position. A mild degree of Trendelenburg tilt is often added. Padding between the support brace at the knee, as well as the leg wrappings, are not shown for the sake of clarity. (From Martin JT. Positioning in Anesthesia and Surgery. Philadelphia: WB Saunders, 1987.)

A pad should be placed between each leg and the corresponding vertical stirrup support bar diminishing the chance of a peroneal nerve injury. Frequently, the surgeon places a sacral pad under the patient, which protects against decubitus injuries and improves surgical exposure of the perineum.

The same sequence but in reverse is followed at the end of the procedure. Care should be taken to protect the fingers from a pinching or a shearing injury that can result when the leg portion of the operating table is returned to the level position at the end of the procedure (see inset, Figure 7–2). Sudden lowering of the legs in a hypovolemic patient after a long procedure can lead to profound hypotension. The hypotension results from decreased cardiac output secondary to venous blood pooling in the newly dependent extremities and the consequent decrement in cardiac filling (preload). The blood pressure and heart rate should be closely monitored as the legs are lowered slowly and together. For longer procedures it is probably preferable to use the more supportive leg brace with foot support shown in Figure 7–3. This relieves pressure on the knee joint; however, it necessitates the placement of protective padding over the ankle and common peroneal nerve (lateral aspect of the knee).

A modified lithotomy position (Fig. 7–4) is frequently employed for abdominal perineal procedures and for ileoanal anastomosis operations. The legs are elevated somewhat less than in the basic lithotomy position. Next, the legs are externally rotated and abducted. The amount of hip flexion is typically greater than in the standard lithotomy position (usually exceeding 90 degrees). Complications of the lithotomy position are shown in Table 7–5.

Prone Jackknife

The prone jackknife position (Fig. 7–5) is usually relegated to anorectal surgery such as anoscopy, fulguration of anal warts, hemorrhoidectomy, and incision and drainage of perirectal abscess. The prone jackknife position has the advantage of allowing patients to position themselves before the beginning of a hypobaric spinal, a caudal epidural, or a local infiltrative (field-block) anesthetic. If general anesthesia is selected, several assistants should be called upon to help position the patient after induction.

The patient is placed prone on the operating room table with the legs extended. A pillow is placed beneath the head, the pelvis, and the ankles. The arms are alongside the head, and the head is turned to one side. The operating room table is reverse-flexed 30 to 40 degrees, forming a reversed V with its apex at the hip joint. The more severe jackknife position (>40-degree reversed V angulation) can introduce hemodynamic

Table 7–5. POSITIONING COMPLICATIONS

Supine position
    Pressure injury to bony prominences
    Stretch injury to flexor tendons and muscles
    Nerve injury, especially brachial plexus

Lithotomy position
    Venous stasis
    Nerve injuries
        Obturator
        Saphenous
        Femoral
        Common peroneal
    Joint damage
        Hip dislocation and knee strain or sprain
    Compartment syndrome

Prone jackknife position
    Ocular and facial nerve injuries in the generally
        anesthetized patient
    Cervical spine and neck muscle spasm
    Scrotal or penile compressive injuries in men
    Breast pain in women

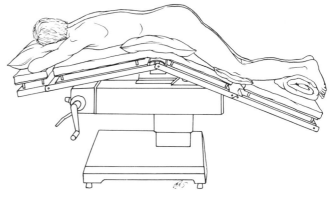

Figure 7–5. Prone jackknife position. The angulation of the reverse V is not severe in this drawing, and can be made more severe as operative exposure requires and table design allows. Gluteal tapes are not shown for the sake of clarity. (From Martin JT. Positioning in Anesthesia and Surgery. Philadelphia: WB Saunders, 1987.)

instability in the frail or obese patient. Once the proper position and anesthetic level are confirmed, gluteal tapes are applied to expose the perianal region. Complications of the prone position are listed in Table 7–5.

CHOICE OF ANESTHETIC TECHNIQUE

During anesthesia for colorectal procedures, our goal, as with all anesthesia, is to ensure the patient's safety and comfort while providing the surgeon with ideal operating conditions. The anesthesiologist selects the anesthetic technique based on the urgency to operate; the region of the colon, rectum, or anus to be operated on; the patient's position; the expected operating time; the extent of the proposed operation; the patient's general condition; the need for postoperative analgesia; the anesthesiologist's personal experience; and the patient's preference.

In emergent colorectal operations and/or in the presence of hypovolemia (e.g., gunshot wound to the abdomen with fecal contamination in a hypotensive patient), general anesthesia with a rapid-sequence induction is indicated. A rapid-sequence induction requires preoxygenation of the lungs; an assistant applies cricoid pressure to protect the airway, and a rapid-acting induction agent and a muscle relaxant are given in sequence. The patient is intubated with a styleted endotracheal tube, without ventilation by mask.

The region of the colon, rectum, or anus operated on is an important factor to consider in selecting an anesthetic technique for elective procedures. General or regional anesthesia can be used for all colorectal procedures; however, local anesthesia and field blocks are appropriate only for well-localized procedures such as anal sphincterotomy or fulguration of anal warts. In the case of regional anesthesia, upper abdominal incisions require a T4 to T2 level. Aitkenhead has been the chief proponent of regional anesthesia for operations on the colon since he demonstrated a significant increase in colonic blood flow following subarachnoid block in the dog.[17] He argues that colonic anastomotic breakdowns occur more frequently when the colonic blood flow is diminished. Regional blood flow with isoflurane and halothane has also been investigated.[18] The splanchnic blood flow is decreased with halothane, whereas it is increased or stable with isoflurane in the range of 1 to 2 minimum alveolar concentration (i.e., MAC). Anastomotic construction may be easier with greater bowel tone, as occurs with high regional anesthesia, and regional anesthesia obviates the potentially harmful use of neostigmine (see discussion under Muscle Relaxants further on). The only outcome data supporting this thesis emanate from a retrospective study in which anastomotic dehiscence was found to occur in 7.4% of patients receiving high spinal anesthesia compared with 23% of patients receiving general anesthesia.[19]

The time and extent of the operation are also major factors in selecting an anesthetic technique. Single-shot spinal anesthesia typically provides operative anesthesia from 1½ (xylocaine) to 3 (bupivacaine) hours. After 3 to 4 hours, even the most cooperative patient becomes restless and uncomfortable. The required level of sedation can often hover on the edge of general anesthesia, which then can deteriorate into loss of the airway and/or aspiration. After major colorectal operations, the fluid shifts and physiologic trespass often lead to increased work in breathing, requiring prolonged mechanical ventilation. When this outcome is anticipated, general anesthesia is indicated. Patients anticipated to have difficult airways, who are undergoing major procedures, should be intubated electively at the start of general anesthesia rather than emergently sometime later during the operation after a regional technique has been abandoned. Patients with full stomachs should receive general anesthesia with a rapid-sequence induction.

The need for postoperative analgesia can encourage the placement of an epidural catheter preoperatively. This catheter can then be used as the sole anesthetic technique, combined with general anesthesia, or used only for postoperative analgesia. "Single-shot" caudal epidural anesthesia in combination with general anesthesia can provide significant postoperative analgesia for 18 to 24 hours when given for perineal procedures.

Patients often have strong preferences for certain types of anesthetics, and their concerns or wishes should be considered. However, patients should not be allowed to over-rule the anesthesiologist's choice for frivolous reasons that might greatly increase perioperative risk. Confusion can be caused by a surgeon who indicates a preferred anesthetic technique to a patient before discussing it with the anesthesiologist.

The major advantages of general anesthesia include the option of protecting the airway with an endotracheal tube, the ability to assist ventilation, the prevention of sudden and undesired movement, and the moment-to-moment titration of anesthetic depth in accord with changing levels of surgical stimulation. The most common disadvantages of general anesthesia include an increased incidence of postoperative nausea, sore throat, and residual anesthetic effects.

General Anesthesia

General anesthesia provides amnesia, loss of consciousness, analgesia, autonomic system modification, and muscle relaxation of various degrees.

Induction Agents

Inhalational induction techniques require a significantly longer period of time than IV techniques, thus exposing the patient to an increased risk of aspiration through the unprotected airway. For an elective procedure in a patient with a low risk of aspiration, an inhalational induction of anesthesia is acceptable. This is the standard method of induction in children. Adults, however, with their proportionally lower blood flow to vessel-rich groups and their markedly larger volume of distribution, require a significantly longer time period for inhalational induction than children; thus, an IV induction agent is preferred in adults. Table 7–6 lists the most common IV induction agents.

Thiopental (4 mg/kg) is the standard IV induction drug utilized by many anesthesiologists. The moderately prompt awakening that occurs following a single bolus is due to redistribution of the drug from brain to inactive tissues (viscera, muscles, fat). Thiopental is 99% metabolized by the liver, but this process is relatively slow (10% to 24%/hr). The major side effects of thiopental are dose-dependent depression of respiration and hypotension secondary to a combination of cardiac depression and systemic vasodilation. Hypotension with thiopental and other induction agents can be life-threatening in volume-depleted patients. The lack of analgesic properties renders barbiturates incomplete general anesthetics.

Propofol is a new hypnotic agent that appears to have several advantages over thiopental for certain procedures.[20] Emergence from brief anesthetics with propofol is extremely rapid because it is cleared more rapidly from the brain than is thiopental. This effect is

Table 7–6. INTRAVENOUS INDUCTION DRUGS

Drug	Major Advantages	Major Side Effects
Thiopental	Widely used, well-understood Moderately prompt awakening	Dose-dependent respiratory depression and cardiovascular depression
Propofol	Prompt, clear-headed emergence Intrinsic antiemetic effect	Dose-dependent respiratory and cardiovascular depression; irritates veins (especially small veins)
Etomidate	Hemodynamic stability	Adrenal supression
Narcotics	Analgesic, hemodynamic stability	Respiratory depression Long duration of action when doses used are large enough to allow induction (except alfentanyl)
Ketamine	Analgesic, amnestic Intrinsic sympathomimetic May support cardiovascular system and relax bronchiole construction	Delayed awakening and possibility of hallucinations during emergence

attributable to propofol's larger volume of distribution and high clearance from the blood (clearance actually exceeds hepatic blood flow). Propofol has some intrinsic antiemetic properties, and patients can emerge from anesthesia hungry, euphoric, and occasionally in a noticeably amorous mood. The hemodynamic side effects of propofol are similar to those of thiopental, except that propofol causes slightly more myocardial depression and very little increase in heart rate. Propofol causes irritation and discomfort during IV administration. Vein irritation can be reduced by administering propofol into larger veins, using a rapidly running intravenous tube, and following pretreatment with IV lidocaine (0.5 mg/kg) or fentanyl. A typical induction dose of propofol (2 mg/kg) may be followed by a continuous infusion (100 to 200 $\mu g \cdot kg^{-1} \cdot min^{-1}$) for maintenance of anesthesia. Because propofol does not have significant analgesic properties, opiates such as morphine sulfate, fentanyl, sufentanil, and inhalational anesthetics are given as supplements.

Etomidate (0.2 mg/kg IV) offers remarkable hemodynamic stability, particularly in the elderly patient. However, it offers no particular benefit for the average patient, and in repeated doses has been reported to cause adrenal suppression.

Ketamine (1 to 2 mg/kg IV) is a unique dissociative anesthetic that produces amnesia and intense analgesia. When very small doses are used, respiration and airway reflexes usually remain intact. Larger doses can cause a release of endogenous catecholamines, often leading to hypertension and tachycardia. Recovery from ketamine can be associated with hallucinations and nightmares, particularly in young people, limiting its usefulness in everyday practice for shorter procedures. However, ketamine (with its sympathomimetic properties) can be a useful induction agent in the hypovolemic patient in whom the emergent need to operate does not allow the time to adequately fluid-resuscitate the patient preoperatively (i.e., in patients with mas-

sive intra-abdominal hemorrhage). However in the hypovolemic patient with maximal sympathetic tone, hypotension can still occur.

Endotracheal Intubation

Guidelines regarding the necessity for endotracheal intubation are controversial. Arguments for routine endotracheal intubation include protection against passive regurgitation (and aspiration) and ensuring adequate ventilation (assuming ventilation is controlled). Arguments against the routine use of endotracheal intubation include avoiding possible injury to the airway and the expectation that less anesthetic is required, thus ensuring a faster recovery. Certainly, healthy nonobese patients who have appropriately fasted and who are undergoing brief colorectal procedures (hemorrhoidectomy, fissurectomy, incision and drainage of perirectal abscess) can be anesthetized safely and expeditiously without intubation. Unfortunately, many patients who present for a colorectal surgical procedure (proctocolectomy, massive tumor debulking, palliative treatment of obstructing lesions) do not fulfill these criteria. Furthermore, these patients sometimes require prolonged postoperative mechanical ventilation. Thus, endotracheal intubation is indicated for most intra-abdominal procedures conducted using general anesthesia.

Maintenance

Anesthesia can be maintained with inhalational drugs such as isoflurane, enflurane, halothane, and nitrous oxide. IV anesthetics are also being selected with increasing frequency as maintenance agents for shorter procedures.

Isoflurane is the most frequently used inhalational anesthetic in adults, because its lower blood solubility allows for a more rapid change in anesthetic depth than either enflurane or halothane. Isoflurane undergoes much less metabolism than enflurane and halothane; however, its airway-irritative pungency makes it far more suitable as a maintenance drug than as an inhalational induction agent. All volatile anesthetics produce dose-dependent bronchodilation to approximately the same degree. Similarly, all inhalational drugs, except nitrous oxide, cause some depression of myocardial contractility. Isoflurane maintains cardiac output more effectively than does enflurane or halothane (mainly through a peripheral vasodilation effect), whereas halothane more effectively maintains blood pressure at the same MAC than does either isoflurane or enflurane.

Enflurane, a chemical isomer of isoflurane, provides a stable cardiac rhythm and excellent skeletal muscle relaxation, but it causes central nervous system excitation and occasionally precipitates seizures.

Halothane produces a rapid and pleasant inhalational induction of anesthesia in children and is frequently used in pediatric anesthesia as the maintenance agent as well. However in adult anesthesia, the induction is typically performed via an IV technique, and thus isoflurane is used for reasons already noted. Halothane is arrhythmogenic in higher concentrations, especially with concomitant hypercarbia, and supplemental local anesthesia with high-dose epinephrine in this setting is relatively contraindicated.

Halothane has very infrequently been associated with the development of fulminant hepatitis. The National Halothane Study was conducted in the mid-1960s to study this association. After investigating over 800,000 anesthetics, the groups found that halothane was not associated with hepatic necrosis, or any other hepatic abnormality, more frequently than was any other anesthetic drug.[21] However, patients with pre-existing liver disease constitute a special group. Halothane is known to decrease hepatic blood flow,[22] whereas isoflurane (which increases hepatic artery blood flow at both 1 and 2 MAC) is probably the maintenance drug of choice for patients with liver dysfunction.

Reductive products of halothane metabolism are increased by hypoxia and are thought to act as antigens with subsequent exposure, resulting in hepatic dysfunction and necrosis.

Nitrous oxide, relatively impotent alone, may be selected as an adjunct to the potent inhalational vapors, because its rapid elimination provides a background for quick emergence from anesthesia. However, routine nitrous oxide is discouraged for prolonged colorectal procedures and is contraindicated when there is known or suspected bowel obstruction. Nitrous oxide preferentially fills gas-containing structures and can cause them to expand. This occurs because the blood-to-gas partition coefficient of nitrous oxide (0.47) is 34 times greater than that of nitrogen (0.014). Thus, the capacity of the blood to bring nitrous oxide to the bowel is greater than the capacity of the blood to remove nitrogen. With time, however, nitrogen is removed, and the bowel gas returns to its previous volume. Nitrous oxide can support combustion and should be avoided if cautery is used to open a distended segment of bowel that contains gas. In order to limit the dose of IV or inhalational drugs near the end of the procedure, nitrous oxide can safely be used during the last 15 to 30 minutes to promote rapid awakening and regaining of protective reflexes.

Desflurane, a relatively new inhalational agent, has the advantages of more rapid induction and emergence, and very low metabolism. It is likely to be most useful in the ambulatory operative setting.

Muscle Relaxants

Adequate relaxation of the abdominal wall is mandatory for all colorectal procedures involving abdominal incisions. This can occasionally be achieved with inhalational anesthetics alone; however, overall operating and physiologic conditions are superior with adjunctive neuromuscular blockade. Muscle relaxants are mandatory when only IV anesthetics are used for intra-abdominal operations. Table 7–7 lists the most frequently employed muscle relaxants.

Mivacurium is a relatively new nondepolarizing neuromuscular blocking drug with a very brief duration (approximately 15 minutes) and is metabolized mainly by plasma pseudocholinesterase. Although mivacurium can release histamine when administered rapidly in large doses, it is hemodynamically stable if administered slowly or as an infusion.

The shorter-acting muscle relaxants, such as vecuronium, atracurium, and mivacurium, are preferable for operations of short duration (1 to 2 hours); operations of greater duration should employ longer-acting muscle relaxants. Vecuronium is often selected when its cardiovascular-sparing properties are desired, and atracurium or mivacurium when circumstances favor a non–hepatorenal-dependent elimination pathway.

Succinylcholine, a depolarizing neuromuscular blocking drug, is spontaneously hydrolized in the plasma by pseudocholinesterase. However, nondepolarizing muscle relaxants generally require reversal with an anticholinesterase in order to ensure return of muscle strength significant enough to protect the airway and maintain ventilation.

Reversal of nondepolarizing neuromuscular blockade with an anticholinesterase may have implications relative to surgical outcome. Anticholinesterase drugs have been implicated in anastomotic breakdown, ostensibly the result of vigorous colonic contractions and diminished colonic blood flow that can occur with their

Table 7–7. NEUROMUSCULAR BLOCKING DRUGS

Drug	Approximate Duration of Action (min)	Intubating Dose (mg/kg)	Histamine Release	Muscarinic Receptor Effect	Approximate Percentage Metabolized via Renal Route
Depolarizing					
Succinylcholine	12	0.7–1.5	–	Stimulating	<20
Nondepolarizing					
d-Tubocurarine	150	0.5	+ + +	None	~50
Metocurine	150	0.4	+ +	None	~50
Atracurium	40	0.4	+	None	<5
Mivacurium	20	0.4	+	None	<10
Pancuronium	120	0.1	–	Blocks	~70
Pipecuronium	180	0.1	–	None	<20
Vecuronium	60	0.1	–	None	<20

administration.[23] Olivieri et al measured pressure in the rectums of 62 patients and found a statistically significant, but probably clinically irrelevant, increase in rectal tone in the neostigmine group compared with patients who had spontaneous recovery of the neuromuscular junction.[24] With appropriate dosing, atracurium, mivacurium, and occasionally vecuronium are used without a reversal agent, thus obviating the anticholinesterase controversy. However, close monitoring of neuromuscular blockade recovery is mandatory in these patients.

Frequently at the end of the procedure, during closure of the fascia, the anesthesiologist is making preparations so that the patient will be able to regain consciousness and be capable of being extubated by the time the dressing is applied at the end of the procedure (providing the circumstances warrant extubation at the end of the procedure). Problems arise when, at this critical time, the patient begins to "buck" (light anesthesia) or otherwise has inadequate muscle relaxation. Frequently, this situation can be rectified by transiently deepening the anesthetic or by adding additional muscle relaxants at the peril of a delayed wakeup or prolonged neuromuscular blockade requiring mechanical ventilation. Adding the rapidly eliminated induction agent propofol at this point is an additional maneuver gaining popularity. Communication between the surgeon and anesthesiologist is critical during this period. Accurate estimates of time to fascial and skin closure are sought, not because of the anesthesiologist's impatience but rather for efficient and safe anesthetic planning.

Regional Anesthesia

Regional anesthesia is indicated for most rectal and perianal procedures. It is also the preferred choice for any patient who wishes to be conscious during the procedure, would like postoperative analgesia (most frequently via continuous epidural catheter), and does not have any contraindications to its use (e.g., emergent full-stomach case and expected massive fluid shifts requiring postoperative mechanical ventilation).

Before beginning regional anesthesia, the anesthesiologist must be prepared to manage the most serious and common complications of regional anesthesia, which include hypotension, local anesthetic–induced seizures, total spinal anesthesia, and rarely cardiac arrest. To compensate for the extensive sympathectomy associated with spinal anesthesia to the level required for abdominal surgery (generally the T4 level), an infusion of 500 to 1,000 ml of crystalloid should immediately precede administration of the regional anesthetic. Vasopressors such as phenylephrine or ephedrine may also be used to treat hypotension. In addition, the anesthesiologist must be prepared to support ventilation and even occasionally to initiate a general anesthetic. There have been reports of unheralded cardiac arrests with subarachnoid blocks[25]; however, these cases probably represent patients who had originally subtle rather than precipitous changes in vital signs (chiefly bradycardia and hypotension) that were not closely monitored and managed by the anesthesiologist.

Innervation of the Abdomen

For success in regional anesthesia or local anesthetic nerve blocks, one must be familiar with the innervation of the abdomen. The skin and muscles of the anterior abdominal wall are supplied by the lower intercostal nerves T7 to T9 above the umbilicus, T10 at the umbilicus, and intercostal and subcostal nerves T11 to L1 below the umbilicus. The inferior portion of the anterior abdominal wall is supplied by the iliohypogastric and ilioinguinal nerves (L1). The dermatomal innervation of the perineum is via sacral roots S2, S3, and S4.

The parietal peritoneum has both somatic and visceral afferents and is thus highly sensitive to mechanical stimulation, especially the anterior abdominal wall. The somatic innervation of the parietal peritoneum is primarily via the spinal nerve fibers, which penetrate from the surface inward. The visceral peritoneum derives its nerve supply solely from the autonomic nervous system and is far less sensitive to mechanical stimulation than is the parietal peritoneum.

Adequate spinal or epidural regional anesthesia can be accomplished with a T4 dermatomal level for upper abdominal procedures, T6 for pelvic, and T10 for perineal procedures. Patients may occasionally complain of dyspnea with high regional anesthetics (if the block reaches above the T2 dermatome, many patients complain of dyspnea secondary to a perceived inability to breathe, probably caused by a loss of sensation of the intercostal dermatomes); this is usually remedied by reassuring patients that they are ventilating adequately. Indeed, Ciofolo et al[26] have demonstrated that there is no significant decrease in ventilation with epidural anesthesia during laparoscopy (even though intra-abdominal pressures are increased because of the pneumoperitoneum), as diaphragmatic action is sufficient to support respiration in the absence of intercostal activity. Dyspnea, nausea, or even regurgitation may occur if the diaphragm is pushed cephalad, as can occur with retractor placement and bowel packing. Nausea and vomiting can also occur when and if the patient becomes hypotensive or when manipulation of the viscera occurs.

Choice of Spinal Versus Epidural Regional Anesthesia

Spinal anesthesia provides a more consistent and often more profound analgesia than does epidural anesthesia. This occurs at the expense of a rapid onset of sympathectomy, which often leads to hypotension due to relative or absolute hypovolemia, and the occasional postoperative spinal headache. The incidence of spinal headache is greater in females than in males; youth and the use of large-gauge needles have also been implicated. Epidural anesthesia has the advantage of limiting the extent and speed of sympathectomy, thus allowing time for intrinsic and extrinsic (fluid administration) compensatory mechanisms to minimize the hemodynamic alterations. However, the total dose of local anesthetic is much larger, adding to the risk of systemic toxicity via epidural vein absorption or inadvertent direct intravascular injection. Additionally, penetration of the dura with the epidural needle leads to an increased risk of spinal headache. Deposition of large quantities of local anesthesia into the subarachnoid space carries the risk of total spinal anesthesia. Both spinal and epidural techniques can incorporate a continuous method of drug delivery through small

indwelling epidural or subarachnoid catheters. Indwelling catheters permit more precise control of the level blocked, provide the means for administering an additional dose during the surgical procedure, and permit postoperative pain control.

After a single dose of hyperbaric lidocaine (100 mg) or bupivacaine (15 mg), spinal analgesia to the T4 dermatome would be expected, lasting 60 to 90 and 90 to 150 minutes, respectively. Similarly, an epidural level of T4 may be achieved using approximately 20 ml of 2% lidocaine or 20 ml of 0.5% bupivacaine, both with and without epinephrine.

Caudal epidural blocks for perineal surgery are technically easy to perform with experience, and they have a high (>90%) success rate.[27] Also, because the perineal area is very sensitive and procedures such as hemorrhoidectomy are highly painful, caudal epidural blocks with bupivacaine (or other long-lasting local anesthetics) provide the added benefit of postoperative analgesia.

Local Infiltration Anesthesia

Bilateral local anesthetic blockade of the intercostal nerves T4 to T12 can provide adequate analgesia for certain abdominal procedures, as well as the muscle relaxation required to distend the peritoneal cavity to improve exposure. The total amount of local anesthetic for this technique can approach the maximum allowable dose (Table 7–8).

This technique is rarely used today and is probably appropriate only when anesthesia is required for a patient who can not be closely monitored (e.g., in time of war). However, Smith et al have described satisfactory postoperative pain control with a rectus sheath nerve block for diagnostic laparoscopy.[28] Clearly, local anesthetic techniques may be successful with short, locally confined procedures; however, most colorectal operations are not amenable to a rectus block. In contrast, certain anal procedures (such as fulguration of anal warts and treatment of anal fissures) are ame-

Table 7–8. LOCAL ANESTHETICS

Drug	Potency	Maximum Dose (mg) for a 70-kg Adult	
		Epinephrine-Containing Solution	Plain Solution
Esters			
Procaine	1	1,000	800
Tetracaine	8	200	150
Amides			
Lidocaine	2	500	300
Bupivacaine	8	200	150

nable to local anesthetic blocks. However, adequate local anesthesia can be difficult to obtain in the posterior midline in the presence of anal fissures[29] and with certain buttock anatomic considerations.[16] Furthermore, Keighley et al found a 50% fissure recurrence rate with local anesthesia compared with a 2.7% fissure recurrence rate for patients treated under general anesthesia.[30] The advantages of a local nerve block technique include lack of residual anesthetic effects and satisfactory postoperative pain control at the cost of increased patient discomfort during the perianal infiltration of the local anesthesia.[31] Local nerve blocks are probably safe in patients with coronary artery disease, because even large volumes (30 to 40 ml) of 0.5% lidocaine with 1:200,000 epinephrine failed to alter heart rate or blood pressure, despite causing a mild increase in plasma epinephrine levels.[32] In summary, local nerve block techniques require the full cooperation of the surgeon, patient, and anesthesiologist experienced in regional anesthesia. The technique of perianal anesthesia is further addressed in Chapter 15.

INTRAOPERATIVE COMPLICATIONS

Intraoperative complications (Table 7–9) can arise from numerous etiologies; however, the most significant for morbidity and mortality involve the pulmonary and cardiovascular systems. Complications related to positioning, including peripheral nerve injuries, have been discussed under positioning and are summarized in Table 7–5.

Pulmonary System

Pre-existing lung disease is common in patients undergoing colorectal surgery, as these patients are frequently elderly and occasionally may present for palliative procedures with established pulmonary metastatic lesions.

Fluid overload can result from intraoperative fluid administration and can lead to large intra- or postoperative alveolar-arterial oxygen gradients. Diaphragmatic elevation caused by abdominal distention or edema can impair ventilation, and this can be acutely exacerbated when the Trendelenburg position is used. Peak inspiratory pressures and adequate chest movement are closely monitored during colorectal surgery. An abrupt increase in peak inspiratory pressure should raise concern that a tension pneumothorax has occurred, especially if subdiaphragmatic tumor debulking is in progress. One should also consider other more common causes of increased inspiratory pressure, such

Table 7–9. COMPLICATIONS OF COLORECTAL SURGICAL PROCEDURES

Operative Complication (and Etiology)	Postoperative Complication (and Therapy)
Hypotension	Nausea and vomiting
Hypovolemia	Metoclopramide
Bleeding	Droperidol
Position	Transdermal scopolamine
Sympathectomy	
Mesenteric traction	
Impairment of ventilation	
Position	
Abdominal packs	
Pneumothorax	
Aspiration	
Position	
Obesity	
Morning admission	
Anxiety	
Bleeding	

as a kinked or occluded endotracheal tube, endotracheal tube migration (to carina or right main stem), light anesthesia, inadequate neuromuscular blockade, and excessively high flow rates or tidal volumes.

Cardiovascular System

Optimization of cardiovascular status is most critical when major colorectal procedures are performed on very ill patients. These patients, therefore, are the focus of this discussion. Hypotension can result from myocardial ischemia, relative anesthetic overdose, arrhythmias, and administration of excess vasodilating substances; nevertheless, hypovolemia should immediately be considered when hypotension occurs in patients undergoing major colorectal operations. Decreased intravascular volume can result from direct blood loss or from indirect means such as evaporative and third-space losses. Similarly, decreased venous return (caval compression or packs) can abruptly lead to hypotension. The combined presence of acute bleeding in the anesthetized and possibly hypovolemic patient, who also has some vena caval compression, can lead to severe hypotension. In this setting transient use of vasopressors is warranted and may be life-saving, while vigorous hydration is required to restore an adequate blood volume. Blood loss is an ever-present source of hypovolemia during colorectal procedures; thus, one or two large-bore intravenous catheters are critically important for these procedures. The most devastating occurrence of sudden (occasionally exsanguinating) intraoperative blood loss occurs during abdominal-perineal resection procedures with large tumors. Exsanguination from the presacral plexus typically occurs late in the procedure when the surgeon enters the wrong plane (deep to the presacral fascia) and bleeding from the presacral plexus occurs.

An additional source of hypotension during colorectal operations is traction of the mesentery, so-called mesenteric traction syndrome.[33] Although this entity has been most clearly studied in patients undergoing thoracoabdominal aneurysm resection, it is also known to occur during routine mesenteric traction. The bowel can liberate a variety of substances including peptides, amines, and lipids; however, there is growing evidence that prostacyclin (PGI$_2$) is the mediator of vasodilation and hypotension in this entity.[34] Therefore, if the patient becomes acutely hypotensive without any other etiology, one should consider changing the orientation of the bowel retractors in such a way as to limit mesenteric stretch.

Finally, legs are elevated and supported with stirrups in the lithotomy position during certain colorectal procedures (such as perirectal incision and drainage, hemorrhoidectomies, fissurectomies, and abdominal-perineal resections). When the legs are lowered at the end of these procedures, blood quickly pools in the now-dependent lower extremities, and the consequent decreased venous return can lead to hypotension.

ENVIRONMENTAL HAZARDS OF THE OPERATING ROOM

The plume of electrocautery and laser smoke, frequently encountered during anal fulguration procedures, is now a recognized *environmental hazard* for both the colorectal surgeon and anesthesiologist. Both human immunodeficiency virus[35] and papillomaviral[36] deoxyribonucleic acid (DNA) have been isolated from cautery smoke emanating from fulgurated anal warts. Thus, during laser or cautery fulguration of anal warts, all operating room personnel should wear protective masks, and the surgeon should employ suction to evacuate the smoke emanating from these warts.

POSTOPERATIVE COMPLICATIONS

The major postoperative complications following colorectal operations are bleeding, nausea and vomiting, atelectasis, and wound infections. Of these, the anesthesiologist has most impact upon control of nausea and vomiting.

Nausea and vomiting can be caused by several mechanisms, including direct drug effects upon the chemoreceptor trigger zone (CTZ), vagal stimulation caused by distention of the peritoneum, hypotension, and possibly direct peritoneal irritation when laparascopic gas is used. Several drugs and techniques can modify postoperative nausea and vomiting. If a nasogastric tube is employed, one first ensures its correct placement and function; subsequently antiemetics are given.

Metoclopramide increases lower esophageal sphincter tone, promotes gastric emptying, and causes central dopaminergic stimulation blocking the CTZ in the medulla.[37, 38] The usual dosage is 10 to 20 mg IV every 2 to 6 hours. Side effects of metoclopramide are rare and include sedation, dysphoria, dry mouth, and extrapyramidal reactions.

Droperidol binds to the dopaminergic sites in the CTZ of the medulla. The dosage for a 70-kg adult is 0.625 to 2.5 mg IV every 6 to 8 hours. Droperidol is also an α-adrenergic receptor antagonist, and in the hypovolemic patient, doses greater than 0.625 mg may lead to hypotension, which can actually increase the nausea.[8, 9] Droperidol tends to be long-lasting and is associated with hallucinations at higher dosages. Transdermal scopolamine has also been shown to be an effective antiemetic; however, the dosage must be significantly reduced in elderly patients in order to avoid postoperative psychosis, and its onset of action is significantly delayed compared with that of other routes of administration.

POSTOPERATIVE ANALGESIA

Systemic narcotic analgesia has been the standard for years; however, with the discovery of opiate receptors in the substantia gelatinosa of the spinal cord, epidural narcotics offer significant advantages over systemic opioid administration and are becoming the analgesic method of choice. For patients who have undergone less extensive procedures or who have refused epidural analgesia, patient-controlled analgesia (PCA) is appropriate and efficacious. Finally ketorolac, a new parenteral nonsteroidal analgesic has become available. In the 30- to 60-mg dose range it provides analgesia equivalent to 6 to 12 mg of morphine without the opioid-induced respiratory depressant side effect. In the presence of severe pain, ketorolac without an opioid is unlikely to provide sufficient pain relief.

Epidural Analgesia

Although opiates can be administered intrathecally at the time of a single-shot spinal anesthetic, this technique provides analgesia for only 18 to 24 hours. Continuous epidural catheters allow for prolonged postoperative dose titration with opiates (typically morphine 3 to 5 mg, or fentanyl 50 to 100 μg), followed by an infusion of opiate (i.e., morphine 0.5 to 1.0

mg/hr or fentanyl 25 to 100 μg/hr) for several days postoperatively. The important side effects include respiratory depression (peak 1 hour with fentanyl, and 4 hours with morphine), sedation, pruritus, and urinary retention. Fentanyl's lipophilic properties are associated more with segmentally controllable side effects, whereas morphine's action spreads over more spinal cord segments owing to its hydrophilicity. This same property (increased cephalad spread) of morphine raises the chance of respiratory depression. However, the incidence of respiratory depression is probably actually greater with intramuscular morphine dosing than with epidural.

Patient-Controlled Analgesia

The major problem with systemic opiates administered by a nurse on an as-needed basis is that the patient must wait (often in acute pain) until the nurse is able to procure and administer the physician-ordered drugs. The typical dose then yields increased side effects with resultant undesirable oscillations from pain to sedation and respiratory depression. In contrast, patient-controlled analgesia (PCA) allows patients to self-administer a small bolus of opiates at a desired frequency. The bolus dose is set by a physician or nurse, and after each dose is administered, a predetermined time interval (lockout) must elapse before the next bolus dose is given. A total amount of opiate over a 4-hour interval is also occasionally selected. Additionally, the PCA device has the capacity to administer a small continuous infusion of analgesic as a background.

Adjunct Analgesics

Nonsteroidal anti-inflammatory drugs (NSAID) are an important adjunct to systemic opiates for analgesic treatment of the postoperative patient. A new nonsteroidal agent (ketorolac) has become available in a parenteral formulation.[39] Thus, patients need no longer await full return of bowel function before gaining the advantage of NSAID therapy. The initial dose for a 70-kg adult is 60 mg intramuscularly (IM), and repeat doses are 30 mg IM every 6 hours thereafter. The chief side effects are the same as those with other NSAID and include gastrointestinal upset, impairment of renal function, and inhibition of platelet function. Patients with a history of aspirin or other NSAID sensitivity and/or asthma with or without nasal polyps can manifest anaphylactoid reactions when given ketorolac.

PEDIATRICS

Although the following discussion focuses on the lower intestinal tract, it also covers the anesthetic implications of some common pediatric upper gastrointestinal entities. These include bowel obstruction, because occasionally it is difficult to know the level of bowel obstruction in pediatric surgical cases, and the anesthetic implications are significant. Certain abdominal wall disorders that may involve the colon are covered as well.

Anesthetic management for pediatric colorectal procedures is similar to that outlined earlier for adults; however, certain points deserve special emphasis. Although inhalational inductions are the standard for most pediatric procedures, those involving trauma to, or obstruction of, the gastrointestinal tract require a rapid-sequence IV induction in order to protect the airway. Attention to fluid and electrolyte status is even more critical than in the adult because the total blood volume is much less in children. In addition to indicators of fluid status described earlier for adults (see Tables 7–2 and 7–3), assessment of fullness of fontanelles is helpful, and close monitoring of vital signs is essential. The hematocrit should be used as a guide to fluid status, and glucose levels may be especially labile in the newborn.

Issues in Pediatrics Fasting

In general, an elective pediatric case should be scheduled as the first case of the day in order to minimize dehydration. For an infant receiving feedings every 3 to 4 hours, most anesthesiologists would require the patient to ingest nothing 4 hours prior to surgery, and relegate the previous feeding to clear liquids. Older children eating every 6 to 8 hours should have an 8-hour fast. Patients with polycythemia may need an IV tube started preoperatively to prevent hemoconcentration, whereas patients with congestive heart failure may not tolerate overzealous hydration preoperatively.

Abdominal Wall Defects (Omphalocele, Gastroschisis)

Although several types of congenital abdominal wall defects can involve the colon, the discussion here is limited to omphalocele and gastroschisis because anesthetic management is similar. In both defects, the neonatal patient can present to the operating room dehydrated and hypothermic, as the exposed bowel and viscera contents act as a heat and moisture "radiator."

Initial management involves prevention of further dehydration and begins intravenous access and fluid resuscitation. An umbilical vein should be considered for access. Baseline electrolyte and glucose levels should be measured, especially if Beckwith's syndrome

Table 7–10. SYNDROMES OR ASSOCIATIONS INVOLVING THE COLON, RECTUM, OR ANUS IN PEDIATRICS: ANESTHETIC IMPLICATIONS

Name	Description	Anesthetic Implication
VATER association	An acronym based on the first letters of the major components of a nonrandom association of congenital defects: V = ventricular septal defect, vertebral anomalies A = anal atresia T = tracheoesophageal fistula E = esophageal atresia R = radial dysplasia, renal and rectal anomalies	Anesthetic management issues pertaining mainly to presence of tracheoesophageal (TE) fistula Increased risk of aspiration, inability to ventilate owing to large TE fistula Overdistention of stomach further impinging on adequate ventilation
Beckwith's syndrome	Infantile gigantism Birthweight >4,000 g Umbilical hernia and omphalocele common Macroglossia	Airway problems common because of large tongue Hypoglycemia common, thus baseline glucose mandatory prior to surgery
Ehlers-Danlos syndrome	Collagen abnormality Frequently gastrointestinal, heart, and pulmonary anomalies Frequently hernias	Difficult intravenous access Spontaneous pneumothorax

is identified (Table 7–10). Most children in this group are able to breathe spontaneously preoperatively. Nearly all require postoperative ventilation, owing to the elevated pulmonary pressures resulting from the tightness of abdominal contents.

Anesthetic monitoring should include temperature and pulse oximetry. A faltering arterial saturation value can alert the anesthesiologist and surgeon to excessively tight abdominal contents during primary abdominal closure.

Rapid-sequence induction is employed because of the full stomach. Typical induction doses of thiopental (Pentothal), 3 to 5 mg/kg, and vecuronium, 0.2 mg/kg, or fentanyl, 20 µg/kg, are appropriate. Maintenance of anesthesia should involve a balanced technique with maximum muscle relaxation and nitrous oxide avoidance, minimizing bowel distention. Nasogastric and rectal decompression may be employed to expedite decompression of the bowel.

Postoperatively, the patient is ventilated until able to do the work of breathing without assistance. Intravascular volume repletion must be ensured, because fluid requirements are amazingly high with this disorder.

Pyloric Stenosis

Pyloric stenosis is a disease that has some very important anesthetic implications. Pyloric stenosis typically occurs in 4- to 6-week-old neonates presenting with nonbilious emesis. These patients frequently manifest severe hypochloremic, hypokalemic metabolic alka-

losis. The need to operate is typically not emergent; however, fluid resuscitation and electrolyte repletion are critical. In some medical centers, a barium upper gastrointestinal study may be used for diagnosis, thereby increasing the risk of particulate matter aspiration.

The anesthetic induction proceeds after the stomach has been emptied with a nasogastric tube. A rapid-sequence induction or an awake intubation is most frequently utilized. Anesthesia is maintained with a volatile agent.

The child remains intubated following the operation, which typically lasts only 15 to 30 minutes, and is taken to the postanesthesia care unit (PACU). Narcotics are relatively contraindicated because these patients tend to retain carbon dioxide postoperatively and breathe slowly because of respiratory compensation of metabolic alkalosis. Narcotic administration can convert hypoventilation to apnea. The child is extubated in the PACU after the procedure, when fully awake—occasionally several hours postoperatively.

Necrotizing Enterocolitis

Ischemia of the bowel occurs because of vascular compromise that may be partially attributed to the presence of a patent ductus arteriosus. The patient presents with metabolic acidosis, sepsis, and abdominal wall discoloration. Anesthetic considerations include fluid repletion; avoidance of nitrous oxide, which causes bowel distention; and occasionally, inotropic support.

Lower Gastrointestinal Bowel Obstruction

Lower gastrointestinal bowel obstructions all produce similar anesthetic considerations. The patient presents with abdominal distention, dehydration, and hypovolemia. Owing to full stomach precautions, rapid-sequence induction is indicated.

Diaphragmatic Hernia

Newborns with diaphragmatic hernias present with respiratory and circulatory distress. Because of congenital diaphragmatic hernias, the abdominal contents gain entry into the chest and the lungs fail to develop properly. The resultant pulmonary hypoplasia manifests as pulmonary artery hypertension and occasionally as pneumothorax. These patients may be diagnosed prenatally and almost always require intubation for respiratory failure immediately after birth. As with procedures for abdominal wall disorders, the repair requires effective muscle relaxation. All should be transported to the neonatal ICU, intubated, and ventilated postoperatively. Because the lungs may be very atretic, many of these children do not survive long.

Syndromes Involving the Lower Gastrointestinal Tract

Several syndromes that involve the colon, rectum, or anus have known anesthetic implications. Several are mentioned within the text of this chapter. Additionally, Table 7–10 lists the few syndromes with the most significant airway, cardiovascular, and venous access implications. These include the VATER (*v*entricular septal defect, vertebral anomalies; *a*nal atresia; *tra*cheoesophageal fistula; *e*sophageal atresia; *r*adial dysplasia, renal and rectal anomalies) association, Beckwith's syndrome, and Ehlers-Danlos syndrome.

SPECIAL ELECTIVE COLORECTAL PROCEDURES

Carcinoid Tumors

Anesthesia for carcinoid tumors of the gastrointestinal tract can be challenging. About 50% of gastrointestinal carcinoid tumors occur in the appendix, and 20% occur in the rectum. These tumors are capable of releasing vasoactive hormones (serotonin, kinins, histamine)

into the bloodstream. The hormones so released travel to the portal vein and are inactivated by the liver. However, once the liver is involved with metastases, the hormones gain access to the systemic circulation and can cause bronchospasm, flushing, hypotension or hypertension, and tachycardia. When planning an anesthetic for a patient with carcinoid tumor, it is essential to obtain a complete history of the patient's symptoms and what triggers them. Pretreatment with bronchodilators (albuterol) and antihistamines (both H_1 and H_2) is probably indicated. The somatostatin analog octreotide has been successfully used to treat carcinoid crisis during anesthesia.[40] Octreotide inhibits the secretion of a variety of hormones. In contrast to somatostatin (which has a half-life measured in minutes), octreotide has a half-life of approximately $1\frac{1}{2}$ hours.

Colonic Interposition for Esophageal Pathology

Patients undergoing colonic interposition procedures require special attention. These patients are typically suffering from esophageal alkali injury or, less frequently, esophageal cancer. They are generally malnourished and may be dehydrated. Depending on the operative technique, there will be either a thoracotomy (necessitating the use of a double-lumen endotracheal tube) or a blunt dissection through the mediastinum, with one incision in the abdomen and a second incision in the neck. In either case, there are frequently periods of hemodynamic compromise resulting from impingement on the venous return to the heart. Thus, these patients should be monitored with an arterial catheter, a central line, and a Foley catheter, and should have two large-bore IV lines.

Patients who have previously had a colonic interposition and require another unrelated operation should be considered at high risk of passive regurgitation, and thus a rapid-sequence induction is indicated.

SUMMARY

Anesthesia for colorectal surgery can be performed safely utilizing current monitoring techniques and drugs. Preoperative preparation should emphasize adequate hydration and a proper period of fasting. General anesthesia and endotracheal intubation are recommended in order to protect the airway, support ventilation, and provide the optimal operative conditions for major colorectal procedures; however, regional techniques are often appropriate for brief perineal procedures. Monitoring should include measurement of end-tidal carbon dioxide, peak inspiratory pressures, oxygen saturation, blood pressure, and an ECG. Major complications include impairment of ventilation and intravascular hypovolemia. The most common postoperative complication attributed to anesthesia is postoperative nausea. As experienced anesthesiologists and surgeons can attest, anesthesia for colorectal surgery requires teamwork and effective communication between both sides of the ether screen. Even "high-risk" patients should be able to benefit from the minimal physiologic insult associated with modern-day anesthetics. They can endure massive operative procedures when prepared properly preoperatively, monitored adequately intraoperatively, and examined frequently postoperatively.

REFERENCES

1. Aitkenhead AR. Anaesthesia and bowel surgery. Br J Anaesth 1984;56:95.
2. Goldberger AL, O'Konski M. Utility of the routine electrocardiogram before surgery and on general hospital admission. Ann Intern Med 1986;105:552–557.
3. Miller RD, ed. Anesthesia. 3rd ed. New York: Churchill Livingstone, 1990.
4. Christopherson R, Frank S, Norris E, et al. Low postoperative hematocrit is associated with cardiac ischemia in high risk patients [Abstract]. Anesthesiology 1991;75:A99.
5. Lunn JN, Mushin WW. Mortality associated with anaesthesia. Nuffeld: Provincial Hospitals' Trust, 1982.
6. Keenan RL, Boyan CP. Cardiac arrest due to anesthesia: A study of incidence and causes. JAMA 1985;253:2373–2377.
7. Nimmo WS. Effect of anaesthesia on gastric motility and emptying. Br J Anaesth 1984;56:29.
8. Gray SJ, Ramsey CG. Adrenal influences upon the stomach and the gastric responses to stress. Recent Prog Hormone Res 1957;13:583.
9. Beaumont W. Gastric juice and the physiology of digestion. New York: Dover Publications, 1959, pp 159–160, 277.
10. Maltby JR, Sutherland AP, Sace JP, et al. Preoperative oral fluids: Is a five hour fast justified prior to elective surgery? Anesth Analg 1986;65:1112.
11. Croughwell ND, Reves JR, Will CJ, et al. Safety of flumazenil in patients with ischemic heart disease. Eur J Anesthesiol 1988;2:177.
12. Feld LH, Urquhart ML, Feaster WW, et al. Premedication in children: Oral vs intramuscular midazolam. Anesthesiology 1988;69:A745.
13. Philip BK, Simpson TH, Hauch MA, Mallampati. Flumazenil reverses sedation after midazolam-induced general anesthesia in ambulatory surgery patients. Anesth Analg 1990;71:371–376.
14. Boey HJ, Way LW. Acute cholangitis. Ann Surg 1980;191:264.
15. Martin JT. Positioning in Anesthesia and Surgery. Philadelphia: WB Saunders, 1987.
16. Nivatvongs S, Fang DT, Kennedy HL. The shape of the buttocks: A useful guide for selection of anesthesia and patient position in anorectal surgery. Dis Colon Rectum 1983;26:85–86.
17. Aitkenhead AR, Gilmour PS, Hothersall AP, et al. Effects of subarachnoid nerve block and arterial pCO2 on colon blood flow. Br J Anaesth 1980;52:1071.
18. Gelman S. Fowler KC, Smith LR. Regional blood flow during isoflurane and halothane anesthesia. Anesth Analg 1986;63:557.
19. Aitkenhead AR, Wishart HY, Pebbles-Brown DA. High spinal nerve block for large bowel anastomosis. Br J Anaesth 1978;50:177–183.
20. Sebel PS, Lowden JD. Propofol: A new intravenous anesthetic. Anesthesiology 1989;71:260–277.
21. The National Halothane Study: Bunker JP, Forrest WH, Mosteller F, eds. A study of the possible association between halothane anesthesia and postoperative hepatic necrosis. Washington, DC: US Government Printing Office, 1969.
22. Therlin L, Andreen M, Inestedt L. Effect of controlled halothane anesthesia on splanchnic blood flow and cardiac output in the dog. Acta Anaesthesol Scand 1975;19:146.
23. Aitkenhead AR. Anaesthesia and bowel surgery. Br J Anaesth 1984;56:95.
24. Olivieri L, Pierdominici S, Testa G, et al. Dehiscence of intestinal anastomoses and anaesthesia. Ital J Surg Sci 1988;18:217–221.
25. Caplan RA, Ward RJ, Posner K, et al. Unexpected cardiac arrest during spinal anesthesia: A closed claims analysis of predisposing factors. Anesthesiology 1988;68:5–11.
26. Ciofolo MJ, Clergue F, Seebacher J, et al. Ventilatory effects of laparoscopy under epidural anesthesia. Anesth Analg 1990;70:357–361.
27. Pentti OM. Bupivacaine in caudal anaesthesia for anal surgery. Anaesthesist 1978;27:74–78.
28. Smith BE, Suchak M, Siggins D, Challands J. Rectus sheath block for diagnostic laparoscopy. Anaesthesia 1988;43:947–948.
29. Courtice ID, MacLeod BA. Ischiorectal space block for anorectal surgery. Can J Anaesth 1990;37:S65.
30. Keighley MRB, Greca F, Nevah E, et al. Treatment of anal fissure by lateral subcutaneous sphincterotomy should be under general anaesthesia. Br J Surg 1981;68:400–401.
31. Smith LE. Ambulatory surgery for anorectal diseases; an update. South Med J 1986;79:163–166.
32. Barber WB, Smith LE, Zaloga GP, et al. Hemodynamic and plasma catecholamine responses to epinephrine-containing perianal lidocaine anesthesia. Anesth Analg 1985;64:924–928.
33. Seltzer JL, Ritter DE, Starsnic MA, Marr AT. The hemodynamic response to traction on the abdominal mesentery. Anesthesiology 1985;63:96–99.
34. Seltzer JL, Goldbert ME, Larijani GE, Ritter DE, et al. Prostacyclin mediation of vasodilation following mesenteric traction. Anesthesiology 1988;68:514–518.
35. Baggish MS, Poiesz BJ, Joret D, et al. Presence of human immunodeficiency virus DNA in laser smoke. Lasers Surg Med 1991;11:197–203.
36. Garden JM, O'Banion MK, Shelnitz LS, et al. Papillomavirus in the vapor of carbon dioxide laser-treated verrucae. JAMA 1988;259:1199–1202.
37. Madej TH, Simpson KH. Comparison of the use of domperidone, droperidol and metoclopramide in the prevention of nausea and vomiting following gynaecological surgery in day cases. Br J Anaesth 1986;58:879.
38. Cohen SE, Woods WA, Wyner J. Antiemetic efficacy of droperidol and metoclopramide. Anesthesiology 1984;60:67.
39. Powell H, Smallman JM, Morgan M. Comparison of intramuscular Ketorolac and morphine in pain control after laparotomy. Anaesthesia 1990;45:538–542.
40. Marsh HM, Martin JK, Krols LK, et al. Carcinoid crisis during anesthesia: Successful treatment with a somatostatin analogue. Anesthesiology 1987;66:89–91.

SECTION II

OPERATIONS ON THE INTRA-ABDOMINAL COLON

Inflammatory Disease

C H A P T E R   8

Ileocolectomy, Total Abdominal Colectomy, and Segmental Resections

Frank J. Harford
Jack Pickleman

ILEOCOLECTOMY FOR CROHN'S DISEASE

Several large longitudinal studies have shown that 70% to 95% of patients with Crohn's disease eventually undergo operations.[1-3] Of the various anatomic patterns of Crohn's disease, the most common is that involving the terminal ileum and a varying amount of the ascending colon.[1] Patients with this anatomic pattern are the ones most likely to require surgical intervention. The indications for operation in this group are usually obstruction, perforation with abscess, or internal fistula. Although surgery is not curative in patients with Crohn's disease, we believe that a patient suffering from a mechanical problem, such as obstruction, abscess, or fistula, should be given the benefit of resection for relief of discomfort, even though it may not effect a permanent cure of the disease.[4]

Elective resection removes the obvious disease, relieves the patient's symptoms, and avoids the side effects of long-term corticosteroid administration. The most common indication for surgery in patients with ileocolonic involvement is obstruction.[1] The site of obstruction is almost always at the terminal ileum. Fistulization often occurs between the terminal ileum and the cecum or right colon, and not uncommonly involves the sigmoid colon if it happens to lie in proximity to the right lower quadrant phlegmon. The presence of an enteroenteric fistula is not by itself an indication for operation, unless it is causing disabilities such as severe diarrhea, weight loss, or discomfort from an associated abscess; phlegmon; or partial obstruction.[5]

Many patients with ileocolonic Crohn's disease have a palpable mass in the right lower quadrant, but usually this represents a phlegmon and not a frank abscess. If there is an abscess, an attempt should be made to drain it percutaneously before operation. Once it is drained and the inflammatory process is allowed to subside, the subsequent resection will be facilitated.

Preoperative Preparation

As in any elective operation involving the gut, mechanical preparation is mandatory, and antibiotic prophylaxis desirable. Patients suffering high-grade partial obstruction from Crohn's disease may not be able to tolerate several liters of oral purgative. These patients, therefore, require several days of fasting, bowel rest, and incremental mechanical preparation. This obligatory preoperative starvation and the expected period of postoperative fasting make parenteral nutrition an attractive adjuvant in the care of these patients. Although data are lacking in support of the beneficial effects of parenteral nutrition preoperatively in the absence of severe malnutrition, the technique allows for "bowel rest" while maintaining adequate nutrition and remedying any acute depletion. Parenteral nutrition is a convenient, and probably helpful, adjuvant in the perioperative period.

Establishment of Site of Resection

When the abdomen has been opened and the pathology assessed, one must decide where the bowel should be resected. The affected bowel typically has a great amount of serosal reaction with erythema, tortuous serosal vessels, and mesenteric fat, which creeps over the bowel. Several studies have been done in an attempt to determine whether a wide resection of the involved bowel is beneficial in preventing recurrence.[6, 7] The most recent studies have focused on the association between microscopic disease at the margins of resection and recurrence, and opinions are sharply divided.[8–10]

We estimate the extent of disease by inspection and by palpation of the bowel at the enteric-mesenteric junction. In normal bowel, one should be able to feel an acute step-off at the angle between the mesentery and the bowel. Where there is some inflammation in the mesentery secondary to active disease, this angle is blunted and no step-off is palpated. We resect the bowel at the point where the angle can be palpated and check the mucosal surface, once the bowel is opened, to ensure that no mucosal ulcerations are present. These ulcerations are typically found on the mesenteric aspect of the lumen. Ideally, margins of a few centimeters of disease-free bowel, both proximally and distally, are sought. Sacrifice of more normal bowel does not protect against recurrence, and because the ileocolic variety of the disease is prone to recurrence, necessitating further resections, conservatism in resection is emphasized to avoid a short-bowel syndrome.

Not infrequently, small aphthous ulcers are present in the mucosa of the proximal small bowel that was found to be normal by inspection and palpation. Their presence alone does not call for extensive resection to obtain a totally normal-appearing margin.

Bowel Mobilization

Once the extent of the resection has been determined, the bowel should be mobilized, starting at the cecum at some distance from the inflammation. Abdominal incisions for Crohn's disease must be planned with the expectation that any patient may be a candidate for future ileostomy. Therefore, all incisions should avoid unnecessary scars on either lower quadrant. Midline incisions and transverse incisions immediately below the umbilicus afford excellent exposure and do not interfere with eventual stoma placement. Paramedian incisions and variations of the McBurney incision are to be avoided.

In the usual ileocolectomy for ileocolic Crohn's disease, dissection is initiated at the proximal ascending colon. The peritoneum is incised at the right gutter and carried up to the hepatic flexure, so that the cecum can be easily mobilized and brought up to the wound edge for convenient resection and anastomosis (Fig. 8–1). The gonadal vessels and the right ureter are identified and avoided, and dissection is continued anterior to these structures (Fig. 8–2).

The gonadal vessels and the ureter may be caught up in an inflammatory mass. If this is the case, the gonadal vessels may be divided above and below the mass, but the ureter can always be dissected free. A peritoneal incision is carried inferiorally and medially around the cecum to the base of the ileum and over the gonadal vessels and ureter. The peritoneal incision is continued at the antimesenteric border of the ileum to the point of normal bowel and the proposed level of transection of the ileum. In some cases, particularly in recurrent disease, extensive lysis of adhesions may be necessary to unfold the small bowel and to identify the transition between normal and diseased bowel.

Before finally determining the level of small bowel transection, it is prudent to estimate the length of small bowel that will remain. This can conveniently be done by counting 4-inch segments of normal small bowel from the ligament of Treitz to the proposed level of resection. Forty such segments indicate that approximately 160 inches of small bowel will remain after resection. A rough rule of thumb is that more than 150 inches of small bowel is adequate; 100 to 150 inches of small bowel does not result in a clinical short-gut syndrome but may require various nutritional supplements, such as folic acid and vitamin B_{12}. Less than 100 inches of small bowel remaining may result in a short-gut syndrome, requiring either enteral or parenteral supplements.

The junction of the small bowel and cecum are dissected free by incising and dividing the underlying fusion fascia. Several small blood vessels course through this fusion fascia and should be clipped prior to division. When this is accomplished, the bowel to be removed with its mesentery is well mobilized and ready for resection.

While mobilizing the ileocecum, the surgeon may encounter a perforation and/or a posterior abscess. If possible, the bowel wall defect is temporarily closed with a running stitch to avoid further contamination, and any abscess cavity is evacuated and irrigated. The duodenum, the right ureter, and the gonadal vessels are frequently reidentified during this dissection to avoid injury.

Mesenteric Division

The mesenteric division may be difficult, particularly when the mesentery is extremely thickened or contains large, hyperplastic lymph nodes. The surgeon may choose to divide the mesentery proximal to the thickening and the enlarged lymph nodes. If this proximal division results in devascularization of a too-long segment of bowel, the thickened mesentery may be at-

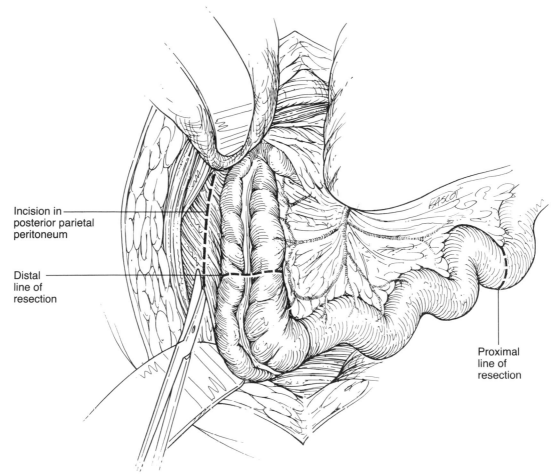

Incision in
posterior parietal
peritoneum

Distal
line of
resection

Proximal
line of
resection

Figure 8–1. Mobilization of the right colon. The dotted lines indicate the limits of resection on the bowel. The posterior parietal peritoneum is incised approximately 1 cm from the colon, and the incision is carried superiorly to the hepatic flexure and inferiorly around the cecum to incise the peritoneal reflection of the terminal ileum. (See Fig. 8–2.)

tacked directly. The inexperienced surgeon should remember that the mesenteric vessels lie at the posterior portion of the mesentery. After the peritoneum of the mesentery is scored with a scalpel, the underlying lymphatic tissue that overlies the vessels may be divided as a separate layer between hemostats and suture-ligated, which vertically divides the thickened mesentery in segments to avoid mass ligature. The underlying blood vessels are individually exposed, divided, and ligated with sutures of stout material.

Resection

In most instances, only the cecum need be removed. This varies, however, with the individual patient, because the disease may sometimes extend in the colon to the hepatic flexure or the transverse colon, necessitating its removal.

The colon and the small bowel are meticulously cleaned of fat so that the serosa is visible for 360

degrees around the viscera. The fat clearance may be accomplished by using electrocautery or by incising the serosa over the fat with a scalpel blade and pushing the fat away, sparing the underlying small vessels.

When operating for recurrent Crohn's disease at or near the previous ileocolic anastomosis, one should remember that the right mesentery that previously protected the duodenum has been sacrificed. Recurrent disease may be complicated by an ileoduodenal fistula, usually passing from the anastomotic site to the junction of the second and third portion of the duodenum. This fistula may have been diagnosed preoperatively by means of contrast radiography, but often it is occult. In these secondary cases, we must assume that any posterior fixation of the ileocolic junction involves a duodenal fistula and proceed accordingly.

The proximal small bowel and the distal colon are mobilized so as to approach the posterior fixation in a V fashion. As dissection proceeds, adherence to the duodenum and pancreas becomes obvious, and care is taken not to damage either structure. If a true fistula

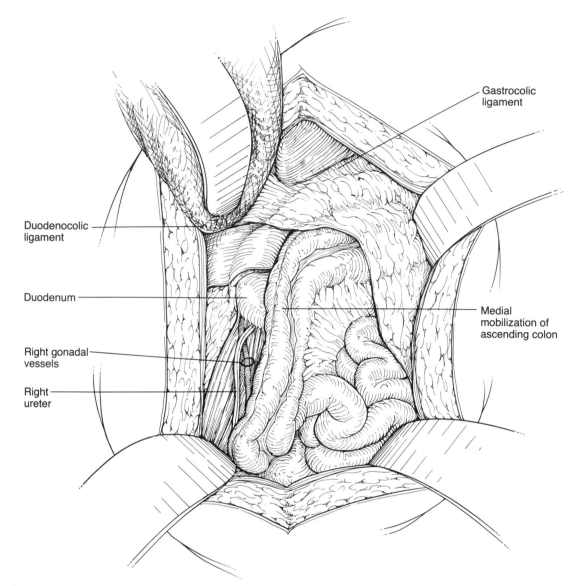

Figure 8–2. Mobilization of the right colon (continued from Fig. 8–1). The right colon is mobilized medially exposing the psoas muscle, the duodenum, the right ureter, and the right gonadal vessels. The area to be resected can be mobilized well into the abdominal wound.

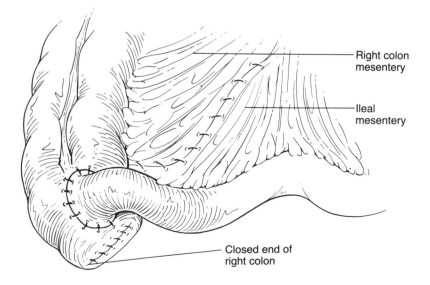

Figure 8–3. Completed end-to-side ileocolectomy. The ileum is anastomosed to the ascending colon with interrupted sutures. The anastomosis is on the anterior surface of the ascending colon and approximately 2 to 3 cm from the closed end of the right colon.

exists, it is transected at the base of the V and the ileocolic specimen removed. In most instances, the fistula is at the anterior or antimesenteric junction of the second and third portion of the duodenum. The fistula is excised and the duodenum repaired in two layers, usually after a Kocher maneuver is performed. If the fistula abuts onto the duodenopancreatic junction, the closure may have to be reinforced by a serosal or omental patch, and the duodenum decompressed by a duodenal catheter introduced as a gastrostomy and inserted through the full length of the duodenum. This tube prevents postoperative distention of the duodenum and is maintained for 7 to 10 days following operation.

In patients in whom there is fistulization from the ileum to the sigmoid colon, which lies in proximity to the inflammatory process, the colon is, in most cases, merely an "innocent bystander," and not involved with Crohn's disease. The fistula may be taken down by simple excision with repair of the sigmoid colon. A segmental resection is unnecessary, unless the sigmoid is extensively involved with dense inflammation.[11]

The anastomosis is usually made by joining the end of the ileum to the side of the colon, because there is usually a considerable size discrepancy between the lumens of these two organs (Fig. 8–3). Alternatively, one may staple the anastomosis in a side-to-side fashion (Fig. 8–4). If an end-to-side anastomosis is selected, the right colon is either amputated by a stapling-cutting device or transected between clamps and closed in two layers. The ileocolic anastomosis is placed no more than 3 cm from the closed end of the colon to avoid a future blind loop syndrome.

There are cases in which, in addition to terminal ileum disease, one finds multiple skip areas in the proximal small bowel that are causing significant obstruction. These are sometimes widely spaced, and their removal would require multiple resections and sacrifice of a considerable amount of bowel. In these situations, a stricturoplasty of the involved lesions is a good solution, whereby relief of the obstruction is obtained while a maximal amount of bowel is preserved. Results of these procedures have been good, with minimal perioperative morbidity and acceptable long-term results.[12, 13] The stricturoplasty is done in a manner similar to that of a Heineke-Mikulicz pyloroplasty (Fig. 8–5). With longer strictures that do not lend themselves to this type of procedure, some authors have described a stricturoplasty resembling a Finney pyloroplasty. We prefer to resect strictures that are too long for a Heineke-Mikulicz type of procedure.

EDITORIAL COMMENT

Preoperative identification of an abscess complicating Crohn's disease as well as its size and location facilitates the planning and execution of any resection. Small abscesses may be conveniently included with the operative specimen, thus avoiding contamination and not precluding a primary anastomosis. Larger abscesses require evacuation or drainage either before or at the time of operation, and significant contamination should preclude a primary anastomosis. In these circumstances, an end-ileostomy is constructed, and the colon is either brought out through a separate stab wound as a mucous fistula or closed and replaced into the peritoneal cavity. The choice between these maneuvers depends on the state of the colon, the degree of contamination, and the condition of the patient. If any of these situations are of concern, a mucous fistula is the safest alternative. A second operation with anastomosis of the ileum to the colon can be accomplished later: usually 6 to 12 weeks after the initial procedure, depending on the amount of peritoneal inflammation encountered or expected.

The method of drainage of attendant abscesses varies with their presentation. Occasionally, large psoas abscesses can be drained primarily by a percutaneous method. In practice, however, most psoas abscesses are chronic and contain little fluid material. Rather, they contain necrotic debris that does not lend itself to percutaneous drainage. These abscesses require evacuation at the time of laparotomy. In these situations, an anastomosis can safely be performed if the anastomotic segment does not lie adjacent to the abscess cavity and/or the cavity can be isolated by an omental or peritoneal flap. Larger psoas abscesses preclude primary anastomosis.

Frequently, an isolated abscess is seen lying between the omentum and the anterior abdominal wall. These collections are conveniently drained by a minimal open approach or by percutaneous routes, to be followed in a few days by elective resection with primary anastomosis. Although anastomosis is possible in these situations, the skin and subcutaneous tissue should be left open to heal by secondary intention.

Large fluid-containing abscesses within the peritoneal cavity may be treated by attempts at percutaneous drainage. These often fail in abscesses of fecal origin, so that the surgeon must resort to open extraperitoneal drainage either prior to laparotomy or at the time of resection, as dictated by the condition of the patient. Any drainage of such an abscess before resection holds the possibility of the development of a fecal fistula, but these are usually minor and do not interfere with the planned procedures.

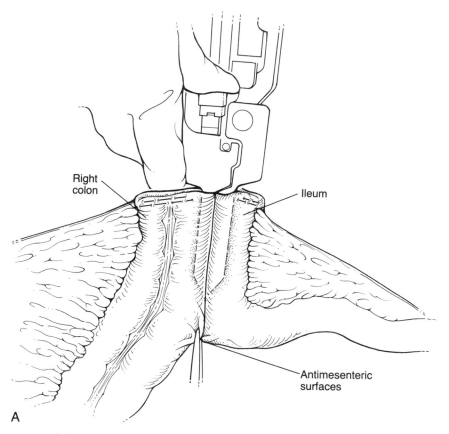

Right
colon

Ileum

Antimesenteric
surfaces

A

Figure 8–4. Stapled anastomosis of the ileum to the cecum. *A,* Construction of a stapled side-to-side (functional end-to-end) anastomosis. The small bowel and ascending colon are approximated at their antimesenteric borders. The lumens of each segment of bowel are partially closed, and a stapling-cutting device is inserted so that one limb of the device is in the lumen of each segment of bowel. The device is then fired, creating a side-to-side anastomosis.

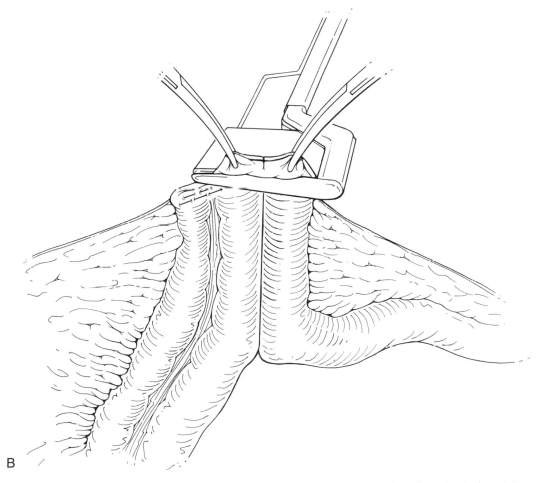

Figure 8–4 *Continued B,* The side-to-side stapled anastomosis between the terminal ileum and right colon. The closure of the ends of the bowel and the anastomosis are depicted.

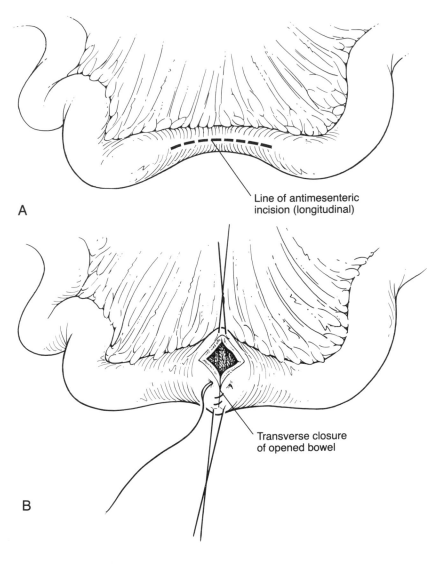

A

Line of antimesenteric
incision (longitudinal)

B

Transverse closure
of opened bowel

Figure 8–5. Technique of stricturoplasty. Stricturoplasty is reserved for short segments of stenosis. *A,* The incision is placed on the antimesenteric portion of the stenotic bowel, and the incision is carried full thickness into the lumen of the bowel. *B,* The bowel is then closed in a transverse fashion with a single layer of stout interrupted suture material. Care is taken to avoid eversion of mucosa in this closure.

SEGMENTAL RESECTION OF THE LEFT COLON

Segmental left colon resection for benign disease is done for diverticulitis, for ischemic colitis confined to a segment of the colon, and very occasionally for colonic Crohn's disease confined to a segment of the left colon. Segmental left colonic Crohn's disease seems to occur more frequently in the older group, and in this population one must distinguish between Crohn's disease and ischemic colitis. The usual indications for operation in these cases are stricture or perforation with abscess. There is little information in the literature about the results of segmental resection of the left colon in Crohn's disease, but the available information suggests that recurrence rates are higher than those found after proctocolectomy or total colectomy with ileorectal anastomosis.[14]

Diverticulitis

The most common indication for segmental resection of the left colon is sigmoid diverticulitis. Surgical intervention is warranted after a second attack of uncomplicated diverticulitis, a single attack in a young person, or an initial attack that does not resolve with bowel rest and parenteral antibiotics. It is also required in cases of diverticulitis complicated by abscess, fistula, free perforation, or large bowel obstruction. In the patient with segmental Crohn's disease, the amount of resection is determined by the gross appearance of the bowel, and the limits of resection are determined nearly as for ileocolonic Crohn's disease.

Preoperative Evaluation

In the case of diverticulitis, the extent of proximal resection should be determined by palpation of the bowel and selection of a point where the bowel wall is supple without muscular hypertrophy. It is not necessary to remove all of the diverticula-bearing colon proximally.[15] However, the distal resection must include all of the sigmoid colon, so that the anastomosis, if one is done, joins the proximal colon to the rectum and not to the sigmoid colon. If distal sigmoid colon is left in place, the recurrence rate is higher than if a colorectal anastomosis is made.[16]

The proximal rectum to which the colon is anastomosed should be normal to palpation. If there is bowel wall thickening in the proximal rectum because of adjacent inflammation, the anastomosis should be made lower in the rectum where the bowel is supple. Great care should be taken to be sure that no diverticula are present at the anastomosis. If the patient is able to be adequately studied preoperatively with contrast radiography or endoscopy and malignancy has been ruled out, the mesentery may be divided adjacent to the bowel wall. There is no reason to perform a wide lymphadenectomy if the diagnosis of diverticulitis is secure. However, it is sometimes impossible to determine with certainty whether the process is benign or malignant. The sigmoid colon is often severely kinked and fixed, making endoscopic examination impossible. In this situation it is often helpful to have a colonoscope available in the operating room, so that with the abdomen open, the scope may be guided through the area in question. If the mucosa appears normal, one may rule out the possibility of colon carcinoma. This endoscopic examination is facilitated by placing the patient in Lloyd-Davis stirrups or simply by placing the colonoscope in the rectum at the time the patient is positioned on the table, so that it can be gently advanced with the help of intra-abdominal manipulation when the abdomen is open.

The presence of malignancy not only necessitates a wide lymphadenectomy but, in addition, requires an en bloc resection of any structure to which the colon is adherent. There are times when neither preoperative nor intraoperative evaluation is successful in ascertaining the presence of malignancy, and one must make a critical judgment on the basis of the appearance of the lesion at the time of operation. In any case, the specimen should be opened at the time of the operation, and the mucosa examined. If a carcinoma is found that was not previously appreciated, a lymphadenectomy should be done at that time, along with resection of parts of any structure to which the tumor was adherent. Although this is not an ideal situation, there is probably some benefit from this remedial maneuver.

Sigmoid Colon Resection

Resection of the sigmoid colon should begin with incision of the reflection of the parietal and visceral peritoneum in the left gutter. The ureter should be identified as soon as possible and traced throughout its course. If the diagnosis of malignancy has been securely ruled out, the colon may then be mobilized with blunt dissection. Often one must pinch off the inflammatory adhesions of the colon to the abdominal wall and sometimes to other structures in the pelvis, such as the bladder or uterus. Once the proximal line of resection has been chosen in a nonthickened, pliable area of descending colon, it may be brought down to the rectum and the anastomosis made at that point. This often requires mobilization of the splenic flexure. The point of proximal resection should be chosen so that no diverticula are included in the anastomosis or immediately adjacent to it, because this would result in early leaks or a later recurrence of diverticulitis at the anastomosis.

In patients who are acutely ill or who have a palpable abdominal mass or fullness, a computed tomographic (CT) scan of the abdomen and pelvis should be done preoperatively. In evaluating a patient with suspected diverticulitis, a CT scan is extraordinarily helpful and is the diagnostic maneuver of choice. The CT scan should be enhanced by contrast. The presence of diverticulitis can be confirmed, as can its location and extent and the presence or absence of abscess or fistula.

In performing a sigmoid resection for diverticular disease, one may encounter extensive inflammation with adherence to the left ureter, bladder, iliac veins, or generative organs. If resection cannot safely be accomplished, it is prudent to abandon it and elect a diverting colostomy. Elective resection can be accomplished at a later date—usually within a period of 2 to 3 months.

If resection appears feasible, it should begin with incision of the junction of parietal and visceral peritoneum at the white line of Toldt. This incision is extended distally well down into the pelvis for future mobilization of the rectum. Superiorly, the peritoneal incision is continued to the splenic flexure, which is often conveniently mobilized at this time beneath the attachment of the omentum.

At the intersigmoid recess, the gonadal vessels are first encountered, and the left ureter is encountered medially. The mesentery of the sigmoid colon is cut free from these structures, so that the plane of dissection frees only the sigmoid colon and its mesentery, with the separation proceeding anterior to the gonadal vessels, ureter, and Gerota's fascia. The sigmoid mesentery can often be easily freed from these structures either by sharp dissection or by gentle posterior wiping with a small gauze sponge.

When sufficient lateral dissection has been accomplished to well mobilize the sigmoid colon and the upper rectum, an incision is made in the sigmoid mesentery, extending parallel to the upper rectum for a few inches. Unless a cancer is suspected, a wide mesenteric lymphadenectomy is not required and only the sigmoid and superior rectal vessels are divided. If an occult cancer is suspected, the mesenteric lymphadenectomy can easily be extended to include the origin of the inferior mesenteric artery, care being taken to preserve the underlying nervi erigentes and the superior pelvic ganglia. These structures can easily be identified posterior and adjacent to the superior rectal vessels, but not within the rectosigmoid mesentery.

After division of the mesentery, the sites of transection of the proximal and distal bowel are scrupulously denuded of fat and areolar tissue. The mesentery of the rectum should be divided between hemostats on the rectal wall, and suture-ligated. Noncrushing Block-Potts clamps are applied, and the specimen is removed.

Anastomosis

Anastomosis can be accomplished in either an end-to-end or a side-to-end fashion. If there is significant disparity between the lumens of the rectum and descending colon, the side-to-end Joel-Baker anastomosis is convenient and safe. If the bowel preparation was not adequate or if there is significant contamination, the prudent surgeon may elect to close the distal segment as a Hartmann pouch and bring out the proximal bowel as a temporary end-colostomy.

Diverticulitis with Abscess

If an abscess is present, it should be drained percutaneously at the time of obtaining the CT scan if possible. Once the abscess has been drained and the inflammation has subsided, the patient may then undergo an elective resection with primary anastomosis.[17] When there is a large abscess in the pelvis or left gutter that cannot be drained percutaneously, the patient should be taken to the operating room for open drainage. We prefer extraperitoneal drainage with the sump drains brought out through the retroperitoneum to avoid contamination of the peritoneal cavity. If it is technically feasible to do so, the diseased sigmoid colon is removed down to the proximal rectum at this time.

A Hartmann pouch should be constructed, and the corners identified with long Prolene sutures so that they can be clearly seen when the second operation is done to anastomose the colon to the rectum. The advantage of making a Hartmann pouch at the first operation is that once the sigmoid colon has been resected, a punch-through technique may be carried out with an endorectal stapling instrument and minimal mobilization of the rectal pouch (Fig. 8–6). In some circumstances, this is a great advantage. If an abscess

has been drained through the peritoneal cavity, one should make an attempt to cover the abscess bed with omentum so as to protect the rest of the peritoneal cavity. If the patient has small abscesses between the leaves of the mesentery, they may be resected along with the colon, and a primary anastomosis made. In patients in whom it is not technically feasible to resect the bowel at the time the abscess is drained, a totally diverting colostomy should be constructed proximal to the inflammatory process, and the affected segment resected when the inflammatory process has subsided.

Diverticulitis with Bleeding

Diverticulitis requiring operation because of bleeding presents problems both in the localization of the bleeding site and in the extent of resection. An elective resection for chronic or occult bleeding may be treated by a segmental resection. In this circumstance an obviously diseased sigmoid colon may be resected empirically. If there is no site of obvious inflammation, a more extensive left colectomy may be required to remove all of the colon bearing diverticula. In this circumstance, the surgeon must be aware that angiodysplasia may be the cause of bleeding. Preoperative endoscopy and superior and inferior mesenteric angiography should be employed.

For catastrophic hemorrhage requiring transfusion to maintain homeostasis, a segmental resection suffices if the site of bleeding has conclusively been demonstrated by angiography before operation. More commonly, the surgeon must manage a colon distended with blood, and the exact site of bleeding cannot be precisely determined. In this circumstance, the operation of choice is total abdominal colectomy with ileoproctostomy. Although it is desirable to preserve all of the terminal ileum in this procedure, care must be taken to ensure that the cause of bleeding is *not* angiodysplasia that may also involve the terminal ileum. If angiodysplasia is confirmed, any obviously diseased ileum must also be resected.

Colovesical Fistula

When the colon must be resected because of a colovesical fistula, one must evaluate the patient preoperatively to rule out malignancy. If colovesical fistula occurs in a premenopausal woman with a normal-size uterus one must be suspicious of a colonic malignancy. The uterus usually interposes between a diverticular process and the bladder to prevent colovesical fistula formation, whereas in the case of malignancy this may not occur. The most sensitive test for detecting a colovesical fistula is the CT scan, because it can dem-

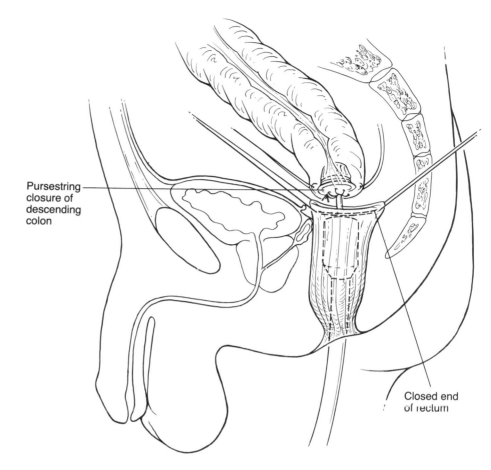

Pursestring
closure of
descending
colon

Closed end
of rectum

Figure 8–6. Coloproctostomy utilizing a stapling technique. An endorectal stapler is utilized through the rectum, effecting an end to end anastomosis through the previously closed (stapled) rectal stump.

onstrate small amounts of air or contrast material in the bladder.[18]

Cystoscopy may be helpful in this situation. Most often, however, the fistula opening is not identified, but bullous edema is seen at the dome of the bladder. In the presence of fecaluria or pneumaturia, this confirms the diagnosis of enterovesical fistula. Cystoscopy has the additional advantage of affording the opportunity to biopsy any suspicious tissue. Although colonoscopy and barium contrast examinations are not particularly valuable investigations for detecting a fistula, they are extremely helpful in determining the nature of the bowel disease that caused the fistula to form.

Colovesical or coloenteric fistula can almost always be resected, and primary anastomosis accomplished, because these processes really represent abscesses that have drained into other organs without a significant residual abscess cavity present at this stage. After resection for diverticulitis in which a fistula was taken down, it is advantageous to interpose the omentum between the closure of the fistula and the colorectal anastomosis (Fig. 8–7).

COLONIC OBSTRUCTION

In the case of large bowel obstruction secondary to diverticulitis, a segmental resection of the sigmoid colon with end-colostomy and Hartmann procedure is the most desirable option. Subtotal colectomy with ileorectal anastomosis is also possible if the rectum is not at all indurated, there is no evidence of peritonitis or abscess, and the small bowel is not edematous.

There are instances of fragile patients with large bowel obstructions in whom a two-stage procedure is still advantageous. The first stage should be a transverse colostomy to relieve the obstruction and to prepare the patient for a subsequent definitive resection with anastomosis. In this situation, we find it advantageous to use a left transverse loop colostomy, instead of the traditional right transverse loop colostomy.

When patients have distal obstruction, the colon is usually large, and a fairly generous aperture in the abdominal wall must be made to bring out the loop. In this situation it is common for a prolapse of the colostomy to occur postoperatively. For reasons not

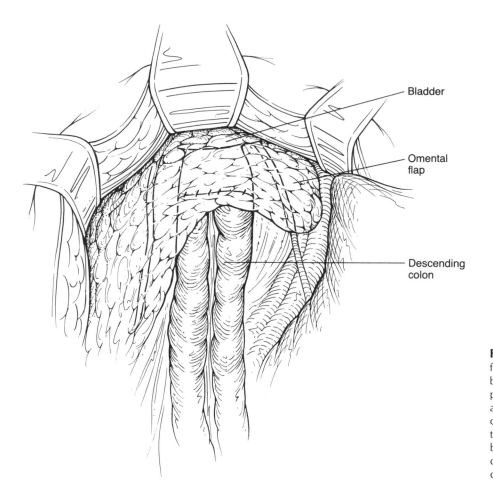

Bladder

Omental
flap

Descending
colon

Figure 8–7. Interposition of omental flap between colorectal anastomosis and bladder closure. The omental flap is placed anterior to the colorectal anastomosis and posterior to the bladder closure. The omental flap is based on the left portion of the omentum supplied by the left gastroepiploic artery and is carried anterolateral to the descending colon.

entirely clear, this is usually a prolapse of the distal rather than the proximal loop. By using a left transverse colostomy one can bring up the loop to a point at which there is no slack distal to the colostomy. This helps prevent the prolapse of the distal loop of the colostomy. Another advantage of the left transverse colostomy is that at the second procedure, the point of proximal resection can include the colostomy site; a primary anastomosis can be done without leaving a colostomy proximal to the colorectal anastomosis, which will require subsequent closure.

EDITORIAL COMMENT

Although the authors' description of a left transverse colostomy is attractive for preventing prolapse of the temporary colostomy, there are sound and compelling reasons to utilize a right-sided stoma. The eventual resection may require mobilization of the splenic flexure, or the surgeon may wish to protect the low anastomosis by the existing colostomy. For these reasons we usually elect to place our diverting colostomy on the right side.

ISCHEMIC COLITIS

Ischemic colitis may occur for the following reasons: as a result of interruption of blood flow through the inferior mesenteric artery during aortic surgery, as a spontaneous event without demonstrable occlusion, as a result of a low-flow state in the critically ill patient, as a result of polycythemia, or as a consequence of vasculitis in diseases such as lupus or polyarteritis. In the first and second circumstances, the ischemic segment is usually in the left colon. In ischemic colitis secondary to a low-flow state, the ischemia often involves the right colon alone or may involve the entire colon.[19] In ischemia resulting from vasculitis, the involvement may be segmental or diffuse.

Ischemic Colitis Following Interruption of the Inferior Mesenteric Artery

Large bowel ischemia following inferior mesenteric artery interruption during aortic surgery occurs in 2%

to 32% of the cases.[20, 21] It is most common following surgery for ruptured aortic aneurysm. The patient presents in the postoperative period with diarrhea, usually containing blood, or with signs of sepsis. Abdominal pain is difficult to evaluate in a patient with a recent laparotomy, but a patient who is septic with peritoneal signs should be considered for immediate reoperation. Flexible endoscopy is extremely helpful in making this diagnosis. On examination the rectum is typically spared and appears normal, although rectal involvement has been described.[22] If one encounters the dusky blue-black color of infarcted bowel in the sigmoid colon on the first examination, immediate laparotomy and resection should be done. The ischemic segment of bowel should be resected up to a point at which there is brisk bleeding from the cut end of the bowel. An end-colostomy and Hartmann pouch should be constructed.

In milder ischemia, one sees patchy areas of edematous, friable hyperemic mucosa alternating with pale areas. The patient may be safely watched and should be re-endoscoped in 24 hours. Over the next 24 to 48 hours small superficial ulcers will appear, and some bluish submucosal hemorrhage may be seen. If the ischemia becomes more severe, as manifested by darkening of the mucosa, the patient should be operated on. If this change does not occur, the patient can be treated expectantly.

The mortality associated with this condition is high.[22] It is hoped that early recognition of impending gangrene and prompt reoperation before perforation will improve the statistics.

Spontaneous Ischemic Colitis

Patients with spontaneous ischemic colitis are usually older and have various associated medical disorders. They typically present with a sudden onset of usually mild, crampy lower abdominal pain, mostly on the left side. They also have some hematochezia within 24 hours of the onset of pain. On physical examination there is usually some tenderness to palpation in the left lower quadrant, and sometimes an accompanying fever or tachycardia. The diagnosis can be made with flexible endoscopy. As with inferior mesenteric ligation, it is highly unusual to have rectal involvement. The endoscopic features of this condition have been documented in detail and are similar to those already described.[23] If a barium contrast study is done soon after the onset of the pain, it shows a typical thumbprinting pattern, which is the result of submucosal edema and hemorrhage. If the patient has peritoneal signs or is septic, these examinations are superfluous

and meddlesome; however, that situation is unusual in this group of patients.

Once a diagnosis of spontaneous ischemic colitis is made, the treatment is expectant. In these patients, progression to full-thickness necrosis is unusual if there is no evidence of gangrenous bowel at the first examination. Resolution of the process is the most common clinical course. Typically, the symptoms subside over a few days or a week. The process may also evolve into an ulcerative stage, which may eventually result in stricture formation. During the ulcerative stage the endoscopic and radiographic findings may mimic Crohn's disease.

Occasionally, the early phases of this disease go unnoticed or undiagnosed, and the patient presents with a stricture. The differential diagnosis in this circumstance includes inflammatory bowel disease and malignancy. Many of these strictures are asymptomatic, and if the strictured area can be adequately examined and biopsied to rule out malignancy, nothing need be done if the patient is without symptoms. If the stricture cannot be completely examined endoscopically or the patient is symptomatic, a resection should be done. At the time of resection, the stricture is excised and care is taken to ensure that there is brisk bleeding from both ends of the bowel before they are anastomosed. If malignancy has not been ruled out a radical resection of the strictured area should be done.

Ischemic Colitis Secondary to Low-Flow States

In patients with ischemic colitis secondary to low-flow states, there is a high incidence of full-thickness necrosis. The mortality associated with colonic infarction in patients who are critically ill from another disease process is extremely high. One must have a high incidence of suspicion in this type of patient who develops abdominal pain. These patients should undergo resection of the infarcted or severely ischemic segment with construction of an end-ileostomy or colostomy and mucous fistula or Hartmann pouch. Primary anastomosis is ill-advised in this setting.

Ischemic Colitis Secondary to Collagen Vascular Disease

Ischemic colitis in patients with collagen vascular disease is not a common occurrence, but it has been described.[24, 25] It is difficult to diagnose, because many patients who have the disorder often have nonspecific abdominal complaints, and they may be receiving corticosteroids, which mask the severity of intra-abdominal processes. A high index of suspicion is necessary if the diagnosis is to be made in a timely fashion. Endoscopy is extremely helpful, as it is in the other types of ischemic colitis. If resection is done, it is generally prudent not to do a primary anastomosis.

EDITORIAL COMMENT

In all but chronically strictured patients, we operate because of impaired perfusion of the bowel. In addition, the setting in which these conditions occur usually implies a compromised patient. Therefore, primary anastomosis is rarely accomplished in the emergency operation for ischemic colitis. Furthermore, the exteriorized segments can indicate the adequacy of the perfusion of the gut. Secondary operations for further resection or a prudent "second look" is common. In general, resection and primary anastomosis in ischemic colitis are reserved for elective resection for chronic strictures.

TOTAL ABDOMINAL COLECTOMY

Total abdominal colectomy with primary anastomosis may be done in selected cases of large bowel obstruction due to neoplastic or inflammatory disease with the purpose of avoiding a two- or three-stage operation. One must be cautious in electing primary anastomosis at the time of emergency abdominal colectomy, as mortalities of 14% to 28% have been reported.[26, 27] The obstructive process must not involve the rectum; there should be no peritonitis or abscess; and anal sphincter function must be adequate to ensure a good functional result. Most important, the patient should be judged to be able to withstand the physiologic insult of total abdominal colectomy.

Ulcerative Colitis

In the case of ulcerative colitis or Crohn's colitis, total abdominal colectomy is done emergently for life-threatening conditions such as massive hemorrhage, toxic megacolon with or without perforation, or perforation in the absence of megacolon. In the elective setting, the indications are usually failure of medical management with continuous diarrhea, abdominal discomfort, or weight loss that is refractory to the usual medications and dietary manipulations. Strictures may also prompt colectomy, if they are symptomatic or simply cannot be adequately evaluated endoscopically with biopsy and brushings to rule out malignancy.

The development of carcinoma in patients with ulcerative colitis far exceeds the incidence found in the general population; this is also true in Crohn's colitis albeit probably to a lesser degree.[28] In the case of ulcerative colitis the risk of carcinoma increases with the extent of colitis and the duration of the disease. It appears to have no relationship to the activity of the disease.[29, 30] In 1967 Morson and Pang demonstrated a relationship between severe dysplasia in ulcerative colitis and the occurrence of carcinoma.[31]

The usual practice is to do periodic surveillance colonoscopy with multiple random biopsies throughout the colon after pancolonic disease has been present for 8 years or left-sided colitis has been present for 15 to 20 years. The frequency with which this needs to be done and the certainty of the relationship between dysplasia and carcinoma in this context are not entirely clear from the data that have been gathered to date. Approximately 50% of the patients undergoing colectomy for dysplasia have an occult invasive carcinoma in the colon. The current practice is to recommend resection if severe dysplasia is found or if any dysplasia associated with a mass or other lesions such as a stricture is found.[32]

Surgical options in the management of ulcerative colitis consist of proctocolectomy with ileostomy, ileoanal pull-through with ileal reservoir, or rarely abdominal colectomy and ileoproctostomy. The first two options are discussed elsewhere. Abdominal colectomy with ileorectal anastomosis has the advantage of removing the majority of diseased bowel and preserving anal sphincter function. The functional result after abdominal colectomy with ileorectal anastomosis appears to be somewhat better than that which follows ileoanal pull-through.[33] After construction of an ileorectal anastomosis, the ileoanal pull-through procedure remains an option if the patient subsequently develops recrudescence of disease in the rectum that necessitates proctectomy. The disadvantage of the procedure in ulcerative colitis is that it leaves the rectum, which may be a source of further symptoms and is also at risk of developing carcinoma. The ileorectal anastomosis is not a feasible option in patients who have an adenocarcinoma of the colon, as the incidence of carcinoma in the remaining rectal segment is higher than if there had been no cancer in the proximal bowel. This appears to also hold true if the resected colon exhibits only dysplasia.[34]

Crohn's Colitis

In the case of Crohn's disease, the risk of adenocarcinoma of the rectum is small. Most proctectomies performed after ileorectal anastomosis for Crohn's disease are done for recurrence in the rectal segment. If the recurrent disease is in the rectum, proctectomy will be necessary if medical treatment fails or for the usual indications, such as fistula. However, recurrence in the ileum proximal to the anastomosis is not uncommon, and in this situation resection of the ileum may be done with reanastomosis, and results may be good if the rectum remains relatively free of disease.

Patient selection for ileorectal anastomosis in the case of inflammatory bowel disease must be done carefully. The rectum should be supple with only mild mucosal changes, if any. Some surgeons do abdominal colectomy with ileorectal anastomosis on patients with a moderate amount of mucosal disease. Even these surgeons require that the rectum be compliant, because if the rectal wall is stiff, the functional results are uniformly bad. Other prerequisites are the absence of anal or perianal disease and good sphincter function. We do not think that any useful information is obtained by rectal biopsy, if the aforementioned criteria are adhered to.

Technique of Abdominal Colectomy

In the patient with ulcerative colitis, the ileum should be transected at the ileocecal valve. In Crohn's disease, if there is associated terminal ileal disease, the point of proximal resection should be selected, as described earlier. If there is a known carcinoma or a stricture that has not been adequately evaluated, the resection of that section of the colon should be a radical one with a complete lymphadenectomy. In the absence of carcinoma or the suspicion thereof, one should try to preserve the omentum by removing it from the transverse colon with cautery. There are no vascular attachments to the colon, and if the proper plane is identified, this should be a relatively bloodless manipulation.

An alternative method involves removal of the omentum. This modification is elected for fulminant colitis, for toxic megacolon, and for instances of walled-off perforations and/or abscesses of the transverse colon. In these situations, dissection of the omentum may lead to a tear of the colon with potentially catastrophic contamination. The right colon is mobilized, as previously described. At the hepatic flexure the duodenocolic ligament is encountered; it is merely the right lateral extension of the gastrocolic ligament. The duodenocolic ligament is divided between hemostats and suture-ligated, and access to the gastrocolic ligament is attained.

Usually the gastrocolic ligament is easily separated from the transverse mesocolon, and the gastrocolic ligament is serially divided between hemostats and suture-ligated. The point of division is inferior to the gastroepiploic vessels. This division is carried past the greater curvature of the stomach. If the gastrocolic ligament is adherent to the transverse mesocolon, these structures may be taken as one layer by utilizing small bites between hemostats and stout suture ligatures.

After the gastrocolic ligament has been divided to a point well to the left of the greater curvature of the stomach, this dissection is temporarily abandoned in favor of mobilization of the left colon, in order to approach the splenic flexure as the apex of a pyramid. The left colon is mobilized to the splenic flexure, and the subcutaneous coli divided. The lienocolic ligament is divided between hemostats and suture-ligated, and the gastrocolic ligament remaining from the previous dissection is encountered and similarly divided. When this dissection is complete, the origin of the omentum will have been completely divided (Fig. 8–8). The underlying transverse mesocolon becomes visible, and its vessels and the vessels of the right and left colon are individually divided and suture-ligated. It is recommended to divide these structures near the colon, so that a relatively long stump of mesentery remains. If a hematoma is observed, the remaining mesentery may be resecured and ligated proximal to the developing hemorrhage.

Experience dictates that the serial division of the omentum or the mesentery should not allow an accumulation of hemostats on the specimen. The weight or points of these instruments can tear a fragile and distended colon. It is preferable, therefore, to apply the hemostats, divide, and suture-ligate and to repeat the performance, so that the operative field will not become cluttered with potentially dangerous hardware.

In the omental sparing procedure the right colon is mobilized by incising the peritoneal reflection in the right gutter. Care is taken to keep the ureter away from danger. The mesentery is mobilized enough to facilitate its transection close to the bowel wall. Once the right colon has been mobilized, a similar incision is made in the left gutter, and the left colon is mobilized. This incision is taken up to the splenic flexure. At that point, gentle traction is put on the distal transverse colon and the proximal descending colon while the peritoneal covering of the mesentery is incised. In this manner, the mesentery can be "peeled away" from the investing peritoneum.

EDITORIAL COMMENT
The editors prefer to remove the omentum for several reasons at the time of colectomy. In the colitic patient, there are often numerous walled-off pericolic abscesses adjacent to the transverse colon. Dissection of the omentum may lead to local contamination or gross fecal spillage. In addition, the preserved omentum may have its blood supply compromised during dissection, leading to adhesions and small bowel obstruction after operation. For these reasons, we usually remove the omentum with the colon.

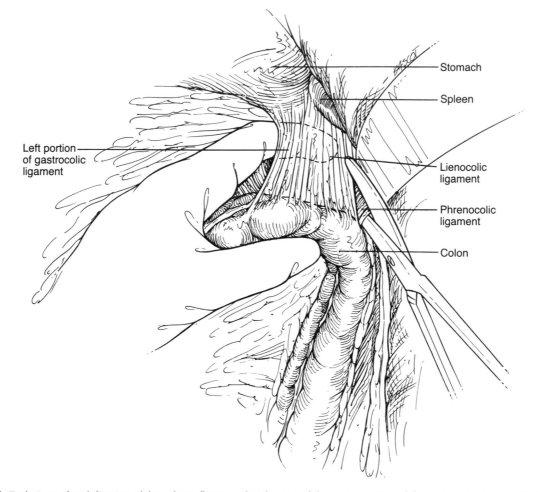

Figure 8–8. Technique of mobilization of the splenic flexure. After division of the major portion of the gastrocolic ligament between the stomach and colon and mobilization of the left colon by incision of the reflection of the parietal peritoneum, the visceral attachments are divided serially. Here the phrenocolic ligament, the lienocolic ligament, and finally the remainder of the gastrocolic ligament are divided, freeing the splenic flexure.

Abdominal colectomy with either enteroproctostomy or an endileostomy is an often-performed operation for a number of diseases. This operation may be discussed from the perspective of being an elective or an emergency procedure.

Colectomy with ileoproctostomy is indicated in Crohn's colitis with rectal sparing, pancolonic diverticulitis, various angiodysplasias, multiple polyposis, multicentric carcinoma, carcinoma of the colon in the young patient, and colonic dysmotility, among other conditions. It is a poor operation for ulcerative colitis, for which it is rarely performed and cannot be recommended. The retained rectum of the ulcerative colitic patient whose symptoms initially required colectomy is usually the site of recurrent disease and rarely a carcinoma.

Total abdominal colectomy performed as an emergency operation may be required for certain subsets of inflammatory bowel disease: fulminant colitis, toxic megacolon, or perforation. These patients are not candidates for either a total proctocolectomy or an endorectal pull-through operation because of the constitutional and local complications of the disease. In these emergency circumstances a total abdominal colectomy is performed, and the distal bowel is either closed as a Hartmann pouch or exteriorized as a mucous fistula. This choice is dictated by the condition of the rectum, the degree of contamination, and the condition of the patient. If the patient is found to have Crohn's disease and a diseased rectum, an eventual proctectomy is performed as a second procedure, usually via the perineal approach. If the rectum is free of disease, an ileorectal anastomosis may be accomplished at a later date. This option is best restricted to the patient who has at least 12 to 14 cm of disease-free rectum from the anal verge and whose terminal ileum has not been resected. A significant ileal resection and/or a short rectal stump will often result in incapacitating diarrhea. A full length of ileum and a long rectal stump are rarely associated with significant diarrhea.

If the patient has ulcerative colitis and has undergone abdominal colectomy as an emergency procedure, the rectum can be removed when the patient has recovered from the initial procedure, or an endorectal pull-through operation can be performed.

Total abdominal colectomy with or without anastomosis is a useful procedure for patients suffering from massive colonic hemorrhage, the exact site of which has not been identified. In this circumstance the surgeon encounters a distended colon filled with blood, and identification of the bleeding site is either impossible or impractical. An expeditious total colectomy is performed, care being taken to inspect the terminal ileum to rule out retained bleeding sites such as arteriovenous abnormalities. The decision to perform an anastomosis is predicated on three conditions: the cause of the bleeding (e.g., ulcerative colitis is a contraindication to anastomosis), the adequacy of preparation of the rectum, and the condition of the patient. The most common disease entities requiring abdominal colectomy for massive hemorrhage are diverticulitis or angiodysplasia in its various forms.

Once the entire colon is mobile, the mesentery is resected in close proximity to the bowel wall. The entire colon is removed down to the rectum. That point is where the bowel becomes circumferentially invested with a complete longitudinal muscle layer. In cases of inflammatory bowel disease, the mucosa of the rectum should be inspected to make sure that only minimal disease is present.

If an anastomosis is to be made, it is convenient to construct it by joining the side of the ileum to the end of the rectum (Fig. 8–9). Alternatively, an end-to-end ileorectal anastomosis may be fashioned. If this is done, it is usually necessary to make an antimesenteric slit in the terminal ileum (Fig. 8–10). If this procedure has been done as an emergency, it may be prudent to fashion an ileostomy rather than ileorectal anastomosis. This would be especially true in cases in which there is perforation with peritonitis or lower gastrointestinal bleeding and the patient has been in shock for any length of time.

Stoma Construction

In any surgical procedures in which there is a possibility of constructing a stoma, the patient's abdominal wall must be marked preoperatively so that the stoma may be placed in the optimal position. Enterocutaneous stomas should be brought through the rectus abdominis muscle, as the rate of parastomal hernia is greater when the stoma is brought out through the abdominal parietes lateral to the rectus muscle. One must bring the stoma through a scar-free part of the abdominal wall, because the scar may make it difficult to obtain a good seal with the faceplate of an ostomy appliance.

The stoma site should be chosen so that the appliance can be placed without abutting on bony prominences, such as the iliac crest or the rib cage. Most people have a fat roll just below the umbilicus, and in most patients a stoma placed on the crest of that roll brought through the outer third of the rectus abdominis muscle sheath will be in a good position. A template of a faceplate or an actual appliance faceplate can be used preoperatively to mark the patient, so that there is maximal contact between the faceplate of the appliance and the skin of the abdominal wall.

The site should be chosen first with the patient in the supine position and then with the patient in a sitting position. Often what appears to be an optimal site while the patient is lying down turns out to be in the middle of a crease or in an area not readily visible when the patient is sitting. In the case of emergency procedures, it is prudent to choose several sites, as one or another may be inaccessible because of the presence of an adjacent abscess or foreshortened mesentery that

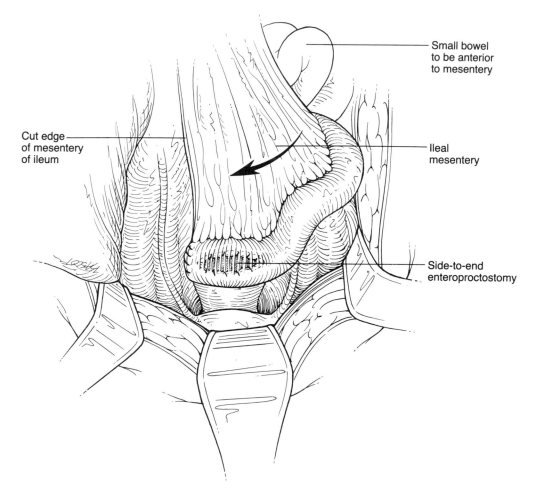

Cut edge of mesentery of ileum

Small bowel to be anterior to mesentery

Ileal mesentery

Side-to-end enteroproctostomy

Figure 8–9. Enteroproctostomy (ileoproctostomy), side-to-end technique. The ileum is closed, and the cut edge of the mesentery of the ileum is in the right lateral position. Upon completion of the side-to-end anastomosis, the small bowel is placed in its natural position anterior to the ileal mesentery.

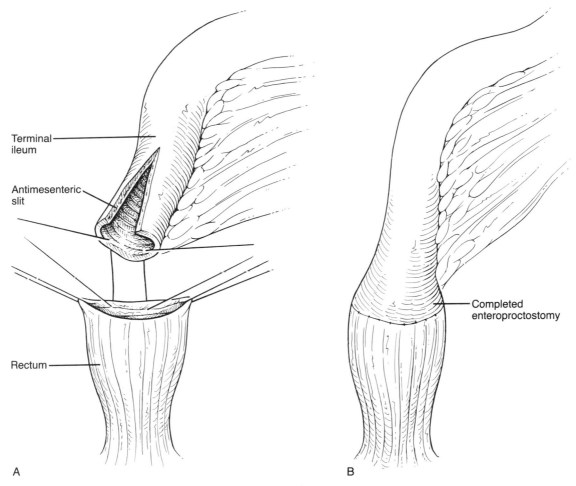

Terminal
ileum

Antimesenteric
slit

Rectum

A

Completed
enteroproctostomy

B

Figure 8–10. End-to-end enteroproctostomy. There is disparity between the lumen of the terminal ileum and the rectum. In order to make the two lumens approximately equal, an antimesenteric slit is fashioned on the antimesenteric portion of the terminal ileum. The corners of the slit are approximated to the edges of the rectum by full-thickness sutures as the first layer. *B,* Completed enteroproctostomy.

does not allow the bowel to be pulled through the abdominal wall. Once the site has been chosen, it should be marked with an indelible marker or a small subcuticular tattoo with methylene blue dye.

The ileostomy should be constructed as follows: a disk of skin no greater than 2 cm in diameter and usually the size of a 5-cent piece is excised at the previously chosen spot. A longitudinal incision is then made in the subcutaneous fat. When the anterior rectus abdominis muscle sheath is reached, the subcutaneous fat is retracted, and an ellipse of the anterior rectus abdominis muscle is excised. The anterior rectus sheath excision equals the diameter of the skin incision, but its width needs to be only about one third to one half of that size. A moist laparotomy pad is then placed underneath the rectus muscle and supported in the left hand while the rectus muscle is split in the direction of its fibers. Retractors are inserted to hold the muscle apart, and the posterior rectus sheath and the perito-

neum are incised again in a longitudinal direction. The laparotomy pad held firmly against the posterior surface of the peritoneum protects the viscera and the surgeon's hand from injury. The aperture should be stretched to easily admit two fingers. Four to five centimeters of ileum should be pulled through the cutaneous opening, so that when the bowel is inverted the ileostomy will be 2 cm in length.

Once the ileum is pulled through, the mesentery of the protruding bowel is trimmed. One should be circumspect about trimming the mesentery of a patient whose bowel has previously been irradiated or who is critically ill and in whom a low-flow state is anticipated. The mesentery is then secured to the posterior rectus sheath (transverse layer), with care taken not to interfere with the vessels within the mesentery. A few sutures may be placed between the seromuscular layer of the ileum and the anterior rectus sheath or Scarpa's fascia to prevent retraction.

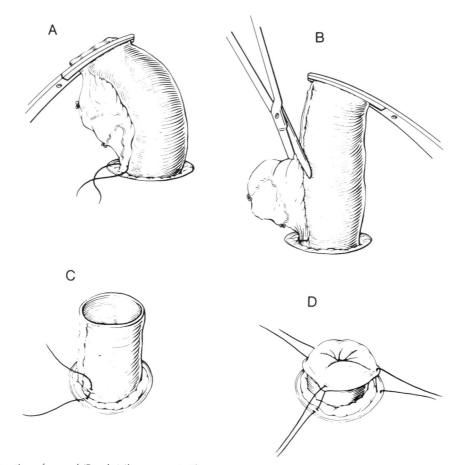

Figure 8–11. Construction of an end (Brooke) ileostomy. *A,* The excess mesentery is trimmed, care being taken not to injure the nutrient vessels of the ileum. *B,* Full-thickness bite of the wall of the terminal ileum is taken, and the second bite includes the muscularis of the terminal ileum at the base of the ileostomy. The final bite is in the subcuticular dermis. *C,* Attention is applied to each suture, serially everting the outer layer of the ileostomy. *D,* Completed eversion for the Brooke ileostomy, which should be approximately 2 cm in height.

EDITORIAL COMMENT

In the description of ileostomy construction, the authors advocate securing the seromuscular layer to either the anterior rectus sheath or Scarpa's fascia. The editors rely only on the fixation of the small bowel mesentery to the transverse layer of the posterior rectus sheath adjacent to the stomal exit. Further suturing is unnecessary and may be meddlesome.

An attractive alternative to the standard ileostomy described in the text is the extraperitoneal ileostomy advocated by Goligher. In this technique the lateral parietal peritoneum on the right is dissected laterally, and the stomal site is made through all layers of the abdominal wall, except the peritoneum. The terminal ileum and its mesentery are tunneled under the elevated peritoneum and made to exit through the stomal wound. This method of ileostomy construction does not lead to a right lateral defect, eliminates the need for closure, and avoids a potential site for internal hernia.

At this point the space between the ileum and the right gutter should be closed. This can be done with a pursestring suture or by sewing the cut edge of the right colon mesentery to the anterior abdominal wall up to the ligamentum terres. After the laparotomy wound is closed, the ileostomy is matured by placing absorbable sutures through the full thickness of the ileum and the subcuticular layer of skin (Fig. 8–11). Occasionally, because of a foreshortened mesentery or a thick abdominal wall, one is not able to bring the ileostomy up to the skin level. In this situation, a loop end-ileostomy may be constructed. This affords several extra centimeters of length, and the stoma can be made without tension. The cutaneous and fascial openings are created in exactly the same way as is done with the end-ileostomy, and a point is chosen several centimeters from the end of the ileum to bring through the abdominal wall aperture. This point should be chosen so that there is maximal length of the mesentery there. A Penrose drain is then put through the mesentery, and the loop is gently brought through the abdominal wall (Fig. 8–12). Once the loop is brought through the abdominal wall, the Penrose drain is replaced with a small plastic ileostomy rod. When the

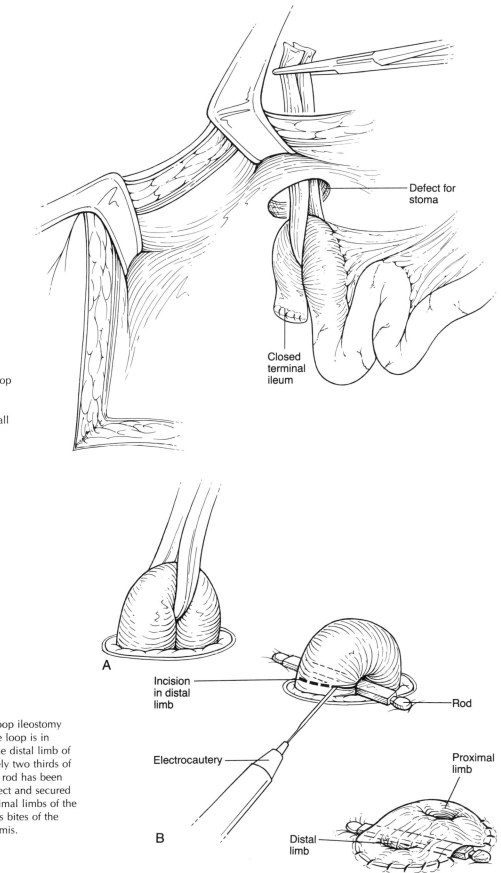

Figure 8–12. Construction of a loop ileostomy. The terminal ileum is closed and brought through the defect in the anterior abdominal wall with a Penrose drain. (See Fig. 8–13.)

Figure 8–13. Construction of a loop ileostomy (continued from Fig. 8–12). *A,* The loop is in place. *B,* An incision is made in the distal limb of the ileostomy incising approximately two thirds of the circumference of the bowel. A rod has been placed through the mesenteric defect and secured to the skin. *C,* The distal and proximal limbs of the stoma are attached as full-thickness bites of the bowel wall to the subcuticular dermis.

rod is in place, a transverse incision is made at the skin level in the distal part of the loop (Fig. 8–13). Sutures are placed between the distal cut edge of the bowel and the skin. The sutures should be placed in the subcuticular layer. When the distal loop is thus secured, sutures are placed through the cut edge of the proximal part of the loop. These sutures are placed in the subcuticular layer of skin as well, thus inverting the proximal part of the stoma and creating a spout. It is important that the transverse incision in the ileum be made over 80% of the circumference of the ileum. If this is not done, the proximal part of the loop will not evert easily. The rod is fastened to the skin with a suture, so it does not become displaced. It is left there usually for a period of 7 days. An appliance is placed over the rod and stoma.

REFERENCES

1. Farmer RG, Whelan G, Fazio VW. Long-term follow-up of patients with Crohn's disease. Gastroenterology 1985;88:1818–1825.
2. Mekhjian HS, Switz DM, Watts HD, et al. National Cooperative Crohn's Disease Study: Factors determining recurrence of Crohn's disease after surgery. Gastroenterology 1979;77:907–913.
3. Bergman L, Krause U. Crohn's disease: A long-term study of the clinical course in 186 patients. Scand J Gastroenterol 1977;12:937–944.
4. Meyers S, Walfish JS, Sachar DB, et al. Quality of life after surgery for Crohn's disease: A psychosocial survey. Gastroenterology 1980;78:1–6.
5. Broe PJ, Bayless TM, Cameron JL. Crohn's disease: Are enteroenteral fistulas an indication for surgery? Surgery 1982;91:249–253.
6. Ellis L, Calhoun P, Kaiser DL, et al. Postoperative recurrence in Crohn's disease. Ann Surg 1984;199:340–347.
7. Trnka YM, Glotzer DJ, Kasdon EJ, et al. The long-term outcome of restorative operation in Crohn's disease: Influence of location, prognostic factors, and surgical guidelines. Ann Surg 1982;196:345–355.
8. Heuman R, Boeryd B, Bolin T, Sjodahl R. The influence of disease at the margin of resection on the outcome of Crohn's disease. Br J Surg 1983;70:519–521.
9. Wolff BG, Beart RW, Frydenberg HB, et al. The importance of disease-free margins in resections for Crohn's disease. Dis Colon Rectum 1983;26:239–243.
10. Hamilton SR, Reese J, Pennington L, et al. The role of resection margin frozen section in the surgical management of Crohn's disease. Surg Gynecol Obstet 1985;160:57–62.
11. Block GE, Schraut WH. The operative treatment of Crohn's enteritis complicated by ileosigmoid fistula. Ann Surg 1982;196:356–360.
12. Fazio VW, Galandiuk S, Jagelman DG, Lavery IC. Strictureplasty in Crohn's disease. Ann Surg 1989;210:621–625.
13. Sayfan J, Wilson DAL, Allan A, et al. Strictureplasty or resection for Crohn's disease. Br J Surg 1989;76:335–338.
14. Allan A, Andrews H, Hiltin CJ, et al. Segmental colonic resection is an appropriate operation for short skip lesions due to Crohn's disease in the colon. World J Surg 1989;13:611–616.
15. Wolff BG, Ready RL, MacCarty RL, et al. Influence of sigmoid resection on progression of diverticular disease of the colon. Dis Colon Rectum 1984;27:645–647.
16. Benn PL, Wolff BG, Ilstrup DM. Level of anastomosis and recurrent colonic diverticulitis. Am J Surg 1986;151:269–271.
17. Stabile BE, Puccio E, van Sonnenberg E, Neff CC. Preoperative percutaneous drainage of diverticular abscesses. Am J Surg 1990;159:99–105.
18. Goldman SM, Fishman EK, Gatewood OMB, et al. CT demonstration of colovesical fistulae secondary to diverticulitis. J Comput Assist Tomogr 1984;8:462–468.
19. Landreneau RJ, Fry WJ. The right colon as a target organ of nonocclusive mesenteric ischemia. Arch Surg 1990;125:591–594.
20. Ottinger LW, Darling RC, Nathan MJ, Linton RR. Left colon ischemia complicating aorto-iliac reconstruction. Arch Surg 1971;105:841–846.
21. Bandyk DF, Florence MG, Johansen KH. Colon ischemia accompanying ruptured abdominal aortic aneurysm. J Surg Res 1981;30:297–303.
22. Schroeder J, Christoffersen JK, Andersen J, et al. Ischemic colitis complicating reconstruction of the abdominal aorta. Surg Gynecol Obstet 1985;160:299–3303.
23. Scowcroft CW, Sanowski RA, Kozarek RA. Colonoscopy in ischemic colitis. Gastrointest Endosc 1981;27:156–161.
24. Kistin MG, Kaplan MM, Harrington JT. Diffuse ischemic colitis associated with systemic lupus erythematosus—response to subtotal colectomy. 1978;75:1147–1151.
25. Wood MK, Read DR, Kraft AR, Barreta TM. A rare cause of ischemic colitis: Polyarteritis nodosa. Dis Colon Rectum 1979;22:428–433.
26. Terry BG, Beart RW. Emergency abdominal colectomy with primary anastomosis. Dis Colon Rectum 1981;24:1–4.
27. Scott HW, Weaver FA, Fletcher JR, et al. Is ileoproctostomy a reasonable procedure after total abdominal colectomy? Ann Surg 1986;203:583–588.
28. Greenstein AJ, Sachar DB, Smith H, et al. Patterns of neoplasia in Crohn's disease and ulcerative colitis. Cancer 1980;46:403–407.
29. Greenstein AJ, Sachar DB, Smith H, et al. Cancer in universal and left-sided ulcerative colitis: Factors determining risk. Gastroenterology 1979;77:290–294.
30. Devroede H, Taylor WF. On calculating cancer risk and survival of ulcerative colitis patients with the life table method. Gastroenterology 1976;71:505–509.
31. Morson BC, Pang LSC. Rectal biopsy as an aid to cancer control in ulcerative colitis. Gut 1967;8:423–434.
32. Dobbins WP. Dysplasia and malignancy in inflammatory bowel disease. Ann Rev 1984;35:33–48.
33. Leijonmarck CE, Lofberg R, Ost A, Hellers G. Long-term results of ileorectal anastomosis in ulcerative colitis in Stockholm County. Dis Colon Rectum 1990;33:195–200.
34. Grundfest SF, Fazio V, Weiss RA, et al. The risk of cancer following colectomy and ileorectal anastomosis for extensive mucosal ulcerative colitis. Ann Surg 1980;193:9–14.

Proctocolectomy

Roland F. Parc
Pierre M. Balladur
George E. Block
A. R. Moossa

The term *inflammatory bowel disease* (IBD) is employed in this chapter in its customary restrictive sense, to include only ulcerative colitis and granulomatous (Crohn's) colitis. However, several other inflammatory disorders of the large bowel, including tuberculous infections, amebic dysentery, parasitic infestations, *Salmonella* colitis, *Campylobacter* infections, antibiotic-associated pseudomembranous colitis due to *Clostridium difficile,* radiation-induced proctocolitis, ischemic colitis, and complicated diverticular disease of the colon, all may share many of the pathologic and clinical features of IBD and must be considered in the differential diagnosis. Indeed, some of these conditions are often mistaken for IBD (or vice versa), and the diagnosis is subsequently reversed.

Until the 1980s, the accepted standard operation for ulcerative colitis or Crohn's colitis was panproctocolectomy with a permanent spout (Brooke) ileostomy. An enormous amount of experience with this procedure, has been accumulated, and it can now be performed very safely with negligible mortality and minimal morbidity in an elective situation. Proper understanding of the management of stomal therapy, advances in stomal therapy, and development of diverse appliances have made the standard spout ileostomy a routine and safe procedure and a satisfactory option for most practicing surgeons.

Patient dissatisfaction with the spout ileostomy has always centered around various cosmetic, social, psychological, and sexual disadvantages and connotations. As a result, in the late 1960s, Kock of Sweden developed a reservoir (Kock) continent ileostomy, which was hailed as a major advance. The continent ileostomy construction can be done in one stage in conjunction with the proctocolectomy or as a later conversion from a Brooke ileostomy. The mortality rate is low, and the main problem with the Kock ileostomy centers on complications resulting from disruption of the nipple valve.[1, 2] A reoperation rate of 10% to 15% over a 5-year period is still reported. In spite of many technical modifications to prevent the nipple valve from sliding, that is, staples across the valve and synthetic mesh around the outlet, valve failure is common. Reservoir ileitis (pouchitis), probably due to stagnant bacterial overgrowth, is also encountered. The operation should not be performed in a patient with Crohn's disease or in an obese patient in whom technical difficulties may pose additional risks. The Kock ileostomy has not retained its popularity; this is because of the relatively high rate of complications and reoperation, the inconvenience of intubation and irrigation, and the mere presence of a stoma, however inconspicuously placed and constructed.

WHEN SHOULD THE RECTUM BE PRESERVED?

Rectal preservation is desirable, whenever feasible, in any patient. In an elective operation, it is applicable only to some 5% to 10% of patients with ulcerative colitis and to some 30% of patients with Crohn's colitis when the rectum is either disease free or only minimally affected. Total abdominal colectomy and ileorectal anastomosis, in one or two stages, is a reasonable choice, provided that the following conditions are satisfied:

1. The rectum is spared as assessed by proctoscopic examination.

2. The patient does not have active perianal disease.

3. There is good anal sphincter function.

4. The patient is young and well motivated.

5. The ileum has not been excised, or only a few centimeters of ileum has been removed.

6. The patient has a reasonable expectation of about three to six bowel movements a day and possibly one bowel movement at night.

7. The patient agrees to careful rectal surveillance for life in order to assess disease recurrence or neoplastic change, which is especially critical for the patient with chronic ulcerative colitis. Thus, patient compliance is paramount.

For Crohn's colitis, the failure rate of ileorectal anastomosis is between 25% and 50%. In our experience, the 5-year actuarial survival rate of ileorectal anastomosis is 74% for Crohn's colitis. For ulcerative colitis, the failure rate after ileorectal anastomosis, in our experience, is 25%.[11] However, the functional results of an ileorectal anastomosis are better than those reported for an ileal pouch–anal anastomosis.

Rectal excision should not be entertained in the emergency setting in cases such as toxic megacolon, colonic perforation, and fulminant colitis. A total abdominal colectomy with the construction of a Brooke ileostomy should be performed. The distal sigmoid colon is preferably brought out as a sigmoid mucous fistula in the left iliac fossa. Alternatively, if the sigmoid colon is severely affected and necrotic, it should be excised, necessitating a Hartmann closure and extraperitonealization of the upper rectum. The rectum's stump is drained transanally. Once the patient has fully recovered from the acute process, a second operation can be performed a few months later to remove the rectum, to perform an ileorectal anastomosis, or to perform a rectal mucosectomy and an ileal pouch–anal anastomosis as a sphincter-saving procedure. These procedures are described in the subchapters by Utsunomiya and Yamamura and by Harford and Pickleman. If a second-stage proctectomy is elected, the Brooke ileostomy may occasionally be converted into a Kock (reservoir) ileostomy, if the patient so desires.

EMERGENCY OPERATIONS FOR COLITIS

The goal of any operative procedure in an urgent or emergency situation is to save the patient's life and to preserve the possibility of a rectal or sphincter-saving procedure in the future. The treatment strategy should encompass diagnosis, appreciation of the disease's severity, and the development of complications.

Diagnosis

In 25% to 75% of patients with severe colitis, the acute colitis may be the first manifestation of the disease before an exact diagnosis has been made. As previously mentioned, infectious causes of colitis, such as *Salmonella* infection, pseudomembranous colitis, *Campylobacter jejuni* colitis, and ischemic colitis, may present with the same clinical features as ulcerative or Crohn's colitis. They must be identified and appropriately treated. Nonetheless, bacteriologic confirmation of these infections may take 48 to 72 hours, and this should not delay the recuscitative and treatment measures described later. The precise differentiation between ulcerative and Crohn's colitis is not important at this stage, because the emergency treatment of both conditions is the same.

Even if the diagnosis of ulcerative or Crohn's colitis is already established, a superinfection with, for example, *Salmonella, Clostridium difficile,* cytomegalovirus (CMV), or amebiasis must be considered and excluded. Again, these situations occur only rarely, and their identification should not delay appropriate therapy.

Appreciation of the Severity of the Disease

Two forms of attack can be clinically recognized. The *mild or moderate attack* is characterized by less than four bloody bowel movements per day, no fever, no tachycardia, and only moderate anemia. If treatment is appropriate, the prognosis is excellent. The criteria generally accepted to define a *severe attack* of colitis are as follows: (a) more than six bowel movements daily, (b) grossly bloody stools, (c) fever greater than 37.8°C, (d) tachycardia greater than 90 beats/min, (e) anemia with a hemoglobin concentration less than 75% of normal, and (f) a sedimentation rate greater than 30 mm/hour.

These criteria, on initial presentation of the patient, are useful parameters for identifying a high-risk group. The progression of these criteria is the indication for surgical intervention.

Quantification of the intensity of these criteria is difficult and variable, because there are many intermediary stages between the simple attack and the fulminant or toxic colitis. Because there is no clear stratification of acute colitis, we have adopted the notion of the most severe acute or fulminant colitis, introduced by others,[22] which includes any four of the following criteria: (1) more than 10 stools per 24 hours, (2) tachycardia in excess of 120 beats/min, (3) fever exceeding 38.5°C for at least 3 days, (4) weight loss of more than 10%, (5) serum cholesterol less than 1 g/l, (6) presence of abdominal tenderness or distention, and (7) radiographic findings of a paralytic ileus or colonic dilatation.

Development of Complications

Several life-threatening complications may supervene as part of an acute fulminant colitis.

Toxic Megacolon

Toxic megacolon is defined as a severe colitis with total or segmental dilatation of the colon. The term "toxic" implies that at least three of the following four criteria are present: (1) fever greater than 38.5°C, (2) tachycardia greater than 120 beats/min, (3) leukocytosis greater than 10,000/mm³, (4) hemoglobin concentration less than 60% of normal. In addition, one of the four following conditions must be present: dehydration, mental changes, electrolyte disturbance, and hypotension.[12] Fazio uses similar criteria for the definition of the term toxic and defines megacolon as the condition in which the diameter of the colon is more than 5 cm with loss of haustral markings.[13] Thus, the clinical picture and the x-ray film of the abdomen are sufficient to make the diagnosis. Proctoscopy *without* air insufflation may show inflammation of the mucosa, pus, and blood and, less frequently, lesions suggestive of Crohn's or ulcerative colitis. A full sigmoidoscopy, colonoscopy, or barium enema is *contraindicated* because of the risk of perforation. Furthermore, none is essential for the diagnosis of toxic megacolon. Anticholinergics and opiates are to be avoided because they may exacerbate any tendency toward colonic dilatation.

Colonic Perforation

Colonic perforation is the most lethal of all complications. In a report from the French Association of Surgery, a series of 697 patients with ulcerative colitis treated between 1960 and 1983 showed that 21% of patients who underwent emergency operations had perforation of the colon (11.4% with free perforation, 6.8% with sealed perforation, and 2.8% with iatrogenic perforation occurring during operation). The mortality rate was 41.6% for free perforation into the peritoneal cavity.[14] Free perforation is less frequent in Crohn's disease, and surgeons are more frequently faced with internal fistulas (to the small bowel or to the bladder) or localized abdominal abscesses.

The diagnosis of perforation and peritonitis may be difficult to achieve, especially in patients who are receiving large amounts of corticosteroids. Thus, any change in the clinical picture or any deterioration of the general condition must immediately be evaluated with an abdominal x-ray film and serious consideration given to emergency operation.

PRINCIPLES OF MEDICAL MANAGEMENT OF ACUTE COLITIS

Moderately Severe Attack

During a moderately severe attack, the treatment is as follows:

1. Hospitalization and rest in bed

2. Low-residue, high-calorie diet, if the patient is able to tolerate oral intake; often, supplemental or total parenteral nutrition

3. Corticosteroid enemas twice a day, with care taken to minimize the risk of perforation

4. Oral corticosteroid therapy 0.5 mg/kg body weight daily

5. Sulfasalazine 4.0 g/24 hr

6. Metronidazole 1.0 g/24 hr

The patient is carefully monitored with emphasis placed on stool frequency and nature (blood, pus); vital signs (pulse, temperature, blood pressure); abdominal examination every 6 hours; flat plate of the abdomen every 24 hours; and a regular check on the white cell count, hemoglobin, and sedimentation rate.

Failure of the patient to improve significantly is an indication for urgent or semiurgent surgical intervention.

Fulminant Attack

During a fulminant attack of colitis, diagnostic and resuscitative measures should be carried out simultaneously and as rapidly as possible. These patients are extremely ill, and the majority require operation on the day of admission. Thus, medical management is synonymous with preoperative resuscitation, and these patients must be admitted to a close observation unit.

Large-bore intravenous catheters, including a central venous pressure line, are inserted for fluid administration and monitoring of right atrial pressure. A nasogastric tube is inserted and connected to suction. A Foley catheter is inserted in the urinary bladder to monitor urine output. A significant extracellular fluid volume deficit invariably exists in this situation and is often accompanied by hypoalbuminemia and decreased oncotic pressure. Infusion of electrolyte solution with salt-free albumin, supplementary potassium, and blood transfusion are often indicated. The goal of fluid administration is to replace the volume deficit and to restore the oncotic pressure. Restoration of circulating blood volume is evident by a rising right atrial pressure, diminution of pulse rate, rise in blood pressure, and a urine output of at least 40 ml/hr. Frequent monitoring of all vital signs is essential for adequate resuscitation without fluid overload, especially in elderly patients. If there is a significant metabolic acidosis, sodium bicarbonate is administered intravenously. Mild to moderate acidosis usually responds to volume replacement alone. *A severe or persistent metabolic acidosis is usually indicative of colon perforation.*

Most patients experiencing a fulminant attack have already received steroid therapy. We prefer to administer 100 mg of intravenous hydrocortisone initially and to replace this dose at least every 4 hours. Blood cultures are drawn prior to starting broad-spectrum antibiotic coverage. A combination of a cephalosporin with metronidazole or an aminoglycoside is usually recommended. Prophylactic low-dose antifungal therapy may be started at this juncture, if it is deemed advisable.

Factors known to precipitate toxic dilatation are carefully avoided. Anticholinergic drugs, opiate derivatives, and diagnostic barium enemas are notorious offenders. If the patient can tolerate a proctoscopy, it can be performed at the bedside without air insufflation. Stools for Gram stains and cultures are obtained at that time.

These intensive resuscitative measures invariably result in an improvement of the patient's general condition within a few hours. *This should not lull the physician into a false sense of security.* The improvement is the direct result of correction of the blood and fluid and electrolyte deficits, and the diseased colon still has a great propensity to dilate and/or to perforate at any time. Even before gross perforation, there is transudation of bacteria across the diseased, thinned wall of the colon into the peritoneal cavity. Thus, the majority of these patients have peritoneal sepsis. Gross perforation tends to occur subtly at a slow pace in this setting and may be difficult to diagnose. It is suggested that one consider urgent operation at this stage. Immediate operative intervention is mandatory if the patient's condition deteriorates, as evidenced by signs of volume deficit, rise in temperature and/or white cell

count, persistence of the metabolic acidosis by arterial blood-gas measurements, and any increase in abdominal tenderness or distention.

When toxic dilatation of the colon supervenes in an attack of fulminant colitis, the exact duration of medical treatment becomes debatable and has to be individualized for each case. Some workers have obtained a remission rate as high as 64% with medical treatment alone, but the mortality rate was 22%. Other authors have reported a mortality rate ranging from 6% to 30% when colectomy was performed *after* failure of medical treatment for a few days. There is no doubt that delaying operation increases the risk of perforation—an operative mortality rate in excess of 80% has been reported in cases of established colonic perforation. In a study from a Mt. Sinai hospital, the operative mortality rate was 2% for toxic megacolon, but increased to 44% in cases of free perforation.[15] Our collective experience in Paris, Chicago, and San Diego confirms the Mt. Sinai experience.

Even when medical management is successful, the long-term outcome is disappointing. In a retrospective study conducted by Grant and Dozois at the Mayo Clinic, 30% of the patients who improved on medical management had a relapse of the toxic megacolon, and 44% needed an emergency operation for a subsequent severe attack.[16] In The Cleveland Clinic experience as reported by Fazio, only 7 of 115 patients with toxic megacolon were successfully treated medically, but 5 of these 7 patients eventually needed colectomy.[12]

Emergency Operation for Fulminant Colitis

We do not recommend the Turnbull "blow-hole" procedure, whereby an ileostomy and two decompressing colostomies are performed.[17] In our experience with toxic megacolon it is an inadequate operation and makes subsequent operations exceedingly difficult. Our preference in these poor-risk patients is to perform a total abdominal colectomy with an ileostomy. A large atraumatic tube inserted through the terminal ileum facilitates the dissection by deflating the colon. The rectosigmoid is brought out as a mucous fistula. If the lower sigmoid colon is friable and necrotic, it is excised, and we oversew the rectum as a Hartmann procedure and extraperitonealize it. These extremely ill, toxic, malnourished, and anemic patients can ill afford the additional stress, operating time, and blood loss of a proctectomy. Hence, we perform a one-stage proctocolectomy in the emergency setting only in *rare* situations such as intractable hemorrhagic proctitis and iatrogenic perforation of a diseased rectum.[18] The Mt. Sinai Hospital in New York suggests that when hemorrhage is the sole indication for subtotal colectomy, there is a 12% risk of continuing bleeding from the

---

EDITORIAL COMMENT

The principles of surgical treatment of colorectal IBD have evolved substantially over the past 2 decades and are now fairly well established, as outlined in this chapter. The operative mortality rate has decreased appreciably to well under 5% in the emergency setting and under 1% in the elective situation.

In the emergency setting rectal preservation is the rule, irrespective of the exact tissue diagnosis (Crohn's disease or ulcerative colitis). This provides the surgeon with the option of rectal and/or sphincter preservation at a later date. In the elective situation the surgeon has five basic operative procedures to choose from: (1) total proctocolectomy with a Brooke ileostomy in one or two stages; (2) total proctocolectomy with a Kock ileostomy in one or two stages; (3) total colectomy with ileorectal anastomosis in one or two stages; (4) total colectomy with mucosal proctectomy and ileal pouch–anal anastomosis in one or two stages; and (5) conversion of a Brooke ileostomy to a Kock reservoir. It is clear that the patient with granulomatous colitis has fewer choices, because the Kock ileostomy and the ileal pouch–anal anastomosis are contraindicated for this disease. For the patient with indeterminate colitis for which an exact histologic label cannot be agreed on, the surgeon may elect to treat the patient as if the diagnosis were ulcerative colitis and wait. It has become mandatory for the surgeon to explain these options and carefully discuss their pros and cons with the patient and/or relatives before designing a surgical strategy. Both the surgeon and patient should remember that although anorectal sphincter preservation is always a desirable goal, it should never become an irrational obsession.

rectum.[19] Irrigation of the rectal stump with adrenaline chloride in saline solution at 4° to 6°C is sometimes successful in controlling the hemorrhage and may help to avoid an emergency proctectomy.[20]

As a result of our policy of early operative intervention, as described, the mortality rate from fulminant colitis has decreased dramatically and no patient has died over the past decade or so. The morbidity rates for emergency operation are still substantial: 7% for a severe attack and 19% for a fulminant attack. Common complications include intraperitoneal fluid collections, peritonitis, wound infection, wound dehiscence and evisceration, and retraction of the mucous fistula. This last complication is avoidable if a sufficient length of the sigmoid is brought out without tension.

ONE-STAGE TOTAL PROCTOCOLECTOMY

Total proctocolectomy with a terminal ileostomy remains the gold standard against which all other operations should be measured. The operation is largely confined to the elective setting for patients with Crohn's colitis and those with ulcerative colitis who are not candidates for a sphincter-saving procedure. The usual indications for elective operation include fear of or development of neoplastic changes, failure of medical management, recurrent flare-ups of bloody diarrhea, chronic debilitation, intolerance of medical management, and the unbearable perineal complications of fistulas, abscesses, and anal incontinence.

The risk of neoplastic transformation often worries the patient with colitis and the physician because of delay in diagnosis. The symptoms of colitic cancer often mimic those of a flare-up of the inflammatory disease. Thus, colorectal cancer in IBD carries a poor prognosis, largely because it is often poorly differentiated and multicentric in origin. The generally quoted five-year survival rate is about 36%. The risk of colorectal cancer is small during the first 10 years of the disease but increases markedly thereafter. Cumulative cancer risk is estimated as 3% at 10 years, 5% to 24% between 10 and 20 years, and 11% to 34% between 20 and 30 years; it can reach 43% after 20 years. Careful and regular surveillance is mandatory for patients with long-standing IBD. If random biopsies of the colorectal mucosa show severe and multiple dysplasia, the patient should be strongly advised to have an operation before frank neoplasia supervenes.

The aim of the operation is to remove the entire diseased colon and rectum and to spare the small intestines. The surgeon should avoid technical complications such as hemorrhage, sepsis (usually by fecal spillage), and damage to the nervi erigentes, which leads to sexual dysfunction in the male patient. The surgeon should preserve abdominal anatomic relationships by appropriate closure of the resulting lateral and inferior defects created by the proctocolectomy.[21]

Patient Positioning

Patient positioning is essential to facilitating access and exposure throughout the operation (Fig. 8–14). We prefer to place the patient in a modified lithotomy position. The hips are flexed no more than 30 degrees in order not to interfere with access to the abdomen. The thighs are abducted no more than 30 degrees because the perineal dissection is limited for benign disease. The coccyx must be easily palpable at the

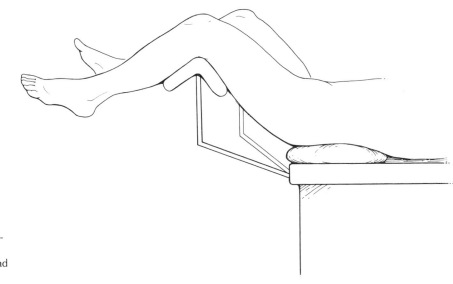

Figure 8–14. Positioning of patient for one-stage proctocolectomy with emphasis on degree of hip and knee flexion and sacral pad to elevate the buttocks and perineum.

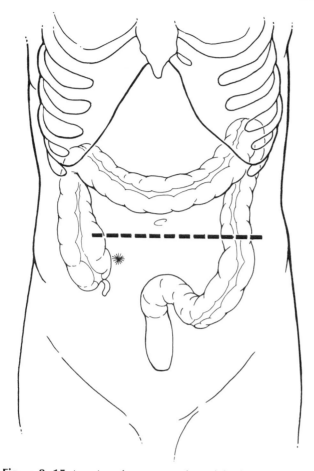

Figure 8–15. Location of transverse infra-umbilical incision and proposed site of ileostomy.

lower edge of the table distal to the pad, which is placed under the sacrum. The fibulas and sacrum are protected to avoid excessive pressure on the peroneal nerves and on the skin.

We routinely fill the rectum with a pack soaked in povidone-iodine (Betadine) solution, and the anus is tightly closed with a pursestring suture. This prevents fecal soilage during the pelvic dissection. The site of the ileostomy, selected often in conjunction with the stoma therapist before the operation is performed, is marked with waterproof ink.

Selection of the stoma site (Fig. 8–15) must be meticulously performed to avoid bony prominences, skin folds, and scars or fistulous orifices, because it must serve the patient for the remainder of his or her life. The ileostomy is usually in the right lower quadrant over the body of the rectus abdominis muscle. It is important to avoid constructing a stoma lateral to the edge of the rectus sheath, because this location is often associated with a parastomal hernia.

The abdominal incision has to be generous and must provide access to all recesses of the abdomen and pelvis. It must not interfere with the eventual stoma placement and must offer security against wound complications, such as dehiscence and hernia. On the basis of the patient's anatomic structure, we choose between a transverse infra-umbilical incision (Fig. 8–15) or a vertical midline incision from xiphisternum to pubic symphysis.

Initial Mobilization

We usually start our dissection on the right side of the abdomen, but depending on the anatomic characteristics encountered at laparotomy, the initial mobilization may be started anywhere along the colon. The cecum and right colon are gently retracted to the left of the patient, and the parietal peritoneum lateral to the cecum and ascending colon is incised along the white line of Toldt. This incision is carried superiorly to the hepatic flexure and inferiorly to free the right lateral portion of the root of the mesentery of the small intestine. In this way, the distal ileum, cecum, and right colon can be freed from the posterior abdominal wall, protecting the right ureter, right gonadal vessels, and inferior vena cava.

The gastrocolic ligament is identified at the superior portion of the ascending colon, and its division allows mobilization of the hepatic flexure and access to the gastrocolic ligament on the right side. Division of this ligament between hemostats avoids troublesome bleeding. With the left hand, the operator retracts the superior portion of the colon and protects it from injury, and with division of the fusion fascia and reflection of the hepatic flexure, identifies and avoids the second portion of the duodenum and head of pancreas. Further division of the fusion fascia by using a mixture of sharp and blunt dissection allows complete mobilization of the right colon and complete separation of the right side of the transverse mesocolon from the duodenum. Throughout the operation, all hemostats, which are serially applied, are immediately and individually ligated, because the weight or the points of the hemostats may tear or perforate a thin, dilated colon and initiate fecal spillage.

Mobilization of the Transverse Colon and Splenic Flexure

The surgeon should decide whether the transverse mesocolon and the gastrocolic ligament can be divided separately or can be taken together as one layer. If the patient is thin with little paracolic and mesenteric fat and inflammation, the surgeon may elect to divide the two layers of the transverse mesocolon and the gastrocolic ligament together as one layer. This has the advantage of rapidity and closure of the lesser sac. If, however, the greater omentum or transverse mesocolon is thickened with fat or local inflammation, the two layers should be taken separately.

The mesenteric window on the right side of the transverse mesocolon is developed and incised between the ileocolic and right branch of the middle colic vessels, and the finger of the surgeon may explore the retromesenteric recess. The ileocolic vessels are preserved until the abdominal portion of the operation is terminated, to prevent ischemic perforation of a diseased cecum.

We prefer to remove the entire greater omentum and leave it wrapped around the transverse colon. Some surgeons preserve the omentum, but we find that its dissection from the transverse colon may result in fecal spillage or opening into a walled-off abscess. In addition, a potentially ischemic omentum may cause small intestinal obstruction during the postoperative period.

The transverse mesocolon or gastrocolic omentum is serially transected from right to left, and the vessels are suture-ligated with nonabsorbable sutures, such as 2-0 or 3-0 silk. We prefer to transect the various mesenteric vessels and leave a 3- to 4-cm stump of mesentery, so that if a hematoma accidentally forms, there is a convenient length of mesentery to religate. This dissection continues to the splenic flexure, where the greater omentum and transverse mesocolon separate from each other. This separation is most apparent at the greater curvature of the stomach, and at this point the two layers *must* be divided and ligated *separately*.

The secret of safe mobilization of the splenic flexure is to be aware of the relative contributions of the transverse mesocolon and the greater omentum to that area. We prefer to approach the splenic flexure as the apex of a pyramid. After mobilizing and freeing the transverse colon close to the splenic flexure, attention is directed to the descending and upper sigmoid colon to free their lateral attachments *before* attacking the splenic flexure proper. The lateral parietal attachment of the sigmoid colon is again incised and divided over the white line of Toldt. Care is taken not to dissect posteriorly to avoid developing a plane posterior to Gerota's fascia. This incision is carried superiorly to the region of the splenic flexure. Small collateral vessels are often encountered beneath the peritoneum of the inflamed colon and should be coagulated or clipped before division is performed.

Thus, with division of the peritoneal attachments of the left colon up to the splenic flexure and completion of the transection of the transverse mesocolon and gastrocolic ligament to the splenic flexure, the splenic flexure can be approached as a triangle of intestine supported at its apex by the anterior and posterior peritoneal ligaments. The understanding of these suspensions and their serial division simplifies the mobilization of the splenic flexure. Excessive traction should not be placed on the splenic flexure during mobilization, to avoid tearing the splenic capsule or rupturing the diseased colon; either complication may have serious consequences.

The anterior ligament of the splenic flexure goes from the left margin of the gastrocolic ligament, which at the lateral aspect of the colon, passes to the diaphragm as the left phrenocolic ligament. After this ligament is divided between hemostats, the posterior attachment of the transverse mesocolon to the pancreas is divided. Here, the inferior mesenteric vein is encountered and should be carefully ligated and divided. The tail of the pancreas and the duodenojejunal junction are identified to avoid injury. The inferior pole of the spleen rests on the phrenocolic ligament, which is known as the supporting ligament of the spleen. This ligament is divided to complete the splenic flexure mobilization.

Descending Colon

After the splenic flexure is freed, the descending colon and sigmoid colon are easily mobilized further by elevating their mesentery from the posterior fusion fascia. The branches of the inferior mesenteric artery are individually ligated and divided at the colonic border. This distal ligation ensures the conservation of adequate left lateral peritoneum for subsequent reperitonealization and also avoids division of the inferior

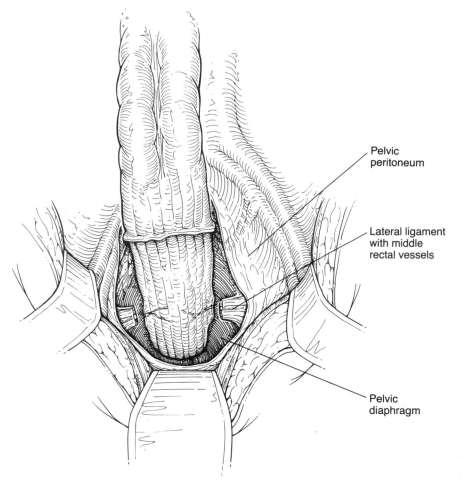

Pelvic
peritoneum

Lateral ligament
with middle
rectal vessels

Pelvic
diaphragm

Figure 8–16. Pelvic dissection of the rectum for inflammatory bowel disease. Note that the dissection is close to the rectal wall, and the pelvic peritoneum is preserved, in contrast to a cancer operation.

mesenteric vessels near the bifurcation of the aorta, where the superior pelvic ganglia may be injured with sexual dysfunction resulting.

Pelvic Dissection

Dissection of the pelvic colon and rectum starts with ligation and division of their vascular pedicle containing the superior rectal vessels close to the bowel wall. This is continued to well below the area of the aortic bifurcation; dissection remains close to the bowel wall in order to avoid damage to both the superior pelvic sympathetic plexus and the sacral parasympathetic nerves. Following this posterior mobilization of the upper rectum, the pelvic peritoneum is incised from the point of ligation of the superior rectal vessels laterally to encompass the rectum. The two lateral peritoneal incisions are joined anteriorly to the rectum into the cul-de-sac between the rectum and bladder or rectum and upper vagina.

The posterior separation of the rectum from the sacrum is achieved by separating the sacral attachments of the rectum with long, fine, curved scissors and keeping close to the rectal wall in order to avoid damage to the nervi erigentes, which are pushed posteriorly. Numerous small communicating vessels can be appropriately clipped and divided.

The anterior pelvic dissection begins at the midline, and the flap of peritoneum between the rectum and bladder or rectum and upper vagina is developed; the dissection is continued inferiorly posterior to Denonvilliers' fascia. This method allows excision of the rectum only and leaves the seminal vesicles or posterior fornix of the vagina undisturbed. This anterior dissection is carried further inferiorly to the level of the prostate gland or lower vagina.

The lateral dissection is not as radical as that for carcinoma of the rectum and does not encroach on the internal obturator muscles. Instead, the lateral ligaments of the rectum with their middle rectal vessels are individually ligated or clipped close to the rectal wall (Fig. 8–16).

In this fashion, the posterior, anterior, and lateral mobilization of the lower rectum is continued to the level of the levator muscles until the endopelvic fascia

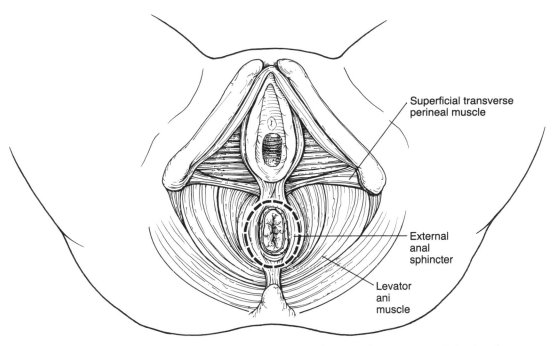

Figure 8–17. Anatomy of the perineum with traditional circumanal incision for proctectomy in benign disease.

covering the levators is clearly visible. This extended superior dissection can be somewhat time consuming, especially in a narrow android pelvis, but it has the advantage of allowing a simple and expedient perineal dissection. Attention is next turned back to the ileocecal junction and the right iliac fossa.

The right colic and ileocolic vessels, which were spared in the beginning of the operation, are now serially divided and ligated. The terminal branches to the distal ileum are carefully preserved, while all the colic branches are sacrificed. It is necessary to preserve as much of the terminal ileum as possible. In cases of ulcerative colitis, the so-called backwash ileitis is, in our opinion, a radiologic mirage and represents only reversible nonspecific inflammation that quickly resolves after the inflamed adjacent colon is removed. We are willing to create an ileostomy through an area of terminal ileum designated as harboring backwash ileitis. However, if the operation is for Crohn's colitis, the site of the proposed ileostomy should be chosen proximal to any *grossly* diseased small intestine. Often, this decision can be made only by multiple resections of small segments of terminal ileum and by inspection of the mucosa. We rely only on gross inspection of the mucosa and serosa. We find frozen-section microscopic examination of the distal ileum to be time consuming, unhelpful, and often confusing. At the appropriate time, the surgeon's assistant uses a linear stapler-cutting device to transect the terminal ileum as close to the ileocecal junction as possible.

Perineal Dissection

The perineal dissection for benign inflammatory disease is much less extensive than the equivalent operation for anorectal cancer (Fig. 8–17). A circular or elliptical incision is made around the anus, encompassing only the voluntary sphincter musculature. The entire perineal dissection is accomplished by means of electrocautery, as this achieves satisfactory hemostasis in an expeditious fashion. One must use the cutting current and avoid the charring of tissues. This circumferential dissection of the anus is carried down to the undersurface of the levator sling, which is exposed laterally and posteriorly, halting anteriorly at the level of the superficial transverse muscle of the perineum. The ischiorectal space is transversed close to the rectal wall, and little or no perirectal fat is excised.

By using Allis or Babcock forceps, the mobilized perianal skin is grasped and gentle traction is applied inferiorly. The posterior median raphe of the levator ani muscle is perforated with Mayo scissors in the midline just anterior to the coccyx. This maneuver allows the surgeon to place an index finger through the created posterior defect into the presacral space. The appearance of serosanguineous fluid collection from this space or the palpation of a previously placed abdominal pack in the presacral space confirms the anatomic landmark. The index finger of the left hand of the surgeon prolapses the levator ani muscle inferiorly, and the muscle is divided on both sides, starting

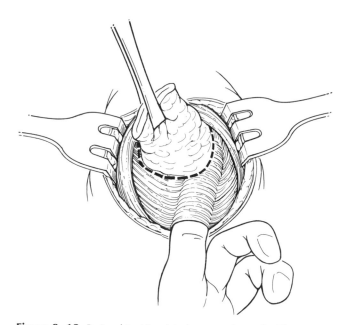

Figure 8–18. Perineal incision into levator ani muscle. The surgeon's finger prolapses the muscle for division as marked.

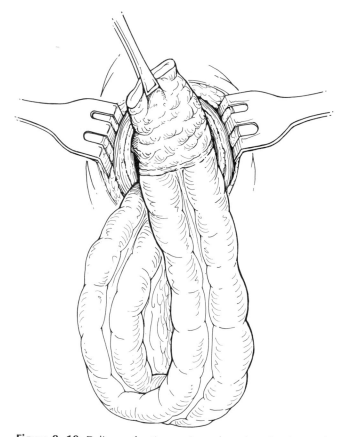

Figure 8–19. Delivery of entire specimen through perineal wound. A few fibers of levator ani muscle remain attached anteriorly.

posteriorly and proceeding laterally, while remaining close to the rectum (Fig. 8–18). At this junction, residual portions of the mesorectum may become apparent and can be serially ligated and divided close to the lower rectal wall. This perineal dissection has now mobilized the posterior three fourths of the anus and rectum. The upper rectum and upper sigmoid colon can now be prolapsed and delivered through the posterior perineal defect. By dividing the terminal ileum close to the cecum, the entire colon is freed and can be gently delivered through the perineal wound into a receptacle (Fig. 8–19). This maneuver reduces the time exposure of the transected intestine to the peritoneal cavity and hence decreases the chances of potential contamination.

Once the entire colon and upper rectum have been delivered through the perineal wound, the lower rectum is attached only to the prostate gland or the posterior vaginal wall. The remaining fibers of the puborectal sling anterolaterally and the Denonvilliers' fascia anteriorly are readily divided by means of electrocautery. A few small bleeding vessels on the surface of the prostate gland or the posterior vaginal wall can be carefully cauterized to ensure hemostasis. Because there is a tendency for the prostatic or vaginal tissue to retract above the perineal incision after the rectum is removed, bleeding points on these structures are serially coagulated as removal of the rectum proceeds. If there is contamination of the perineum by fistulas, these tracts are excised with the specimen.

Closure of the Pelvic Floor and the Perineal Wound

There are several methods of pelvic and perineal wound closure or nonclosure, depending largely on the surgeon's personal preferences. Our procedure of choice is the intrasphincteric amputation, conducted to the plane of the abdominal dissection. We adhere to a policy of precise and complete anatomic closure of layers of the pelvis and perineum using suction drains. The pelvic space is drained with two soft suction drains brought out through the abdominal wall. In our experience with our last 100 operations, we observed that failure to achieve primary healing of the perineal wound was largely associated with either sepsis or hemorrhage, which necessitated packing and eventual use of the open method.

After the proctocolectomy is completed, the entire pelvis and perineum are copiously irrigated and inspected. Points of occult hemorrhage are identified and coagulated. Devitalized and foreign material are washed away. We do not routinely use antibiotic solutions.

Because the levator muscles are divided close to the rectal wall, they are almost entirely preserved and can be approximated with interrupted stout absorbable sutures from the coccyx to the prostate gland or vagina. The medial margins of the gluteus maximus are closed in similar fashion, and the skin and subcutaneous tissues are carefully approximated with interrupted sutures. If there has been any preoperative or intraoperative contamination of the perineal wound, the skin and subcutaneous tissues are left open to heal by secondary intention. A soft Jackson-Pratt–type suction drain is placed in the presacral space above the levator muscles and brought out through a separate stab wound in the buttock. It is our experience that drains coming out in the midline through the main wound have a tendency to produce a persistent perineal sinus.

While the surgeon is completing the perineal part of the operation, the assistant carefully closes the peritoneum of the pelvic floor with interrupted sutures. The complete closure of the preserved pelvic peritoneum obliterates the supralevator and presacral curve dead space. When suction drainage is applied as already described, the closed pelvic peritoneum can be seen to mold to the new pelvic contour. The avoidance of dead space appears to be a major factor in preventing a persistently unhealed perineal wound.

Attention returns to the abdominal cavity, where the lateral peritoneal gutter may or may not be closed. Although its closure may contribute to hemostasis, closure under tension is to be avoided at all costs.

Construction of the Brooke "Spout" or Kock "Reservoir" Ileostomy

Techniques of the construction of a Brooke or a Kock ileostomy are amply described in Chapter 18. We employ either of two types of Brooke ileostomy: the classic transperitoneal Brooke (Figs. 8–20 and 8–21) and the extraperitoneal modification described by Goligher (Fig. 8–22). For chronic ulcerative colitis, we prefer the Goligher modification. However, we do not recommend it in patients with Crohn's colitis or in patients in whom the rectal stump has been left in situ with the expectation of a possible sphincter-saving second-stage operation. If appropriate, we also offer patients with chronic ulcerative colitis who undergo a total proctocolectomy the option of a Kock reservoir ileostomy. We do not advocate this procedure for patients with Crohn's colitis because of the possibility of recurrent Crohn's disease in the pouch.

Postoperative Care

Depending on the general condition of the patient at the end of the operative procedure, the patient is

EDITORIAL COMMENT

The perineal dissection described in this discussion is that of an extrasphincteric resection. An attractive alternative is the intrasphincteric resection. In this technique the pelvic dissection is on the muscular wall of the rectum and is continued to or even through the pelvic diaphragm. This frees the rectum to the perineum. In the perineal phase a circular incision is made between the internal and external sphincter and is continued at this plane through the pelvic diaphragm to join the supralevator dissection. The specimen is removed, and the perineum is closed by approximation of the external sphincter.

Although appealing in concept, this technique has limited applications today. The majority of ulcerative colitic patients are now treated by some variation of an ileoanal anastomosis. Total proctocolectomy is, in substance, reserved for patients suffering from Crohn's colitis. A substantial majority of these patients suffer from perineal fistula, which must be excised with the specimen or at least laid open, thus obviating the advantages of the intrasphincteric resection.

transferred either to the surgical intensive care unit for close monitoring or directly to the ward. A temporary stomal appliance is placed over the Brooke ileostomy, and a permanent appliance is not employed until 2 to 3 weeks when all the edema has disappeared. If a Kock ileostomy has been performed, continuous catheter drainage into a bag is maintained for 1 week to 10 days. Suction drainage is continuously applied to the perineal drains for about 48 hours or until any serum or blood disappears. The urinary catheter is removed early in women, because the bladder is usually well supported by the uterus and appendages. In men, especially the elderly, catheter drainage is maintained until the patient is fully ambulant and normal bladder function is demonstrated by cytometric examination. Corticosteroid therapy is tapered as rapidly as possible to a maintainence level of hydrocortisone 35 to 50 mg/day. This is further weaned during the subsequent 3 to 4 weeks after discharge. If the patient is in a high-risk category for postoperative thromboembolic disease, as exhibited by a previous history of thrombophlebitis or pulmonary embolus, a prophylactic caval interruption is adopted at the time of the operation. Prophylactic anticoagulation is dangerous in this setting, because the extensive retroperitoneal and pelvic wounds are prone to develop large retroperitoneal hematomas. Oral feeding is resumed as soon as gastrointestinal activity is back to normal. In the emergency setting, especially in the presence of intra-abdominal sepsis, when the resumption of gastrointestinal activity is likely to be delayed, we employ a period of total parenteral nutrition but this is discontinued as soon as the patient is able to eat normally.

After being discharged from hospital, the patient is regularly followed by the surgeon to ensure proper

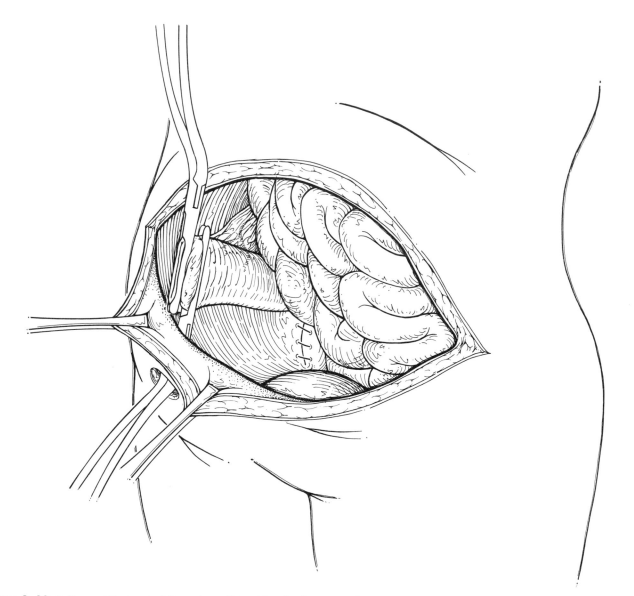

Figure 8–20. Delivery of the terminal ileum for traditional Brooke ileostomy. The cut edge of the mesentery is placed in the right oblique position in the abdominal cavity.

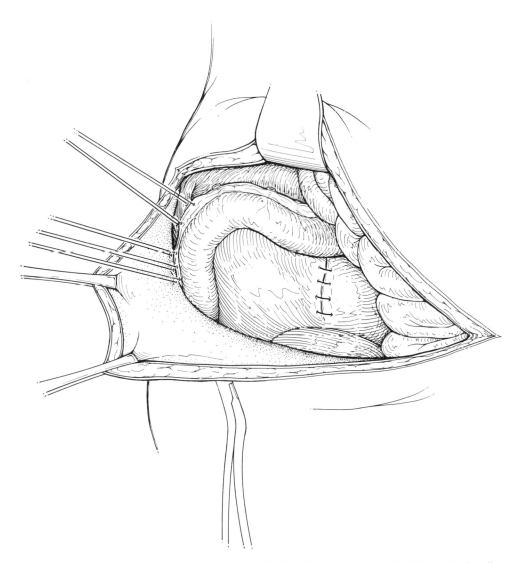

Figure 8–21. Suture of ileal mesentery to peritoneum and transversalis fascia of right anterior and lateral abdominal wall, starting at site of stoma exit. This closes the lateral gutter and prevents parastomal internal herniation.

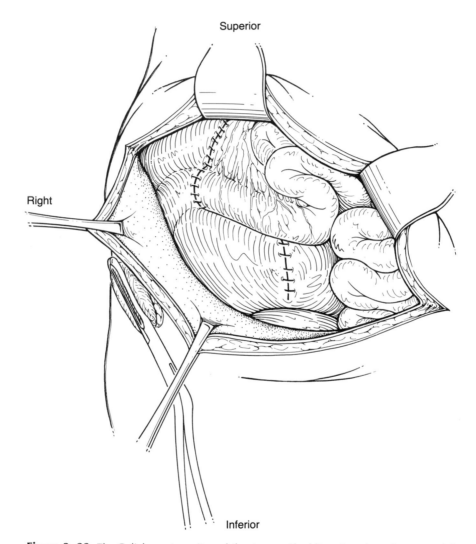

Superior

Right

Inferior

Figure 8–22. The Goligher extraperitoneal ileostomy with obliteration of paraileostomy defect.

wound healing, stomal care, and general counseling. Even after the patient has totally adapted and has been completely rehabilitated, we do not abrogate our responsibilities to the gastroenterologists; with them, we jointly follow the patient at regular intervals.

REFERENCES

1. Kock NG. Intra-abdominal "reservoir" in patients with permanent ileostomy: Preliminary observations on a procedure resulting in fecal "continence" in 5 ileostomy patients. Arch Surg 1969;99:223.
2. Kock NG, Myrvold HE, Nilsson LO, et al. Continent ileostomy: An account of 314 patients. Acta Chir Scand 1981;147:67.
3. Farnell MB, Van Heerden JA, Beart RW Jr, et al. Rectal preservation in nonspecific inflammatory disease of the colon. Ann Surg 1981;192:249.
4. Hughes ESR, McDermott FT, Masterston JP. Ileorectal anastomosis for IBD: 15 year follow-up. Dis Colon Rectum 1979;22:399.
5. Johnson WR, McDermott FT, Hughes ESR, et al. The risk of rectal carcinoma following colectomy in ulcerative colitis. Dis Colon Rectum 1983;26:44.
6. Jones PF, Bevan PG, Hawley PR. Ileostomy or ileorectal anastomosis for ulcerative colitis. Br Med J 1978;1:1459.
7. Khubchandani IT, Sandfort MR, Rosen L, et al. Current status of ileorectal anastomosis for inflammatory bowel disease. Dis Colon Rectum 1989;32:400.
8. Leijonmarck CE, Lofberg R, Ost A, et al. Long term results of ileorectal anastomosis in ulcerative colitis in Stockholm County. Dis Colon Rectum 1990;33:195.
9. Oakley JR, Jagelman DG, Fazio VW, et al. Complications and quality of life after ileorectal anastomosis for ulcerative colitis. Am J Surg 1985;28:394.
10. Aylett SO. 300 cases of diffuse ulcerative colitis treated by total colectomy and ileorectal anastomosis. Br Med J 1966;1:1001.
11. Parc R, Legrand M, Frileux P. Comparative clinical results of ileal pouch–anal anastomosis and ileo-rectal anastomosis in ulcerative colitis. Hepatogastroenterology 1989;36:235.
12. Mungas J, Moossa AR, Block GE. Treatment of toxic megacolon. Surg Clin North Am 1976;56:95.
13. Fazio VW. Toxic megacolon in ulcerative colitis and Crohn's colitis. Clin Gastroenterol 1980;9:389.
14. Berard P, Parc R. Le Traitement de la Rectolite Ulcerohemorragique. Rapport Presente au 86 eme Congres Francais de Chirurgie [Monographie]. Paris: A.F.C. Masson, 1984.
15. Greenstein AJ, Sachar DB, Gibas A, et al. Outcome of toxic dilatation in ulcerative colitis and Crohn's colitis. J Clin Gastroenterol 1985;7:137.
16. Grant CS, Dozois RR. Toxic megacolon: Ultimate fate of patients after successful medical management. Am J Surg 1984;147:106.
17. Turnbull RB Jr, Hawk WA, Weakley FL. Surgical treatment of toxic megacolon: Ileostomy and colostomy to prepare patients for colectomy. Am J Surg 1971;122:325.
18. Block GE, Moossa AR, Simonowitz D, et al. Emergency colectomy for inflammatory bowel disease. Surgery 1977;82:531.
19. Robert JH, Sacchar DB, Aufses AH Jr, et al. Management of severe hemorrhage in ulcerative colitis. Am J Surg 1991;159:550.
20. Pesce G, Geccarino R. Treatment of severe hemorrhage from a defunctionalized rectum with adrenaline chloride in ulcerative colitis. Dis Colon Rectum 1991;34:1139.
21. Block GE. Total proctocolectomy for inflammatory bowel disease. In: Nyhus LM, Baker RJ, eds. Mastery of Surgery. 2nd ed. Boston: Little, Brown and Co, 1992.
22. Levy E, Cosnes J, et al. Le syndrome de colite aiguë grave et ses elements pronostics. Gastroenterol Clin Biol 1972; 637–646.

Total Colectomy, Mucosal Proctectomy, and Ileoanal Anastomosis

Joji Utsunomiya

Takehira Yamamura

The surgical procedure that aims for the total removal of the large bowel mucosa while preserving the anal fecal function has been called *total colectomy, mucosal proctectomy, and ileoanal anastomosis* (IAA) by Utsunomiya et al.[1] It had previously been termed *anal ileostomy,*[2] *ileoproctostomy,*[3] *endorectal ileal pull-through,*[4] *proctocolectomy without ileostomy,*[5] or *rectal mucosal replacement.*[6] More recently the term *restorative proctocolectomy* has been used.[7] As Best has already indicated, the use of the term IAA should be restricted to the anastomosis of the ileum adjacent to the dentate line with the rectal and transition zone mucosa removed and should be distinguished from an operation to create an anastomosis above the anorectal line that leaves the anal canal mucosa intact.[3] The latter operation was previously termed *ileoanal channel stomy,*[8] and more recently *conservative proctocolectomy.*[9] This operation cannot adequately eradicate the large bowel mucosa, because it involves an anastomosis outside the sphincteric zone. Therefore, these operations might be regarded as variants of ileorectal anastomosis (IRA). The term *subtotal proctocolectomy and ileoanal canal anastomosis* (IACA) is used in this chapter in order to avoid confusion in discussing the technique of the true IAA.

HISTORY

Nissen has been credited with the first attempt at IAA in 1932 on a boy with adenomatous polyposis coli by anastomosing a loop of the ileum to the anus through a sacral approach by the Hochenegg method.[10] However, it was not known whether the anal mucosa was removed, and its functional outcome was not exactly defined. The initial clinical study on IAA was made by Ravitch and Sabiston in 1947, who reported the first clinical success in patients with ulcerative colitis (UC).[2] Devine and Webb independently performed it by using the original technique on the patients with familial adenomatous polyposis (FAP)[11]: according to personal correspondence from Dr. Rowan Webb of Melbourne to the author (J.U.) in 1982, they performed this operation in a total of four patients; two progressed well, but two failed and had to have ileostomies. The main problem was said to be severe sepsis around the anus.

In 1951, Best found the overall success rate of IAA performed in the United States to be 59%.[3] Accordingly, he had difficulty in convincing himself that "facing the issues (many complications and technical difficulties) is not worth the sweat and tears of both patient and surgeon" and believed that improving the technique to limit the complications would lead to its wider acceptance. Thus, IAA did not achieve favorable status in surgical treatment for polyposis and colitis.

Since the beginning of the 1970s, surgeons' interest in IAA surgery has been rekindled by the sporadic clinical successes of Safaie-Shirazi and Soper (1973) in treating patients with polyposis[4] and of Martin et al (1977) in treating patients with ulcerative colitis.[12] IAA had become more practical after the introduction of the pelvic pouch, which had developed by way of two independent ideas. One idea involved pooling the intestinal content in the ileal reservoir, which was experimentally initiated by Valiente and Bacon in 1955.[13] It had been clinically introduced by the abdominal pouch of Kock in 1969,[14] and it was finally applied to the pelvic pouch by Parks and Nicholls in 1978.[5] The other idea, attempted by Peck, was to replace the rectal mucosa by the ileal mucosa.[6] This approach inspired Utsunomiya to introduce the concept of a direct connection of an ileal pouch to the anal sphincter mechanism, resulting in the first success in consistent voluntary evacuation.[1]

Our procedure, which has evolved with improvements in certain technical details based on 125 cases since the first trial, is described here, and the rationales for it are elucidated. Although the number of cases is not large, this discussion represents the personal experiences of the author (J.U.) over a 12-year period, and the procedure is presented as the most feasible and safest method of IAA.

STRATEGIC CONSIDERATIONS

The final success of surgery depends not only on technical skill and tactics but also on strategy, which includes appropriate selection of the patients (indication), choice of appropriate procedures (surgical options), and timing of implementation (staged surgery).

Indications

Of the patients who underwent IAA, 90% had UC and 10% had FAP; a rarer indication was severe constipation. The author's total personal experience consists of 54 patients with UC and 69 with FAP, excluding two misjudged cases, one each of Crohn's disease and amyloidosis.

Ulcerative Colitis

It is well known that in patients with UC the symptoms are dramatically relieved when the colorectal mucosa is eradicated by proctocolectomy but that if any mucosa remains, the disease often recurs at that site. Having witnessed the happy patients who had been spending much of their lives in hospitals and who after operation were able to return to normal life without a permanent abdominal stoma, the surgeon can never doubt the effectiveness of IAA for UC. All the patients with UC for whom total colectomy with IRA or proctocolectomy with an abdominal ileostomy (AIS) were previously selected are now candidates for IAA.

In our series, 35.4% of patients experienced major side effects of steroid therapy, some of which never reversed after operation. This finding suggests that surgical treatment for UC should be performed much earlier than it is currently done. Compared with the polyposis patients, the colitis patients had a higher daily stool frequency and poorer continence after operation, and pouchitis occurred exclusively in UC patients. As similar findings are now reported in patients who have undergone IRA,[16] some UC-specific extracolonic predispositions may persist after IAA, suggesting that this operation does not end the treatment for the colitic patient.

Familial Adenomatous Polyposis Coli

IRA followed by surveillance, as popularized by Lockhart-Mummery in 1956, is still a subject of dispute.[17] In our personal series of IRA, the appearance of remnant rectal cancer was 18% at 6 postoperative years, during which period about one half of the colectomized patients had dropped out of the follow-up surveillance. As a result, the author (J.U.) decided to establish a practical technique of IAA. A patient with FAP has a 1% risk of colorectal cancer at 15 years of age, and the risk rises to 10% at 25 years of age.[18] Therefore, prophylactic surgery has generally been advised for this age group. We maintain our policy of utilizing IAA for prophylactic surgery in consonance with the Mayo Clinic.[19] Jagelman recommended IRA for this disease because the extracolonic tumors, such as desmoid tumors and foregut cancers, caused death more frequently than did the remnant rectal cancer.[20]

In general, the safer and less mutilative procedures, such as IRA or IACA, may be appropriate for certain selected asymptomatic and active FAP gene carriers with no or few polyps in the rectum. Rectal mucosa, however, should not be retained in the patient with profuse polyposis, in whom the cancer risk is much higher than average and in whom the remnant mucosa after IACA may regenerate[21]; in the patient of 40 or older whose colorectal cancer risk is assumed to be 60% or more[18]; and in the patient who is unlikely to comply with life-long postoperative surveillance.

For the patient with colorectal cancer (56% of the total at diagnosis),[18] IAA is strongly recommended as the *therapy of choice*, because 38% of this group were found to have multiple cancers in the large bowel. Even patients with cancer of the rectum are candidates for IAA, if the lesion is well differentiated and above 4 cm from the anal margin. All patients who have undergone IRA and IAA must be followed for the development of extracolonic tumors.

Constipation

Nicholls and Kamm reported on IAA for treating two patients with severe idiopathic constipation and described dramatic improvement in one.[22] Hosie et al, on the basis of their experiences with 13 cases, concluded that IAS may be an acceptable alternative to stoma formation in patients with failed IRA for slow transit constipation and in patients with primary megacolon associated with megarectum.[23]

Previous Colorectal Surgery

Some patients with IRA were converted to IAA because the rectum became cancerous. Their bowel function quickly recovered after IAA to equal that of their previous IRA, presumably because their terminal ileum had already been colonized. Also the ileostomies of the Brooke type[24, 25] or Kock type[26] were reported to be successfully converted to IAA if the anal sphincter had been preserved.

Contraindications

IAA for *Crohn's disease* is contraindicated because this disease is transmural, tends to recur in the intestinal pouch, and often is complicated by persisting anal fistulas. If Crohn's disease is suspected, a three-stage approach is advocated to eliminate the disease without commitment to an ill-advised IAA. The patient with indeterminate colitis may tolerate an IAA.[27] Internal hemorrhoids and non-Crohn's anal fistula are not specific contraindications to IAA; however, a sphincteric muscle damaged by previous surgery, pre-existing incontinence, or a reduced maximum resting pressure of 40 H_2O mm or less all are reasons to exclude this operation. Additionally, most elderly patients may be excluded from candidacy for IAA.

Other Surgical Options

In the era of IAA, the frequency of the other surgical options has been greatly reduced, but the proper indication and performance of these operations have greatly improved the success rate of IAA. The performance of a conventional proctocolectomy is now only one tenth as frequent as in the previous era, but the proper technique of ileostomy and the strict discipline of stoma care are still essential to success. The experience with the Kock pouch gives support to the IAA surgeons who are confronted with various pouch pathologies and who may have to convert the failed pouch to the abdominal type.

The postoperative mortality and morbidity rates for the IRA and the IAA were about the same, and the postoperative bowel functions did not differ significantly.[28] Stool frequency per day (SFD) for IRA was 4.2 for UC and 3.6 for FAP, and 17% of the patients with IRA were reported to have experienced major incontinence.[16] According to the cooperative study group of inflammatory bowel disease in Japan, after 1 year the percentage of patients with five or more stools per day was 84.6% with IRA versus 73.3% with IAA. The IRA series inevitably excluded cases with severely diseased rectums, which can be managed with IAA.

Pouchitis occurred after IAA, but it was much less frequent and more manageable than the colitis seen in the remaining rectum after IRA. Nevertheless, IRA is still a useful option for mild cases of UC and FAP, as the initial operation of a staged IAA program, and as a palliative measure for indeterminate colitis or FAP with far-advanced cancer.

The author previously attempted subtotal proctocolectomy and IACA in several patients and obtained excellent bowel function, even without a pouch, in young patients with FAP. However, in UC patients persistent bloody mucous discharges from the retained mucosa disturbed bowel functions. Therefore, we decided always to remove the entire rectal mucosa. Since the circular stapler anastomosis technique was introduced[30] and since, more recently, the improved PC-EEA model of stapler (U.S. Surgical Co.) became available for the double-stapler technique, an anastomosis between the ileal pouch and the upper end of the anal canal without mucosectomy has become popular.[9, 31, 32] It provides better continence, is apparently simpler and quicker to perform, and is safer than a true IAA. Therefore, the necessity of a diverting ileostomy has been substantially reduced in these operations. Use of the stapler, however, has never guaranteed the total removal of the anal canal mucosa (transition zone and lower rectum).

The amount of the anal canal mucosa that remained after these techniques were implemented varied from 2 to 3 cm above the dentate line[9] or from 0.2 to 4.0

cm (median 2.0 cm) above it.[33] The clinical significance of the retained anal canal mucosa has often been underestimated. One study of the anal mucosa showed that 87% had inflammation, 25% contained dysplasia, and 1 of 16 specimens demonstrated adenocarcinoma.[34] We are not opposed to IACA but insist that it must be distinguished from IAA to avoid confusion in technical discussion and that the criteria for its indication be given for each of these options, since IACA may have indications similar to IRA.

Staged Surgery

For an acute obstruction from colon cancer, the trend has changed from staged procedures to primary resection. For IAA, however, we do not hesitate to perform staged surgery in order to minimize any danger that might disturb the postoperative quality of life, because patients undergoing IAA are usually young and the disease is essentially benign. The routine employment of the temporary proximal diverting ileostomy to protect the anastomosis, advocated by Schneider[35] and Martin et al,[12] has been one of the most significant contributions and adopted by most surgeons. The anastomosis in the mucosectomized anal canal is fragile, and there is often a septic reaction around the anastomosis that adversely affects the eventual functional result. Some surgeons have questioned the need for the diverting ileostomy,[31, 36] although they used a stapler for the anastomosis. With IAA a major leakage or perforation occurred more frequently when an ileostomy was not employed, even when strict selection criteria were used.[37, 38]

The staged surgery with ileostomy places some economic and physical burdens on the patient and has led to some increase in complications related to the ileostomy per se. However, these are not life threatening and do not preclude a long and high-quality life after surgery. In our institution, the diverting ileostomy is now a common and important procedure when IAA is performed.

In patients with UC, IAA has frequently (in 80% of patients in our series) been performed in three or more stages, not only for emergency procedures but also for elective procedures, when the patient has major steroid side effects, is nutritionally compromised, or is suspected of having Crohn's disease. The three-stage procedure initiated with total abdominal colectomy, ileostomy, and colonic mucous fistula (Schneider's procedure) is generally recommended (Fig. 8–23).[35] The distal sigmoid colon is always kept open as a suprapubic mucous fistula through which irrigation can be performed to treat the rectal disease. It is never closed as in the Hartmann method, to avoid leakage and pelvic sepsis at the stump. For temporary stomas, the colonic

type, which we previously attempted, was abandoned because of cecal perforation and bleeding and because the end-loop ileostomy was found not to interfere with the later creation of the J-pouch.

After the first-stage operation, steroid therapy can be withdrawn in almost all cases within the 3 months prior to IAA. If Crohn's disease is confirmed in the resected specimen, the intestine may be reconstructed by IRA. The initial ileostomy and blow-holes of the colon (Turnbull's procedure) have not been utilized in our more recent practice.[39] An initial IRA as the first-stage operation may be considered for selected patients.

TECHNICAL CONSIDERATIONS

Approach and Positioning of Patient

The selection of the best approach and position is one of the most important factors for facilitating the operation. Initially (1978 to 1981), the operation was colectomy, rectal mucosectomy, and pouch construction from the abdomen with the patient in the lithotomy position. It was completed by the anal mucosectomy and pouch-anal anastomosis per anus (abdominoanal approach).[1] After 1981, our procedure changed, to start with rectal mucosectomy initially performed per anus while the patient was in the prone jackknife position. This was followed by the abdominal phase in the lithotomy position (prone jackknife, anoabdominal approach),[15, 40, 41] also recommended by others,[42, 43] in order to facilitate mucosectomy with a much greater exposure than was possible with the lithotomy position. The time lost during the position change can be minimized to 15 minutes or less. A decrease in venous return of the inferior vena cava by an increase in pressure on the abdominal cavity in the prone position is well compensated for by elevating the hips in the jackknife position.[44]

Mucosectomy

This is an old and unique technique that has been infrequently used in other gastrointestinal operations. In IAA, an adequate mucosectomy is essential, and it is the most tedious and difficult aspect of the procedure. The problem has been how to minimize its extent while obtaining the best functional result (and how to perform it more easily).

There are three types of mucosectomy, each starting at a different level in the anorectal canal. The starting distal dissection at the upper border of the dentate line (DL), that is, at the level of the top of the pectens (the DL preserving IAA) is appropriate (Fig. 8–24C).

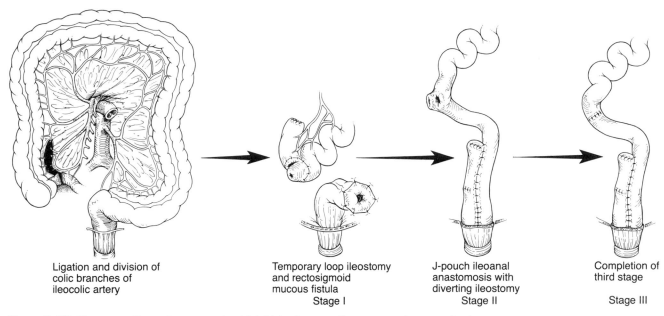

Ligation and division of colic branches of ileocolic artery

Temporary loop ileostomy and rectosigmoid mucous fistula
Stage I

J-pouch ileoanal anastomosis with diverting ileostomy
Stage II

Completion of third stage
Stage III

Figure 8–23. Three-stage ileoanal anastomosis with initial colectomy, ileostomy, and mucous fistula.

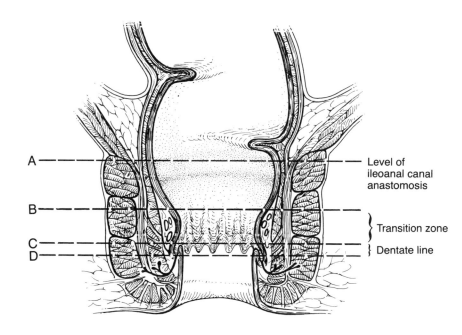

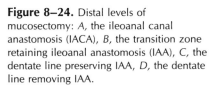

Figure 8–24. Distal levels of mucosectomy: *A*, the ileoanal canal anastomosis (IACA), *B*, the transition zone retaining ileoanal anastomosis (IAA), *C*, the dentate line preserving IAA, *D*, the dentate line removing IAA.

A — Level of ileoanal canal anastomosis

B — } Transition zone

C — } Dentate line

D —

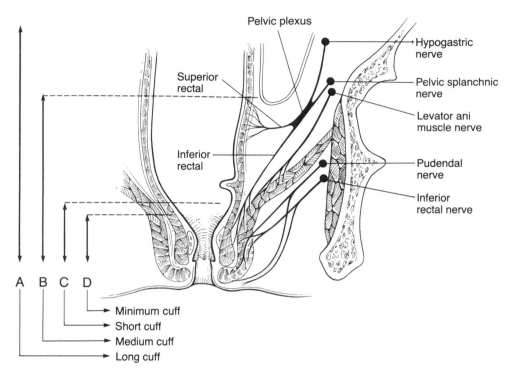

A B C D

→ Minimum cuff
→ Short cuff
→ Medium cuff
→ Long cuff

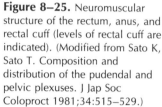

Figure 8–25. Neuromuscular structure of the rectum, anus, and rectal cuff (levels of rectal cuff are indicated). (Modified from Sato K, Sato T. Composition and distribution of the pudendal and pelvic plexuses. J Jap Soc Coloproct 1981;34:515–529.)

Many surgeons have adopted this method, and function has been found to decrease with the DL removed (Fig. 8–24D).[1, 5, 45–47] Some investigators have recommended a dissection line of 1 cm above the DL to preserve the anal transition zone (ATZ), which ranged from 4 to 25 mm (mean 8.5 mm) in histologic specimens (the ATZ preserving IAA) (Fig. 8–24D).[9] The importance of the ATZ for anal sensation and continence was shown in normal subjects.[49] However, despite a significant impairment in threshold sensation in the patient whose ATZ was excised, no functional differences in either discrimination or continence were detected, irrespective of whether the ATZ had been excised or preserved.[50]

The clinical significance of the retained transition zone for malignant risk and sustained inflammation at the anastomosis cannot be neglected. We observed adenomatous crypts often invading beneath the transitional epithelium in FAP patients; in some patients, this zone was totally abolished.[34] The ATZ-preserving operation may have no merit either functionally or therapeutically. As in IACA, when mucosectomy was initiated at the *anorectal line* (ARL) to preserve the entire anal canal mucosa 2 to 3 cm above the DL, the anal function was naturally well preserved (Fig. 8–24 A). In IAA with mucosectomy, however, after operation a temporary decrease in resting anal pressure and minor incontinence were observed in most patients. This defect was probably attributable to several factors, such as the interruption of Meissner's intramural plexus, on which the dynamic properties of the internal

sphincter depend; removal of the sampling zone in the upper canal; and presence of a full-thickness ileum within the anal canal.[9] All efforts to improve IAA surgical technique have been devoted to compensating for the functional disadvantage produced by removal of even such a small amount of anal canal mucosa.

Rectal Cuff

This is the rectoanal neuromuscular structure created after mucosectomy and consists of the muscular rectal stump above the levator ani muscle and denuded canal. The trend has been a gradual move toward shortening the rectal cuff. There have been four general categories of cuff length. Originally, Devine and Webb performed mucosectomy starting at the level of the rectosigmoidal junction in order to preserve the whole rectal muscular layer with the intrinsic nerve plexus and connections to the sacral segment of the spinal cord (the long cuff method) (Fig. 8–25).[11] This method was practiced by many surgeons.[1, 4, 6] The author (J.U.) initially created a long rectal muscular cuff of about 15 cm in length, in which the mucosal layer was to be replaced with the ileal wall, as proposed by Peck.[6] Later we and others started the mucosectomy just below the peritoneal reflection (to be called the medium cuff method) to preserve the muscular cuff of the lower 8 to 10 cm of rectum (see Fig. 8–25).[5, 42] More recently, many surgeons (except the authors) abandoned the long or medium cuff method because it was considered not to have functional merit and to have the disadvantages of a higher frequency of cuff abscess, longer time to construct, increased blood loss, and restriction of compliance of the pouch placed within the cuff. In the short cuff method, currently the most popular one, the mobilized rectum is divided just proximal to the levator ani muscle (pelvic floor) or at the anorectal junction, leaving the anorectal cuff of only about 3 to 5 cm in length with the mucosa removed only per anus (see Fig. 8–25).[45, 47, 51]

We have found that when the rectal stumps were totally excised above the levator ani muscles per anus with the anal canal mucosa removed (minimum cuff), the patient was not sufficiently continent (see Fig. 8–25).[52] The internal and even external sphincteric functions are impaired after total removal of the rectal stump with a stapler for either a coloanal anastomosis[53] or the IACA technique.[54] In IAA, the maximum resting and voluntary squeeze pressures of the anal canal are reduced in the patients with a short (2- to 5-cm) cuff, compared with those with a long (8- to 10-cm) cuff.[51] These results indicated that, contrary to the general clinical impressions that have led to shortening of the cuff, the retained denuded rectal wall may play a significant role in the internal and external sphincter functions (see Fig. 8–25).

In the medium cuff, the superior rectal branches that enter into the rectal muscular wall in an area within 2 cm below the peritoneal reflection can be partially preserved.[55] With the short cuff method, however, only the inferior rectal branches of the visceral nervi, including the pudendal nerves that emerge into the rectum approximately 2 cm above the dentate line, can be retained.[55, 56] Anatomically, the preserved rectal wall can form the "protective wall" for obviating urogenital functional sequelae and also for the structural enforcement of the vagina and urethra against fistula formation. Our technique, as discussed further on, can make such an extensive mucosectomy feasible with preservation of the rectal neuromuscular structure. A posterior longitudinal incision on the cuff removes the disadvantages of a longer cuff. In fact, we have not experienced cuff abscesses in our more recent cases and have found the distensibility and compliance of the pouch not to be restricted.[52] Our results suggest that in the patient who has undergone IAA with the mucosa totally removed, the neuromuscular coat of the lower rectum should be preserved, if technically feasible.

Mucosectomy Technique

The number of aids to rectal mucosectomy that have been tried experimentally or clinically, such as chemical débridement,[57] curettage,[58] and surgical ultrasonic aspiration, are evidence of its technical difficulty.[60] Actually, none of these devices seems more effective than a manual dissection of the mucosa elevated with an isotonic saline solution containing adrenaline. Parks and Nicholls stripped out the mucosa divided into three sheets (sheet mucosectomy) within the anal canal (endocavitary technique) using special retractors[5]; surgeons at the Mayo Clinic recommended everting the anal orifice with two sets of Gelpi retractors to avoid stretching fibers of the muscle.[45] Goligher performed mucosectomy on the everted rectal wall outside of the anus (extra-anal everted technique).[61] However, because these techniques are not suitable for preserving the medium rectal cuff, we strip out the mucosa as a tube (cylindrical mucosectomy) under the specific precautions to be described, including the "forceps electrocoagulation technique," which was devised for bloodless separation of the submucosal space (see Fig. 8–27).[40, 41] With our method an inflamed mucosa can be separated up to 10 cm or more to reach the subperitoneal level.

Ileal Pouch

Pioneering surgeons, including one of us (J.U.), performed IAA without a reservoir and found that it was successful in children.[12, 62] However, in adults it produced frequent stools, and about 20 months were needed to achieve a stool frequency of six or more per day, which never decreased thereafter.[15] These results provoked our initial decision to create a substitute for reservoir continence. Currently, many types of ileal pelvic pouches are used (Fig. 8–26). Other attempts to preserve the ileal content, such as myotomy of the ileal segment, grafting of an antiperistaltic ileal segment, or ileal dilatation by a balloon,[62] have not been clinically popular.

S- or Triple-Loop Pouch

This was the first clinically applied pelvic pouch, made from the terminal 50 cm of the small bowel folded into an S-shaped configuration, each limb being about 15 cm long and a length of distal ileum projecting 5 cm beyond the third limb, which was anastomosed end-to-end to the anal canal.[5] About one half of these patients were reported to require self-catheterization to evacuate stool.[63] The problem has largely been improved by shortening the spout to 2 cm from the original 5 cm or more, which could become kinked or spastic with straining.[64–66]

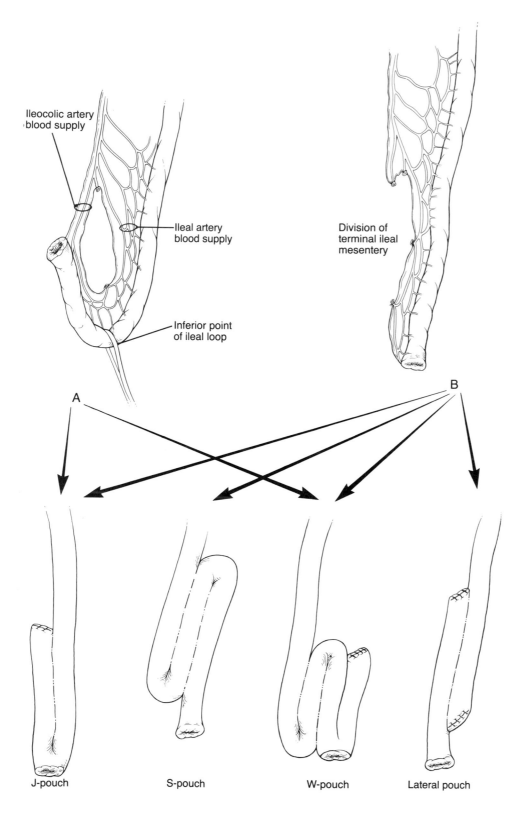

Ileocolic artery blood supply

Ileal artery blood supply

Inferior point of ileal loop

Division of terminal ileal mesentery

A

B

J-pouch

S-pouch

W-pouch

Lateral pouch

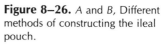

Figure 8–26. *A* and *B,* Different methods of constructing the ileal pouch.

H- or Lateral Isoperistaltic Pouch

Peck first started his study with the idea of replacing rectal mucosa by an ileal mucosal pedicle graft on the preserved rectal muscular cuff.[6] After finding that the grafted rectum shrunk, he created a reservoir by a long side-to-side anastomosis between the grafted neorectum and a segment of ileum at a second laparotomy. Fonkalsrud[67] and Utsunomiya et al[1] independently devised a similar pouch (see Fig. 8–26). The author (J.U.) abandoned this method after he found that patients experienced difficulty in evacuation associated with abdominal distention.

J- or Antiperistaltic Double-Loop Pouch

With the aim of eliminating the evacuation difficulty associated with the H-pouch, the looped pouch was devised by Utsunomiya et al in order to install a reservoir neorectum, which would be located, like the natural rectal ampulla, with direct communication to the anal sphincteric mechanisms and without creation of a spout.[1] The procedure later called the J-pouch was originally called the Type B, whereas the nonpouch was the Type A 1 and the H-pouch was the Type A-2.[1] Our concern at that time was preservation of circulation in the pouch that was brought to the anus. The superior mesenteric vessels (SMA) were divided in the terminal trunk to offer mesenteric elongation and to preserve the marginal artery for providing bilateral blood flow from both the ileal and the ileocolic arteries (ICA) to the pouch (standard J-pouch) (see Figs. 8–25 and 8–29).[69, 70]

This pouch, constructed with bilateral blood supplies, had a 23% increment of blood flow, compared with the short J-pouch, with the ICA divided and giving only a unilateral blood supply to the pouch.[63] The most inferior point of the terminal ileal loop that always reached the dentate line was located at a distance of about 20 cm or more from the ileocecal junction. The short J-pouch gave a slightly longer reach (by 1 or 2 cm) than the standard J-pouch, but the distal limb of the short J-pouch was shorter by about 4 cm than the 20 cm of the standard method.[70] We usually use the standard J-pouch because of its superior blood supply and larger capacity, except in the patient who has undergone a prior total colectomy. Although we never failed to bring down the standard J-pouch to the anus in Japanese patients, in Caucasian patients with a fatty mesentery the short J-pouch could be suitable for an easier transfer of the pouch. The J-pouch can easily be constructed by using staplers, whereas the S- or W-pouch requires manual sewing.

Use of the stapler resulted in a twofold increase in capacity of the J-pouch with a shorter construction time (one fifth of the time) than the handsewn technique.[71] Two or three applications by the GIA 90 stapler can now accomplish lateral anastomosis to produce a pouch of 18 or 27 cm, which had previously required four or more applications by the GIA 50 stapler. The GIA stapler is inserted from the apex of the pouch by some surgeons, but we insert it on the body of the loop in order to leave the apex intact until just before the anastomosis is made. A bridge thus created with an unsplit septum in the apical portion of the pouch might help to provide a better blood supply to the area of anastomosis where mucosal blood flow is considerably reduced.[72] However because the apical bridge, albeit rarely, could prolapse into the anal canal to interfere with evacuation, its width should be minimized.

W- or Quadrupled Pouch

In order to combine the spontaneous evacuation of the J-pouch with the greater capacity of the S-pouch, the W-pouch was designed by placing two J-pouches side by side.[73] The terminal 50 cm of the small bowel is folded into four loops, each 12 cm long, forming a W-shaped configuration. As with the J-pouch, a side-to-end anastomosis is made directly between the anal canal and reservoir at its most dependent part. It is claimed that the W-pouch is not more difficult to construct than the J-pouch and that better function results than with the other pouch.[47]

Anti-H-Pouch or Lateral Antiperistaltic or Modified J-Pouch

One of the limbs of the J-loop is divided at 3 cm from the apex using the GIA 50 stapler, and the two limbs are anastomosed side-to-side in an isoantiperistaltic manner, leaving a 2-cm efferent conduit on either the isoperistaltic limb[74] or the antiperistaltic limb.[36] This method has not been popular, but it may be useful in extending the J-pouch when it is difficult to bring it down to the anus, although its function is reported to be somewhat inferior to the J-pouch.

K- or Kock-Type Pouch

The Kock abdominal pouch has been utilized as a pelvic pouch.[75] Its functional superiority to the J-pouch has not been established.[75] Currently, the three types of pouches, the S-, J-, and W-pouches, are in general use. The J-pouch constituted 55% of the 1,600 cases that had appeared in the literature until 1989. Comparative studies have been done functionally, technically, and metabolically by different investigators. No significant functional differences between the S-pouch and J-pouch have been found,[76–78] although the former was judged to be slightly superior to the latter.[74, 79]

The W-pouch was attributed to its larger initial capacity (about 300 ml), compared with that of the J-pouch (about 200 ml). A randomized study, however, revealed that compared with the W-pouch, the J-pouch was quicker (by 20%) to perform and produced almost identical bowel functions.[81] In the long-range follow-up periods after operation, function improved with time, even after 3 years with the J-pouch.[82]

Technical problems may depend more on the surgeon's familiarity and experience than on the theoretical advantages of any pouch; the learning curve may provide a better result, regardless of theory. The J-pouch is the simplest one to construct and functions as well as, if not better than, the other types.

Anal Anastomosis and Drainage

Initially Ravitch used a three-layer anastomosis, and Best modified it to a secondary pull-through anastomosis, which resulted in imperfect continence in our early cases. The use of a few interrupted sutures as is usually done in anal surgery, theoretically to allow for drainage of blood and fluid and to rely on the secondary healing, was abandoned; this is because the primary, clean healing of an anal anastomosis was found to be essential for achieving good continence in an anastomosis within the anal canal, where the lumen is usually closed by the sphincter tone. Absorbable fine synthetic sutures may be one of the major aids to successful IAAs. Silk that can cause persistent infection and catgut that is absorbed too quickly should never be used.

By following Parks' endocavity method, one can place the sutures to achieve a well-tailored anastomosis. A side-to-end anastomosis in the J-pouch or W-pouch design is advantageous for sealing off the cuff cavity from the intestinal content during anastomosis. It is performed easily and in a cleaner fashion than the end-to-end anastomosis used in the other pouches, because the size of the opening in the ileal wall can be adjusted to the size of the anal canal. Drainage of the cuff is regarded as being of little importance and may be harmful. A transanastomotic drain can lead to ascending infection into the cuff, whereas the transperineal drain may result in a fistula. A well-functioning transperineal sump drain into the deep pelvis for several days is our drainage method of choice.

Diverting Ileostomy

Although loop ileostomy by Turnbull's method has generally been used, some prefer a Brooke-type ileostomy because the former method is more likely to be associated with peristomal complications than the latter.[83, 84] Most of our patients with an ileostomy underwent stomal closure in 8 to 12 weeks.[83] By this time the reduced sphincteric tone can recover, and the patient can return to normal activity. For uneventful closures of the ileostomy, the essential technical goal is the mobilization and exteriorization of an intestinal loop of sufficient length to facilitate suturing. An ileostomy closure using staplers[86] appears superior to the handsewn technique.[37] In our series, the stapler has reduced operating time by 23%, reduced blood loss by 37%, and, more importantly, resulted in fewer intestinal obstructions (reduced from 37.9% to 13.6%) and fewer anastomotic leaks (reduced from 4.5% to 0.0%).[87] Instead of the linear cutaneous closure, point closure with the pursestring suture is valuable in anticipation of a possible reopening of the stoma.

CURRENT OPERATIVE TECHNIQUE

The practical details of our present procedures, the J-pouch medium-cuff IAA, which is usually performed by the three-stage method for UC patients is described (see Fig. 8–23). The reader is encouraged to consult publications for discussion of other popular procedures that have been established in specialized centers, such as the J-pouch short-cuff procedure of the Mayo Clinic,[45, 46] the S-pouch short-cuff procedure of University of Minnesota,[64] the W-pouch short-cuff procedure of St. Marks Hospital.[47]

Abdominal Colectomy with End-Loop Ileostomy and Suprapubic Mucous Fistula (First-Stage Operation)

Before surgery, a proper stoma site is selected, as recommended by Turnbull. Although no bowel preparation is necessary, broad-spectrum antibiotics effective for both aerobes and anaerobes are infused intravenously immediately before and during the operation. Steroid coverage is done in the usual manner.

With the patient in the supine position, the abdominal cavity is widely opened with an extended left paramedian incision, and the wound is sealed off using a plastic Ring Drape. The small intestine is never enveloped in an intestinal bag, because the mesenteric root is easily rotated by this maneuver with resultant intestinal ischemia after the mesocolon is totally divided. After the ascending colon is mobilized from its lateral attachment, the ileum is divided close to the ileocecal junction with careful preservation of the ileal branches of the ileocolic vessels by using a suturing stapler-cutter (GIA 50 or PLC). The entire colon with the major omentum attached is devascularized by dividing the three colic and sigmoid colic vessels, but the superior rectal vessels are preserved.

The colon is exteriorized from the abdominal cavity and removed by dividing the sigmoid colon at a level of 2 to 3 cm above the abdominal surface using a GIA 50 or PLC stapler-cutter. If a toxic megacolon is associated, the colon is deflated first through a large balloon catheter (no. 32) inserted and fixed on the transverse colon before any manipulation on the colon is started. An end-loop ileostomy is fashioned at the previously marked stoma site by using a portion of the ileal loop 10 cm from the end by Turnbull's method. The exteriorized sigmoid colon stump is fixed with several serocutaneous sutures at the suprapubic end of the incision. The peritoneal cavity is fully irrigated with a large volume of saline solution.

The abdomen is closed by using a running suture of 1-0 Vicryl for the peritoneal layer, doubled running sutures with 2-0 Prolene for the fascial layer, and by interrupted suture with silk or a stapler for the skin. A triple-lumen sump drain is placed in the left subphrenic space to monitor postoperative bleeding. The closed stump of the sigmoid colon is secondarily opened by using an electrocoagulator to create a mucous fistula on the fourth or fifth postoperative day, after the abdominal wall has completely adhered to the colonic serosa so as to seal off the wound.

When the stoma begins to function, oral intake is initiated as usual. The dosage of the systemically administered steroid is tapered, and the rectal stump is irrigated daily with 500 ml of saline solution containing 100 mg hydrocortisone and 250 mg metronidazole. When the general condition of the patient has improved (usually in months), the patient is readmitted to undergo ileoanal anastomosis.

Mucosal Proctectomy and J-Pouch Anal Anastomosis (Second-Stage Operation)

For patients who are undergoing a primary IAA for FAP, a lavage bowel preparation with oral administration of 400 ml of a polyethylene glycol solution is given. In addition, Latamoxef Natorium at a dose of 1.0 g is infused intravenously immediately before and during the operation. The patient is usually placed in the prone jackknife position, and the buttocks are spread with wide adhesive tapes. The anal canal is carefully dilated by using a pediatric Parks retractor (Fig. 8–27A). The anal orifice is everted by holding the anal edge together with the skin and the external sphincter with Allis clamps (Glassman model) to expose the mucosal surface of the anal canal.

After a saline solution containing adrenaline (1:200,000) is injected submucosally to elevate the mucosal layer, the mucosa is cut circumferentially with an electrocoagulator at the level of the apex of the pectens of the dentate line. While gently holding the cut edge with mucosal forceps (Glassman model), the mucosa is elevated to expose the submucosal connective tissue and bridging vessels (the mucosa elevating phase) (Fig. 8–27A). These vessels are severed by picking them up with vascular forceps (Glassman model), to which a blended current is introduced from an electrocoagulator in order to separate the submucosal layer from the muscular layer selectively and bloodlessly with either scissors or a scalpel (forceps coagulating technique) (see Fig. 8–27A).

When initial circumferential submucosal separation is completed to create a mucosal tube of 1 to 2 cm in length, the intact fibers of the internal sphincter are exposed. Six stay sutures of 3-0 Vicryl are placed with an atraumatic needle between the perianal skin and anal margin, including the external sphincter, to evert the anal orifice; special attention is paid not to damage the internal sphincter. The open end of the created mucosal tube is closed by several 3-0 Vicryl interrupted sutures and with the mucosal tube gently stretched by tension on the threads, the muscle layer is everted with the aid of muscle retractors to expose the submucosal structures (the muscle layer everting phase), which are continuously separated in a dry field by using the forceps-coagulating technique (Fig. 8–27B).

All small bleeders on the muscle are meticulously coagulated, and any holes in the mucosal tube, if created, are immediately closed by using 4-0 Vicryl to prevent their enlargement. If the mucosa is completely fused with the muscle, which may occur in the rectum above the anorectal line in patients with long-standing colitis, the superficial fibers of the muscle attached to the mucosal layer are usually removed.

When a length of mucosal tube of about 8 cm or more is achieved, which indicates a mucosectomy up to the level of the seminal vesicles in male patients and the upper vagina in female patients, the created mucosal tube is ligated to prevent soiling by intestinal contents. The denuded anorectal cuff is packed with a series of connected gauze sheets to maximally extend the separated submucosal space toward the peritoneal floor. The patient is placed in the lithotomy position to allow simultaneous access to the abdomen and the perineum (Lloyd-Davis position).

Proctosigmoidectomy

Prior to laparotomy, the ileostomy stoma and the colonic mucous fistula are separated at their margins

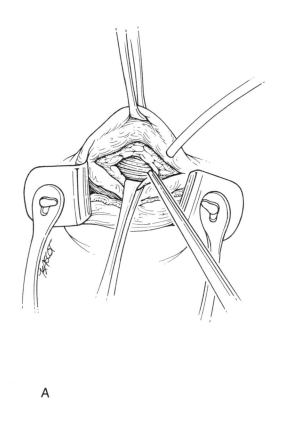

A

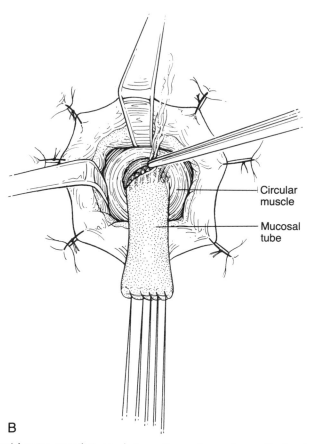

B

Figure 8–27. Mucosectomy per anum: *A*, mucosa elevating method and forceps coagulating technique, *B*, muscle everting method and forceps coagulating technique.

from the skin and subcutaneous tissue by using the cutting current of the electrocoagulator. The sites are closed with several interrupted sutures. The peritoneal adhesions, which are usually minimal if the precautions already mentioned were followed in the preceding operation, are carefully dissected. The end-loop ileostomy is detached from the abdominal wall by dissection from the peritoneal side, and a clean skin hole is preserved for later use in the diverting ileostomy construction.

The sigmoid colon and rectum are separated from the surrounding structures with dissection as close as possible to the rectal wall to avoid injury to the hypogastric and parasympathetic nerves. After the inferior mesenteric vessels are divided, the presacral space is bluntly dissected down to the levator ani muscle and laterally to the lateral ligaments while preserving the middle rectal vessels. Anteriorly, the peritoneal floor, which is elevated by the mass of gauze packed from the anus, is opened at the base by an electrocoagulator. The exposed rectal muscular layer is cut transversely by using an electrocoagulator at the level of the seminal vesicles or at the vaginal apex to enter the rectal submucosal space previously separated

through the anal approach (Fig. 8–28). The space can easily be identified by the gauze packing, which is removed through the abdominal cavity to observe the rectal cuff space.

The rectal mucosal tube, already created by the anal mucosectomy, is brought out through an opening on the cuff to expose the posterior inner surface of the rectal muscular wall. This is divided circumferentially to remove the sigmoid colon and upper rectum together with the lower rectal mucosa. The rectum is thus quickly and bloodlessly removed, leaving a medium rectal muscle cuff with a length of 6 to 8 cm covering the pararectal pelvic structures (see Fig. 8–28). The posterior wall of the cuff is cut longitudinally for 2 to 3 cm to enlarge the capacity inside the cuff.

Construction of Ileal J-Pouch

The ileal mesentery is detached from the retroperitoneum up to the lower duodenal margin, and the serosal sheath covering the superior mesenteric artery is relaxed by making several transverse cuttings on it to increase the mesenteric length. The most inferior por-

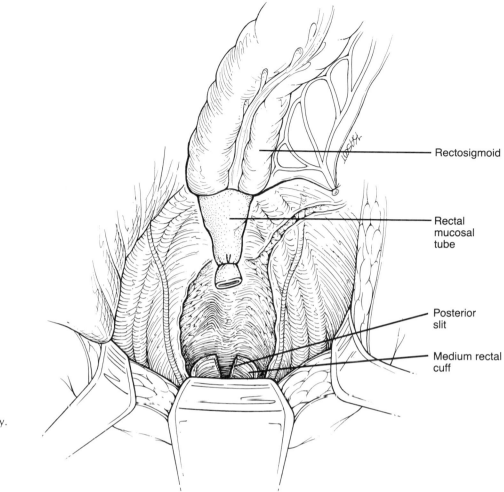

Rectosigmoid

Rectal
mucosal
tube

Posterior
slit

Medium rectal
cuff

Figure 8–28. Rectosigmoidectomy.
The upper rectum attached to the
lower rectal mucosa is removed,
leaving the medium rectal cuff,
which is enlarged by a posterior
incision.

tion (the apex) of the ileal loop that can be brought down in close proximity to the pubic bone is carefully selected, and a Nélaton catheter is inserted through the mesentery for traction on the apex of the loop, which is usually found at about 20 cm from the ileal end (Fig. 8–29).

The vessels in the mesentery are examined by palpation and transillumination, and the incision point that will result in the maximal extension of the loop is determined. This point is usually found on a main trunk of the superior mesenteric vessels near the fourth or fifth distal subdivision; typically, this is the common trunk of the two large vascular arches, called the major and minor arches, in the mesentery (see Fig. 8–29A and B). The artery and vein are independently divided between double 3-0 Vicryl ligatures, and the avascular area of the mesentery is transversely cut out with care taken to preserve the ileocolic vessels (see Fig. 8–29A). In this fashion the ileal mesentery can be extended by about 5 to 8 cm. The extended ileal loop has bilateral blood supplies from both the ileocolic

and the ileal arteries. If the ileocolic vessels have been previously divided, as in the patient with a previous IRA, the ileal vessels are cut more distally to preserve the mesenteric vascular arcade (see Fig. 8–29B).

Before pouch construction is begun, the reach of the pouch is tested by the pull-through maneuver, as described further on. After it is confirmed that the apex of the loop reaches the anal margin, a side-to-side anastomosis is performed between both limbs of the ileal loop by using two applications of the GIA 90 stapler-cutter (Fig. 8–30). The stapler is introduced from the opening previously used for the stoma on the distal limb and through small holes created by a coagulator at the midportion of the proximal limb; it is fired both distally and proximally to perform the lateral anastomosis. The apical bridge is maintained. The holes are closed transversely with a continuous suture covered by seromuscular sutures (the previously used stapled closure was abandoned because it may invite chronic sepsis around the pouch).

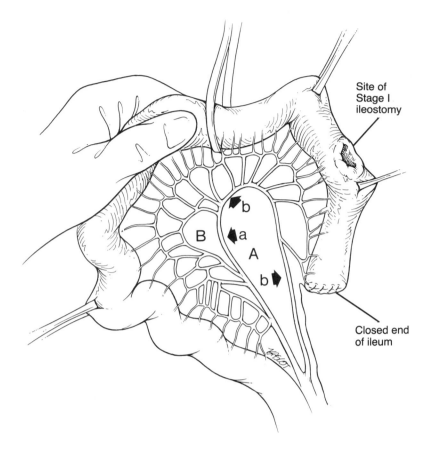

Site of
Stage I
ileostomy

Closed end
of ileum

Figure 8–29. Location of the vessel division points for elongation of the ileal mesentery: *A*, "major arch," *B*, "minor arch," *a*, division point for the standard J-pouch, *b*, division point for the short J-pouch.

Pouch-Anal Anastomosis

The right side of the peritoneal cavity is emptied by removing all the small intestinal loops to expose the mesenteric root up to the lower margin of the duodenum in order to avoid improper rotation of the root. While the patient is in the exaggerated lithotomy position, the pouch is brought through the anal canal by pulling down on the Allis mucosal clamps, which are attached to the apex of the pouch. The pouch is rotated 180 degrees counterclockwise so as to place the antimesenteric side of the pouch against the sacral surface, forming a neorectum similar to the normal rectal configuration and obtaining an additional few centimeters in reach (Fig. 8–31).

With the anal orifice already exposed by the six perianal stay sutures, the pouch is anchored to the denuded anal canal at the level of the anorectal line with approximately eight seromuscular 4-0 polyglycolic acid sutures. The apex of the pouch is then punched out under Kelly forceps to create a round hole with a diameter of 1.5 cm (Fig. 8–32 *A*). The reservoir is then directly anastomosed to the anal canal at the dentate line using 24 to 32 interrupted 4-0 polyglycolic acid sutures attached to an atraumatic needle. These sutures incorporate the mucosa of the anal canal, a deep bite

of the internal sphincter, and the full thickness of the ileal wall (Fig. 8–32 *B*).

The sutures for the pouch-anal anastomosis are serially tied after all sutures are placed, so as to obtain a uniform distance between the stitches and to achieve the clean, circular, anastomotic line that is essential to good fecal function. A cardiac surgery thread holder is convenient for this anastomosis.

Construction of Diverting Ileostomy and Closure of Abdomen

The most distal ileal loop that leaves no tension on the mesentery of the transposed loop is selected, and a Nélaton catheter is placed through the mesentery for traction. A marking suture is placed to identify the efferent loop. This site is usually 15 cm above the pouch, that is, 60 cm from the end. We never suture the mesentery to the retroperitoneum in order to avoid tension on the mesentery. The loop is exteriorized through the abdominal tunnel used for the previous ileostomy, and the catheter is replaced by a supporting rod. The loop is rotated 90 degrees counterclockwise to place the distal mucous fistula medially. The nipple is created by Turnbull's technique as usual, and the

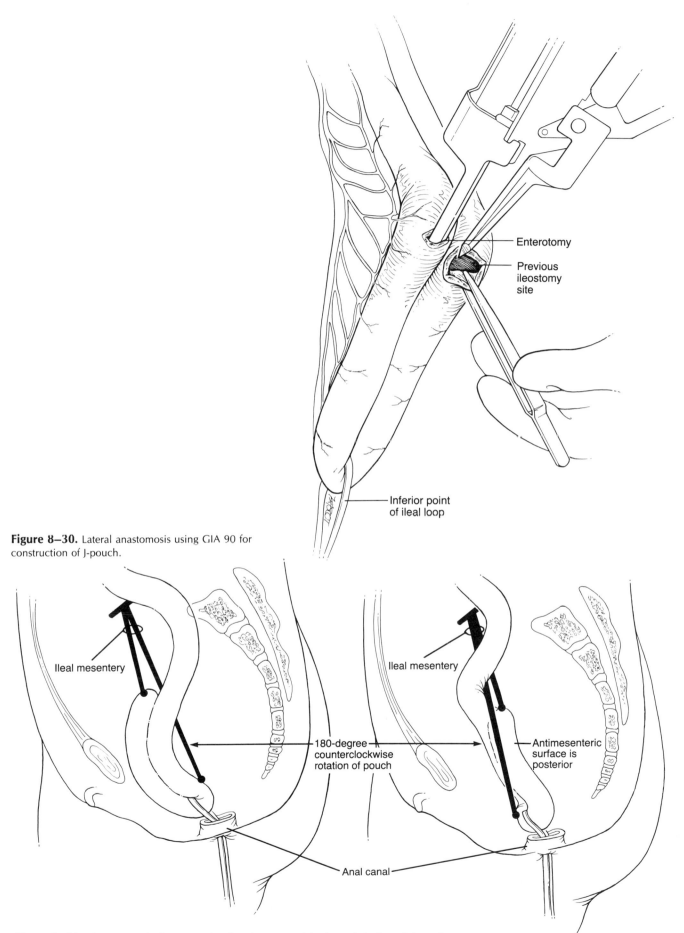

Figure 8–30. Lateral anastomosis using GIA 90 for construction of J-pouch.

Figure 8–31. The counterclockwise rotation for placement of the J-pouch in the pelvic cavity.

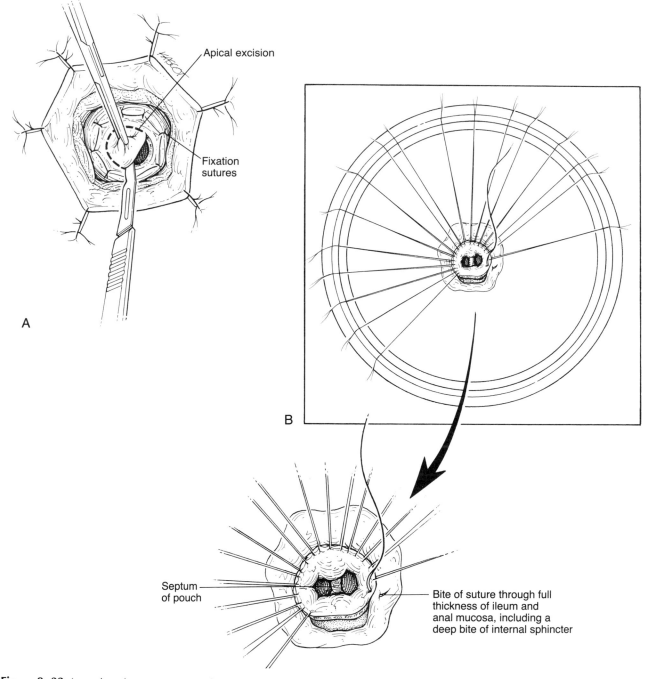

Figure 8–32. J-pouch and anastomosis. *A,* The apex is circularly incised after the pouch is fixed to the rectal cuff. *B,* The wall of the pouch is sutured to the internal sphincter and anal mucosa at the dentate line by using a cardiovascular surgery thread holder.

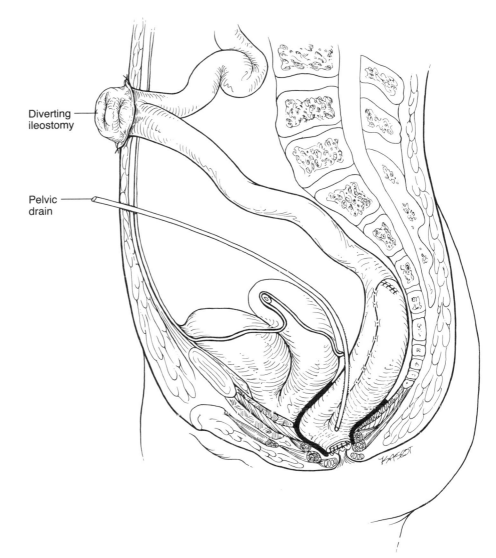

Figure 8–33. Completion of ileoanal anastomosis.

intestinal loop is not fixed to the peritoneum or fascia in order to avoid injury on the intestinal serosa during closure of the stoma at a later operation (Fig. 8–33).

After the peritoneal cavity is thoroughly irrigated with saline, a triple sump drain is placed in the presacral area behind the pouch and brought out through the left lower abdominal wall. A stomal appliance with a synthetic skin barrier (Varicare System 2) is immediately attached to the abdomen around the stoma. A no. 30 Malecot catheter is inserted through the anus to decompress the excluded J-pouch, in which considerable amounts of intestinal secretions may accumulate during the period immediately after the operation.

Immediate Postoperative Care

When the abdominal stoma begins to function, usually in the second to third postoperative day, oral intake is allowed, with gradual increases in solidity and amount of food. The transanal catheter in the pouch and the transabdominal pelvic drains are removed on the second and fifth postoperative days, respectively. Ileostomy care is performed using the standard discipline by an enterostomal therapist. The patient is discharged on recovery and returns to normal social activity. Three months later, when endoscopy shows the ileoanal anastomosis to be clearly healed, contrast radiography shows no fistula or sinus at either the anastomosis or the pouch, and the maximum anal resting pressure is recovered to 40% or more, the patient is admitted for closure of the ileostomy to complete the procedure.

Closure of Ileostomy (Third-Stage Operation)

The operation is done under general anesthesia. The stoma is freed by incising the peristomal mucocutaneous junction with a scalpel, followed by cutting with an electrocoagulator, and is temporarily closed by placing several interrupted sutures. While the sutured threads are held, the intestinal loop is completely mobilized from the surrounding subcutaneous fat and fascia, and the free peritoneal cavity is entered. The loop is exteriorized to a length of about 5 to 7 cm. After the everted nipple is dissected free and the stomal edge is trimmed, the intestinal wall is reconstructed by placing a double layer of fine interrupted sutures. A functional anastomosis using the PLC 50 or the GIA stapler-cutter is an alternative method. After the fascia layer is sutured, the abdominal tunnel is closed with a subcutaneous pursestring suture using 3-0 Vicryl to minimize the scar tissue.

Postoperative Care

Watery stooling usually begins within 48 hours after the operation. The frequency is often as high as 10 times in 24 hours, and the stool soils the perianal skin, which must be rinsed and carefully cleaned to avoid the development of anal ulcers. Oral loperamide is administered at a dose of 2 to 3 mg/day. The frequency of stooling typically rapidly decreases to six times a day or less, and anal fecal leakage usually resolves within 3 months.

POSTOPERATIVE COMPLICATIONS

Diverse and specific postoperative complications may often occur: we observed complications in 75% of the patients in our early series. These complications were usually not life threatening, but some of them, such as pelvic sepsis, could defeat the purpose of the operation by causing inflammation of the reservoir. Therefore, surgeons must be aware of potential complications.

Early Complications

Cuff abscesses can form inside the rectal cuff, between it and the wall of the ileum, in the absence of an apparent anastomotic leak.[11] The patient becomes febrile, complains of anal pain, notes a purulent discharge from the anus, and occasionally has lower abdominal pain and dysuria. It usually (80% of our patients with cuff abscess) is manifest within 1 month after the operation (the early abscess), but may also occur as late as 8 months postoperatively (the late abscess). Anoscopy may disclose a small fistula discharging pus to the anastomotic line. A contrast radiograph may demonstrate tracts coursing upward from the anastomosis. These abscesses may be caused by

intraoperative contamination of pooled blood within the rectal cuff or by an ascending infection from the anastomotic line.[88] Abscesses occurred more frequently (26.0% in our series) with the long cuff and were rare in the shorter cuff (3.9% of our series). The fistula should be laid open under spinal or local anesthesia and the pouch irrigated with an antibiotic solution combined with systemic administration of antibiotics.

A disrupted ileoanal anastomosis occurs rarely. It is due to excessive tension at the suture line, impaired circulation of the pouch, or necrosis at a fragile, inflamed ileal wall.

Intestinal Obstruction

This is the most common complication and has diverse causes that must be identified for treatment. In patients with polyposis, simple mechanical obstruction was more frequent in our series (43.3%) than in the patients with colitis (8.3%). An excessive fibroproductive reaction specific to the polyposis patient may be responsible for this finding. All of the general precautions to minimize peritoneal adhesions should be stressed. A superior mesenteric artery (SMA) syndrome was assumed to be a cause of the high rate of intestinal obstruction or prolonged ileus following this operation.[91] The stretched SMA may compress the horizontal duodenal portion over the aorta following J-pouch anal anastomosis. The patient manifests belching, prolonged high output from the nasogastric tube with a silent stoma, and acute gastroduodenal dilatation seen on radiograph. All four of our patients were successfully treated with effective nasogastric decompression and by encouragement of the patient to turn onto the abdomen or side. For prevention, a postoperative nasogastric tube should be maintained until function returns. Ischemic change of the J-pouch has reportedly been produced by an intussuscepted proximal ileal segment.[32]

Diverting Ileostomy–Related Complications

The diverting ileostomy with IAA is usually about 60 cm from the ileal end and has some specific problems. Mucous overflow from the efferent loop of the loop ileostomy was found to cause peristomal irritation, and the resultant loose fixation led to stomal recession and breakdown. This can be prevented by proper construction at operation. For treatment, conversion to an endileostomy is the method of choice. The first evacuation usually occurs within 48 hours following IAA, but it may be delayed when the closure site of the stoma is inflamed. Mild transitional intestinal obstruction symptoms may occur several days after oral intake. The program of a graded increase in diet should be individualized, depending on intestinal activity. In one of our patients, an intussusception formed in the ileal segment proximal to the stoma.

Metabolic Disorders

Patients who have a delay in the ileostomy closure because of slow recovery of anal function may become dehydrated. According to our data they evacuate about 1,000 ml of intestinal effluent per day, which is six times the volume of fluid in normal feces and twice as much as from an end-ileostomy; their urinary volume is decreased by 40% from the preoperative state and by 30% from that seen with a terminal ileostomy.[92] Their urinary sodium-to-potassium ratio (0.8) was slightly below 1.0, which is the lower limit for normal individuals. Medication such as loperamide or somatostatin may be effective in patients with a particularly high output.[93, 94] Urolithiasis was found in 1.7% of patients in our series.

The mean bile acid output in the ileal effluent of the diverting ileostomy was eight times that of the preoperative level and four times that with terminal ileostomy.[95] The decrease of serum cholesterol levels by 20% to 30% in patients with stomas and their return to a normal level after the closure of the stoma have suggested that the hepatic synthesis of bile acids was abnormally increased in these patients. Transient liver dysfunction associated with an increase of glutamic oxaloacetic transaminese (GOT), glutamyl transpeptidase (GTP), and lactate dehydrogenase (LDH) during the diverting period has been observed in some patients.[96] The incidence of gallstones increased threefold in patients with ileal resection,[97] because the cholesterol saturation index was increased by a decrease of the acid concentration in bile.[98] Periodic examination using ultrasonography for stone disease and preventive oral administration of ursodeoxycholic acid may be necessary in such patients with a long-standing diverting ileostomy.

Late Complications and Sequelae

Pouchitis Syndrome

Pouchitis syndrome is a common, and the most important, late complication. Its incidence varies from 10% to 40%, averaging 14% in patients with colitis in some reports[99] and increases with the length of follow-up.[77] When the patient with IAA complains of malaise, slight fever, increased stooling, and hematochezia after a period of good bowel function and when the other

types of enteritis are excluded, pouchitis must be considered as the most likely diagnosis. Some degree of inflammation in the pouch is common; nevertheless, some patients manifest such a syndrome the etiology of which has not been fully understood. The type and size of the pouch were reported not to be related to pouchitis.[100]

Bacterial overgrowth in the pouch has been suggested as a possible causal factor, because it is known to occur in the Kock abdominal pouch.[101] Additionally, the host factors common with colitis itself may play a role, because this condition has rarely occurred in polyposis.[102] In our series, 10% of our colitis patients develop pouchitis, but we have not encountered it in the polyposis patients. So-called backwash ileitis, is not related to pouchitis.[103] Endoscopy usually discloses a diffusely fragile and edematous mucosa with multiple erosions and occasionally ulcers. Histologically, nonspecific acute or chronic ileal mucosal inflammation is present.[100] Oral administration of metronidazole usually relieves the syndrome within a few weeks.

Steroids may be effective, but the result is not definitive when they are taken without antibiotics.[99] In some cases, hospitalization may be required for diarrhea, dehydration, malnutrition, and anemia. Patients with recurrent attacks are instructed to take metronidazole immediately when they begin to experience the symptoms in order to control the progress of pouchitis.

Other Forms of Enteritis

Several similar syndromes must be differentiated from true pouchitis: a deep solitary ulcer surrounded by noninflamed mucosa in the pouch was reported in a polyposis patient with a similar syndrome.[104] We have also seen solitary ulcer in one patient with colitis. Solitary ulcers responded slowly to metronidazole. If the anastomotic ring is stenotic and noncompliant and a necrotic mucosal cast is evacuated, obstructive enteritis should be considered. Delayed abscesses in the pelvis are also manifested by fever, frequent diarrhea, and loss of continence and may be associated with peritonitis.

Salmonella typhimurium enteritis has been reported in some patients.[105, 106] They exhibit fever, distended abdomen, and diarrhea, symptoms that should be differentiated both from pouchitis and intestinal obstruction. These patients may require broad-spectrum antibiotics because metronidazole is not effective.

Crohn's disease in the ileoanal pouch should also be kept in mind.[107] Fistulas that occur in 1% to 5% of the cases from the pouch or from the anastomosis to the vagina, urinary tract, vulva, or anterior abdominal wall are serious complications that can devastate the patient.[106] The pouch-vaginal fistula is formed after severe pelvic sepsis, but it may occur several months after the ileostomy closure in patients without pelvic sepsis.[108] The principles to follow in preventing these fistulas are the avoidance of pelvic soilage and the preservation of the anterior rectal muscular wall in order to cover the posterior vaginal wall, which may be injured during anterior pararectal dissection. For management of the rectovaginal fistula, repair with a muscle flap such as the gracilis may be effective.[108]

Functional Disturbance of Urogenital Organs

Bladder dysfunctions have been reported, and Neal et al reported a significant increase in bladder capacity following IAA.[109] Because most of the surgical candidates are in the reproductive age group, sexual functional disturbances are serious complications. Although retrograde ejaculation does not occur with long rectal cuffs,[60] this is reported in 9% of the male patients with the short cuff in whom injury to the pudendal nerve was implicated.[56] The female sexual function is less commonly disturbed by IAA. Dyspareunia was common in the women who underwent IRA for colitis,[110] but it was less frequent in women with IAA, presumably because the inflammation in the rectum was removed.[111] Women who have undergone IAA are able to deliver vaginally without impairment of anorectal function.[112]

Late Metabolic Disorders of Pouch

Functional improvement immediately after the operation is now achieved because of the technical details mentioned earlier. However, there are potential late consequences associated with metabolic alterations and pathology of the colonized ileum, such as a stagnant loop syndrome or adenomatous change of the ileal mucosa of the pouch, which have also been reported in the Kock pouch.[113] In general, water-electrolyte[92] and bile acid metabolism[95] return nearly to the preoperative state in the IAA patient. The secondary and less conjugated bile acids are increased in the IAA excreta, compared with patients who have an end-ileostomy, suggesting a relative increase in anaerobic organisms in the former group.[95] Iron-deficiency anemia was observed in some of our patients with a marginally low Schilling test.[7] The patients with IAA who had less frequent stools tended to excrete more secondary bile acids.[95] The evacuation of stool with some increased frequency in the patient with IAA may be necessary in order to maintain a decolonized pouch. After IAA, some patients may manifest symptoms of steroid withdrawal, such as malaise, diarrhea, fever, anemia, and extracolonic manifestations such as rheumatoid arthritis.

Bowel Functional Disturbance

Very frequent liquid stooling and incomplete continence associated with nocturnal soiling and perianal skin irritation seen after IAA can be called the post-IAA bowel dysfunction syndrome, which is the result of the loss of anal canal (transitional) mucosa, loss of the colonic reservoir, and increased amounts of liquid stool. In fact, the history of IAA has been one of attempts to avoid this postoperative syndrome.

Clinical Assessment

Several criteria have been used to describe the bowel functional disorder. The stool frequency per day (SFD) expressed by the average number of stools passed in 24 hours is the most widely used criterion. Usually the patient evacuates stools less frequently while working, traveling, performing sports, and sleeping, and they desire to use the toilet more often after meals or at rest.

Nighttime (nocturnal) stool frequency (NSF) has been regarded as being independent of lifestyle but greatly influences the quality of life. NSF has been expressed either as the average frequency per night or as the percentage of patients needing to defecate during the night. The degree of urgency is assessed, ascertaining how long defecation can be deferred after need is first experienced. Inability to defer evacuation for 30 minutes or more was regarded as positive urgency.[75]

Soiling of underclothing is more distressing to the patient than frequent stooling. This problem has been described by investigators in various ways, such as "soiling" or "minor leakage" (leakage sufficient to cause staining of a pad or underwear, but not social embarrassment)[74] or spotting (one or two episodes per week with an undergarment stain not exceeding 3 cm in diameter).[102] Perianal soreness is an objective sign of soiling, but its severity may not always correlate with the grade of incontinence, because it is found to depend largely on the quality of perianal care. A perineal pad can indicate the existence of soiling, but it is sex specific; although 90% of women with minor soiling in our series wore pads, only 50% of men with the same grade of soiling did so. The need to use antidiarrheal agents also depends on the personality of the patient.

In order to compare the results of different investigators, we have devised a continence disturbance grade (CDG) system, which was expressed essentially by the frequency of soiling.[114] The state of continence (CO) was divided into two classes. Normal continence (CO-1) refers to patients who had never experienced soiling in the last several months, and nearly normal continence (CO-2) refers to those who had no soiling in the

Table 8–1. CONTINENCE DISTURBANCE GRADE AND OTHER PARAMETERS

	Continence Disturbance Grade										
Parameter	**Total** 56	100.0%	**CO-1** 25	44.6%	**CO-2** 14	25.0%	**DC-1** 8	14.3%	**DC-2** 5	8.9%	**IC** 4	7.1%
SFD	5.4 (4.8)*		4.1		5.0		5.6		6.3		14.5	
NSF	18	32.1%	1	4.0%	6	42.9%	4	50.0%	3	60.0%	4	100.0%
Sensation	5	8.9%	0	0.0%	0	0.0%	1	12.5%	1	20.0%	3	75.0%
Pad	22	39.3%	0	0.0%	8	57.1%	5	62.5%	5	100.0%	4	100.0%
Loperamide	16	28.6%	2	8.0%	2	14.3%	4	50.0%	4	80.0%	4	100.0%
Sore	14	25.0%	1	4.0%	2	14.3%	4	50.0%	3	60.0%	4	100.0%
Period (month)	28.4		30		35		23		17		37	
Social	5	8.9%	0	0.0%	0	0.0%	0	0.0%	1	20.0%	4	100.0%

SFD = stool frequency per day; NSF = nocturnal stool frequency (%); social = restricted social life.
*Parenthesis indicates data excluding IC.

last few weeks but occasionally experienced it with diarrhea.

The state of incomplete continence, which we termed dyscontinent (DC), has also been divided into two classes including mild dyscontinence (DC-1), which refers to soiling that occurs for 3 days or less in the last few weeks, and marked dyscontinence, which refers to continuous soiling day and night with severe social embarrassment, because of which the patient might prefer to have an abdominal ileostomy rather than an IAA. The correlation of each category of CDG to the other categories is presented in Table 8–1.

The ability to discriminate gas and feces (sensation or discrimination) was not abolished in most of the cases of IAA in which the transition zone was removed.[50] The habitual need for self-catheterization per anus indicated the inability of spontaneous evacuation, which was frequently seen in pouches with a long spout. The J-pouch may rarely show evacuation difficulty because of a prolapsed apical bridge.[128]

The grading system of patient satisfaction expressed as excellent, fair, good, and poor by Peck,[6] which was modified by us as shown in Table 8–2, was applied to the study of a small number of patients. The scoring system in the University of Goteborg, designed to quantify overall function,[115] may be used in analysis using a large number of patients. Performance status for quality of life was termed "improved" or "re-stricted" by comparing the pre- and postoperative states in five categories: social activity, sports, sexual activity, recreation, and work.[82]

Functional Tests

Bowel function is regulated through multiple complementary components, such as sphincteric reservoir functions and the amount and viscosity of the intestinal content. The tests for assessing functional efficacy of these components are essential to identifying the etiology of bowel dysfunction after IAA and to deciding about the timing of surgery and the selection of candidates. The test methods have been standardized.[116]

The maximum resting anal pressure (MRP) represents the combined tonus, 80% of which is contributed by the internal sphincter, and 20% by the external sphincter, and is mainly responsible for controlling leakage of liquid during unconsciousness. MRP was reduced by 50% of the preoperative value after IAA, but it gradually recovered to 80% or 90% within 12 months after closure of the stoma. Among the anal manometry parameters, MRP correlated most strongly with clinical assessments such as grade of continence and stooling frequency[117–120] and thus proved to be a useful diagnostic procedure. The maximum squeeze pressure represents the voluntary contractibility of the external sphincter muscle. In most patients, MRP was well maintained after IAA, but it was reduced with incontinence.[56] MRP abnormality represents either the injury of the external muscle or the neural control to the muscle through the pudendal nerves. The length of the high-pressure zone, which represents structural derangement of the internal sphincter, is always somewhat reduced after IAA, but this does not affect bowel function.

The positive rectoanal inhibitory reflex implies an active presence of the extramural reflex arcs between the rectal wall and the internal sphincters. Although some investigators found it was abolished in all patients who had undergone IAA,[56, 109] 37.5% of our patients

Table 8–2. GRADING SYSTEM FOR PATIENT SATISFACTION

	Daily Stooling Frequency		
Soiling	**~6**	**~7–10**	**~11**
No soiling	Excellent	Good	Fair
Occasional minor soiling (≤3/wk)	Good	Good	Fair
Frequent minor soiling (<4/wk)	Fair	Fair	Poor
Continuous soiling	Poor	Poor	Poor

Modified from Peck DA. Rectal mucosal replacement. Ann Surg 1980; 191:294–303.

retained the positive reflex. This finding is similar to data reported by Pescatori and colleagues.[121] The variations may be due to the different lengths of the preserved cuff. Electromyography was useful in assessing injury to the pudendal nerve.[56]

The pouch is visualized by barium contrast examination to verify that no fistula, sinus, or leakage from the anastomosis exists, before the ileostomy is closed. The examination is also indicated to assess bowel functional disturbance and to demonstrate adequate size and shape of the pouch. The width of the pouch was considered to be the most significant factor correlating to function.[123] We found that the pouch-anal angle was not a significant indicator for IAA dyscontinence.[124] Special evacuation pouchography was useful for the study of difficult evacuation with an S-pouch.[122] The pouch manovolumetry is performed by the balloon method with a stepwise bolus injection of air[118] or by a continuous injection under isobaric pressure.[115] The maximum pouch capacity is identified as the volume at which the subject experiences continuous discomfort and the urge to evacuate. The distensibility (or compliance) of the pouch is the pressure exerted by the pouch, which is evaluated by the change in volume divided by the change in pressure expressed as milliliters per centimeters H_2O or Hg. The volume of pouch that incites the urge is expressed by the threshold volume, which is determined by the volume at which large-amplitude pressure waves appear and corresponds to 45% to 50% of the maximum capacity.[119] Both the capacity or volume and the compliance are inversely correlated with stool frequency[78] and with continence.[115] The efficacy of emptying is not related to the number of stools, pouchitis, or design of the reservoir.[73, 78]

An excessive amount of stool produces incontinence, even under normal sphincteric pressure,[125] whereas an aged person, even with a reduced sphincteric pressure, may not soil when the feces are sufficiently consolidated. According to our study, immediately after the ileostomy closure 400 to 500 ml of feces were evacuated daily from IAAs. Within several weeks the daily volume was reduced to 320 to 420 ml, about one third of the amount excreted from diverting ileostomies and 70% of that excreted from terminal ileostomies. An average amount of excreta from the S-pouch in the St. Marks series was reported to be 660 g,[7] whereas that of the J-pouch from the Mayo Clinic series was 776 ml, which included the high-output patients.[119] The stool frequency is directly related to the daily stool volume.[119]

The consistency of the stool after IAA is performed changes from an initial watery liquid to a mushy and then a semiformed state. This increasing consistency of the intestinal contents may significantly help fecal continence. Although the water content of the stool decreased only slightly (from 85% to 75%), its viscosity increased markedly within 8 weeks after the ileostomy closure; this change was found to correlate with the prolongation of the ileal transit time and with the characteristic change from the aerobic-dominant bacterial pattern of the ileostomy excreta to an anaerobic-dominant pattern with a remarkable increase of total bacterial count similar to feces in the colon.[79, 127] Measuring the amount of evacuation and assessing the stool consistency are helpful in evaluating bowel dysfunction after IAA.[127]

Before a comparative analysis of the technical factors is conducted, many factors that could independently influence the functional result should be considered. Bowel functions gradually recover during the 12 months following the ileostomy closure (the adaptive phase) and stabilize thereafter (the stabilized phase), According to our studies, in the initial 3 months volume reduction and consolidation of stool occur; SFD is about 6.3, which is still 34% more frequent than the stabilized state (SFD of 4.6), and the continence rate is about 50%, compared with 70% in the stabilized phase. In the sixth month, SFD improves to within 5% to 10% of the stabilized state, and the continence rate reaches 60%, which is nearly 90% of the stabilized state. Anal sphincter manometry and pouch volumetry studies at this stage reveal that the functional adaptation by the sixth month is still incomplete, but it markedly improves thereafter.[52]

Severe pelvic sepsis is catastrophic to pouch function. Even with mild sepsis, the continence rate was found to be reduced[114]; no significant difference was demonstrated following mild sepsis in the Mayo series.[82] Age also determined the quality of bowel function.[128] Older patients had more stools during the day than did the younger patient.[82] SFD did not differ between sexes, but women had more fecal spotting,[82] although we did not demonstrate a difference in the continence rate (68.9% in men versus 78.4% in women). Underlying disease was also a determinant. The patient with polyposis showed significantly better results (continence rate of 70%) than patients with colitis (56%).[100] The effect of race and eating habits is unknown.

Care and Management

Patients should be followed by the surgeon and enterostomal therapist, if one is available. The first choice of antidiarrheal agent is loperamide (Imodium); 4.6 mg of this agent reduces stool frequency with the same effectiveness as 12.5 mg of diphenoxylate with atropine (Lomotil) or 104 mg of codeine sulfate. It also increases anal resting pressure, which improves continence. A bulk-forming agent such as psyllium hydrophilic mucilloid (Metamucil) may be used in combination. The

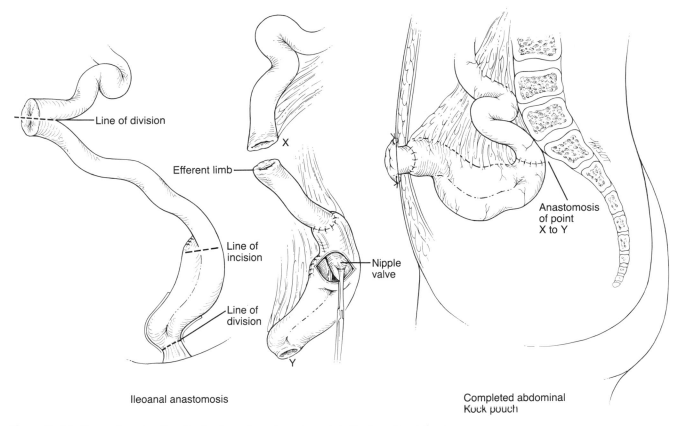

Line of division

Efferent limb

Line of incision

Line of division

X

Nipple valve

Y

Ileoanal anastomosis

Anastomosis of point X to Y

Completed abdominal Kock pouch

Figure 8–34. Conversion of malfunctioning J-pouch anal anastomosis to Kock continent ileostomy.

patient is instructed about diet and toileting: take a meal regularly three times a day; chew food well; avoid spicy, fatty, and cold food; avoid alcohol; avoid eating a large meal before bedtime; and evacuate before going to bed.[129]

For patients with dyscontinence, anal sphincter exercises and rope skipping have proved helpful. Exercise is started about 1 month before the loop ileostomy closure and is performed three times a day. Perianal care has proven effectiveness in accelerating the functional recovery. Immediately after the ileostomy is closed, almost 70% of the patients experience perianal soreness. The soreness has an etiology in common with the peristomal dermatitis of abdominal ileostomy, and it may progress, in a vicious circle, to dermatitis and weakening of the sphincter muscles. The patients who remain severely dyscontinent after the 12 months have abnormal function and require further management. If the incontinent patient with previous pelvic sepsis has a tender and strictured anus (stiff anus), dilation may be attempted, but the results are not satisfactory. When daily amounts of feces are liquid and excessive and septic complications such as pouchitis or late pelvic sepsis are excluded, H_2 antagonists for gastric hypersecretion and antibiotics for bacterial overgrowth in the pouch are recommended, as is somatostatin, which reduces ileostomy effluent by 23%.[94]

An abnormally low sphincteric resting pressure associated with a reduced squeeze pressure suggests a neural origin with injury to the pudendal nerves during operation. In such cases, biofeedback conditioning[130] or valproate sodium of γ-aminobutyric acid (GABA) could be effective in combination with other general management.[131] For intractable continence disturbance, surgical measures are ultimately indicated. Initially, the diverting ileostomy is reopened on the pointed scar of the abdominal wall of the previous stoma to palliate the problems while the etiology is analyzed. Aggressive diagnosis and therapy to save the pouch and to maintain function are attempted.[132] If sphincteric continence is finally abandoned, the metabolically valuable ileum used for the pouch should be salvaged.[133] We have successfully converted a J-pouch to a modified Kock pouch (Fig. 8–34).[134]

CONCLUSIONS

Forty years after the initial clinical study by Ravitch and Sabiston, the practical surgical procedures of ileoanal anastomosis have been established to provide a nearly natural anal function to 90% of the patients with colitis and polyposis. Although there are several schools using different techniques, methods, and procedures, there is unanimous agreement about the necessity of a pelvic pouch. The extent and method of mucosectomy are still debated, and the trend has been moving toward a gradual shortening of the rectal cuff. However, we still prefer the medium cuff, which may work as the functional support for the sphincter muscles and as a protective wall for the neighboring pelvic organs. The technique and rationale of the authors' J-pouch medium-cuff procedure have been described and discussed. The result of IAA should be evaluated by bowel function as measured by objective criteria and also by quality of life, by socioeconomic profiles, and by any late metabolic sequelae.

The stapled anastomosis, which is easier to perform but neglects removal of the anal canal mucosa, is termed the IACA (as a variant of IRA) to distinguish it from IAA with mucosectomy and to avoid confusion in technical discussion. Therefore, IACA has been discussed as an alternative surgical option of IAA. Patients with either colitis or polyposis who undergo IAA must agree to life-long surveillance of metabolic outcome and cancer risk.

REFERENCES

1. Utsunomiya J, Iwama T, Imajo M, et al. Total colectomy, mucosal proctectomy and ileoanal anastomosis. Dis Colon Rectum 1980;23:459–466.
2. Ravitch MM, Sabiston DC. Anal ileostomy with preservation of the sphincter: A proposed operation in patients requiring total colectomy for benign lesions. Surg Gynecol Obstet 1947;84:1095–1099.
3. Best RR. Evaluations of ileoproctostomy to avoid ileostomy in various colonic lesions. JAMA 1951;150:637–642.
4. Safaie-Shirazi S, Soper RT. Endorectal pull-through procedure in the surgical treatment of familial polyposis coli. J Pediatr Surg 1973;8:711–715.
5. Parks AG, Nicholls RJ. Proctocolectomy without ileostomy for ulcerative colitis. Br Med J 1978;2:85–88.
6. Peck DA. Rectal mucosal replacement. Ann Surg 1980;191:294–303.
7. Nicholls RJ, Belleveau P, Neill M, et al. Restorative proctocolectomy with ileal reservoir: A pathophysiological assessment. Gut 1981;22:462–468.
8. Tosatti E. The ileo-anal-channel-stomy. Surg Italy 1973;3:201–205.
9. Johnston D, Holdsworth PJ, Nasmyth DG, et al. Preservation of the entire anal canal in conservative proctocolectomy for ulcerative colitis: A pilot study comparing end-to-end ileoanal anastomosis without mucosal resection with mucosal proctectomy and endo-anal anastomosis. Br J Surg 1987;74:940–944.
10. Nissen R. Berliner Gesellschaft für Chirurgie. Zentralbl Chir 1933;15:888.
11. Devine J, Webb R. Resection of the rectal mucosa, colectomy and anal ileostomy with normal continence. Surg Gynecol Obstet 1951;92:437–442.
12. Martin LW, Le Caultre C, Schubert WK. Total colectomy and mucosal proctectomy with preservation of continence in ulcerative colitis. Ann Surg 1977;186:477–479.
13. Valiente MA, Bacon HE. Construction of pouch using "pantaloon" technique for pull-through of ileum following total colectomy. Am J Surg 1955;90:742–750.
14. Kock NG. Intra-abdominal "reservoir" in patients with permanent ileostomy. Arch Surg 1969;94:223–231.
15. Utsunomiya J, Iwama T. The J ileal pouch-anal anastomosis: The Japanese experience. In: Dozois RR, ed. Alternatives to Conventional Ileostomy. Chicago: Medical Year Book, 1985, pp 371–383.
16. Newton CR, Baker WNW. Comparison of bowel function after ileorectal anastomosis for ulcerative colitis and colonic polyposis. Gut 1975;16:785–791.

17. Lockhart-Mummery HF, Dukes CE, Bussey HJR. The surgical treatment of familial polyposis of the colon. Br J Surg 1956;43:436–481.

18. Utsunomiya J. Pathology, genetics and management of hereditary gastrointestinal polyposes. In: Lynch H, Hirayama T, ed. Genetic Epidemiology of Cancer. Boca Raton: CRC press, 1989;220–249.

19. Beart W, Welling DR. Surgical alternatives in the treatment of familial adenomatous polyposis. In: Herrera L, ed. Familial Adenomatous Polyposis. New York: Alan R Liss, 1990: pp 199–208.

20. Jagelman DG. Choice of operation in familial adenomatous coli. Ann Chir Gynecol 1986;75:71–74.

21. Wolfstein IH, Dreznik AJ, Avigaid S. Total colectomy and anal ileostomy in multiple polyposis coli. Arch Surg 1978;113:1101–1106.

22. Nicholls RJ, Kamm MA. Proctocolectomy with restorative ileoanal reservoir for severe idiopathic constipation: Reports of two cases. Dis Colon Rectum 1988;31:968–969.

23. Hosie KB, Kimot WA, Keighley MRB. Constipation: Another indication for restorative proctocolectomy. Br J Surg 1990;77:801–802.

24. Pearl RK, Nelson RN, Prasad L, et al. Ileoanal anastomosis 24 years after total proctocolectomy for ulcerative colitis. Dis Colon Rectum 1984;28:180–182.

25. Fasth S, Scaglia M, Nordgrew S, et al. Restoration of intestinal continuity (pelvic pouch) after previous proctocolectomy with distal mucosal proctectomy. J Colorect Dis 1986;1:256–258.

26. Hulten L, Fasth S, Nordgren S, Bresland T. Kock's pouch converted to a pelvic pouch—report of a case. Dis Colon Rectum 1988;31:467–469.

27. Pezim ME, Pemberton JH, Beart RW, et al. Outcome of "Indeterminant" colitis following ileal pouch-anal anastomosis. Dis Colon Rectum 1989;32:653–656.

28. Parc P, Legrand P, Frileux E, et al. Comparative clinical results of ileal-pouch anal anastomosis and ileorectal anastomosis in ulcerative colitis. Hepatogastroenterology 1989;36:235–239.

29. Trem TM, Jagelman DG, Fazio VW, et al. A price to pay for an ileal pouch anal anastomosis. Presented at the 84th Annual Meeting of the Society of Colon Rectum Surgeons, 1987, p 91.

30. Heald RJ, Allen DR. Stapled ileoanal anastomosis: A technique to avoid mucosal proctectomy in the ileal pouch operation. Br J Surg 1986;73:571–572.

31. Peck AD. Stapled ileal reservoir to anal anastomosis. Surg Gynecol Obstet 1988;116:562–564.

32. Kimot WA, Keighley MRB. Totally stapled abdominal restorative proctocolectomy. Br J Surg 1989;76:961–964.

33. Tsunoda A, Nicholls RJ. A randomized trial comparing hand sutured ileoanal anastomosis with excision of the anorectal mucosa with stapled ileoanal anastomosis with preservation of the anorectal mucosa. Submitted for publication, 1990.

34. King DW, Lubowski DZ, Cook TA. Anal canal mucosa in restorative proctocolectomy for ulcerative colitis. Br J Surg 1989;76:970–972.

35. Schneider S. Anal ileostomy: Experience with new three-stage procedure. Arch Surg 1955;70:539–574.

36. Thow CB. Single stage colectomy and mucosal proctectomy with stapled antiperistaltic ileal reservoir. In: Dozois RR, ed. Alternatives to Conventional Ileostomy. Chicago: Year Book, pp 420–433.

37. Feinberg SM, Robin SM, Cohen Z. Complications of loop ileostomy. Am J Surg 1987;153:102–107.

38. Everett WG, Pollard SG. Restorative proctocolectomy without temporary ileostomy. Br J Surg 1990;77:621–622.

39. Turnbull RG Jr, Hawk WA, Weakley FL. The surgical treatment of toxic megacolon. Ileostomy and colostomy to prepare patient for colectomy. Am J Surg 1971;122:325–331.

40. Utsunomiya J, Yamamura T, Kusunoki M, Iwama T. The current technique of ileoanal anastomosis. Dig Surg 1988;5:207–214.

41. Utsunomiya J, Yamamura T. Radikale Chirurgie der Schwerer Colitis Ulcerosa. Chirurg 1989;60:565–572.

42. Sullivan E, Garnjorst WM. Advantage of initial transanal mucosal stripping in ileoanal pull-through procedures. Dis Colon Rectum 1982;25:170–172.

43. Rothenberger DA, Vermeulen FD, Christiensen CE, et al. Restorative proctocolectomy with ileal reservoir and ileoanal anastomosis. Am J Surg 1983;145:82–88.

44. Hatada T, Kusunoki M, Yamamura T, et al. Hemodynamics in the prone jackknife during surgery. Am J Surg 1990;162:55–58.

45. Ballentyne GH, Pemberton JH, Beart RW, et al. Ileal J-pouch-anal anastomosis, current technique. Dis Colon Rectum 1985;28:197–202.

46. Dozois RR. Ileal (J) pouch-anal anastomosis. Br J Surg 1985;72(suppl):80–82.

47. Nicholls RJ, Lubowski DZ. Restorative proctocolectomy the four loop (W) reservoir. Br J Surg 1987;74:504–566.

48. Deasy JM, Quarke P, Dixon M, et al. The surgical importance of the anal transitional zone in ulcerative colitis. Br J Surg 1987;74:533–534.

49. Duthie HL, Bennett RC. The relation of sensation in the anal canal to the functional anal sphincter: A possible factor in anal continence. Gut 1960;4:179–182.

50. Keighly MRB, Winslet MC, Yoshioka K, Lightwood R. Discrimination is not impaired by excision of the anal transition zone after restorative proctocolectomy. Br J Surg 1987;74:1118–1121.

51. Grant D, Cohen Z, McHugh S, et al. Restorative proctocolectomy. Clinical results and manometric findings with long and short rectal cuffs. Dis Colon Rectum 1986;29:27–32.

52. Shoji Y, Kusunoki M, Fujita S, et al. Functional role of the preserved rectal cuff in the ileoanal anastomosis. Surgery 1990;111:266–273.

53. Williams NS, Price R, Johnston D. The long-term effect of sphincter preserving operations for rectal carcinoma on function of the anal sphincter. Br J Surg 1980;67:203–208.

54. Williams NS, Marzouk DEM, Hallan RI, Waldron DJ. Function after ileal pouch and stapled pouch-anal anastomosis for ulcerative colitis. Br J Surg 1989;76:1168–1171.

55. Sato K, Sato T. Composition and distribution of the pudendal and pelvic plexuses [Japanese text with English abstract]. J Jap Soc Coloproct 1981;34:515–529.

56. Stryker SJ, Daube JR, Kelly KA, et al. Anal sphincter electromyography after colectomy, mucosal retectomy, and ileoanal anastomosis. Arch Surg 1985;120:713–716.

57. Fujiwara T, Kawarasaki H, Fonkalsrud EW. Endorectal ileal pull-through procedure after chemical debridement of the rectal mucosa. Surg Gynecol Obstet 1984;158:437–442.

58. Hampton JM. Rectal mucosal stripping: A technique for preservation of the rectum after total colectomy for chronic ulcerative colitis. Dis Colon Rectum 1976;19:133–135.

59. Hodgson WTB, Funkelstein JL, Woodriffe P, Aufses AH Jr. Continent anal ileostomy with mucosal proctectomy: A bloodless technique using a surgical ultrasonic aspirator in dog. Br J Surg 1979;66:857–860.

60. Rohner A. Ileoanal anastomosis. In: Lee ECG, ed. Surgery of Inflammatory Bowel Disease. Edinburgh: Churchill Livingstone, pp 125–132.

61. Goligher JG. Eversion technique for distal mucosal proctectomy in ulcerative colitis: A preliminary report. Br J Surg 1984;71:26–28.

62. Telander RJ, Perrault J. Total colectomy with rectal mucosectomy and ileoanal anastomosis for chronic ulcerative colitis in children and young adults. Mayo Clin Proc 1980;55:420–425.

63. Parks AG, Nicholls RJ, Belliveau P. Proctocolectomy with ileal reservoir and anal anastomosis. Br J Surg 1980;67:533–538.

64. Rothenberger DA, Buls JG, Nivatvongs S, Goldberg SM. The Parks S ileal pouch and anal anastomosis after colectomy and mucosal proctectomy. Am J Surg 1985;149:390–394.

65. Bubrick MP, Jacobs DM, Levy M. Experience with the endorectal pull-through and S pouch for ulcerative colitis and familial polyposis in adult. Surgery 1985;98:689–698.

66. Cohen Z, McLeod RS, Sterm H, et al. The pelvic pouch and ileoanal anastomosis. Procedures: Surgical technique and initial results. Am J Surg 1985;150:601–609.

67. Fonkalsrud EW. Total colectomy and endo-rectal ileal pull-through with ileal reservoir for ulcerative colitis. Surg Gynecol Obstet 1980;150:1–9.

68. Fujimoto Y, Utsunomiya J, Yamamura T, Kusunoki M. Study on blood supply to the J shape ileal pouch. Unpublished data, 1989.
69. Smith L, Friend WG, Medwell SJ. The superior mesenteric artery. The critical factor in the pouch pull-through procedure. Dis Colon Rectum 1984;27:791–794.
70. Cherqui D, Valleur P, Perniceni T, Hautefeuille P. Inferior reach of ileal reservoir in ileoanal anastomosis, experimental anatomic and angiographic study. Dis Colon Rectum 1987;30:365–371.
71. Soper NJ, Kestenburg A, Becker JM. Ileal J pouch: Sutured versus stapled construction. Surg Forum 1986;37:193–194.
72. Perbeck L, Lindquist K, Liljeqvist L. The mucosal blood flow in pelvic pouches in man. A methodologic study of fluorescein flowmetry. Dis Colon Rectum 1985;28:931–936.
73. Nicholls RJ, Pezim ME. Restorative proctocolectomy with ileal reservoir for ulcerative colitis and familial adenomatous polyposis: A comparison of three reservoir designs. Br J Surg 1985;72:470–474.
74. Nasmyth DG, Johnston D, Williams NS. Comparison of the function of triplicated and duplicated pelvic ileal reservoirs after mucosal proctectomy and ileo-anal anastomosis for ulcerative colitis and adenomatous polyposis. Br J Surg 1986;73:361–366.
75. Öresland T, Fasth S, Nordgren S, et al. A prospective randomized comparison of two different pelvic pouch designs. Scand J Gastroenterol 1990;25:986–996.
76. McHugh SM, Diamant NE, McLeod R, Cohen Z. S-pouches vs. J-pouches. A comparison of functional outcomes. Dis Colon Rectum 1987;30:1–677.
77. Wexner SD, Gensen L, Rothenberger DA, et al. Long-term functional analysis of the ileal reservoir. Dis Colon Rectum 1989;32:275–281.
78. Heppel J, Belliveau P, Taillefer R, et al. Quantitative assessment of pelvic ileal reservoir emptying with a semisolid radionuclide enema. Dis Colon Rectum 1987;30:81–85.
79. Nasmyth DG, Johnston D, Gowin PGR, et al. Factors influencing bowel function after ileal pouch-anal anastomosis. Br J Surg 1986;73:469–473.
80. Nicholls J, Pescatori M, Motson RW, Pezim ME. Restorative proctocolectomy with a three-loop ileal reservoir for ulcerative colitis and familial adenomatous polyposis: Clinical results in 66 patients followed for up to six years. Ann Surg 1984;199:383–388.
81. Keighly MRB, Yoshioka K, Kimot W. Prospective randomized trial to compare the stapled double lumen pouch and the sutured quadruple pouch for restorative proctocolectomy. Br J Surg 1988-a;75:1008–1011.
82. Pemberton JH, Kelly KA, Beart RW, et al. Ileal pouch-anal anastomosis for chronic ulcerative colitis. Long-term results. Ann Surg 1987;206:504–513.
83. Metcalf AM, Dozois RR, Beart Jr RW, et al. Temporary ileostomy for ileal pouch-anal anastomosis, function and complications. Dis Colon Rectum 1986;29:300–303.
84. Fasth S, Hulten L. Loop ileostomy a superior diverting stoma in colorectal surgery. World J Surg 1984;8:401–405.
85. Dozois RR. Surgical treatment of chronic ulcerative colitis. Hepatogastroenterology 1989-a;36:227–234.
86. Kestenberg A, Becker JM. A new technique of loop ileostomy closure after endorectal ileoanal anastomosis. Surgery 1985;109–111.
87. Yamamura T, Kusuhara K, Shoji Y, et al. Diverting ileostomy [in Japanese]. Operation 1989;43:541–548.
88. Lindquist K, Nilsell K, Liljeqvist L. Cuff abscess and ileoanal anastomotic separation in pelvic pouch surgery: An analysis of possible etiologic factor. Dis Colon Rectum 1987;30:355–359.
89. Pezim ME, Taylor BA, Davis C, Beart RW. Perforation of terminal ileal appendage of J-pelvic ileal reservoir. Dis Colon Rectum 1987;30:161–163.
90. Ballentyne GH, Graham SM, Hammers L, Modlin JM. Superior mesenteric artery syndrome following ileal J-pouch anal anastomosis. An iatrogenic cause of early postoperative obstruction. Dis Colon Rectum 1987;30:772–779.
91. Kimot WA, Keighly MRB. Intussusception presenting as ileal reservoir proctocolectomy. Br J Surg 1989;76:148.

92. Okamoto T, Utsunomiya J. Water-electrolite metabolism in patient with ileoanal anastomosis. Proceedings of the International Symposium for Ileal-Pouch Anal Anastomosis, Versailles, September, 1992.
93. Cooper JC, Williams NS, King RFGJ, Barker MCJ. Effect of a long acting somatostatin analogue in patients with severe ileostomy diarrhoea. Br J Surg 1986;73:128–131.
94. Kusuhara K, Kusunoki M, Sakanoue Y, et al. The effect of somatostatin analog (SMS 201-205) on the management of ileostomy. Unpublished data, 1990.
95. Natori H, Utsunomiya J, Yamamura T, et al. Fecal and stomal bile acid after ileostomy and ileoanal anastomosis in patients with chronic ulcerative colitis and adenomatous coli. Gastroenterology 1992;102:1278–1288.
96. Max E, Trabanino G, Reznick R, et al. Metabolic changes during the defunctionalized stage after ileal pouch-anal anastomosis. Dis Colon Rectum 1987;30:508–513.
97. Hill GL, Mair WSJ, Goligher JC. Gall stones after ileostomy and ileal resection. Gut 1975;16:932–936.
98. Dowling RH, Bell GD, White J. Lithogenic bile in patients with ileal dysfunction. Gut 1972;13:415–420.
99. Shepherd NA, Hultén L, Tytgat GNJ, et al. Workshop: Pouchitis. J Colorect Dis 1989;4:205–229.
100. Moskowitz RL, Shepherd NA, Nicholls RJ. Histopathological grading of inflammation in the reservoir after restorative proctocolectomy with ileal reservoir. Int J Colorect Dis 1986;1:167–174.
101. Luukkonen P, Valtonen V, Sivonen A, et al. Fecal bacteriology and reservoir ileitis in patients operated on for ulcerative colitis. Dis Colon Rectum 1988;31:364–367.
102. Dozois RR, Kelly KA, Welling DR, et al. Ileal pouch-anal anastomosis: Comparison of results in familial adenomatous polyposis and chronic ulcerative colitis. Ann Surg 1989-b;210:268–271.
103. Gustavsson S, Weiland LH, Kelly KA. Relationship of backwash ileitis to ileal pouchitis after ileal pouch anal anastomosis. Dis Colon Rectum 1987;30:25–28.
104. Franceschi D, Chen PF, Yen-Nan Y. Solitary J-pouch ulcer causing pouchitis-like syndrome. Dis Colon Rectum 1986;29:515–517.
105. Løntoft E. *Salmonella typhimurium* infection after colectomy with a mucosal proctectomy pouch, and ileoanal anastomosis. Dis Colon Rectum 1986;29:671–672.
106. Kusunoki M, Tanaka T, Sakanoue Y, et al. *Salmonella* injection after ileoanal anastomosis. Lancet 1989;2:113.
107. Sakanoue Y, Kusunoki M, Yamamura T, Utsunomiya J. Crohn's disease in ileal J-pouch. Dis Colon Rectum 1990;33:541.
108. Gorenstein L, Boyd JB, Ross TM. Gracilis muscle repair of rectovaginal fistula after restorative proctocolectomy. Report of two cases. Dis Colon Rectum 1988;31:730–734.
109. Neal DE, Williams NS, Johnston D. Rectal bladder and sexual function with and without a pelvic reservoir. Br J Surg 1982;69:599–604.
110. Grüner OPN, Naas R, Fretheim B, Gjone E. Marital status and sexual adjustment after colectomy: Result of 178 patients operated on for ulcerative colitis. Scand J Gastroenterol 1977;12:193–197.
111. Metcalf AM, Dozois RR, Kelly KA. Sexual function in women after proctocolectomy. Ann Surg 1986;204:624–627.
112. Metcalf AM, Dozois RR, Beart RW Jr, Wolff BG. Pregnancy-following ileal pouch-anal anastomosis. Dis Colon Rectum 1985;28:854–861.
113. Beart RW, Fleming CR, Banks PM. Tubulovillous adenomas in a continent ileostomy after proctocolectomy for familial polyposis. Dig Dis Sci 1982;27:553–556.
114. Fujita S, Kusunoki M, Shoji Y, et al. Quality of life after total proctocolectomy and ileal J-pouch-anal anastomosis. Dis Colon Rectum. 1992;35:1030–1039.
115. Öresland T, Fasth S, Nordgren S, et al. Pouch size: The important functional determinant after restorative proctocolectomy. Br J Surg 1990;77:265–269.
116. Keighly MRB, Henry MM, Bartolo DCC, Mortensen NJMC. Anorectal physiology measurement: Report of a working party. Br J Surg 1989;76:356–357.

117. Matsuo S. Anorectal function after total colectomy, mucosal proctectomy and ileoanal anastomosis [in Japanese with English abstract]. J Jap Surg Soc 1981;82:1366–1376.
118. Stryker SJ, Philips SF, Dozois RR, et al. Anal and neorectal function after ileal pouch anal anastomosis. Ann Surg 1986;203:55–61.
119. O'Connell PR, Pemberton JH, Brown ML, Kelly KA. Determinants of stool frequency after ileal pouch-anal anastomosis. Am J Surg 1987;153:157–163.
120. Kusunoki M, Shoji Y, Fujita S, et al. Characteristics of anal canal motility after ileoanal anastomosis. Surg Gynecol Obstet 1992;174:22–26.
121. Pescatori M, Mattana D, Castagneto M. Clinical and functional results after restorative proctocolectomy. Br J Surg 1988;75:321–324.
122. Pescatori M, Manhire A, Bartram CI. Evacuation pouchography in the evaluation of ileoanal reservoir function. Dis Colon Rectum 1983;26:365–368.
123. Hatakeyama K, Yamai K, Muto T. Evaluation of ileal W pouch-anal anastomosis for restorative proctocolectomy. Int J Colorect Dis 1989;4:150–155.
124. Parks AG. Anorectal incontinence. Proc R Soc Med 1975;68:681–690.
125. Read NW, Harford WV, Schulen AC, et al. A clinical study of patients with fecal incontinence and diarrhea. Gastroenterology 1978;76:747–757.
126. Read M, Read W, Barber DC, Duthie HL. Effect of loperamide on anal sphincter function in patient complaining of chronic diarrhea with incontinence and urgency. Dig Dis Sci 1982;27:807–814.
127. Imajo M. Study of the small bowel transit time and physiochemical characteristics of the ileal excreta in abdominal and anal ileostomy [in Japanese with English abstract]. J Jap Surg Soc 1981;82:546–565.
128. Öresland T, Fasth S, Nordgren S, Hulten L. The clinical and functional outcome after restorative proctocolectomy. A prospective study in 100 patients. Int J Colorectal Dis 1989;4:50–56.
129. Harada T, Utsunomiya J. To make more improvement of "quality of life" after restorative proctocolectomy with J pouch. Toronto: World Council of Enterostomal Therapists (an association of nurses), Eighth Biennial Congress, 1990;7:15–20.
130. Cerulli MA, Nikoomanesh P, Schulta MM. Progress in biofeedback conditioning for fecal continence. Gastroenterology 1978;76:742–746.
131. Kusunoki M, Shoji Y, Ikeuchi H, et al. Usefulness of valproate sodium for treatment of incontinence after ileoanal anastomosis. Surgery 1990;107:311–315.
132. Schoetz DJ, Coller JA, Veidenbermer MC. Can the pouch be saved? Dis Colon Rectum 1988;31:671–675.
133. Thompson WHF, O'Kelly TJ. Ileal salvage from failed pouches. Surgery 1988;75:1227–1229.
134. Kusunoki M, Sakanoue Y, Shoji Y, et al. Conversion of malfunctioning J pouch to Kock's pouch. Case report. Acta Chir Scand 1989;30:113–115.

Neoplastic Diseases of the Colon, Rectum, and Anus

C H A P T E R 9

Operative Treatment for Carcinoma of the Abdominal Colon

Warren E. Enker

The proper operative treatment of abdominal colon carcinoma is rewarded by a high cure rate, compared with cure rates of many diseases, in particular, other cancers.

Proper operative treatment is characterized by anatomic resection, a complete resection of the mesentery based on the total arterial blood supply to the affected segment. This technique contrasts sharply with the too-common practice of segmental resection, which focuses on the colonic margins on either side of the primary tumor with little regard for the anatomy or the pathophysiology of potential mesenteric lymph node spread (Fig. 9–1).

A growing body of literature over the past 2 decades attests to the significantly higher cure rates achieved by anatomic resections. This is especially apparent in patients with regional disease, that is, mural penetration or nodal involvement, in which the pattern and the extent of resection appear responsible for differences in outcome. Thus, details of operative treatment for this disease are critical.

This chapter provides those details as well as the general principles for treatment of colon adenocarcinoma and the pathophysiology on which it is based. Remarks are limited to the management of primary tumors affecting the intra-abdominal or intraperitoneal colon. This portion of the large bowel is defined by the limits of the peritoneal cavity; the distal limit of this colon lies approximately 12 cm from the anal verge.

HISTORICAL DEVELOPMENT

Despite 80 years of modern history of the operative treatment of colorectal cancer, there are no controlled trials comparing time spans from treatment to survival. The historical data constitute a convincing body of literature based on the pathophysiology of the disease. The majority of patients, that is, approximately 85% of all curable patients, present with the regional spread of disease, that is, complete penetration of the bowel wall or involvement of regional lymph nodes. Operations must be designed to cure a majority of these patients; those that focus on the length of the resected bowel, rather than on the potential for regional lymph node metastases, fail to address the needs of most patients.

Before 1900, operations for rectal cancer were based on excision of the primary tumor without regard for patterns of spread. In 1908 Mr. Ernest W. Miles described the "upward zone of spread," the lymph node metastases from primary rectal cancer along the superior hemorrhoidal artery. He argued that the appropriate operation for rectal cancer would involve ligation and division of the superior hemorrhoidal artery with en bloc proctectomy to remove the primary tumor and its array of lymph node metastases.

In 1909 Professors Jamieson and Dobson from the University of Leeds reported evidence of the same pattern of spread, that is, to lymph nodes along the main named arterial blood supply to the affected bowel segment, for all colon cancers at any site (see Fig. 9–1). They argued that the appropriate operative treatment of colon carcinoma involved ligation of the total arterial blood supply at its origin ("high ligation") and removal of the total area of mesentery, which could harbor actual or potential lymph node metastases.

The principle of high ligation was also supported by Mr. B.G. Moynihan, who also advocated mobilization of the splenic flexure in order to reconstruct any defect resulting from "adequate" resections of the left colon. By 1913 Mr. Drummond described the marginal artery

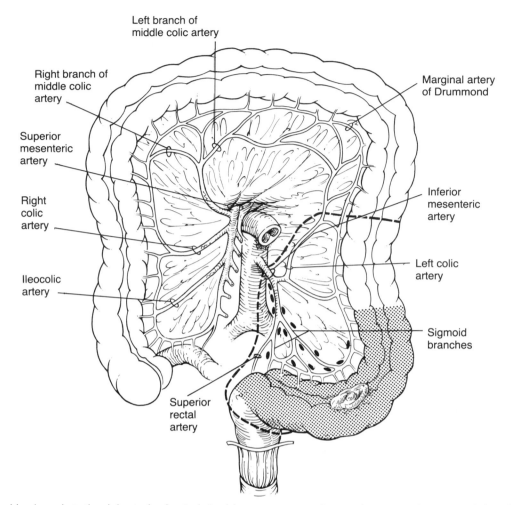

Left branch of
middle colic artery

Right branch of
middle colic
artery

Superior
mesenteric
artery

Right
colic
artery

Ileocolic
artery

Marginal artery
of Drummond

Inferior
mesenteric
artery

Left colic
artery

Sigmoid
branches

Superior
rectal
artery

Figure 9–1. The blood supply to the abdominal colon is derived from two sources: the superior mesenteric artery and the inferior mesenteric artery. Identified here are the ileocolic artery, the right colic artery, and the right and left branches of the middle colic artery, all of which are derived from the superior mesenteric artery. The left branch of the middle colic artery anastomoses with the left colic artery via the marginal artery of Drummond, which supplies arterial circulation to the descending-sigmoid junction. Branches of the inferior mesenteric artery include the left colic artery, the sigmoid branches, and the superior rectal (hemorrhoidal) artery. The latter becomes the main blood supply to the rectum.

The difference between an anatomic resection and a segmental resection is shown. A segmental resection (as indicated by stippling) focuses on the resection of a length of bowel to either side of a primary tumor, whereas an anatomic resection focuses on a resection of the mesentery that contains the predictable pathways of lymph node spread. The anatomic resection is outlined by a broken line.

based on the left branch of the middle colic artery and demonstrated that the marginal artery alone provided adequate blood supply to at least the descending colon–sigmoid colon junction. By 1913 all of the principles for adequate resection and primary reconstruction were in the literature.

Few advances followed immediately because of the limitations of anesthesia and surgery in the early twentieth century. Although the recommendations of Moynihan and others in the early part of the twentieth century were correct in principle, it was difficult to implement such practices in the absence of techniques such as fluid management and transfusions. The 1930s witnessed advances that corroborated the patterns of spread first outlined by Jamieson, Dobson, and Miles. Unique among these was the contribution of J. Kennedy Gilchrist, who demonstrated at autopsy that segmental resections of the colon failed to remove all regional curable lymph node metastases that could be incorporated by anatomic resection.

In 1941 Coller and associates demonstrated that abdominal colon carcinomas spread first to epicolic nodes, then to paracolic lymph nodes, then to intermediate or centrally located lymph nodes, and finally to apical or principal lymph nodes at the origin of the named arteries (Fig. 9–2). Coller emphasized the fact that this relatively orderly pattern of spread allowed for the cure of a high percentage of patients with the regional spread of disease in contrast to those with most other visceral cancers. Early figures reflecting these higher cure rates were published by Grinnell in 1952 and by Rosi in 1954. Rosi demonstrated that by changing his practice from segmental resection of the colon to high ligation and anatomic resection, he increased the relative cure rate from cancer resections by 18% (from 55% to 73%) and diminished his local recurrence rates from 18% to 2.8%. The latter observation was most persuasive.

In 1967 Rupert B. Turnbull of The Cleveland Clinic reported on the "no-touch" isolation technique. On the basis of Warren Cole's observation of tumor cells in the portal circulation, Turnbull suggested that the interruption of embolic venous spread or of the spread of cancer along the lumen of the bowel would play an important role in the cure rates for the treatment of colon cancer. Initial high ligation and luminal interruption were followed by mobilization of the colon and resection. Turnbull's resections produced an overall cure rate of 69% for Dukes A, B, and C tumors, and 58% for Dukes C, node-positive, colon cancer.

During this same period, Turnbull's colleagues achieved a 30% 5-year survival for Dukes C disease, continuing their practice of segmental resection at the same institution. Most contemporaries, including Edward Ellison and Maus W. Stearns, Jr., attributed the results of his operation to adequate mesenteric resection, that is, anatomic resection, or to high ligation, the resection of regional carcinoma based on removal of the total arterial blood supply in cases of actual or potential lymph node spread along the primary vascular distribution.

Enker and coworkers demonstrated in 1979 that the disciplined adherence to the principles of anatomic resection alone, with no adjuvant therapy, resulted in

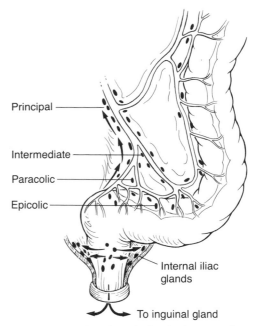

Figure 9–2. Patterns of lymph node distribution according to Dr. F. A. Coller (1941). Regional lymph nodes along the colon and within the mesentery are identified as epicolic, paracolic, intermediate, and principal, or main, lymph nodes. Intermediate lymph nodes are located along the secondary branches of the sigmoid blood vessels. Principal (main) lymph nodes can be found along the origin of the inferior mesenteric artery.

65% to 70% 5-year survival rates for patients with node-positive colon cancer. Four of every five patients with a curable stage of colon cancer could be cured by resection alone. Again, during that same decade, national figures derived from surveys by the American College of Surgeons, the Surveillance, Epidemiology, and End Results Program (SEER) group of the National Cancer Institute, the American Cancer Society, and others, confirmed the ubiquitous but inadequate 30% survival achieved by segmental resection for the same extent of disease.

Until modern times, the historical development has consistently supported the most important principle for the resection of colon cancer, namely, resection of the mesentery based on the total arterial blood supply to the affected bowel segment. In all cases, this is accomplished by ligation of the arterial blood supply at its origin.

PATHOPHYSIOLOGY OF LYMPHATIC SPREAD IN CARCINOMA OF THE COLON

Numerous authors have contributed to our knowledge of the lymphatic spread of colorectal cancer. A noteworthy modern thesis on this subject is that of Herter and Slanetz. Their work summarizes the meticulous pathologic studies of Dr. Robert Grinnell, who between 1938 and 1965 cleared and studied over 1,000 surgical specimens, plotting the location of involved and uninvolved lymph nodes among many other important pathologic features. Although certainly not the only sources of this information, their work summarizes best the current understanding of the lymphatic spread of primary colon cancer.

There are no lymphatic capillaries superficial to the muscularis mucosa. For this reason, carcinoma in situ or intraepithelial or intramucosal carcinoma cannot spread from the colon. Lymphoid capillaries can be observed at the junction of the mucosa and submucosa, along with lymphoid follicles. These capillaries flow into an extensive submucosal lymphatic plexus, which progresses through the bowel wall in a circumferential fashion. Lymphatic flow is primarily radial or circumferential; hence cancers tend to grow circumferentially, rather than longitudinally, along the axis of the colon. Lymphatic spread of cancer beyond the bowel wall itself may affect the surgeon's approach to circumventing the primary tumor, either at the paracolic gutters or at any other organ site immediately adjacent to the primary tumor.

In the colon itself, distal intramural spread of cancer along the submucosa is a less significant issue than in the rectum. In general, colon cancer averages less than 2 cm of distal intramural spread, and rarely does the cancer spread beyond 4 cm. When such is the case, the cancers are almost always poorly differentiated, and the survival or death of the patient is the result of multiple adverse features, not strictly the result of the extent of distal intramural spread of cancer.

Aside from multiple pathologic features, such as poor differentiation, mucinous component, extracapsular metastases to lymph nodes, extranodal mesenteric implants, and vascular invasion, two aspects of lymphatic spread defy the concept that regional spread is strictly anatomically definable. The first is the presence of numerous communications between the venous and lymphatic channels at all levels of the lymphatic circulation. Thus, tumor emboli that have entered the lymphatic circulation through open junctions between lymphatic endothelial cells may ultimately become responsible for the hematogenous spread of cancer through venolymphatic interconnections. Second, some cancers of the colon spread by "skip metastases." Grinnell cites a 12% incidence of lymphatic metastases bypassing the epicolic or paracolic lymph nodes and directly affecting the intermediate or more centrally located mesenteric lymph nodes, or the principal nodes at the mesenteric apex.

Despite these two unusual findings, the goal of the surgeon is to resect effectively the regional spread of disease, which for the majority of patients is defined by the traditional patterns of lymph node spread. Coller was the first to demonstrate that colon cancers spread first to epicolic, then to paracolic, then to intermediate, and finally to high, main, or principal lymph nodes at the apex of the mesentery along the origin of the blood supply in question. These lymph nodes are all found along the branches of the arterial and venous blood supply, enabling the surgeon to design regional anatomic resections. When the primary colon cancer is situated immediately opposite the artery in question, one can expect that virtually all nodal metastases will be found along the primary arterial pathway.

In the few instances in which lymph node metastases can be found outside the primary arterial distribution, such aberrant findings have been explained by extensive tumor blockade of lymphatic pathways in association with poorly differentiated disease. For tumors between major vascular arcades or between two primary vascular pedicles, lymphatic flow may drain to either pedicle or, more typically, to both pedicles.

Grinnell pointed to the many "watershed areas" of the colon in which the distribution of lymph node metastases was common to two or more major vascular pedicles. Thus, for example, cancers of the hepatic flexure stood an equal chance of spreading to either the middle colic or to the right colic lymph node distribution and, in some cases, even to the ileocolic distribution (Fig. 9–3). Cancers of the transverse colon directly opposite the middle colic distribution would more often than not spread directly to lymph nodes along the middle colic artery alone. The need to consider the watershed areas of the colon is addressed under guidelines to resection for each individual site. Following these guidelines ensures that the individual situations of most curable patients will be appropriately addressed.

GENERAL GUIDELINES OF OPERATIVE MANAGEMENT

Exposure

There can be no compromise of complete exposure of the operative field. The patient should be positioned and retraction accomplished in order to provide adequate lighting for the entire operative field with light concentrated on the immediate site of dissection.

Position of Patient

Most patients should be in the supine position. For lesions of the distal sigmoid colon 12 to 18 cm from the anal verge, it is often advantageous to place the patient in the Trendelenburg lithotomy position on Lloyd-Davis stirrups. When this position is used, padding at the peroneal nerves and sacral support both are appropriate.

Traction and Countertraction

In all instances, the operating surgeon and the assistant must provide local traction and countertraction at the site of dissection. The operative field should, in all cases, resemble the illustrations of an atlas, the assistant providing traction and the surgeon providing countertraction simultaneous with dissection.

Retraction

Self-retaining retractors assist with proper exposure and with retraction of the small bowel for cases in which evisceration into a plastic bag is not possible. The Balfour retractor (with or without additional extensions), the Goligher retractor, and the Thompson Elite retractor all are adequate and flexible systems

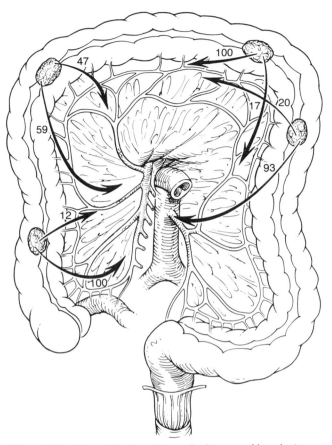

Figure 9–3. The predominant "watershed" areas of lymphatic spread for tumors situated between, as opposed to immediately opposite, the major vascular pedicles. Lymph node spread may occur along the main vascular pedicles to either side of the primary tumor, as illustrated. (Adapted from Herter FP, Slanetz CA. Patterns and significance of lymphatic spread from cancer of the colon and rectum. In: Weiss L, Gilbert HA, Ballon SC, eds. Lymphatic System Metastases. Boston: GK Hall Medical Publishers, 1980, p 275.)

that place a minimum amount of hardware between the operating surgeon and the operative field.

Restoration of Anatomy to Normal

Before the onset of any resection, all anatomy is restored to normal. In patients who have undergone previous resections, extensive lysis of adhesions may be necessary. *Any adhesions or anatomic distortions that may interfere with the adequacy of mesenteric resection must be dealt with fully at the outset.*

Prevention of Deep Venous Thrombosis

Intermittent compression devices are applied to the calves in order to minimize deep vein thrombophlebitis. Obese patients and those with congestive heart failure, supraventricular arrythmias, hypercoagulable states, and immobility or debilitated and/or sedentary patients all may benefit from perioperative heparin administered as 5,000 units preoperatively and continued postoperatively every 8 to 12 hours for a minimum of 7 days or until discharge.

Prevention of Contamination

All operative sites are irrigated, and gloves are changed to avoid bacterial wound contamination during closure.

Impermeable Barriers

In resections of the right colon, moist laparotomy pads with an added impermeable barrier of plastic or rubber should be applied to the wound edges. The small bowel must be left in situ for resections of the right colon, the transverse colon, and the hepatic flexure.

For resections of the left colon, similar protective waterproof wound towels or other wound barriers should be employed, and the small bowel is isolated in a Lahey bag when possible. This frequently requires minimal mobilization of the peritoneum overlying the root of the small bowel mesentery, the cecum, and the right paracolic gutter.

Gastrostomy

A temporary gastrostomy is employed in all patients undergoing major colonic resection. This avoids the discomfort associated with the nasogastric tube in the 15% to 20% of patients who experience early absence of nasogastric decompression. If early postoperative

bowel obstruction ensues, a temporary gastrostomy is of extraordinary benefit, both to the patient and to the surgeon. When the length of nasogastric decompression is indeterminate, gastrostomy eliminates the patient's discomfort and allows the surgeon to treat the condition by decompression for the advisable period of time without regard for nonsurgical dynamics. In over 400 such cases, I have encountered only two minor and easily correctable problems: a suture catching one limb of a Malecot catheter and an episode of minor infection.

PRINCIPLES OF OPERATIVE MANAGEMENT

Resection of Mesentery

The single most important principle for the resection of colon cancer is resection of the mesentery based on the total arterial blood supply to the affected bowel segment.

Ligation of Arterial Blood Supply

Resection of the mesentery is based on ligation of the involved arterial blood supply at its origin. The involved venous blood supply is divided, either parallel to the artery or at its own apex. The mesentery is divided along lines that are *secondary* to the anatomy of the vessels. The bowel is divided after the mesentery and its arcade vessels have been divided.

Planes of Dissection

The surgeon must be aware of the appropriate planes of dissection. These planes are areolar in nature, and there is a minor presence of superimposed perforating vessels between the mesentery and retroperitoneum. These generally avascular planes guide the surgeon to the appropriate mobilization of the colon. Dissection of the colonic mesentery from the adjacent retroperitoneal structures requires a knowledge of the planes of dissection to be followed after division of the lateral peritoneum.

Complete Mobilization

The affected segment of the bowel should be completely mobilized by sharp dissection along the appropriate planes. Care must be exercised to minimize manipulation of the primary tumor. I do not practice the specific steps of the no-touch isolation technique, although some surgeons do, in addition to high ligation and wide mesenteric resection. In all cases, as the affected segment of the bowel is mobilized, one must respect the primary tumor by widely circumventing it in clearly normal tissues.

Complete mobilization of the affected segment and of the colon needed for reconstruction generally is accomplished at the outset of the operation. For example, in a sigmoid resection requiring takedown of the splenic flexure, complete mobilization of the colon from the retroperitoneum along Gerota's fascia, division of all ligaments of the splenic flexure, and mobilization of the gastrocolic ligament precede division of the arterial and venous distribution.

Sharp Dissection

Sharp dissection throughout the entire operation is essential. Blunt dissection may be expedient but is far more likely to result in bleeding, in inadequate mobilization of the colon, in incomplete development of the mesentery, and in injury of the portion of the mesentery not to be resected or injury to sites of adherence from past operations.

Intraoperative Staging

Primary Tumor

At the time of an elective operation, all areas of potential spread must be examined before the resection proceeds. The primary tumor itself must be examined for the involvement of either adjacent peritoneum or adjacent organs. Any adjacent organ involvement must be taken into consideration in the planning of the resection with appropriate reconstruction.

Questionable Margins

Wider-than-average direct extension or involvement of the peritoneum can be managed by designing the operation to circumvent any margins of potential involvement by the primary tumor. Intraoperative radiation, such as brachytherapy and afterloading, may be useful for patients in whom margins are questionable (i.e., those with psoas involvement).

Distant Metastases

Distant metastases beyond conventional cure include hepatic metastases, para-aortic or paracaval nodal metastases, celiac or portal lymph node metastases, or peritoneal seeding. Although some surgeons make

extraordinary efforts to cure such spread of disease, the far larger yield of rewarding results is in the appropriate mesenteric resection of regional disease (in which cure rates are high) in contrast to the extraordinary resection of distant disease (in which cure is anecdotal).

Any and all metastatic disease should be documented histologically for future therapeutic considerations. In cases in which the gross observation of hepatic metastases is problematic, intraoperative ultrasound as well as ultrasound-directed needle biopsy may prove helpful. In the case of peritoneal implants, by either metastases or seeding, the extent of such disease should be documented. When peritoneal implants can be reduced to lesions smaller than 1 cm, in the appropriate cancer treatment setting, peritoneal catheters for intraperitoneal chemotherapy can be placed.

As a rule, the resection of aortocaval, para-aortic, celiac, or portal nodal disease is not curative. Such disease invariably represents the presence of other metastatic disease, which usually presents as disseminated disease at some future point. Such resection should not be undertaken for cure but may occasionally offer palliation, as in the prevention of extrahepatic biliary disease.

RESECTION OF CARCINOMA OF THE COLON

Right Colon

For cancers of the right and transverse colon, and some cancers of the splenic flexure, resection through a transverse abdominal incision is recommended. A transverse supraumbilical incision, extending approximately from the tenth rib on the right to the tenth rib on the left, provides intra-abdominal exposure and access to all such primary tumors, sites of vascular dissection, and sites of anastomoses. In addition, exposure of the liver and pelvis may be adequately achieved through this incision.

A mechanical retractor, such as the Goligher, the Thompson, or the Balfour, is employed. Mobilization of the colon proceeds just lateral to the white line of Toldt. The paracolic gutter is developed by sharp dissection along Gerota's fascia. The ligament of the hepatic flexure is encountered (Fig. 9–4). This ligament is generally associated with numerous small vessels and is best divided and ligated. As the right colon is retracted toward the midline, dissection continues in the areolar plane anterior to Gerota's fascia and posterior to the mesentery. During this dissection, the right gonadal vessels and duodenum become apparent.

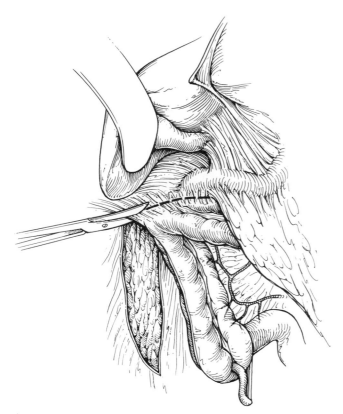

Figure 9–4. Ligaments of hepatic flexure. The right paracolic gutter is generally more vascular than the left one. As one approaches the hepatic flexure, the ligament of the hepatic flexure itself can be variable. Thus, a fixed ligamentous structure infiltrated by fat can be present and is generally divided into two bands stretching from the middle of the right kidney to the edge of the biliary tree. In each case, division and ligation, cautery or hemoclips can be used, as indicated, to divide this ligament. The medial end of the ligament of the hepatic flexure, or the gastroduodenal ligament, is a space situated caudad between the greater omentum and the subpyloric nodes (gastric). Occasionally, the lesser sac may be entered at this point in the dissection.

The gonadal vessels are reflected laterally and posteriorly, and the mesentery of the right colon is sharply dissected anteriorly from the duodenum. At this point, vulnerable branches of the right or middle colic veins may join the portal circulation via the uncinate process, and care must be taken to avoid injury to these vessels while the right colon is mobilized away from the pancreas.

Failure to mobilize these vessels adequately results in the failure to resect mesenteric lymphatic pathways that are responsible for recurrence of disease at the junction of the superior mesenteric vein and the third portion of the duodenum. Recurrent disease at this site is responsible for incurable disease, bleeding via erosion of the duodenum, and obstruction. Virtually no palliative treatment is rewarding, and such recurrence should be prevented, even if resection is palliative.

The right ureter, medial to the gonadal vessels, is identified and is similarly reflected laterally and posteriorly while dissection of the small bowel mesentery continues in association with the right colon (Fig. 9–5).

Once the limits of the right colon are fully reflected medially, the ileum and cecum are elevated, and the peritoneum overlying the small bowel mesentery is incised along its origins up to the root of the superior mesenteric vessels. This procedure frees the ileum and right colon for resection.

The gastrocolic ligament is divided, and the lesser sac is entered; the stomach is reflected upward. The middle colic vessels are identified, and the right branch of the middle colic artery and vein are divided at their origin. The right colic artery and vein may be absent in 15% to 20% of patients. Under these circumstances, careful identification of the right branch of the middle colic vessels is more important to the resection.

The ileocolic vessels are divided, at their origin, from the superior mesenteric vessels. The amount of ileum to be resected generally conforms to the anatomy of the patient. As a rule, any resection that approaches the ileocecal valve is inappropriate. The distal arcade of the superior mesenteric artery to the terminal ileum is the appropriate site for division of the small bowel mesentery, which generally results in the resection of approximately 15 cm of small bowel and attached mesentery (Fig. 9–6).

After the mesentery is divided, all terminal vessels issuing from the final arcade to the surface of the bowel are obliterated. This is most effectively accomplished by outlining each vessel over a fine hemostat and by individually cauterizing each vessel between the tips of DeBakey forceps (Fig. 9–7). The identification, obliteration, and division of each vessel provide a bowel surface free of any fat or other peritoneal attachment that might interfere with a safe anastomosis.

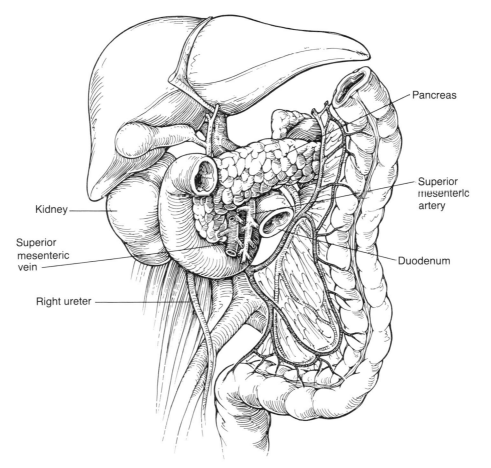

Figure 9–5. Following complete resection of the right colon, including the distal arcade of the terminal ileum, the cecum, the ascending colon, and the right transverse colon, the retroperitoneal structures are visible.

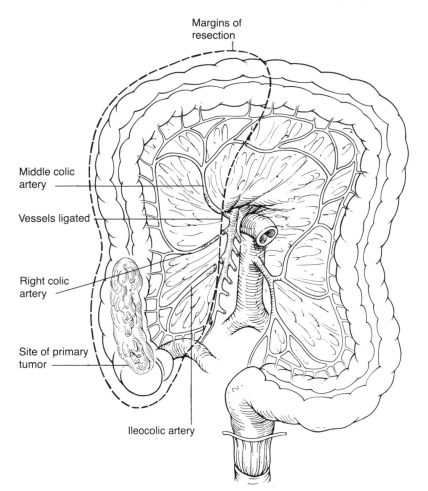

Margins of resection

Middle colic artery

Vessels ligated

Right colic artery

Site of primary tumor

Ileocolic artery

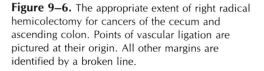

Figure 9–6. The appropriate extent of right radical hemicolectomy for cancers of the cecum and ascending colon. Points of vascular ligation are pictured at their origin. All other margins are identified by a broken line.

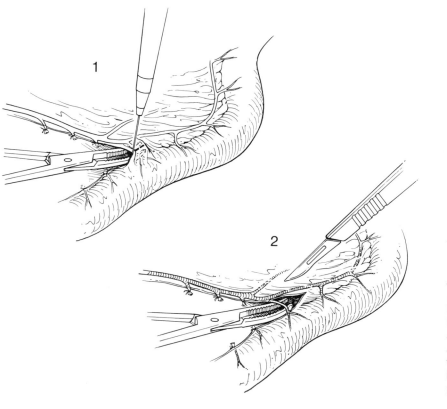

Figure 9–7. Preparing a clean bowel edge for anastomosis: *Step #1:* Division and ligation of all mesenteric vessels. A fine pointed hemostat, that is, a Coller hemostat or a mosquito, is used to open the peritoneum overlying the junction of the bowel and the mesentery. *Step #2:* A fine hemostat is used to identify each small vessel again. DeBakey forceps are used to isolate and cauterize the vessel. *Step #3:* The thrombosed vessels are divided and a clean bowel edge left for several centimeters (not pictured).

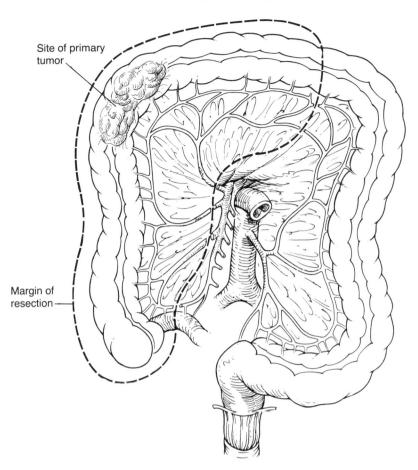

Site of primary tumor

Margin of resection

Figure 9–8. Cancer of the hepatic flexure. The ileocolic, right colic, and middle colic vessels are all ligated at their origins. The left branch of the middle colic artery is divided along the left transverse colon; adequacy of the mesenteric resection is ensured. All margins of resection are outlined by the broken line.

In general an end-to-end ileocolic anastomosis between the end of the ileum and the transverse colon is favored. This can be accomplished in two layers, by using an outer layer of 3-0 or 4-0 interrupted silk sutures and an inner running layer of chromic catgut. It can also be accomplished by utilizing a single layer of Lembert sutures. A minor discrepancy in the size of the bowel can be accommodated by a small antimesenteric slit of the ileum. Significant discrepancy in bowel size requires either a side-to-side or end-to-side anastomosis. Side-to-side anastomosis with straight stapling devices may also be employed and is currently popular. In this case, the ileum and the colon are divided by using a straight stapling device at the elected sites. Care is taken to apply the automatic stapling device at right angles to the bowel, leaving the antimesenteric edges free for the anastomosis.

Several interrupted silk sutures are applied to the antimesenteric surfaces of the ileum and transverse colon. Small defects are created in the bowel wall immediately adjacent to the antimesenteric edges of the stapled closure line. The straight stapling device is introduced separately into the ileal and colonic segments, and the anastomosis is lined up so that no mesenteric or epiploic fat is in the suture line. A side-to-side anastomosis is accomplished. The suture line is checked for bleeding via the defect created by the anastomotic stapling device. The defect is then closed either by a handsewn technique or by application of a nonanastomotic staple line. The mesenteric defect is closed by approximating the peritoneal surfaces either with interrupted or with running suture material.

Hepatic Flexure

Cancers of the hepatic flexure represent a so-called watershed of lymphatic spread. There is an equal chance of lymph node spread, either to the right colic or to the middle colic distribution. For this reason, a resection for cancer of the hepatic flexure involves division of the right, middle, and ileocolic vessels at their origin (Fig. 9–8).

The operation is performed through a transverse incision. After it has been determined that the tumor is not adherent to the liver, kidney, or gallbladder, the right colon is mobilized to identify the vessels and divide the mesentery. The gastrocolic ligament is divided by interruption of the individual branches caudal to the gastroepiploic artery. This approach necessitates en bloc resection of the right half of the omentum with the colon and its mesentery.

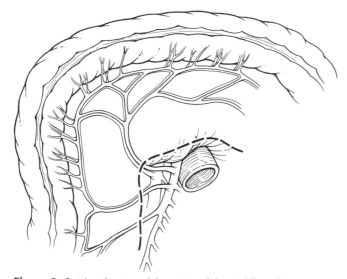

Figure 9–9. Identification of the origin of the middle colic artery and vein for complete resection of the transverse mesocolon. In cancers of the transverse colon, the middle colic artery and vein are divided at their origin. The gastrocolic ligament has been divided, and the stomach is reflected cephalad. Caudal traction on the transverse colon helps identify the middle colic vein and artery at their origin and apex, respectively. The colon is reflected upward, allowing incision of the peritoneum overlying the middle colic and vein, approximately 1 cm above the small bowel mesentery and the superior mesenteric artery and vein. In this way, the latter vessels are identified and protected. Depending on the circumstances, the middle colic artery and vein may be divided and ligated with the colon reflected cephalad or caudad.

The gastrocolic ligament is liberally opened, and the stomach is reflected upward. Careful dissection identifies the inferior edge of the pancreas and superior mesenteric artery and vein with the origins of the middle colic arteries. Elevation of the transverse colon at this point allows for incision of the peritoneum 1 cm above the small bowel mesentery. In this way, the middle colic vessels are identified, and the pancreas and superior mesenteric vessels are protected from injury (Fig. 9–9).

At this point, one can either isolate and divide these vessels at their origin or mobilize the right colon and complete the resection, as previously described for cancers of the right colon. The extent of the ileal resection is the same as in right colonic resections, making it possible to divide the right colic vessels at their origin as well as the ileocolic vessels. Mobilization of the right colon is completed, and a point well along the left branch of the middle colic artery is chosen for division of the colon. Care is taken to leave adequate peritoneum overlying the left transverse colonic mesentery to enable a proper repair of the peritoneal defect. This means not leaving a defect at the ligament of Treitz.

The anastomosis is accomplished, as described, after the right colonic resection. End-to-end ileocolic anastomosis, end-to-side ileocolic anastomosis, or functional end-to-end (side-to-side) anastomosis can be accomplished. If a primary anastomosis is being accomplished after resection of an obstructing right colic or hepatic flexure carcinoma, a side-to-side anastomosis is recommended, because it avoids any mesenteric defect within the anastomosis.

Transverse Colon

The operation begins with division of the entire gastrocolic ligament just below the gastroepiploic vessels. The object is the resection of the entire transverse colon, based on the middle colic vessels. The ligaments of the hepatic and splenic flexures are completely divided. The stomach is reflected upward to reveal the pancreas and the superior mesenteric vessels at their origin (see Fig. 9–9). As in the case of the hepatic flexure, the transverse colon can be reflected upward to reveal the origin of the middle colic vessels just beneath the peritoneum. The transverse mesocolon is incised 1 cm above the small bowel mesentery, and the middle colic vessels are isolated at their origin from the superior mesenteric vessels just beneath the pancreas.

The ligament of the hepatic flexure is easiest to divide. At various points between the pancreas and the ligament of the hepatic flexure, the gastroduodenal ligament variably thickens and thins. The edge of the transverse mesocolon begins at the juncture of the gastroepiploic vessels, the inferior or subpyloric lymph nodes, and the first portion of the duodenum.

On the left side, the ligaments of the splenic flexure are divided. The gastrocolic ligament is serially divided up to the short gastric vessels to define the splenocolic ligament, the ligament of the splenic flexure, and the splenorenal ligament, which are the remaining structures to be divided. In general, it is preferable to divide these ligaments after partially mobilizing the left colon (see Fig. 9–11). It is often possible to divide these ligaments in discrete planes. Depending on the obesity of the patient, these ligaments may require either division and ligation or simple cautery for small vessels. When these ligaments are divided, the left edge of the transverse mesocolon becomes visible caudal to the inferior edge of the pancreas. At this point, all attachments of the transverse mesocolon are divided caudal to the pancreas.

After the ligaments of both flexures are completely divided and the right and left paracolic gutters have been mobilized, the transverse colon is completely resected en bloc with its mesentery and the greater omentum.

Under many circumstances, a colocolic anastomosis can be performed without resection of the right colon. This requires complete absence of tension on the anastomosis after resection of the transverse colon. With appropriate mobilization of the right and left colon, both structures become "midline organs." Anastomosis of the right colon to the upper portion of the descending colon becomes possible with primary repair of the peritoneal defect.

Just as often, it is necessary to resect the remaining right colon in order to complete the anastomosis. A colocolic anastomosis or an ileocolic anastomosis can be performed by utilizing any of the methods previously described.

Splenic Flexure and Left Transverse Colon

The choice of incision for cancers of the splenic flexure requires individualization based on the patient's body habitus. On many occasions, a transverse incision extended to the midaxillary line on the left provides the best exposure. In the extremely deep, barrel-chested male patient, a midline incision with a "hockey stick" to the apex of the costal margin (the midpoint between the tenth rib and the xiphoid) may provide exposure and flexibility that cannot be found in either the midline or the transverse incision. This incision should be used only in limited circumstances.

Cancers of the left transverse colon and the splenic flexure represent a second major watershed for lym-

phatic metastases. Cancers of the left transverse colon invariably metastasize to the lymph nodes along the middle colic artery, and in 20% of cases, metastases also occur along the left colic distribution. The ratio of lymph node metastases is reversed in lesions of the splenic flexure; nearly 100% of cancers spread via the paracolic nodes to the left colic distribution. For these reasons, cancers of the left transverse colon and the splenic flexure must be treated by high ligation and resection of the middle colic distribution and the entire left colic distribution.

Beyond these boundaries, there appears to be no cancer-related rationale for resections of either the sigmoid distribution or the right colic distribution. Resection should involve high ligation of the middle and left colic vessels and resection of all mesentery from the hepatic flexure to the descending colon–sigmoid colon junction. Three options for resection and reconstruction of cancers of the left transverse colon and splenic flexure are presented (Fig. 9–10A to C).

Ligaments of Splenic Flexure

Resection of lesions of the left transverse colon and splenic flexure requires a knowledge of the ligaments of the splenic flexure. These include the ligament of the splenic flexure proper, the gastrocolic ligament as it approaches the short gastric vessels, the splenocolic ligament, and the splenorenal ligament. In order to identify these ligaments properly, exposure must be excellent (Fig. 9–11).

Depending on the obesity of the patient, each ligament may be isolated and divided as a discrete anatomic structure. Areolar spaces frequently divide one ligament from another. In the lean patient, an occasional series of nearly avascular ligaments can be taken down sharply without need for much hemostasis. In the obese patient, long, large clamps may be required to gain access for anatomic identification and division.

Mobilization of Left and Transverse Colon

Central to all approaches to the splenic flexure and the left transverse colon is the proper mobilization of the left and transverse colon. The splenic flexure should be approached with complete control, both from the left paracolic gutter and from the lesser sac. After abdominal exploration is completed, the gastrocolic ligament is divided to the short gastric vessels until it is evident that the splenic flexure remains attached via the splenocolic ligaments, the splenorenal ligaments, and the ligament of the splenic flexure itself. The lateral peritoneal reflection of the descending colon is incised by sharp dissection. The entire left colon is reflected away from Gerota's fascia overlying the left

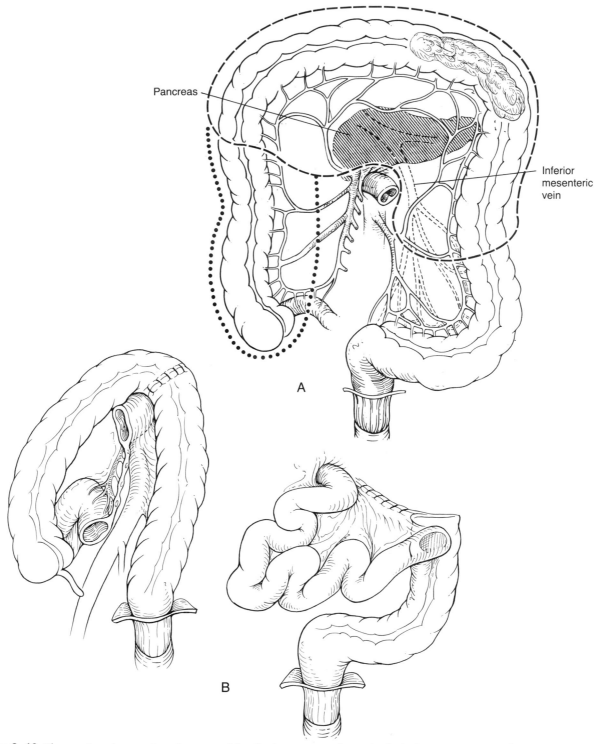

Pancreas

Inferior mesenteric vein

A

B

Figure 9–10. Three options for resection of cancers of the distal transverse colon and splenic flexure are presented.

A, The extent of resection is based on the origin of the middle colic arteries (see Fig. 9–9) and the origin of the left colic artery. The inferior mesenteric vein is ligated at its apex. The ascending colon is preserved and a colocolic anastomosis is performed from the ascending colon to the upper sigmoid colon.

B, Although the landmarks of resection for cancer are the same as those pictured in *A,* the anastomosis between the right and left colon is deemed impractical or unsafe. The ascending colon and cecum are resected, and the ileum is anastomosed to the sigmoid colon. If the ileum is reflected to the midline, the divided edges of the mesentery are easy to approximate. It is not necessary to divide either the right colic or the ileocolic arteries at their origins, because this portion of the operation plays no role in the resection for cancer.

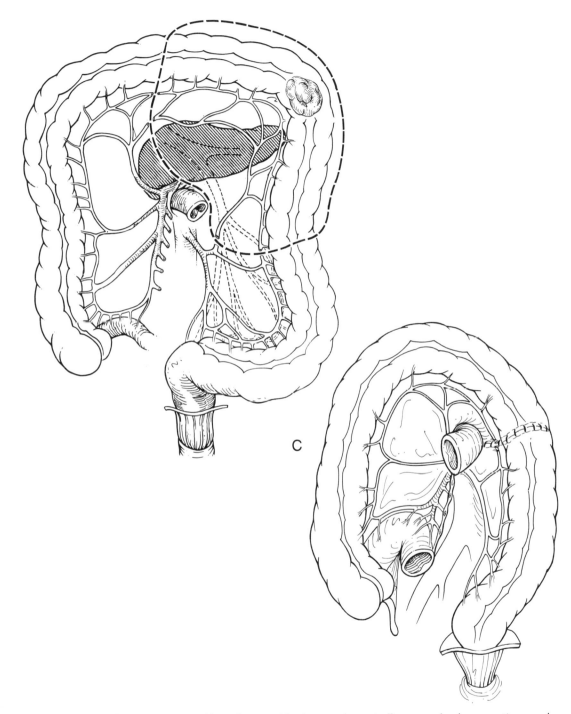

C

Figure 9–10 *Continued C,* For early cancers of the splenic flexure arising in an endoscopically removed polyp, resection may be accomplished from the origin of the left branch of the middle colic artery to the origin of the left colic artery. Anastomosis is accomplished from the right transverse colon to the proximal sigmoid colon.

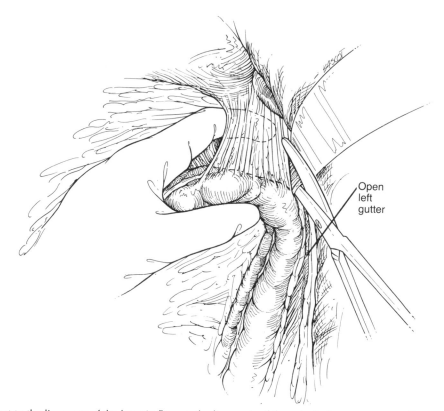

Figure 9–11. In contrast to the ligaments of the hepatic flexure, the ligaments of the splenic flexure are generally more well defined. One ligament comes from the abdominal wall, whereas the second comes from the spleen and, for practical purposes, is identified as the splenocolic ligament. The stomach is reflected upward, and the gastroepiploic vessels have been divided. The short gastric vessels are preserved. The left paracolic gutter is opened, and the ligaments of the splenic flexure are identified, from both the medial and lateral aspects. Communication between the left paracolic gutter and the lesser sac behind these ligaments is generally easy to find. Depending on the vessel and fat content of the ligaments, they can be clamped, divided, and ligated; cauterized; or clipped and divided.

Within the image: Open left gutter

kidney. The dissection is complete when the left colic mesentery has been freed from the retroperitoneum to the aorta and to the transverse portion of the duodenum. Often, the completion of this mobilization is deferred until the ligaments of the splenic flexure have been divided.

Once the transverse colon and descending colon are mobilized, the splenic flexure remains attached only by its ligaments. These may be divided between clamps, or individual vessels may be ligated or clipped; the technique is selected to suit the individual patient. Following division of the gastrocolic ligament and splenocolic ligament, the splenorenal ligament is divided as the colon is reflected away from the retroperitoneum toward the midline. The dissection is complete when the gonadal vessels, the left ureter, and the left renal vein have been identified laterally and posteriorly; the pancreas identified cephalad; and the aorta and duodenum identified medially.

Division and Ligation of Arteries and Veins

The entire left colon is mobilized in preparation for resection. The peritoneum overlying the ligament of Treitz is incised, revealing again the middle colic vessels. The superior mesenteric vessels and pancreas are protected from injury. The middle colic vessels are ligated at their origin. The large and reproducible vein from the splenic flexure is identified as it courses toward the inferior mesenteric vein. The inferior mesenteric vein is ligated at its apex. The left colic artery is identified at its takeoff; while damage to the blood supply to the sigmoid colon is avoided, the left colic artery is divided at its origin from the inferior mesenteric artery. The peritoneum and underlying mesentery are resected in the midline along the aortoduodenal junction.

In unusually early cases, only the left branch of the middle colic artery need be taken with the left colic artery at its origin. This more limited resection is appropriate for early carcinoma (i.e., sessile adenoma) or for operations in which carcinoma has been diagnosed in an endoscopically removed (i.e., pedunculated) adenoma for which the histology or margins dictate the need for a resection. Division and ligation of the middle colic arteries at their origin do not indicate an obligatory right hemicolectomy. Despite division of the middle colic arteries at their origin, blood supply to the hepatic flexure and the right transverse colon from the right colic distribution may be entirely adequate. On this basis, reconstruction is individualized.

Anastomosis

Patients undergoing anatomic resection for lesions of the left transverse colon and splenic flexure may have reconstruction via anastomosis of the ascending colon to the upper sigmoid or descending colon–sigmoid colon junction (see Fig. 9–10A). Complete mobilization of the ascending colon, the cecum, and the ileum with appropriate rotation of these structures allows for complete lack of tension on the anastomosis and complete repair of the mesenteric defect.

A cecosigmoid or cecodescending anastomosis is possible under rarer circumstances. Approximation of the mesentery is more difficult with these anastomoses. In the event that it is not possible to reapproximate the mesentery safely, any attempt to perform a colocolic anastomosis should be abandoned in favor of a subtotal colectomy with ileosigmoid anastomosis (see Fig. 9–10B). There appears to be no rationale for the removal of sigmoid mesentery for lesions of the left transverse colon and splenic flexure.

Adjacent Organ Involvement

Adjacent organ involvement is relatively common at this site. Involvement of the greater curvature of the stomach, the spleen, the ligaments of the splenic flexure, the tail of the pancreas, or of Gerota's fascia, is not an unusual finding. In the event of such involvement, en bloc resection of the contiguous organ with reconstruction is appropriate. There is no role for splenectomy in the absence of direct involvement. Rarely, involvement of the most proximal jejunum, even up to the duodenojejunal junction, presents technical difficulties requiring creative reconstruction. Options for reconstruction following en bloc resection of the proximal jejunum include end-to-end jejunojejunostomy, end-to-end duodenojejunostomy, or gastrojejunostomy with Roux-en-Y duodenojejunostomy, depending on the amount and location of the jejunum to be resected.

Descending Colon

Cancers of the descending and sigmoid colons are best operated on through a full-length midline incision extending from the symphysis pubis to the xiphoid process.

Sigmoid colon cancers, although most commonly resected through a full-length midline incision, can occasionally be resected via a transverse infraumbilical incision, which offers a cosmetic benefit for the young female patient.

Cancers of the descending colon and descending colon–sigmoid colon junction are treated by anatomic left hemicolectomy. Cancers of the upper descending colon, just distal to the splenic flexure, may occasionally spread to lymph nodes along the left branch of the middle colic artery. Cancers of the upper descending colon and the descending colon–sigmoid colon junction spread to lymph nodes located directly along the left colic distribution with principal or main nodes at the inferior mesenteric artery. Left radical hemicolectomy is based on this vessel.

Mobilization of Left Colon

The entire left colon is mobilized by sharp dissection. The usual limits of mobilization are the midtransverse colon proximally and the sigmoid colon opposite the sacral promontory distally. Mobilization of the left colon begins with an incision just lateral to the white line of Toldt. The left colon itself is placed on steady traction medially, and sharp dissection separates the entire left colic mesentery from the retroperitoneal structures. Dissection proceeds along Gerota's fascia with identification of the left gonadal vessels. The mesentery itself forms the first plane of dissection. The gonadal vessels constitute a second discrete plane and are recognizable while one proceeds inferolaterally toward the internal inguinal ring. The third and deepest retroperitoneal plane is the left ureter. A knowledge of the anatomy of the left ureter is critical to safe operation on the left colon.

Mobilization of the Left Ureter

The left ureter is usually observed first as the most medial margins of the retroperitoneal dissection (i.e., mobilization) are approached. Frequently, the left ureter is first recognized by its distinctive blood supply. A prominent venous plexus courses along the medial aspect of the ureter. Once this blood supply has been identified, the ureter itself is visible immediately lateral to these veins. Gentle lateral traction on the areolar tissue just medial to the blood supply retracts the ureter laterally, providing an avascular areolar plane in which to mobilize the ureter further. The ureter is neither skeletonized nor mobilized circumferentially. Instead, it is dissected free of any medial tissues to allow the ureter to fall away laterally from any mesenteric dissection.

For abdominal operations, identification of the ureter rarely needs to proceed beyond the iliac bifurcation. The longitudinal venous plexus along the medial aspect of the ureter must remain intact, whereas any other

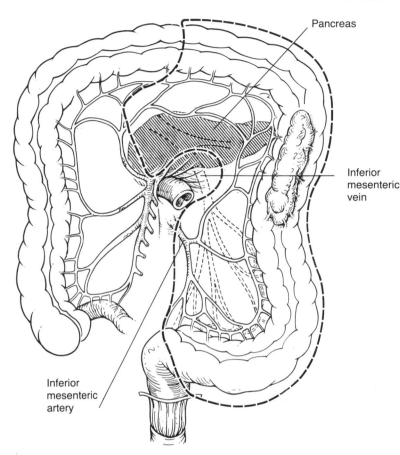

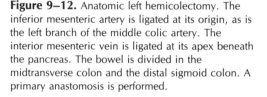

Pancreas

Inferior
mesenteric
vein

Inferior
mesenteric
artery

Figure 9–12. Anatomic left hemicolectomy. The inferior mesenteric artery is ligated at its origin, as is the left branch of the middle colic artery. The interior mesenteric vein is ligated at its apex beneath the pancreas. The bowel is divided in the midtransverse colon and the distal sigmoid colon. A primary anastomosis is performed.

perforator or small retroperitoneal vessels may be divided to enhance mobilization. Small perforator or retroperitoneal vessels should be divided between hemoclips. The use of the cautery for this purpose is ill conceived and may aggravate bleeding if the longitudinal venous plexus of the ureter is violated. Fine sutures may also be appropriate, but the use of hemostats in this location is decried, because injury to the ureter may result.

Dissection of the Splenic Flexure

With steady medial retraction on the colonic mesentery, the paracolic gutter is incised to the splenic flexure. Depending on the patient's build and weight, it may be profitable to open the left side of the gastrocolic ligament at this point. This allows for bimanual, gentle traction on the splenic flexure and facilitates identification of the ligaments of the splenic flexure outlined in the preceding discussion (see Fig. 9–11). These ligaments are divided in the manner elected by the surgeon, and mobilization of the left colon proceeds to the midline.

Sharp dissection is employed throughout mobilization. The areolar plane is anterior to Gerota's fascia, the left gonadal vessels, and the left ureter; cephalad, sharp dissection proceeds along the caudal or inferior

margin of the pancreas. The hypogastric nerves are identified medially and reflected posteriorly to avoid injury. When this dissection is completed, the entire left colon has become a "midline organ," and a laparotomy pad is placed beneath the entire extent of the dissection (Fig. 9–12).

Peritoneal Incision

The medial peritoneal incision begins along the anterior or right surface of the aorta. For convenience, the incision in the peritoneum is performed while the mobilized left colon is steadily retracted laterally. This retraction creates slight tension on the peritoneum, and with the first incision in the peritoneum, air fills the retroperitoneal space and outlines the course and plane for the peritoneal incision and the ensuing mobilization. The incision begins just below the duodenum. The duodenum may need to be reflected to the right, because it frequently covers the aorta and the inferior mesenteric artery. Once this is accomplished and the duodenum is retracted laterally, the peritoneal incision is begun caudad and proceeds to the distal sigmoid colon.

In the course of this dissection, it is generally a simple matter to separate the sigmoid mesentery from the retroperitoneal structures; this step is essential to

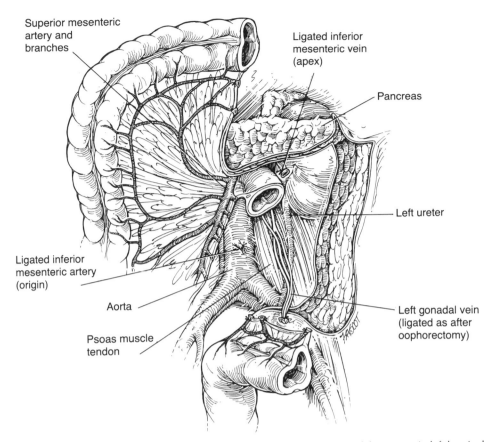

Superior mesenteric
artery and
branches

Ligated inferior
mesenteric vein
(apex)

Pancreas

Left ureter

Ligated inferior
mesenteric artery
(origin)

Aorta

Psoas muscle
tendon

Left gonadal vein
(ligated as after
oophorectomy)

Figure 9–13. The retroperitoneal structures identified during the course of the anatomic left hemicolectomy.

avoid inappropriate damage to the hypogastric nerves. The first assistant maintains steady traction on the left colon for the operating surgeon, who continues the sharp dissection cephalad. The midline peritoneum is incised at least to the junction of the ligament of Treitz, the pancreas, and the transverse mesocolon. By gentle dissection of the retroperitoneal areolar tissue, an easy communication with the previously entered retroperitoneal space is effected (Fig. 9–13).

Division of Inferior Mesenteric Artery and Vein, and Middle Colic Artery

The inferior mesenteric artery is identified, heading directly upward from the retroperitoneum into the mobilized left colic mesentery. Its origin is located, on average, 4.5 cm cephalad to the aortic bifurcation. Generally, it is possible to identify the left colic artery at its takeoff from the inferior mesenteric artery. The inferior mesenteric artery is surrounded by dense nerves and lymphatics, which are best isolated by dissection with a fine instrument and divided between either ligatures or clips. When the inferior mesenteric artery is cleaned in this manner, it is a simple matter to accomplish either clamping and division or ligation

in continuity. In addition, the hypogastric nerves pass extremely close to the origin of the inferior mesenteric artery, and cleaning of the inferior mesenteric artery while it remains on gentle tension usually prevents inappropriate nerve damage.

The inferior mesenteric artery may be divided anywhere above the origin of the left colic artery. Several centimeters to the left, one can identify the inferior mesenteric vein, which, under tension, is now easily identifiable. The inferior mesenteric vein is joined by a little-recognized but generally present significant tributary from the splenic flexure. The peritoneum and underlying tissues surrounding the inferior mesenteric vein are cleaned, and the vein is ligated and divided at its apex just beneath the inferior or caudal edge of the pancreas. An ascending branch of the left colic artery frequently accompanies the inferior mesenteric vein. It may be divided separately or together with the vein. The appropriate outline of the left hemicolectomy has now been determined.

If one is resecting a cancer of the upper descending colon, the left branch of the middle colic artery is divided at its origin. If one is resecting a cancer of the true descending colon or of the descending colon–sigmoid colon junction, this vessel may be spared or

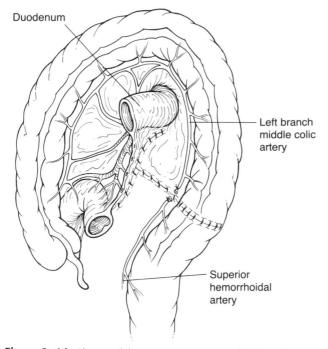

Duodenum

Left branch middle colic artery

Superior hemorrhoidal artery

Figure 9–14. Closure of the mesenteric peritoneal defect after left anatomic hemicolectomy. Closure is done mainly along the edge of the small bowel–right colic mesentery. Only a small interface of the colonic mesentery requires primary repair.

divided closer to the splenic flexure. Such a move facilitates reconstruction, because a greater portion of the sigmoid mesentery is included in the more distal resection.

Resection of Sigmoid Mesentery

For resection of a cancer of the upper descending colon, one may be satisfied to resect the sigmoid mesentery to a point opposite the aortic bifurcation. However, for resection of a cancer of the descending colon–sigmoid colon junction, the entire upper sigmoid mesentery is resected and the bowel is divided opposite the sacral promontory. In either event, the decision about either a more proximal or a more distal set of boundaries for the resection is made after the inferior mesenteric artery and the inferior mesenteric vein have been ligated and divided and the left colic mesentery is entirely movable in the hands of the operating surgeon.

Anastomosis

As in all previously discussed resections, the edges of the bowel are cleaned in preparation for an anastomosis. The anastomosis is almost invariably handsewn and consists of either two layers or a single layer of sutures. A two-layer anastomosis with an outer layer of interrupted silk sutures and an inner running layer of absorbable suture material is traditional. Depending on the preference and training of the surgeon, a single-layer anastomosis may be accomplished.

Repair of Mesenteric Defect and Adjacent Organ Involvement

Reapproximation of the peritoneum, that is, repair of the mesenteric defect, is less simply accomplished after this resection than in some of the resections previously described. Instead of approximating one edge of the mesentery to the other, the proximal colon's mesenteric edge is generally approximated through the incised peritoneum along the duodenum and right colon while the distal sigmoid is similarly approximated to the cut edge of the right colic mesentery. Actually, only a small defect exists between the mesenteries of the proximal and distal ends of the anastomosis, which accepts direct suturing from one side of the mesentery to the other (Fig. 9–14).

Cancers of the upper descending colon and the descending colon–sigmoid colon junction rarely involve adjacent organs. The principles of resection and reconstruction are the same as those described under Cancers of the Splenic Flexure, should adjacent organ involvement be found.

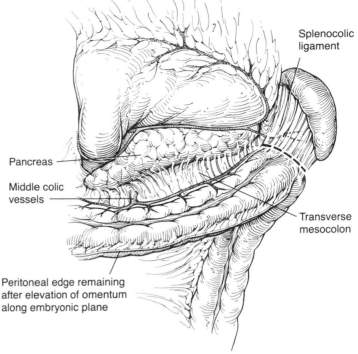

Figure 9–15. Infraomental mobilization of the splenic flexure. The omentum and stomach are reflected upward after division of the omentum along the edge of the transverse colon or entry of the lesser omental space. The left paracolic space has been opened. A communication exists between the left paracolic gutter and the lesser omentum. While the ligaments are approached from the lesser space, the surgeon's left hand is inserted posteriorly, and the ligaments are divided from right to left. Alternatively, the surgeon's right hand may be inserted via the left paracolic gutter, and the approach from the lesser sac to the left paracolic gutter. Infraomental mobilization of the splenic flexure is generally avascular and is most useful in cases in which the omentum itself need not be sacrificed.

The greater omentum is left intact whenever the anatomy of a resection does not dictate the need to resect the omentum en bloc. In many instances, in which cancers of the descending colon and sigmoid colon are sufficiently distant from the splenic flexure, the flexure may be mobilized by utilizing an infraomental technique. This is described further on in the discussion of sigmoid resection in which an infraomental mobilization of the splenic flexure is more appropriate and more common.

Sigmoid Colon

This discussion refers to carcinomas of the intraperitoneal sigmoid colon, that portion of the classically envisioned sigmoid colon with a long, free, intraperitoneal mesentery. All cancers of the sigmoid colon are treated in a similar fashion. Although some may be more proximal, that is, closer to the descending colon–sigmoid colon junction, and some may be more distal, that is, closer to the distal sigmoid colon or rectosigmoid colon, the principles remain the same. Only the proximal or distal margins of the bowel resected vary in accordance with the location of the primary tumor.

Mobilization of Sigmoid Colon and Left Colon

The entire sigmoid colon and the entire left colon are mobilized. All dissection is accomplished sharply with steady traction on the sigmoid mesentery. Care is taken not to manipulate or unnecessarily handle the primary tumor itself. The sigmoid mesentery is steadily drawn toward the midline. The three planes previously described in the discussion of the descending colon—the mesentery, the gonadal vessels, and the left ureter—all are identified as the dissection continues, freeing the mesentery from all retroperitoneal structures (see Fig. 9–13). Occasionally, a patient with a sigmoid cancer may not require taking down the splenic flexure. Such a gratuitous situation allows for anatomic resection of the entire sigmoid mesentery with division of all retroperitoneal attachments and paracolic gutters to, but not including, the splenic flexure.

More commonly, the splenic flexure should be taken down either partially or completely. It is here that the infraomental mobilization of the splenic flexure is most helpful (Fig. 9–15).

With appropriate retraction in the left upper quadrant, the operating surgeon may proceed from either the right or the left side of the table. If the surgeon proceeds from the right side of the table, the left paracolic gutter is incised and the left colon is separated from the retroperitoneum, to the extent possible, up to the splenic flexure. The greater omentum is then reflected upward as the ligament of the splenic flexure is identified by the surgeon's right hand. While the ligament of the splenic flexure is outlined and the omentum is reflected upward under mild tension, the embryologic plane that separates the greater omentum from the transverse mesocolon becomes evident as a

Labels on figure: Splenocolic ligament; Pancreas; Middle colic vessels; Transverse mesocolon; Peritoneal edge remaining after elevation of omentum along embryonic plane

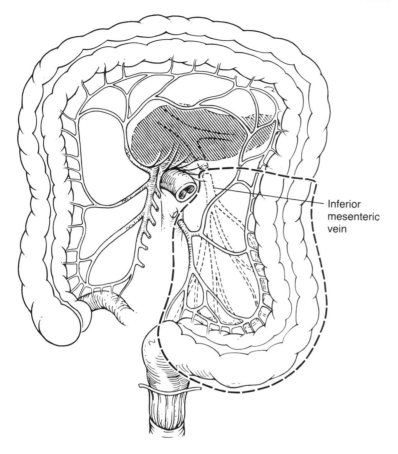

Inferior mesenteric vein

Figure 9–16. Anatomic sigmoid resection. The inferior mesenteric artery is ligated at its origin. The inferior mesenteric vein is ligated at its apex beneath the pancreas or parallel to the inferior mesenteric artery. The entire sigmoid mesentery is resected, and the bowel is resected from the descending sigmoid junction to the distal sigmoid or rectosigmoid junction. Depending on the location of the primary tumor, the bowel is resected along a more proximal or distal set of vectors.

relatively avascular and areolar space *immediately adjacent* to the left transverse colon.

The peritoneum on the posterior surface of the greater omentum, which is now reflected cephalad, is incised immediately adjacent to the colon, and this areolar avascular space is entered. By further dissection of this space, the entire greater omentum can be elevated from the colon and from the transverse mesocolon, as one would do in a radical gastrectomy for carcinoma of the stomach. Instead, however, the omentum is spared, and the splenic flexure of the colon is further identified immediately along the colon itself. All ligaments are divided where they insert onto the colon, and the colon becomes free from any of the surrounding ligaments while the omentum remains intact. This method allows the small bowel to be resurfaced with an intact omentum at the end of the operation. This method does not alter the extent to which the transverse mesocolon can be divided or the entire left colon mobilized.

The dissection proceeds caudad with further division of the white line of Toldt. The gonadal vessels and left ureter are identified along their course, and the ureter is identified and dissected away from the sigmoid mesentery to a point well below the sacral promontory.

The medial incision of the peritoneum proceeds as described previously in the discussion of the descending colon (Fig. 9–16).

The inferior mesenteric artery is identified under traction and is cleaned and divided near its origin, as described previously. The inferior mesenteric vein is identified and divided just beneath the pancreas. In early cases, for example, in cancer arising in an adenoma, the inferior mesenteric vein may be divided just opposite the inferior mesenteric artery. The higher ligation of the vein has other technical advantages, especially in patients with a short, fat mesentery.

The bowel is divided at the descending colon–sigmoid colon junction, and the "specimen side" is retracted caudad. Any connections between the mesentery and retroperitoneum are usually few in number, and these are sharply divided. The hypogastric nerves are generally identified at this time. The sigmoid colon is dissected away from the ureters, nerves, and other structures until the sacral promontory of the primary tumor is situated in the mid sigmoid colon. If the primary tumor is situated more distally, dissection and mobilization may proceed into the true pelvis.

The superior hemorrhoidal artery and vein are divided. Division of these vessels generally leaves two pedicles of fat and vessels anterolaterally, covering the bowel wall. These pedicles are cleaned by using fine right-angle clamps, or hemostats, and the bowel is prepared for an anastomosis.

Types of Anastomosis

Depending on the circumstances, any of a number of different anastomoses may be employed. Most commonly, a handsewn end-to-end anastomosis will be utilized. A traditional outer layer of interrupted silk sutures is combined with an inner layer of running absorbable suture material. Other options exist. Especially in the presence of diverticular disease, these options may be important.

One of these options is the side-to-end anastomosis between the proximal descending colon and the distal sigmoid colon. This is especially useful if either residual diverticular disease or muscular hypertrophy of diverticular disease may compromise an end-to-end anastomosis.

The anastomosis itself is performed between the antimesenteric surface of the descending colon and the end of the distal sigmoid colon. If the anastomosis is handsewn, the traditional two-layer type is chosen. The end of the descending colon may be closed with either one or two layers. If preferred, a running absorbable suture can precede the placement of a row of nonabsorbable Lembert sutures.

Staple Technique for Side-to-End Anastomosis

A circular stapling device is well suited to the side-to-end anastomosis constructed at this level. If a staple technique is elected, the following guidelines are employed (Fig. 9–17).

A whipstitch of 1-0 polypropylene suture material is placed along the edge of the distal sigmoid colon. Sutures are placed approximately 4 mm apart and 4 mm from the mucosal edge. It is not important to include the serosa in every stitch. In fact, reaching back for serosa generally everts the mucosa unnecessarily. Muscular and mucosal bite are more important.

Following the placement of this pursestring suture, four Allis clamps are applied to the open edge of the proximal descending colon. Sizers are used to determine the size of the appropriate circular stapling device. An appropriately sized circular stapling device, either 28 or 31 mm, is selected for the procedure. The circular stapling instrument is opened, and the anvil, along with the shaft, is inserted into the distal sigmoid colon where the pursestring suture is tied down into a predetermined groove. This act prevents further contamination. A sharp, penetrating plastic point is placed in the center of the cartridge shaft and is withdrawn deeply into the instrument.

Using the appropriately sized instrument, the circular stapling device, which is generously lubricated, is introduced into the end of the distal descending colon. The instrument is introduced to the point to where the anastomosis itself will be constructed, approximately 5 to 7 cm from the cut edge of the bowel. The instrument is turned at right angles so that the anastomosis will be constructed along the free edge, or antimesenteric edge, of the colon. Generally, as in handsewn anastomoses, this anastomosis should take advantage of the taenia libera of the sigmoid colon. Turning the wing nut causes the plastic penetrating device to gently push the bowel wall ahead. At the earliest sign of penetration, a 3-0 silk pursestring suture is applied around the tip. This prevents unnecessary widening of the defect as the instrument is manipulated during the course of the anastomosis. After the pursestring suture is placed, it is tied down along the shaft of the instrument, once the plastic penetrating device and the shaft have completely emerged.

While the clamps and the device are in hand, the shaft of the anvil is seated in the shaft of the cartridge; the circular stapling device is closed and fired, and the anastomosis is performed. Before these steps are executed, one must be certain that the mesentery is properly aligned.

After the instrument is fired, the edges of the cartridge are opened by turning the wing nut, and the surgeon ensures that the cartridge is not caught on any of the staples. The cartridge is withdrawn from the anastomosis via the open end of the descending colon. At this point, care must be taken not to pull too hard because the broad surface of mucosa in contact with the cartridge, the thick lubricant jelly, and the anvil all work against the ease with which the cartridge can be withdrawn. Withdrawing the cartridge is easier said than done.

Once the cartridge has been withdrawn, the anastomosis may be checked under direct vision by using long forceps and gentle spreading of the lumen. Allis clamps are placed along the edges and the center of the remaining distal portion of the descending colon. The operation is completed by closing the distal end by using a gastrointestinal anastomotic stapling device.

The stapled side-to-end anastomosis following sigmoid resection has been especially useful under difficult circumstances, specifically, for the obese male patient with a short fatty mesentery and a narrow pelvic inlet. In such patients, whose fat encroaches on the antimesenteric edge of the bowel, the taenia libera or the antimesenteric surface may be the only safe site for anastomosis. In other patients, the same circumstances caused by diverticular disease—in some, ischemia that accompanies diverticular disease—may make an end-to-end anastomosis unsafe, whereas the gastrointestinal

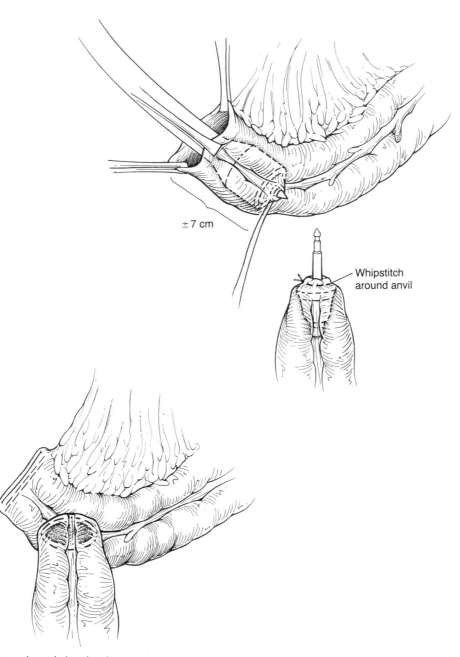

±7 cm

Whipstitch around anvil

Figure 9–17. A side-to-end, stapled, colocolic or colorectal anastomosis, using the circular stapling device.

Step #1: A whipstitch is placed along the edge of the distal segment by using nonabsorbable suture material. Sutures are placed 4 mm apart and 4 mm from the cut edge of the bowel. The anvil of the circular stapling device is inserted into the distal segment, and the pursestring whipstitch is ligated.

Step #2: The appropriate-size circular stapling device is inserted via the opened end of the colon, which is held with four long Allis clamps. The plastic penetrating spike is brought out through the taenia libera of the colon, approximately 7 cm from the bowel opening. A pursestring suture of 3-0 silk is placed around the spike as it penetrates the bowel wall to ensure that the opening in the bowel does not widen unnecessarily.

Step #3: The circular stapling cartridge and anvil are joined, and the device is fired to create the anastomosis. The device is withdrawn, and the anastomosis is checked.

Step #4: A gastrointestinal anastomosis straight stapling device is used to close the open end of the bowel by dividing it where the bowel is clean and where there is evidence of good blood supply.

stapling device can be applied at the exact junction of the mesentery where vascular demarcation is evident.

Distal Sigmoid Colon

This discussion refers to the portion of the intraperitoneal sigmoid colon that is approximately 12 to 18 cm from the anal verge. In general, it occupies the false pelvis in the area that is junctional between the free sigmoid colon and the extraperitoneal rectum.

Above 12 cm, cancers of the large bowel assume a pattern of recurrence and metastasis that closely resembles all other portions of the abdominal colon and differs significantly from the local recurrence rate of the rectum. Tumors of this region must be classified as tumors of the colon and not as tumors of the "upper rectum." The rectosigmoid colon is so named only because of its junctional location. In reality, it has no rectal anatomy, blood supply, or function.

From the surgical standpoint, cancers of the rectosigmoid colon are notorious for adjacent organ involvement but of a highly treatable and curable nature. Early works on the curative resection of pelvic tumors with extraordinary adjacent organ involvement published by Van Prohaska and by Brunschwig generally referred to primary cancers of the rectosigmoid colon. In the female patient, common sites of adjacent organ involvement include the body of the uterus, the ovary and fallopian tubes, and the broad ligament. In the male patient, they include the dome of the urinary bladder, which is otherwise protected in the female. The appendix, small bowel, omentum, ileum, and even other portions of the intraperitoneal colon may be involved in both sexes. Ureteral encroachment by the primary tumor or by inflammation or fibrosis surrounding the tumor is common. Although tradition teaches that direct extension of the primary tumor or its surrounding inflammation more commonly involves the left ureter, the right ureter may frequently be involved.

These patients are best operated on in the Trendelenburg lithotomy position. Bimanual examination under anesthesia (with or without proctoscopy) is often the most instructive assessment of the extent of primary tumor. Cystoscopy with placement of bilateral ureteral catheters is frequently helpful, and although not a substitute for knowledge of anatomy, ureteral catheters may obviate problems created by dense fibrosis, inflammation, or the mass created by a large tumor of the pelvic inlet. At the very least, ureteral catheters may reduce the time of a technically difficult, tedious, and potentially dangerous operation.

Pelvic inlet tumors combine the needs of surgery for sigmoid cancers with surgery for cancers of the upper rectum. In all respects, the principles of resection that apply to cancers of the sigmoid colon are the same, whether applied to the distal sigmoid colon or the rectosigmoid colon. Changes in anatomy dictate changes in technique. Thus, an intraperitoneal cancer may be located in the portion of the sigmoid colon that is a midline structure *before* any mobilization of the colon is done. While still located in the peritoneal cavity, the cancer may be closer to the cul-de-sac within the true pelvis requiring dissection in order to circumvent all potential margins of spread and in order to mobilize an adequate length of distal colon and mesentery for appropriate resection. The peritoneum is commonly incised as for resection of a rectal carcinoma.

Any adjacent organ involvement is managed before the segment of colon to be resected is completely mobilized and divided. Whether it be en bloc hysterectomy, oophorectomy, appendectomy, small bowel resection, omentectomy, or simple cystectomy, this phase of the operation must precede resection of the colon in order to ensure adequate margins and to prevent dissection in inappropriate planes.

The peritoneum is incised to the cul-de-sac. The retroperitoneum is entered, and the colonic segment is mobilized as described previously for the sigmoid colon. The gonadal vessels and the ureters are reflected away from the mesenteric resection to a point well distal to any resection. The inferior mesenteric artery and vein are divided and ligated as in any sigmoid resection.

Generally, on the right side, in the transverse colon, and in the descending colon, the extent of the distal margin of resection plane is so wide that it need not be measured in centimeters. In the distal sigmoid, however, especially in a male patient with a narrow pelvic inlet, it is necessary to define a distal margin of at least 5 cm. In some cases, this may lead to entry of the extraperitoneal pelvis and mobilization of the upper rectum. The object of dissection is not the length of the distal margin so much as the distance of distal dissection necessary to develop a distal margin of resection well away from the primary tumor and in completely normal bowel. The mistaken impression that one must dissect the mesentery and the colon for only a distance of 5 cm past the lowest edge of the primary tumor must be abandoned in favor of distal dissection continued until the colon is mobile, free, and can be divided in an area that is normal. At this level, a bowel clamp may be applied after the bowel has been cleaned, as already described.

The anastomosis can be performed by any of the techniques previously described: end-to-end handsewn or side-to-end, either handsewn or stapled. In addition, an end-to-end anastomosis may be performed in the vicinity of the peritoneal reflection by using a circular stapling device that has been passed transanally. This latter technique is described in the discussion of rectal cancer.

SPECIAL ISSUES IN SURGICAL MANAGEMENT OF CARCINOMA OF THE COLON

Obstructing or Perforating Carcinoma of the Colon

Obstructing cancer of the colon may be dealt with in a variety of ways. Generally, the clinical condition of the patient, the extent of intraperitoneal inflammation, the extent of distal contamination, and the presence or absence of peritonitis all influence one's operative decisions.

For cancers of the proximal colon, those proximal to and even including the splenic flexure, abdominal colectomy is advised. In cases of subacute obstruction in which bowel preparation including distal preparation has been possible, and in an optimally healthy young patient, ileocolic anastomosis can be performed at the level of the descending colon–sigmoid colon junction or beyond. A side-to-side anastomosis is advised.

For cancers of the left colon, the clinical condition of the patient dictates the initial approach to management. The young and healthy patient may be treated by primary resection, whereas the elderly, frail, or medically suboptimal patient may be treated by initial diverting colostomy. If the patient is capable of undergoing resection, the safest operation is a definitive primary resection combined with an end-colostomy. This operation obviates the reported poorer survival rate for staged procedures and avoids the highest risk inherent in primary resection and anastomosis—anastomotic failure, and death due to septic complications. Favoring resection is a 15% incidence of missed perforations when the treatment is diverting colostomy alone, the death of patients treated by diverting colostomy alone, the need of the patient to undergo multiple operations, and the repeatedly observed poorer survival rates in patients not treated by primary resection at the outset.

The only factor favoring a staged procedure is the medical condition of the patient. In order to obviate septic complications, a two-stage procedure—resection followed by internal laparotomy and colocolic anastomosis—accomplishes resection from the outset, eliminates most major septic complications, and reduces the number of stages of the so-called staged operations. In no case shall the resection be compromised. Either the patient is capable of undergoing resection or the procedure should be staged. If the patient is capable of undergoing resection, the same operation that would have been done under elective circumstances should be attempted and accomplished, barring any unforeseen intraoperative complications.

Perforation of the carcinoma significantly reduces the chances of long-term survival. This is true whether perforation is due to obstruction, direct perforation of the carcinoma, or iatrogenic perforation of the carcinoma or the adjacent colon. Perforated carcinomas are relatively rare, but when they are seen, adjacent peritoneal seeding or implants are common. Rarely, mucinous intra-abdominal content results from perforation.

Most perforated carcinomas are treated as obstructing carcinomas. In various cancer centers, trials of intraperitoneal chemotherapy are under way in patients with documented perforation, in whom all gross tumor can be reduced to masses smaller than 1 cm in diameter. No known benefit from adjuvant intraperitoneal chemotherapy in the setting of either obstruction or perforation has yet been reported. Instances of perforation, specifically, penetration of the psoas muscles by a primary cancer, may be addressed by resection and by intraoperative radiotherapy. Depending on the institution and the methods available for treatment, this can be electron beam treatment or brachytherapy utilizing either permanent implants or afterloading. Intraoperative afterloading brachytherapy is currently under investigation.

Oophorectomy

Oophorectomy is generally performed in the postmenopausal female. In various studies, the benefit of oophorectomy is reflected either in the detection of a small percentage of patients with metastatic disease in the ovaries from primary colon cancer or in the discovery of previously unsuspected primary ovarian cancer. To date, there has been no proof of a statistical advantage affecting the survival of postmenopausal patients with colon cancer in whom oophorectomy is routinely performed. Nevertheless, certain observations do apply:

1. Bilateral oophorectomy prevents the development of ovarian cancer in a population slightly more prone to develop ovarian cancer than the population at large.

2. Anecdotal reports of cure and/or long-term survival exist for patients who underwent concomitant oophorectomy at the time of colonic resection and in whom metastatic disease in the ovaries was detected.

3. In a series reported from Memorial Sloan-Kettering Cancer Center, 6.7% of women developing sys-

temic metastatic disease required a subsequent second laparotomy for the removal of painful large ovarian metastases. Patients with advanced disease represent a high-risk group for the development of ovarian metastases and can benefit from concomitant oophorectomy performed at the time of colonic resection.

4. Of patients who developed ovarian metastases, two survived for 7 years or longer following oophorectomy, and the median survival per patient with recurrent disease limited to the pelvis who was rendered surgically free of disease was 48 months. If oophorectomy in the presence of advanced recurrent cancer can dramatically help a small percentage of patients, concomitant oophorectomy may also contribute to diminished morbidity and long-term survival for a select group of patients. It remains unlikely that this will be proved statistically.

BIBLIOGRAPHY

1. Coller FA, Kay EB, MacIntyre RS. Regional lymphatic metastases of carcinoma of the colon. Ann Surg 1941;114:56.
2. Turnbull RB, Kyle K, Watson FR, Spratt J. Cancer of the colon: The influence of the "no-touch isolation" technique on survival rates. Ann Surg 1967;166:420.
3. Enker WE. Surgical treatment of large bowel cancer. In: Enker WE, ed. Carcinoma of the Colon and Rectum. Chicago: Year Book, 1978, p 73.
4. Herter FP, Slanetz CA. Patterns and significance of lymphatic spread from cancer of the colon and rectum. In: Weiss L, Gilbert HA, Ballon SC, eds. Lymphatic System Metastases. Boston: GK Hall, 1980, p 275.
5. Hardy TG. Cancer of the colon. In: Fazio VW, ed. Current Therapy in Colon and Rectal Surgery. Toronto: BC Decker, 1990, p 301.
6. Philipshen SJ, Heilweil M, Quan SHQ, et al. Patterns of pelvic recurrence following definitive resections of rectal cancer. Cancer 1984;53:1354.

ACKNOWLEDGMENT. The author is grateful to Ms. Milicent L. Cranor for her critical review and editorial assistance in the preparation of this manuscript.

Operative Treatment for Carcinoma of the Rectum

Takashi Takahashi
George E. Block
A.R. Moossa

Since Ernest Miles described the abdominoperineal resection of the rectum in 1908, surgeons have debated the technique and the extent of the ideal operation for rectal cancer. The "minimalists" describe extended resections by using the pejorative term "radical." This implies excessive, extensive, or extreme operative procedures usually not appropriate to the disease. The resections that we describe and endorse may be reasonably described as "standard": appropriate, conservative, or tested.

What constitutes an adequate operation for rectal cancer centers around two main questions: (1) Can the anal sphincter be preserved and colorectal or coloanal continuity re-established without compromising the chances of cure? (2) What extent of perirectal soft tissue (including lymphatic tissue) excision is necessary to provide the greatest chance of cure?

Clearly these two issues are interrelated, and it is not unusual for the so-called suture line recurrence to be just the "tip of the iceberg," indicative of a more extensive perirectal pelvic recurrence. Numerous factors must often be taken into consideration by the surgeon in choosing between a low anterior resection versus an abdominoperineal resection of the rectum.

Level of the Cancer. This is, without doubt, the most important parameter that the surgeon must assess. Careful digital examination coupled with a rigid proctoscopic examination is essential. The distance of the distal tumor margin from the *anal verge* (*not* the buttocks) must be carefully measured. The old dictum "If the entire lesion can be completely felt with the index finger, the patient should have an abdominoperineal resection" is still valuable, especially for an obese male patient. In general, tumors in the low rectum (5 cm or less from the anal verge) are best treated by an abdominoperineal resection. Tumors at or above 12 cm from the anal verge can usually be managed by an appropriate low anterior resection. Tumors between 5 and 12 cm (i.e., in the midrectum) are in a "no man's land," and careful consideration must be given to other parameters discussed further on.

The question "What is a safe distal rectal margin of resection?" should be individualized, depending on multiple factors. A 3-cm margin below the tumor may be adequate for a small localized polypoid tumor, whereas a 7-cm margin may be necessary for an ulcerative, infiltrating tumor. The *general* guideline of an *average* of 5 cm distal to the tumor is still useful. Controversy in the literature exists, because the exact conditions of measurement of the distal margin are never stated. Is it measured in the intact rectum at operation (stretched or unstretched)? Is it measured in the fresh resected specimen (stretched or unstretched)? Is it measured in the fixed pathologic specimen in the laboratory?

Macrosopic Appearance of the Lesion. The distance of distal intramural spread of tumor in resected specimens is extremely variable and depends on the type of tumor—whether it is polypoid, ulcerated, or infiltrative.

Extent of Circumferential Involvement of the Tumor and Its Fixity. Highly aggressive or advanced lesions usually involve a greater circumference of the rectal wall at the time of diagnosis and may be a contraindication to a low anterior resection. Fixity of the tumor in the pelvis also implies a bad prognosis, and an abdominoperineal resection, although it provides no guarantee of cure, may be a more effective palliation in the long run. A fixed circumferential tumor is also the type of clinical situation in which one should consider preoperative radiotherapy before resorting to surgical extirpation.

Histologic Differentiation and DNA Content of the Tumor. Broder's classification of tumor differentiation coupled with the presence or absence of perineural, lymphatic, or venous invasion is information that helps the surgeon assess the aggressiveness of the tumor. Lesions that stimulate a pronounced lymphocytic infiltration seem to carry a more favorable prognosis than those that do not. Thus, the surgeon should communicate with the pathologist about these microscopic findings.

The chromosomal composition of normal colon epithelium, as seen on a DNA histogram, reveals that over 90% of the cells have a single diploid peak. Near-diploid carcinomas are clinically less aggressive and thus have a better prognosis than aneuploid carcinomas.[1]

Newer Imaging Techniques. Endorectal ultrasound examination, computed tomography, and magnetic resonance imaging can help evaluate the extent of the tumor through the rectal wall and perirectal or presacral adenopathy.[2] Any of these investigations could be used to supplement the information obtained by a careful rectal digital examination and proctoscopy.

Other Considerations. *Body habitus* of the patient is a major consideration, because a standard rectal excision and a low rectal or anal anastomosis can be more easily and satisfactorily performed, from the technical point of view, in the thin than in the obese patient. *Gender* is another factor. A wide female pelvis permits a wider resection (a more successful cancer operation) and a greater chance for a low anastomosis.

Chronologic age, per se, is not a contraindication to either abdominoperineal resection or low anterior resection. A resection that involves a low anastomosis has, clearly, a higher risk of complications. Elderly patients, especially if they are frail with multiple comorbid diseases, may not tolerate a major complication such as anastomotic leak. Furthermore, a second operation, such as colostomy closure, always carries its inherent potential risks, especially in elderly patients.

The patient with *metastatic disease* often poses a dilemma. Obsession with preserving the anal sphincter and with avoiding a colostomy at all costs in the terminal phase of life may not always be in the patient's best interest. The operative mortality and complication rates are much higher in palliative resections, either low anterior resection or abdominoperineal resection. If the patient's life expectancy is limited, a terminal colostomy and a Hartmann resection may be the most judicious and kindest procedure to offer to prevent the distressing symptoms of tenesmus and bleeding in the last months of life.

Several other practical issues must be addressed during the decision to choose between low anterior resection and abdominoperineal resection. A patient who is blind, who has severe arthritis of the hands, or who has significant mental illness cannot take adequate care of a colostomy.

Comorbid Disease. Numerous preoperative risk factors have been evaluated and found to have an influence on operative outcome. Factors shown to be statistically significant as predictors of mortality and morbidity include age (75 years or older), congestive heart failure, previous abdominal and/or pelvic radiotherapy, serum albumin less than 2.7 g/dl, chronic obstructive pulmonary disease, previous myocardial infarction, diabetes mellitus, cirrhosis, renal insufficiency, and chronic use of corticosteroids.

Thus, the surgeon must assess numerous parameters before making a recommendation to the patient. In many cases of midrectal tumors, the ultimate decision (left anterior resection versus abdominoperineal resec-tion) may not be possible until the entire rectum has been fully mobilized and all of its ligaments divided. The surgeon must treat each patient as an individual, taking into consideration all the risk factors as well as the pros and cons of each procedure. A tumor in a specific location may require different treatments in different patients.

Extent of Perirectal Excision. In order to perform a curative operation for rectal cancer, several retroperitoneal and extraperitoneal structures must be dissected; careful attention must be paid to their close anatomic relationships to the lymphatic vessels and nodes draining the rectum. Underneath the posterior parietal peritoneum, a dense but thin sheet of connective tissue is spread all over, extending laterally over the kidneys on both sides. It is called the retroperitoneal fascia, and its lateral extent encompassing the kidneys is often known as Gerota's fascia. This fascia is a significant landmark in delineating the depth of dissection in the retroperitoneal space and should be recognized as soon as the posterior parietal peritoneum is incised. This fascia also envelopes the main structures and organs in the retroperitoneal space, including the kidneys, ureters, aorta, and vena cava, and it extends inferiorly into the retroperitoneal part of the pelvis, where it is given the name endopelvic fascia. An important anatomic rule is that no vessel (artery, vein, or lymphatic channel) or nerve fiber penetrates this endopelvic fascia anywhere except in the area around the origin of the inferior mesenteric artery and its accompanying autonomic nerves and lymphatic chains.

The lymphatic channels draining the rectum follow three different directions. One direction is toward the inguinal nodes from the lower anal canal. This is only pertinent in the discussion of anal or anorectal cancer (see subchapter Tumors of the Anal Canal). The two other flows are important in the surgical treatment of rectal cancer and lymphatics originating in the rectal wall that travel in the extraperitoneal space. The main lymphatic flow of the rectum ascends along the inferior mesenteric artery and terminates in lymph nodes in front of and behind the retroperitoneal fascia. The third route of lymphatic drainage is via several lymphatic vessels that depart from the rectal wall through the lateral ligaments and climb along the internal and common iliac arteries and veins, maintaining close contact with their vascular sheaths. Some of these lymphatics separate from the main flows and enter the lateral vesical space. In addition, several lymphatic chains travel further proximally along the iliac arteries and up the aorta, keeping close contact with the autonomic nerve fibers.

Thus, in order to carry out a *complete* lymphatic dissection, total excision of the retroperitoneal fascia and exposure of the abdominal aorta from the origin of the inferior mesenteric artery downward have to be

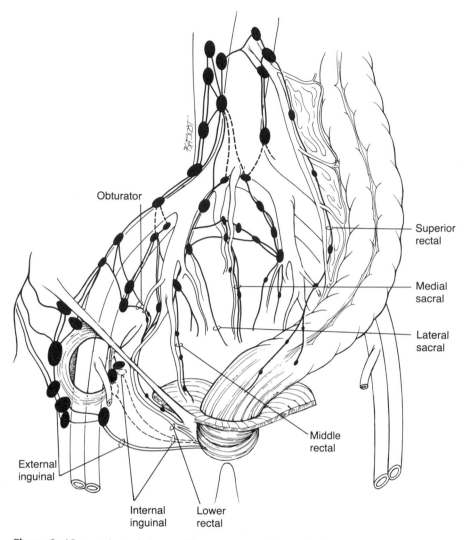

Figure 9–18. Lymphatic drainage of the rectum according to Senba.

carried out. In addition, total excision of the lateral ligaments and peeling of the vascular sheaths to "skeletonize" the iliac vessels are required. Finally, the space lateral to the iliac vessels must be opened and dissected. Figure 9–18 shows a schema of the lymphatic drainage of the rectum that was done primarily by Yoshikiyo Senba, a Japanese surgeon and anatomist, as early as 1927. Obviously, a "radical" operation to remove all the possible lymphatic drainage from the rectum implies the sacrifice of a great number of autonomic nerve fibers to the left colon and to the pelvic organs. This inevitably leads to motility disorders in the distal colon and to disturbances in micturition and sexual function in the male. Thus, the surgeon must choose between the higher cure rate and the greater complication rate of the radical operation for rectal cancer and the prospects of avoiding postoperative dysfunction.

The *standard* (radical) operation to be described involves *excision* of the retroperitoneal fascia and en-

dopelvic fascia from the origin of the superior mesenteric artery downward (plane B in Fig. 9–19). From the aortic bifurcation, the dissection moves down to the sacral promontory posteriorly and proceeds inferiorly along the curve of the sacral bone to excise the entire mesorectum and the rectosacral ligament at the bottom of the pelvis. Anteriorly, the scissors should excise Denonvilliers' fascia, exposing the posterior part of the prostate gland or the posterior vaginal wall. Laterally, the scissors should be advanced closely along the common iliac, then to the internal iliac arteries and veins; the sheaths of these vessels together with the endopelvic fascia are excised. The lateral ligament is excised in toto until the levator ani muscles are reached. Thus, in the standard operation the rectum is isolated in such a way that every element of its lymphatic network, as well as the autonomic nervous system to the pelvic organs, is excised. The destruction of autonomic nervous control of the intrapelvic organs results in several kinds of disorders, such as difficulty of micturition, irregular defecation, and, more seriously, sexual dysfunction in the male patient.

The *limited* operation entails dissection *superficial* to the retroperitoneal fascia (plane A in Fig. 9–19) and *above* the endopelvic fascia in the pelvis. In this way, most elements of the autonomic nervous system, hypogastric plexus, and pelvic nervous plexuses are preserved. The rectosacral ligament is preserved on the posterior side of the rectum, and Denonvilliers' fascia is also left intact anteriorly. Laterally, the lateral ligaments are divided along the inner border of the pelvic plexus. This limited operation should *only be adopted for a small cancer that has not penetrated deeply through the rectal wall.*

A third operation, appropriately called the "nerve-preserving procedure," is a combination of the *limited* and *standard* operations in that only part of the retroperitoneal and endopelvic fascia is excised, and the autonomic nerve fibers and plexuses supplying the pelvic organs are left intact.

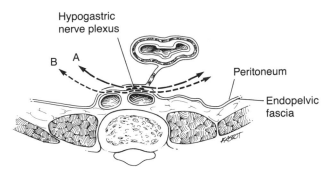

Figure 9–19. Transverse section just above the level of the sacral promontory to show the relationship of the aorta and inferior vena cava with the posterior peritoneum, the posterior retroperitoneal fascia (endopelvic fascia), and the hypogastric nerves. Two possible planes of dissection (*A* and *B*) are shown.

LOW ANTERIOR RESECTION VERSUS ABDOMINOPERINEAL RESECTION

Position and Skin Incision

The patient is placed in a Trendelenburg lithotomy position with legs apart and hip and knee joints bent. The position is similar to that described in the second subchapter of Chapter 8, Proctocolectomy, with the exception that the hips are relatively extended and the thighs are widely abducted in order to allow unlimited and simultaneous access to both the abdomen and the perineum. Too much hip flexure interferes with the abdominal operator's access to the abdominal organs. The right-handed surgeon usually prefers to stand on the left side of the patient, and, once again, the choice of incision depends on the patient's body habitus. In most instances, we perform a long vertical midline incision starting at the symphysis pubis and ending close to the xiphisternum. An alternative incision is a transverse infraumbilical one, as described in Chapter 8.

Self-retaining retractors of the Balfour type are inserted to keep the abdominal wound open. The whole peritoneal cavity is carefully examined, and special attention is paid to the presence or absence of liver metastasis and/or peritoneal nodules. The condition of the serosal surface around the tumor site in the pelvis provides information that helps in designing the extent of the operative procedure.

For a low anterior resection, the line of transection of the rectum distal to the tumor establishes the distal clearance margin of the tumor. This can be empirically determined as a *minimum* of 3 cm from the lower margin of the tumor with a shorter or longer margin,

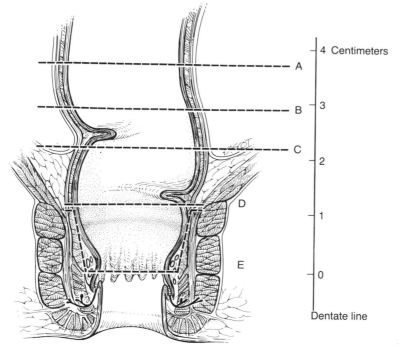

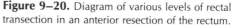

Figure 9–20. Diagram of various levels of rectal transection in an anterior resection of the rectum.

according to stage of the lesion. Therefore, we can visualize several possible lines of rectal transection, as indicated in Figure 9–20.

Incision of the Mesosigmoid Colon

All loops of small bowel are packed with large moist pads and concealed in the upper abdomen. Alternatively, all the small bowel may be wrapped in a large transparent bag, moistened with normal saline, and placed outside the operative field. The sigmoid colon is gently pulled out of the abdomen to extend the mesosigmoid. Developmental adhesions, if present, are gently lysed on the left side. The peritoneum on the left lateral side is incised at the base of the mesosigmoid colon, and the retroperitoneal space is entered. The retroperitoneal fascia should be identified in this space. In so doing, the left ureter and gonadal vessels are exposed in the same plane as the fascia. The ureter must always be visualized at this stage, because it can easily be injured at this phase of the dissection. A similar incision is made in the peritoneum of the mesosigmoid colon on the right side.

Determination of the Plane of Dissection

At the level of the aortic bifurcation, the peritoneal incisions on both sides of the mesosigmoid colon are joined, and at this moment, a decision needs to be made about the extent of the dissection in the retroperitoneal space. The hypogastric nerve plexus can at this stage be recognized as a fine white string in front of the aortic bifurcation in the same plane as the retroperitoneal fascia. By incising the fascia and passing a ligature behind the plexus, one can isolate the entire plexus to expose the adventitia of the abdominal aorta at its bifurcation (Fig. 9–21). At the discretion of the surgeon, an appropriate depth of dissection is selected: (1) *standard,* (2) *limited,* or (3) *standard with nerve preservation.*

Identification and Control of the Inferior Mesenteric Artery

By exerting traction on the string around the hypogastric nerve plexus, curved scissors are used to dissect tissue in a cephalic direction.

In the limited operation, the dissection reaches the origin of the inferior mesenteric artery from the aorta without sacrificing any of the elements of the nerve fibers (plane A, Fig. 9–22). In the standard operation, the scissors are advanced behind the nerve fibers and retroperitoneal fascia (plane C, Fig. 9–22). When the dissection moves cephalad, every element of the nerve fibers and fascia is excised to expose fully the adventitia of the abdominal aorta until the origin of the inferior mesenteric artery is reached. The depth of the dissection, that is, the choice of the plane of dissection (limited operation versus standard operation versus standard operation with nerve preservation), is clearly determined by considering the stage of the tumor as well as other factors discussed previously. The inferior mesenteric artery is ligated and divided at its origin.

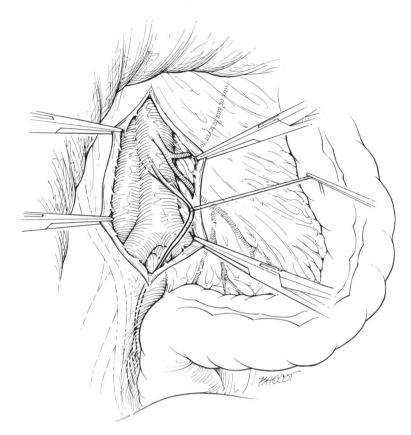

Figure 9–21. The posterior peritoneum has been incised in front of the abdominal aorta.
The origin of the inferior mesenteric artery is identified.
The hypogastric nerves are retracted by a ligature.

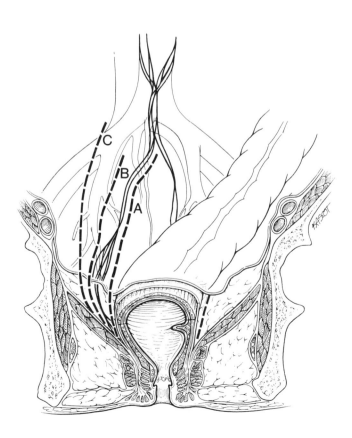

Figure 9–22. The aortoiliac vessels and the hypogastric nerves are depicted with three possible incision lines in the right posterior peritoneum. Line C is used for the standard operation, line A for the limited excision, and line B for the standard procedure with nerve preservation.

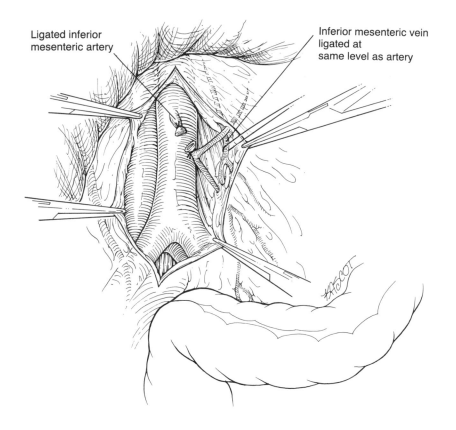

Ligated inferior mesenteric artery

Inferior mesenteric vein ligated at same level as artery

Figure 9–23. High ligation and division of the inferior mesenteric artery. The aorta has been cleaned of the retroperitoneal fascia and the hypogastric nerves.

The inferior mesenteric vein is also ligated and divided at the same level as the artery, usually proximal to the crossing of the left colic artery in the standard operation and distal to it in the limited or nerve-preserving operation (Fig. 9–23).

Incision of the Mesosigmoid Along the Marginal Vessels

Starting at the site of division of the inferior mesenteric artery, the peritoneum of the mesosigmoid colon is incised in the line that continues toward the estimated site at which the descending colon will be transected. The incision is advanced close to the marginal vessels while care is taken not to damage the blood supply to the upper descending colon, which will be used for an anastomosis or a terminal colostomy. Division and ligature of several branches of sigmoid vessels will be necessary. At this point, the distal descending colon is transected with a linear stapler to prevent leakage of colon contents into the operative field.

Dissection of the Posterior Side of the Rectum

Traction on the divided distal sigmoid colon and upper rectum opens the retroperitoneal space around the

aortic bifurcation, where the hypogastric nerve plexus can be lifted with a ligature.

In the limited or nerve-preserving procedure, the plane of dissection is started directly superficial to the hypogastric plexus. As the nerve moves downward and enters the pelvis beyond the sacral promontory, the plexus starts to divide into two branches—left and right hypogastric nerve fibers (Fig. 9–24). The dissection proceeds inferiorly along both branches and moves to the lateral side of the midrectum on both sides. Finally, the hypogastric nerves on each side merge with dense, fibrotic tissue in the lateral ligament, which can be recognized as the upper limit of the pelvic plexus (Fig. 9–25).

In the standard procedure, the dissecting plane is located at a much deeper level than the nerve fibers and plexus. The aortic bifurcation has already been exposed as a consequence of the excision of the retroperitoneal fascia and hypogastric plexus, and the dissecting scissors continue to excise fascia and nerves downward to expose the left common iliac vein and then the sacral promontory next to the bifurcation (Fig. 9–26).

The scissors are advanced closely along the natural curve of the sacral bone until the fifth sacral vertebra or the coccyx is reached. A long and stout retractor placed on the posterior wall of the rectum can provide direct vision for the surgeon, and sharp dissection of

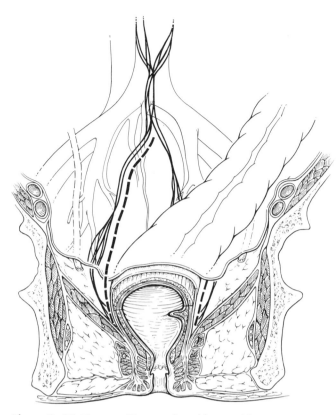

Figure 9–24. The aortoiliac vessels and hypogastric nerves are depicted. The dotted line indicates the initial pelvic peritoneal incision for the limited operation.

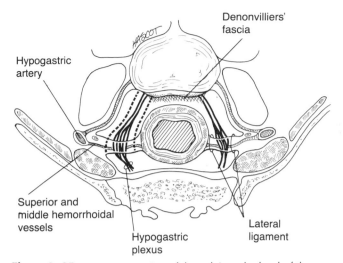

Figure 9–25. Transverse section of the pelvis at the level of the midrectum. The two dotted lines indicate the possible sites of division of the lateral ligament for the standard operation and for the nerve preservation procedure respectively.

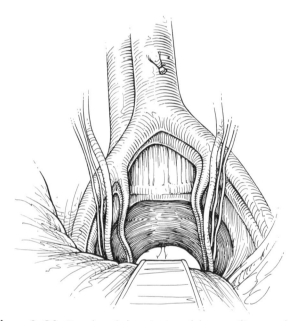

Figure 9–26. Complete skeletonization of the aortoiliac vessels and their secondary branches following rectal excision by the standard approach.

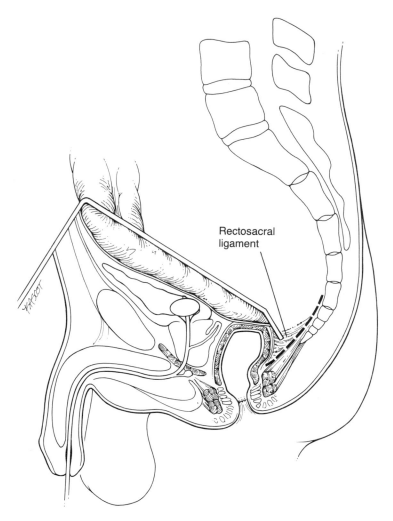

Rectosacral
ligament

Figure 9–27. Posterior dissection along the sacral curve, showing the incision line in the rectosacral ligament during the standard operation.

the presacral space is essential to maintaining the correct dissection plane (Fig. 9–27).

Mobilization of the Anterior Wall of the Rectum

The rectum is retracted superiorly, and a retractor is placed on the posterior surface of the urinary bladder or the uterus. The peritoneum is incised about 1 cm above the pouch of Douglas (Fig. 9–28). In the standard operation, Denonvilliers' fascia and the rectum should be excised together. In the case of the limited procedure, the fascia may be preserved. This fascia can easily be recognized as a whitish fine sheet, and the scissors should dissect into the space anterior to it. It is necessary to excise Denonvilliers' fascia farther downward in the midline first before dissecting toward the lateral sides (Fig. 9–29). The scissors should reach the level of the lower part of the prostate gland in the male or the upper vagina in the female. Further dissection in this space may be difficult because of the

presence of thick adhesions and numerous small veins, which need to be exposed and carefully coagulated (Fig. 9–30).

As the rectovaginal or rectoprostatic space is opened more laterally, thick bundles of fibrous tissue can be seen on both sides. These are accumulations of nerve fibers that have separated from the pelvic plexus and run toward the neck of the urinary bladder. The scissors can be advanced between these nerve fibers and the rectum to reach the space of the levator ani muscles containing loose fatty tissue.

Dissection of the Lateral Ligaments

The lateral ligament extends between the lateral pelvic wall and the lateral side of the midrectum on a horizontal plane and shows a stout and thick bundle of fibrous tissue. The pelvic nerve plexus penetrates the lateral ligament near its midpoint. At operation, the nerve plexus can be recognized as a slightly denser

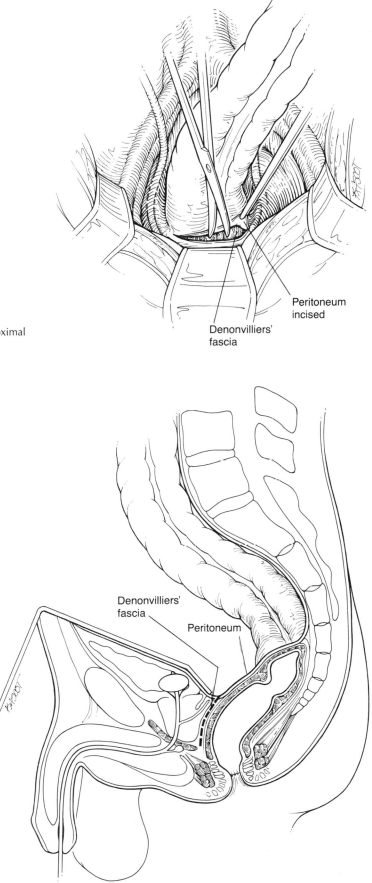

Figure 9–28. Incision of the anterior rectal peritoneum just proximal to the pouch of Douglas.

Figure 9–29. Plane of anterior dissection anterior to Denonvilliers' fascia.

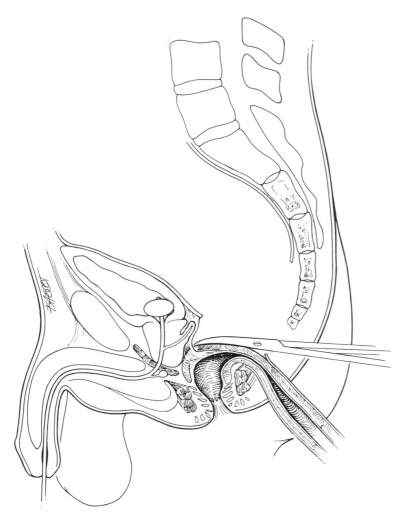

Figure 9–30. Excision of Denonvilliers' fascia posterior to the prostate gland and seminal vesicles.

part of the lateral ligament and has the appearance of an almost-square plate of dense tissue.

When the dissection along the hypogastric nerve fiber reaches the end of the pelvic plexus, the plane of dissection in the limited operation is on the inner side of the pelvic plexus (Fig. 9–31). The vessels of the lateral ligaments are either ligated or hemoclipped and divided. The dissecting scissors will then reach the space above the levator ani muscle, which had already been opened anteriorly and posteriorly.

At about this stage of the procedure, one must confirm and isolate the pelvic nerves arising from the lateral side of the sacral bones. For this purpose, the space dissected on the posterior side of the rectum should be opened more laterally, where two or three pelvic autonomic nerves, mostly from the third and fourth sacral vertebrae, can be identified as whitish strong fibers running toward the anterior side and uniting with the pelvic plexus (Figs. 9–32 and 9–33).

In the standard operation, the dissecting procedure is carried out in a wider plane and starts by excising the vascular sheath on the common iliac artery as a continuation of the dissection of the endopelvic fascia

on the posterior side (Fig. 9–34). The excision process moves downward toward the iliac bifurcation and exposes the internal iliac vessels to reach the origin of the lateral ligament. In this case the scissors excise the lateral ligament, after the vessels are individually ligated, to enter the space above the levator ani muscle (Fig. 9–35). In this standard dissection, the dissection plane passes laterally and behind the pelvic plexus; the nerve fibers running toward the urinary bladder and the pelvic nerves coming up from the sacral bone are excised both anteriorly and posteriorly in a "radical" fashion. The entire rectum down to the levator ani muscle is now completely mobilized.

LOW ANTERIOR RESECTION

Preparation of the Rectum for Transection and Anastomosis

The entire rectum has been isolated by a mobilization procedure that leaves the rectum wrapped anteriorly

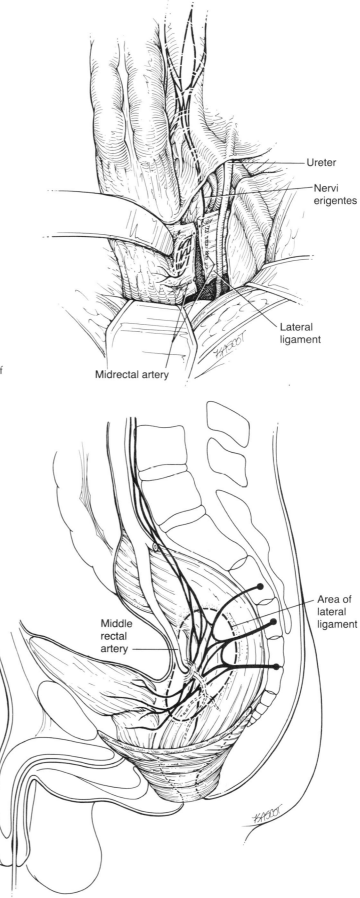

Figure 9–31. Division of the lateral ligament with preservation of the pelvic autonomic nerve plexus.

Figure 9–32. Sagittal section showing the relationship between the lateral ligament and the pelvic autonomic nerve plexus.

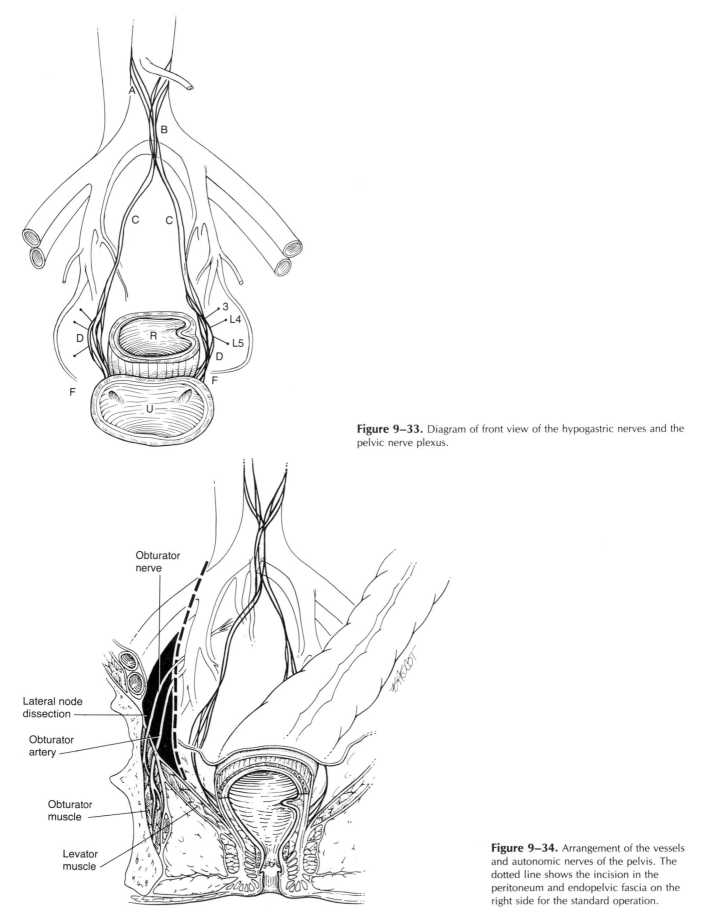

Figure 9–33. Diagram of front view of the hypogastric nerves and the pelvic nerve plexus.

Obturator nerve

Lateral node dissection

Obturator artery

Obturator muscle

Levator muscle

Figure 9–34. Arrangement of the vessels and autonomic nerves of the pelvis. The dotted line shows the incision in the peritoneum and endopelvic fascia on the right side for the standard operation.

in Denonvilliers' fascia, posteriorly by the mesorectum and endopelvic fascia, and laterally by the lateral ligament on both sides. This type of isolation of the rectum is indicated by a U-shaped dissection, in contrast to a V-shaped one with tapering from the top. The U-shaped dissection is distinctive not only in maintaining a sufficient margin around the depth of possible tumor invasion but also in providing a complete dissection of the regional lymphatic chains, a majority of which travel up within these fasciae (Fig. 9–36).

At the site of the proposed transection line distal from the tumor, these fascia are incised, and the fatty tissues inside them are dissected together with the draining lymphatic vessels of the rectum. This dissecting process begins on the anterior side by incising Denonvilliers' fascia and dissecting all the perirectal tissues superiorly to reveal the muscle coat of the rectum. All areolar and fatty tissues are dissected off at this level along *the entire circumference* of the rectal tube (Fig. 9–37). As the process proceeds posteriorly, the perirectal tissues become thicker and the mesorectum contains the right and left branches of the superior rectal artery, which can be ligated and divided.

The way in which the rectum is divided and the anastomosis performed depends on multiple anatomic and technical factors, such as the level of the transection, the size of the pelvis, and the surgeon's personal preference. At the site of the proposed transection, all the perirectal fatty tissues are excised, as discussed, until the muscle coat of the rectum becomes exposed. The rectum can now be divided after an appropriately sized right-angle clamp is placed. The rectum is divided distal to this clamp, and the specimen is removed (Fig. 9–38). The excised specimen is immediately sent to the pathology laboratory, where it is opened, orientated, and pinned on a corkboard for fixation. Frozen-section histology of any suspicious area may be performed, if indicated. In this fashion, an open anastomosis between the distal colon and the divided rectum will be performed. Before this is done, the remaining distal rectum must be carefully washed in order to free it from any remaining feces and any exfoliated cancer cells before construction of the anastomosis proceeds. Similarly, the descending colon must be milked of its contents proximally, and an intestinal clamp must be applied to prevent fecal spillage of its contents into the area of the anastomosis. End-to-end or side-to-end anastomosis of the lower descending colon to the rectum can be performed by conventional suturing in two layers (Fig. 9–39) or by using a circular stapling device, as described in Chapter 5.

An alternative method of restoring colorectal continuity is to perform the Dixon type of anastomosis. After the right-angle clamp is placed just above the proposed line of rectal division, the inside of the distal

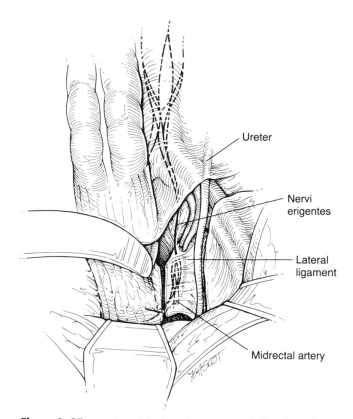

Figure 9–35. Excision of the lateral ligament including the pelvic plexus in the standard operation.

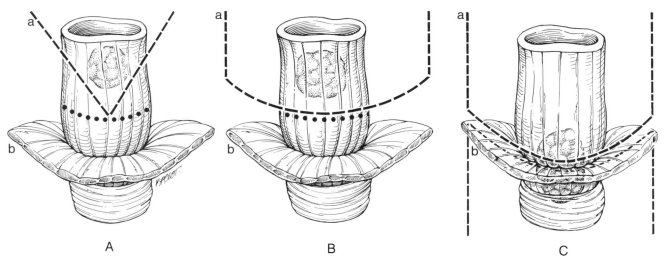

A   B   C

Figure 9–36. *A* to *C*, U-shaped rectal and perirectal dissection and transection is a much better cancer operation than the V-shaped dissection.

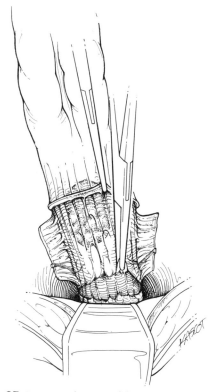

Figure 9–37. Excision of perirectal fatty tissues to expose the muscle coat of the rectum at the proposed line of transection.

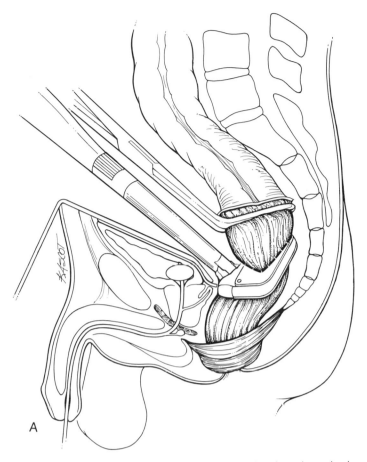

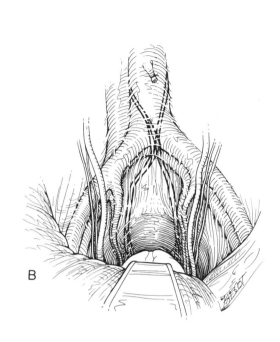

Figure 9–38. *A* and *B,* Division of the rectum distal to the right-angle clamp.

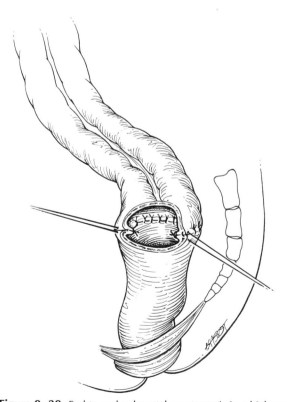

Figure 9–39. End-to-end colorectal anastomosis in which two layers of interrupted sutures are used.

rectum is washed from the perineum in order to free it from remaining feces or exfoliated cancer cells, as previously described. Similarly, the contents of the descending colon are prevented from leaking by the use of a proximal intestinal clamp on the distal colon. The anastomosis is started *before* the rectum is completely divided.

By lifting up the angled forceps to extend the distal rectum, an incision is made in the muscle layer just distal to the clamp. The submucosal layer is exposed for approximately 2 to 3 cm in width. On the posterior cut end of the descending colon, which will be approximated to the rectal stump, a similar incision is made in the muscle layer in exactly the same way as done on the distal rectum. An outer layer of sutures is placed on the posterior side by using 4-0 silk sutures in interrupted fashion. Each stitch "bites" the entire muscle layer and some of the subserosal layer to prevent any tearing of the muscle; 8 to 10 sutures are necessary. They are carefully placed before being individually tied.

After a good apposition on the posterior wall is obtained, the lumens on both stumps are opened by incising the submucosal layer and excising the edges of the stumps. The anterior wall of the rectum is left in place with the clamp, and this helps keep the anastomotic orifice open and facilitates the inner suture layer of the posterior row. The inner suture layer is made by utilizing an absorbable suture material in interrupted fashion, approximating the mucosal and submucosal layers. After completing the posterior row of sutures, the anterior wall of the rectum is divided below the right-angle clamp, and the specimen is thus removed. The anterior row of sutures is placed and the mucosa and submucosal layers are inverted using 4-0 absorbable sutures. Finally, the outer layer of suture on the anterior wall is completed by using interrupted 4-0 silk sutures. During this phase of the operation, the surgeon moves to the right side of the patient and bites the rectal muscle layer and then the wall of the descending colon with the same suture material. For the right-handed surgeon, this is the most natural and easiest way of placing those sutures.

Several other methods can be useful for restoring colorectal continuity. In the Baker type of anastomosis, the divided end of the sigmoid colon is closed with interrupted 4-0 silk sutures to invaginate the stapled line by using seromuscular apposition. A side-to-end anastomosis is performed in exactly the same way as the end-to-end, using the antimesenteric wall of the sigmoid colon. In this way, the size of the orifice in the descending colon can be tailored to suit the size of the stoma of the rectal stump (Fig. 9–40).

Stapled Anastomosis

Instead of an angle clamp being placed at the site of proposed transection of the rectum, specialized clamp forceps designed for easy application of a pursestring suture is applied. Before the rectum is divided, a stout suture material to be used for a pursestring suture is inserted into the forceps. The rectum is divided between the applicator, and a right-angle clamp placed superiorly. After the rectal stump is thoroughly cleaned, the stapler apparatus is inserted through the anus. Occasionally, it is necessary to dilate the sphincter muscles gently by using four to six fingers to facilitate access.

When the tip of the stapler reaches the rectal stump, the forceps are released and the anvil of the apparatus is advanced until the full length of the shaft clears the edge of the rectal stump. The pursestring suture on the rectal stump is tied to fix the stump to the apparatus.

The sigmoid colon with the pursestring suture material at the edge is eased over the anvil, and the proximal pursestring suture is secured. As the dial of the apparatus is turned from the perineal end, the two edges of the bowel tied to the apparatus are joined together. The abdominal surgeon must be careful that no tissue comes between the two faces of bowel that are approximated. The apparatus should be gently withdrawn to give the rectal stump a little relaxation at the time of approximation. It is essential not to apply excessive tension on the mesentery of the descending colon. It is also mandatory to avoid malrotation of the proximal segment colon. The excised cut edges (doughnuts) of the anastomosis should be carefully examined to ensure that the rings are intact. If not, the anastomosis must be appropriately reinforced with sutures or be totally reconstructed.

Stapler Anastomosis: Modification 1

When the anastomosis is planned much lower in the pelvis or at a level much nearer the anal canal, within 1 to 2 cm above the anal canal, it is often difficult to place the pursestring applicator at the line of transection. In this case, the pursestring suture must be placed by hand. After the proximal right-angle clamp is placed just above the planned transection line, division of the rectum is started on the rectal wall just distal to the clamp, while 1 cm or so of the wall is cut off at a time. At the cut edge, a "start" suture is fixed by hand. The rectal wall is divided 1 cm at a time by using scissors or electrocautery. At each incision site, the stitch is repeated in a continuing over-and-over fashion from

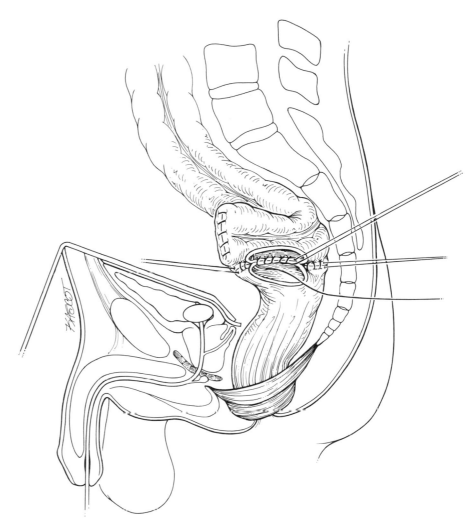

Figure 9–40. Side-to-end colorectal anastomosis in which two layers of interrupted sutures are used.

inside to outside. Gentle and steady traction of the proximal clamp is essential to ensure a good view of the site of anastomosis.

Stapled Anastomosis: Modification 2— Double-Stapler Method

In place of the pursestring applicator, a linear stapler apparatus is placed to close the distal end at the site of transection. The angle of the head to the shaft of the apparatus can be changed to obtain easy access to the transection site. Once the stapler is successfully placed at the appropriate site, the rectum is ready to be divided between it and a proximally placed, angled clamp.

The distal rectum is washed, as discussed previously, and an instrument for stapled anastomosis with a detachable needle shaft on top of it is inserted through the anus. As the instrument is gently advanced through the anus, the needle shaft appears out of the closed stump through a puncture hole in the center of the staple line. An anvil shaft, which has already been attached to the stump of the descending colon (as described previously), is inserted into the main shaft in place of the needle shaft. The handle of the stapler apparatus is rotated to approximate the two ends of the bowel together. Both sides of the rectal stump may be grasped by Allis-like forceps to extend over the entire surface to allow good apposition of the two ends of the bowel.

Coloanal Anastomosis

Coloanal anastomosis is defined as a method of restoring bowel continuity by uniting the descending colon to the anal canal. At the anorectal junction, the muscular layer of the rectum becomes thicker, and as it proceeds downward, it surrounds the anal canal to become the external sphincter muscle. This is fully encircled by the puborectal muscle, which is also known as the external sphincter.

Once the transection line is designed to be just at the upper limit of the anal canal or on the dentate line

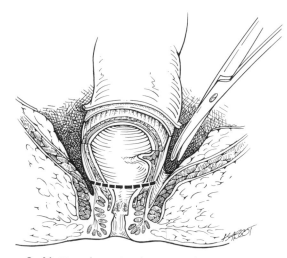

Figure 9–41. Line of resection for near-total rectal excision and coloanal anastomosis.

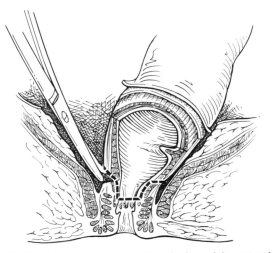

Figure 9–42. Total rectal excision. Note the line of dissection for total extirpation of rectal mucosa.

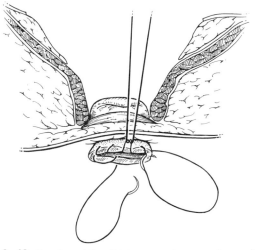

Figure 9–43. Eversion of the distal anorectal stump after anal dilatation for application of the pursestring suture. The anorectum can be pushed back for stapled anastomosis.

(Fig. 9–41), there remains virtually no margin for the construction of a safe and satisfactory anastomosis.

In order to save a margin of the anorectum, it is essential to dissect the tissues between the internal and external muscles. A "peeling" process for a few centimeters distal to the anorectal junction is required before the rectum is transected (Fig. 9–42). In order to achieve this, the rectum must be pulled up strongly. With the application of deep pelvic retractors, the scissors can be advanced along the border of the muscular layer under direct vision. In these circumstances, it is impossible to place any pursestring applicator or any angled forceps for closure; hence, suturing of the pursestring becomes mandatory.

Two methods of placing the pursestring suture at the anal stump should be considered. One is the continuing "cut and sew" process, employed in the low anterior resection. The other method is designing the distal stump with preservation of a piece of rectum. This dividend end is inverted and pulled out through the anus after full dilatation of the anal sphincter (Fig. 9–43). The pursestring suture can be placed outside the anus and pushed back for the stapled anastomosis (Fig. 9–44).

A low anastomosis in the pelvis must be tension free. This often entails mobilization of the entire descending colon, splenic flexure, and left half of the transverse colon. Division of the peritoneal attachment along the left paracolic gutter and separation of the splenic flexure and transverse colon from the greater omentum become necessary.

ABDOMINOPERINEAL RESECTION OF THE RECTUM

Regardless of whether an abdominoperineal resection or low anterior resection is performed, the abdominal phase of the dissection remains the same. The extent of the posterior, lateral, and anterior dissection is identical for both operations. Posteriorly, the scissors being employed for the dissection reach the surface of the levator ani muscles and allow easy access to the attachment site of the puborectalis bundle by excision of the sacrorectal ligament. On both lateral sides, the dissection approaches the levator ani muscles by appropriately separating the lateral ligament as far out as possible, and this dissection terminates on the lateral bundle of the puborectal muscle. Anteriorly, Denonvilliers' fascia is peeled off the prostate or posterior vaginal wall to just above the perineal body. At this stage of the operation, the rectum has been fully isolated from surrounding tissues to the upper limit of the anal canal.

Shape and Size of the Ischiorectal Space

Before the perineal phase of the operation begins, it is necessary to have a clear picture of the shape and size of the ischiorectal space (Fig. 9–45). At the center of this picture, a small circle represents the orifice of the anus. Around this circle, four distinctive points must be identified as landmarks. Each pair of points is positioned separately on a straight line; the two straight lines, horizontal and vertical, cross at a right angle at the center of the perineum. The horizontal line is constituted by joining the two ischial tuberosities (C) on either side. The vertical line joins the perineal body (A) anteriorly and the coccyx (B) posteriorly. When we draw a line to join these four points, it forms a diamond that represents the outline of the ischiorectal space as seen in the lithotomy position. Each line has two corresponding structures. The upper two lines from the ischial tuberosities to the perineal body indicate the course of the superficial perineal muscles (D), and the lower two lines from the ischial tuberosities to the tip of the coccyx identify the border of the gluteal muscles (E).

In order to visualize the image of the perineum in the coronal plane, the capital letter M is a good symbol, and the column of the center of the M indicates the rectum. The bases of the two legs of the M are the ischial tuberosities, and the center intersection of the two bars of the M indicates the location of the perineal body anteriorly and the coccyx posteriorly.

Incision and Excision of Ischiorectal Space

Once a decision has been made to perform an abdominoperineal resection, the anus is packed with gauze (Kerlix) soaked in povidone-iodine (Betadine) and is closed shut with a stout suture through the perianal skin. The perineum is appropriately prepared and redraped as deemed necessary. A skin incision is made in the shape of a diamond, but within the margins of the diamond already described. The subcutaneous fat is dissected to enter the inside of the perineal diamond or the ischiorectal space from the perineal side. The landmarks to be identified first are the lower margins of the diamond or the inner border of the gluteal muscles on both sides. Because most of the superficial perineal muscles are not fully developed, it is sometimes difficult to identify them in the dissecting field; therefore, we have to look for these muscle fibers after confirming the correct location of the ischial tuberosities from which these muscles originate.

The dissection is continued along the legs of the M. At the top of the each vertical limb, in the deepest

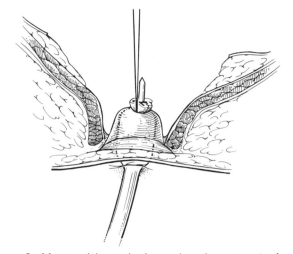

Figure 9–44. Use of the stapler for a coloanal anastomosis after pursestring application, as shown in Figure 9–43.

EDITORIAL COMMENT

Professor Takahashi properly emphasizes the importance of complete lymphadenectomy as well as a wide, cylindric, 360-degrees excision of perirectal tissue for the adequate operative treatment of carcinoma of the rectum. These principles pertain whether an anterior or abdominoperineal resection is performed. Any adherent structures are excised en bloc. It is of particular importance to excise the posterior vaginal wall (with or without an en bloc hysterectomy) when treating anterior or circumferential tumors that are fixed or that give any indication of invasion of the rectovaginal septum. The vaginal defect is easily repaired at the end of the procedure with excellent functional results. In the male patient, the seminal vesicles and/or the prostatic capsule should be excised en bloc when adherence or invasion by the tumor exists.

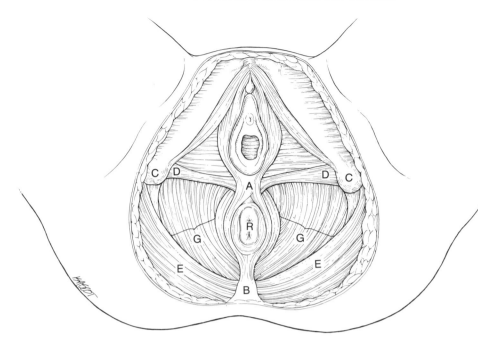

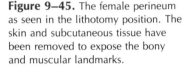

Figure 9–45. The female perineum as seen in the lithotomy position. The skin and subcutaneous tissue have been removed to expose the bony and muscular landmarks.

parts of the space, the inferior rectal vessels accompanied by nerve fibers and lymphatics appear as a bundle of "strong strings" along the fatty tissues. Because these structures originate from the Alcock canal, which traverses along the bars toward the center of the M, we have to be cautious to avoid damaging the Alcock canal in the process of dividing the vessels. This dissection leads to the lateral attachment of the levator ani muscle (Fig. 9–46).

Excision of the Levator Ani Muscle and Dissection of the Perineal Body

Excision of the levator ani muscle starts at the tip of the coccyx. Occasionally, it may be necessary to excise the lower two pieces of the coccyx. By inserting the index finger of the left hand through an incision in the median raphe of the levator ani muscle at the tip of the coccyx, the levator ani muscle can be gently retracted toward the perineum, and excision of the muscle fibers can be achieved along the lateral pelvic wall by means of electrocautery. The surgeon reaches the puborectalis bundle on both sides; these can also be divided. At this juncture, the divided distal sigmoid colon and rectum, which have already been fully mobilized by the abdominal dissection, can be pulled out through the perineal wound in such a way that the distal cut end of the sigmoid colon prolapses out of the perineal wound posteriorly. Traction on the colon allows dissection of the adhesions between the anterior wall of the rectum and the prostate or vaginal wall

under direct vision, where Denonvilliers' fascia can easily be peeled off and the specimen freed anteriorly.

At this moment, the perineal body becomes the only structure that connects the rectum to the patient, and it can be carefully separated while care is taken not to injure the urethra anteriorly in the male and the posterior vaginal wall in the female. There is no landmark indicating the correct dissection plane in the perineal body. Therefore, this dissection must be the last phase of the operation so that the appropriate plane can be estimated as a continuation of the previous perineal and abdominal dissection.

Colostomy, Drainage, and Wound Closure

The most troublesome parts of the operation concern operative and postoperative bleeding. The most common areas of bleeding are the presacral space, the lateral walls of the pelvis, and the posterior wall of the prostate gland, where small venous plexuses are exposed on the peeled surfaces. A judicious and careful combination of electrocautery and suture-ligature with fine silk may be necessary to control the bleeding. An end-colostomy is made in the left lower quadrant by using the extraperitoneal approach of John Goligher. This approach prevents many complications, such as colostomy prolapse, peristomal hernias, and small bowel obstruction.

The perineal wound is closed with interrupted nonabsorbable nylon sutures that bite both the skin and

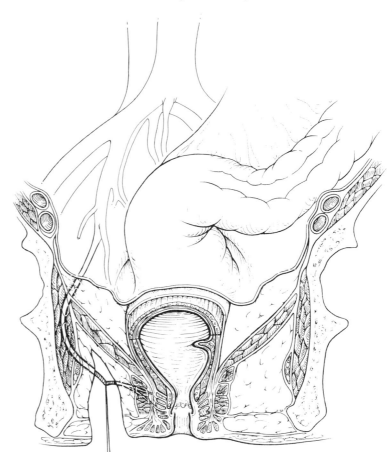

Figure 9–46. Coronal section of the lower pelvis and perineum showing the plane of dissection in the ischiorectal space and ligation of the inferior rectal vessels.

the subcutaneous tissues. The presacral space is drained by using two Jackson-Pratt type suction drains placed in the pelvis and brought out either on the lateral sides of the abdominal wall or on the lateral sides of the perineal wound.

Closure of Pelvic Dead Space and Repair of Pelvic Floor

The dead space resulting from a wide excision of the rectum and perirectal tissues (abdominoperineal resection or low anterior resection) needs to be managed. We routinely bring down an omental pedicle along the left paracolic gutter to fill in this dead space. This maneuver has the advantage of preventing small bowel from getting caught in the pelvis. If postoperative radiotherapy is needed, this omental pedicle graft protects the small bowel from the dangers of severe radiation enteritis.[3] The greater omentum is fully detached from the transverse colon along its entire length. The right gastroepiploic vessels are doubly ligated and divided close to the first part of the duodenum. The gastric branches of the gastroepiploic vessels are serially and individually ligated with 3-0 silk and divided

from right to left. In this way, the entire greater omentum can be mobilized from right to left, its blood supply from the short gastric and left gastroepiploic vessels remaining intact. The greater omentum can easily be brought down along the left paracolic gutter to fill in the pelvic dead space.

Another method of excluding the small bowel from the pelvis is by reconstructing a new floor at the pelvic brim made of synthetic nonabsorbable or absorbable mesh or an appropriate size silicone breast prosthesis or even a synthetic polymer mold.[4] The dangers of secondary infection and other complications, such as fistula formation, cannot be overemphasized in this setting. The fear of pelvic tumor recurrence may be reduced by using high-dose postoperative radiotherapy of the lesser pelvis, which must be balanced against the fear of severe radiation enteritis.[5]

INDICATIONS AND TECHNIQUES FOR LATERAL LYMPH NODE DISSECTION

The lateral lymph node dissection constitutes the widest dimension of perirectal dissection and implies dissection beyond the level of the internal iliac vessels. In other words, the lateral node dissection means the complete excision of all lymphatic chains in the lateral flow from the rectum. In addition to the standard clearance of the aortoiliac, middle rectal, internal iliac, and mesorectal soft tissues and lymphatics, *lateral node dissection implies excision of the obturator nodes and the fatty tissues of the lateral vesical space.*[6, 7]

The lateral lymphatic channels drain from the lower half of the rectum and the upper part of the anal canal. Therefore, lateral node dissection is *only* indicated for a low rectal tumor that is *below the level of the peritoneal reflection.*

The first step of the lateral node dissection has already been completed in the process. The standard excision of the rectum is as previously described. Dissection of the lateral vesical space now remains.

Dissection of the Lateral Vesical Space

By excision of the vascular sheath of the iliac vessels, the dissection now enters the lateral vesical space, which is mainly composed of fatty tissue containing several lymph nodes. At the center of the space, the obturator nerve traverses toward the anterior side. Dissection along the internal iliac vessels leads to the origin of the superior vesical artery, which is gently hooked with a small retractor in order to widen the space. The fatty tissue is dissected first from the true pelvic wall, second from the obturator nerve, and finally from the tributaries of the internal iliac artery and vein.

As the dissection proceeds deeper, the obturator artery and vein are seen traversing the space. They may be isolated and retracted or may have to be ligated and divided. At the bottom of the space, the dissection reaches the level of the levator ani muscle.

Excision of the Internal Iliac Artery and Vein

Most of the lymph nodes in the lateral lymphatic flow from the rectum are situated closely along the internal iliac vessels and their branches, that is, in their vascular sheath. In order to achieve a complete eradication of the lateral nodal basin, excision of the internal iliac vessels may be considered, especially when involvement of any nodes is confirmed during the operation by frozen-section histologic findings.

In this case, the level of ligation and division of the iliac vessels should be set up distal to the branching of the superior vesical artery. This ensures that the blood supply to the urinary bladder is preserved, even if the internal iliac vessels are to be excised on both sides.

A valuable technique for obturator node clearance is carefully isolating and dividing the internal iliac artery distal to the origin of the superior vesical artery. The distal cut end of the internal iliac artery is lifted to achieve good access to the internal iliac vein, which is tightly adherent to the pelvic wall. Isolation and division of the vein require careful dissection in order not to injure it. When the dissection behind these vessels proceeds inferiorly, the biggest branch of the internal iliac vessels—the superior gluteal artery and vein—comes into view. These two vessels enter the pelvic wall with a very short stem, and their ligation and division have to be carried out with great care so that the distal cut end does not retract and disappear. As the dissection proceeds further inferiorly, several somatic branches of the internal iliac vessels are ligated and divided as they enter the pelvic walls. Finally, the most peripheral branch of the internal iliac vessels—the pudendal artery and vein—need to be ligated directly on the levator ani muscles.

At this stage, the dissection is completed, and the pyriform muscle and ischial nerve plexus can be seen on the side wall of the pelvis. Occasionally, division and excision of the internal iliac artery and vein may be planned, starting at the iliac bifurcation. However, this procedure can only be safely performed on one side of the pelvis.

Results of Surgical Treatment

Many surgeons of notable repute do not practice the high ligation of the inferior mesenteric artery and the extended lymphadenectomy, as described in the standard operation.[8] We, in conjunction with others, believe in the superiority of the operation described. A good prognosis can be expected when the regional lymph nodes are free from cancer spread. Enker, at Memorial Sloan-Kettering Hospital, analyzed 412 cases and reported a 5-year survival rate of 84.4% for Dukes A and 59.6% for Dukes B patients. The 5-year survival rate for Dukes B rectal cancer is lower than that in colon cancer, and this is explained by the difficulty of wide dissection of tumor in the pelvis.[9]

Once the regional nodes are involved (i.e., in Dukes C cases), the question of whether the limit of the resection should be extended is still debated. Stearns and Deddish and Bacon independently tried to find out the superiority, if any, of an extended nodal dissection over the conventional operation.[10, 11] They defined the extended operation as ligating the inferior mesenteric artery at its origin, dissecting the para-aortic lymph nodes, and peeling off all the tissues from the iliac vessels on the lateral side of the rectum. They termed the procedure an "abdominopelvic lymphadenectomy," but they did not perform an obturator node dissection. Both reports show a benefit for the extended operation: 54% 5-year survival versus 46% in the Stearns series, and 54% versus 49% in the Bacon series. In contrast, Glass and Mann, at St. Mark's Hospital in London, failed to demonstrate the effectiveness of regional lymphadenectomy in improving the 5-year survival rate: 54% for extended versus 52% for conventional dissection.[12]

In Enker's series, the overall 5-year survival rate for Dukes' C tumors was reported to be 37%, but when the figures are broken down, they demonstrate the superiority of pelvic lymphadenectomy for patients' survival rates: 48% 5-year survival rate for the extended dissection compared with 28% for the conventional dissection. His data provide ample evidence of the value of lymphadenectomy combined with wide excision of the tissues surrounding the rectum. In other words, he strictly performed the U-shaped dissection around the rectum, as described.

None of the foregoing authors extended the dissection into the paravesical space (lateral lymphatic flow is also located). A series of patients at the Cancer Institute Hospital in Tokyo underwent wide excision of the perirectal tissues and abdominopelvic lymphadenectomy with a complete excision of the lateral lymph nodes, including the paravesical space (obturator nodes), for a low-lying rectal cancer. This extensive dissection appears to confer additional benefit to Dukes' C cases with a spectacular 58% 5-year survival rate. Even when the levels of intermediate node group in the upward lymphatic flow and the peripheral node group in the lateral lymphatic flow are involved, a 5-year survival rate of more than 40% is reported. Once the cancer spread has reached the main proximal nodal group around the origin of the inferior mesenteric artery or at the bifurcation of the iliac arteries, the survival rate drops sharply, but a few patients (13.8% to 16.9%) can still be expected to be cured of cancer.[6]

The distressing problem of local tumor recurrence following excision of rectal cancer needs emphasis. The mechanism of local recurrence is simply failure to remove completely all the primary tumor and its foci of local or regional lymph node metastases. Suzuki and colleagues from Tokyo have reduced the incidence of local recurrence from 18% to 8% by performing lateral node dissection.[7] It is also generally accepted that patients with Dukes B2, C1, or C2 rectal cancer should be *considered* for postoperative adjuvant radiotherapy to decrease the likelihood of local pelvic or perineal recurrence following abdominoperineal resection or low anterior resection.[13–15]

When local recurrence develops at the anastomotic site after a low anterior resection, the patient may simply have local regional disease that may be amenable to further excision. The level of tumor markers (carcinoembryonic antigen, CA-19-9) may not be ele-

vated. Computed tomography scan and proctoscopic biopsies are essential to evaluate the extent of the disease and obtain tissue confirmation of the diagnosis. The only chance of cure is an abdominoperineal resection with postoperative radiotherapy.[16]

MULTIPLE ORGAN RESECTION

About 5% to 10% of patients with rectal cancer present when the tumor has already invaded adjacent organs. Uterus and vagina in the female and the bladder in the male are the structures most commonly involved. Such adhesions must be treated as malignant, rather than inflammatory, in nature. Clinical experience suggests that if the primary tumor with its lymphatic basin and adherent structures can be encompassed in an en bloc resection, the survival rate is comparable to that of the general population with rectal cancer. The surgeon should still proceed with an appropriate excision according to the halstedian principles in such situations, provided that the patient is carefully selected.

The incidence of ovarian metastasis in women with rectal cancer is usually low but may be as high as 8% in some series. Furthermore, there is a relatively high frequency of unsuspected primary ovarian cancers in these women. Therefore, prophylactic oophorectomy should always be considered and discussed with the patients preoperatively, especially if they are already postmenopausal.

POSTOPERATIVE CARE

The postoperative course of a patient who underwent an ALR is exactly the same as that of an abdominoperineal resection. Continuous nasogastric suction is recommended for a few days, the number depending on the amount of postoperative ileus that develops. The indwelling urinary catheter needs to be left in place for 5 to 7 days, until bladder function returns. Oral intake is started as soon as the patient has passed flatus and is gradually increased. The average length of hospitalization is usually about 7 days.

Intraoperative and Early Postoperative Complications

Several complications may occur during the performance of a low anterior resection or an abdominoperineal resection of the rectum. As previously mentioned, intraoperative hemorrhage may be a problem. However, careful ligation or hemoclipping of individual vessels can usually prevent excessive blood loss. Bleeding from the perineal wound after abdominoperineal resection can usually continue in the form of oozing from the presacral or prostatic venous plexuses. Adequate visualization, judicious use of suture ligation, and electrocautery can usually help achieve adequate hemostasis. However, if the bleeding is so diffuse that a specific bleeding point cannot be identified, the perineum should be packed and the pack gradually removed 3 or 4 days later.

If perineal bleeding becomes evident during the early postoperative period, it is essential to return the patient to the operating room, where the patient is placed in the lithotomy position and the perineal wound reopened. All clots must be carefully evacuated and hemostasis achieved by conventional techniques. A slipped ligature or dislodged hemoclip is occasionally found to be the source of the hemorrhage. Once again, if no discrete bleeding point is found, generalized oozing is controlled by appropriate packing.

Anastomotic bleeding is a rare complication (<1.0%) of anterior resection. It is usually due to inadequate hemostasis at the suture line and occurred more frequently when the early Russian instrument with the single row of staples was employed.

Pelvic hematoma rupturing into the posterior wall of the anastomosis may also manifest itself in the early postoperative period. If severe, this can easily result in an anastomotic dehiscence. In both instances, the bleeding usually subsides spontaneously, and an initial conservative approach is recommended.

Urologic Complications

Injury to the ureter or the bladder is largely preventable by utilizing proper surgical technique, including adequate access, exposure, and assistance. The ureter must be *visualized,* and one should not rely on palpation to identify the course of this structure.

The ureter can usually be damaged at three different points during the operation. First, as mentioned, mobilization of the peritoneum of the mesosigmoid colon early in the operation may endanger the ureter if it is not properly and carefully visualized. Second, during high ligation of the inferior mesenteric vessels, the left ureter must be carefully identified and mobilized laterally away from the vascular pedicles. Third, the ureter can be damaged during division of the lateral ligaments deep in the pelvis. The ureter is particularly at risk if a synchronous hysterectomy is being performed. It is essential to retract both ureters laterally and to *visualize* them throughout their entire course.

Once a ureteric injury has occurred, the most important factor is immediate recognition and appropriate repair according to well-established urologic principles. The various techniques are adequately covered in several urologic texts.

Occasionally, bladder injury and damage to the small bowel may inadvertently occur; it should be recognized at the time of the operation and appropriately repaired.

REFERENCES

1. Chang KJ, Enker WE, Melamad M. Influence of tumor cell DNA ploidy on the natural history of rectal cancer. Am J Surg 1987;153:184–187.
2. Fleshman JW, Myerson RJ, Frye RD. Accuracy of transrectal ultrasound in predicting pathologic stage of rectal cancer before and after preoperative radiation therapy. Dis Colon Rectum 1992;35:H23–H26.
3. DeLuca FR, Riggins H. Construction of an omental envelope as a method of excluding the small intestine from the field of postoperative irradiation to the pelvis. Surg Gynecol Obstet 1985;160:365–367.
4. Deutsch AA, Stern HS. Technique of insertion of pelvic Vicryl mesh sling to avoid postradiation enteritis. Dis Colon Rectum 1989;32:628–630.
5. Krook JE, Moertel CG, Gunderson LL, et al. Effective surgical adjuvant therapy for high-risk rectal carcinoma. N Engl J Med 1991;324:709–713.
6. Takahashi T, Mori T, Moossa AR. Tumors of the colon and rectum: Clinical features and surgical management. In: Moossa AR, Robson M, Schimpff S, eds. Comprehensive Textbook of Oncology. 2nd ed. Vol 1. Baltimore: Williams & Wilkins, 1991, pp 904–933.
7. Suzuki K, Sawada T, Muto T, et al. Prevention of local recurrence by lateral node dissection for rectal cancer. Cancer 1993. In press.
8. Corman ML. Tumors of the rectum. In: Colon and Rectal Surgery. 3rd ed. Philadelphia: JB Lippincott, 1993.
9. Enker WE, Heilweil ML, Hertz RL, et al. En bloc lymphadenectomy and sphincter preservation in the surgical management of rectal cancer. Ann Surg 1986;203:426–433.
10. Stearns MVV Jr, Deddish MR. Five-year results of abdominopelvic lymph node dissection for carcinoma of the rectum. Dis Colon Rectum 1959;2:169–172.
11. Bacon HE. Abdomino-perineal proctosigmoidectomy with sphincter preservation: 5 year and 10 year survival after "pull-through" operation for cancer of the rectum. JAMA 1956;160:628–632.
12. Glass RE, Ritchie JK, Thompson HR, et al. The result of surgical treatment of cancer of the rectum by radical resection and extended abdomino-iliac lymphadenectomy. Br J Surg 1985;72:599–601.
13. Cawthorn SJ, Parums DV, Gibbs NM, et al. Extent of mesorectal spread and involvement of lateral resection margins as prognostic factors after surgery for rectal cancer. Lancet 1990;335:1055–1058.
14. Moossa AR, Ree PC, Marks JE, et al. Factors influencing local recurrence after abdomino-perineal resection for cancer of the rectum and rectosigmoid. Br J Surg 1975;62:727–730.
15. Douglass, HO. Adjuvant therapy of colorectal cancer. In: Moossa AR, Robson M, Schimpff S, eds. Comprehensive Textbook of Oncology. 2nd ed. Vol 1. Baltimore: Williams & Wilkins, 1991.
16. Kodner IJ, Shemesh EI, Fry RD, et al. Preoperative irradiation for rectal cancer improved local control and long-term survival. Ann Surg 1989;209:194–198.

Abdominosacral Resection

Kenneth Eng
S. Arthur Localio

RATIONALE

Sphincter-saving operations have been playing an increasing role in the treatment of cancer of the rectum. The technical problems of radical resection of low-lying cancers and restoration of intestinal continuity deep within the pelvis have led to abdominal, trans-sphincteric, perianal, and trans-sacral approaches and various methods of sutured and stapled anastomoses. Sphincter function is adequate if structures below the puborectalis muscle and their sensory and motor innervation are preserved. However, there should be no complacency about adequate radical resection of the cancer. The current role of abdominosacral resection is assessed here in the context of the other sphincter-saving operations.

Anterior Resection

Most surgeons use anterior resection for tumors as low as they consider technically feasible to approach this way, and they resort to abdominoperineal resection for the rest. The availability of staplers that allow end-to-end colorectal anastomosis has extended the range of anterior resection for some surgeons.[1, 3, 4] Although the stapler facilitates performing low anastomoses, the problem of exposure for adequate radical resection remains. Despite the use of ingenious newer versions of these devices and new techniques that facilitate the most awkward anastomoses in the depths of the pelvis, the resection is limited to that which is visible from the abdominal incision.[5] Clearance of the tumor must not be jeopardized to save the sphincter.

Even in the hands of experienced surgeons, the abdominal approach alone cannot provide sufficient exposure for reliable resection of many midrectal cancers. The abdominal exposure in men is limited to the level of the seminal vesicles. The anterior wall of the rectum below this level is obscured by the pubis. After thorough mobilization of the rectum, a midrectal tumor may be barely in view, and determination of an adequate distal margin will be in doubt. In women, the wider pelvis may permit mobilization under direct vision to the levators, but obesity, an enlarged uterus, or previous inflammation and scarring may compromise this exposure.

Abdominoanal Resection

The coloanal pull-through operation described by Parks provides for anastomosis within the anal canal.[8] After abdominal mobilization and resection of the rectum are done, the anus is dilated and the mucosa stripped from the remaining anorectal stump. The proximal colon is pulled through the muscular cuff and sutured at the dentate line perianally. Although the anastomosis is constructed as low as at the dentate line, mobilization and resection of the cancer are carried out entirely by the abdominal route. Exposure is no different from that for anterior resection. The distal margin is at the level of the rectal transection and not at the dentate line. Unless one is willing to accept blind mobilization and transection of the lower rectum, the method cannot allow radical resection to the levators in every case.

Abdominotrans-sphincteric Resection

One method of enhancing the exposure for resection of midrectal tumors is the trans-sphincteric approach.[7] The levators and the anal sphincters are serially incised and tagged with sutures for later reapproximation. This approach was initially used for local excision of benign tumors and early cancers, but Mason later described a combined abdominal and trans-sphincteric approach for radical resection of midrectal cancers. Although the method provides the necessary exposure for wide resection, it results in two intersecting suture lines when a radical resection and end-to-end anastomosis are performed. Anastomotic failure and pelvic sepsis might cause failure of the sphincteric repair, even when a protective colostomy is employed.

Abdominosacral Resection

In our opinion, only abdominosacral resection consistently provides the necessary exposure for resection of

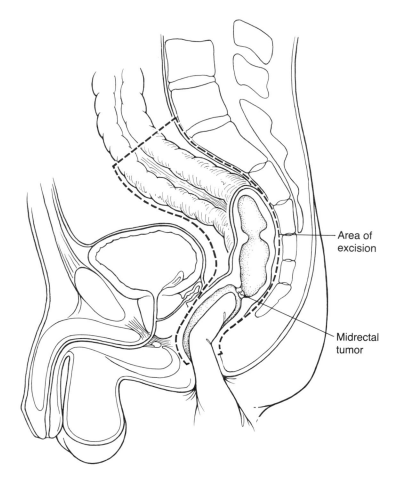

Area of
excision

Midrectal
tumor

Figure 9–47. The sagittal section shows the extent of resection, including entire mesorectum and perirectal fat within the fascia propria to the levator ani muscles. Feasibility of abdominosacral resection is assessed by digital examination.

the rectum to the levator ani muscles and anastomosis under direct vision without disturbing the anal sphincters. Removal of the coccyx allows direct view of the pelvis and radical resection in every case in which it is theoretically feasible (Fig. 9–47). This exposure is possible, despite obesity or a narrow pelvis. The rectosigmoid stump is delivered through the posterior wound with an intact fascia propria containing perirectal fat and lymphatics. The lowest portions of the lateral ligaments are divided by this posterior approach.

The distal limit of the tumor is identified by palpation or sigmoidoscopy through the rectosigmoid stump. The distal margin is measured with a ruler and no tension on the bowel. The rectum is cleared only after this distal site is determined. Denonvillier's fascia is incised, and the anterior wall of the rectum is cleared to bare longitudinal muscle. The entire rectal mesentery is swept upward from the levators posteriorly and included in the specimen. In this way, the widest-possible clearance around the tumor is achieved.

PATIENT SELECTION

The level of the cancer is initially determined by sigmoidoscopy in the knee-chest position. The distance is measured from the anal verge to the lowest gross extension of the tumor. Patients with lesions 5 to 10 cm from the anal verge are candidates for abdominosacral resection. Lesions above these limits are treated by anterior resection. Lesions below the midrectal level are treated by abdominoperineal resection. Choice of operation according to sigmoidoscopic measurement has certain limitations, including variations in mobility of the tumor and length of the anal canal. A patient with a tumor that prolapses into the lower rectum or a patient with a short anal canal may be a suitable candidate for sphincter-saving resection, despite a low measurement on sigmoidoscopy.

The feasibility of abdominosacral resection may be assessed most accurately by digital examination (see Fig. 9–47). The lower limit of the operation is at or just below the puborectalis sling. The limiting distance is actually the distance from the puborectalis to the point of attachment of the tumor. This distance can be accurately estimated by palpating the tumor while hooking the proximal interphalangeal joint on the puborectalis. The intraluminal extension of an exophytic tumor suitable for sphincter preservation may actually reach the top of the anal canal. The examining finger may initially encounter the tumor at the top of the anal canal, but the finger can then slide into a sulcus between the tumor and the rectal wall. If this attachment lies 2 to 3 cm above the puborectalis on digital examination, a 3-cm or wider margin is usually obtainable after mobilization.

Candidates for abdominosacral resection are explored in the lateral position. In about 20% of cases of midrectal cancers, after the rectum is mobilized, the exposure is adequate to complete the resection and anastomosis entirely through the abdominal approach. Only rarely has abdominosacral resection been abandoned in favor of abdominoperineal resection because an adequate distal margin could not be obtained. Preoperative assessment predicts quite accurately whether a sphincter-saving operation is possible. Anterior resection or abdominoperineal resection may be performed without repositioning and redraping the patient.

RESULTS OF TREATMENT

Abdominosacral resection has been evaluated over the past 25 years in the treatment of 926 consecutive patients with primary adenocarcinoma of the rectum. The operation was anterior resection in 456, abdominosacral resection in 272, and abdominoperineal resection in 195. Three high-risk elderly patients had local excision only.

Mortality and Morbidity

The risk of abdominosacral resection is comparable to the risks of anterior resection and abdominoperineal resection. The mortality rates were 2.4% after anterior resection, 1.5% after abdominosacral resection, and 1.5% after abdominoperineal resection. Morbidity rates following each of the three operations were also comparable with the exception of anastomotic complications.

Anastomotic leaks were detected in 3.8% of the 728 patients undergoing anterior resection or abdominosacral resection. There were five leaks after 456 anterior resections (1.1%) and 23 after 272 abdominosacral resections (8.5%). The anastomotic leak rate has im-

proved from 12% of the first 100 patients to 3.5% currently.

Continence

Sphincter function following abdominosacral resection is normal in every case. As in all low rectal resections, the loss of the rectosigmoid reservoir results in frequent small stools in the early postoperative period. However, the ultimate functional results of abdominosacral resection are indistinguishable from those of anterior resection.

Long-Term Survival

The crude 5-year survival rate for 553 patients after curative operations done from 1966 to 1981 was 63.8%. The individual 5-year survival rates were 67.8% for anterior resection, 67.9% for abdominosacral resection, and 51.4% for abdominoperineal resection (Table 9–1). The long-term survival rate for abdominosacral resection was comparable to that for anterior resection and better than that for abdominoperineal resection. For all stages of tumor, the survival rate for abdominosacral resection paralleled that for anterior resection.

Pelvic recurrence rate was 10.7% after anterior resection, 12.8% after abdominosacral resection, and 12.5% after abdominoperineal resection (Table 9–2). Pelvic recurrence rate was 3.6% for Dukes A lesions, 9.4% for Dukes B lesions, and 22.3% for Dukes C lesions. There was no increase in pelvic recurrence rate in patients undergoing sphincter-saving operation. Pelvic recurrence rate like survival rate was determined by the stage of disease and not by the operation performed.

OPERATIVE TECHNIQUE

Position

The patient is placed on his right side with his back at the edge of the operating table (Fig. 9–48). The rectum is irrigated with normal saline until clear. The incisions are marked (Fig. 9–49), the skin is prepared, and the patient is draped to provide simultaneous access to the abdominal and posterior wounds. Placement of a pillow between the knees of the patient allows access to the anus for digital evaluation of the anastomosis or insertion of a stapler.

This approach facilitates mobilization and delivery of the rectosigmoid stump and proximal colon through the posterior wound and obviates the need for turning

Table 9–1. CRUDE FIVE-YEAR SURVIVAL AFTER 553 CURATIVE RESECTIONS FOR RECTAL CANCER (1966 TO 1981)

Operation	Dukes Classification	No. of Patients	Five-Year Survivors	Percentage Five-Year Survivors
Anterior resection (AR)	A	82	75	91.4*
	B	108	70	64.8
	C	71	32	45.0
	All	261	177	67.8†
Abdominosacral resection (ASR)	A	49	42	85.7
	B	56	42	75.0‡
	C	51	22	43.1
	All	156	106	67.9†
Abdominoperineal resection (APR)	A	35	27	77.1*
	B	48	25	52.1‡
	C	53	18	33.9
	All	136	70	51.4†

*Dukes A: APR vs. AR p < .03.
†Overall: APR vs. AR p < .001.
  APR vs. ASR p < .004.
‡Dukes B: APR vs. ASR p < .015.

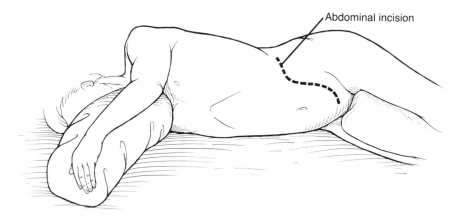

Figure 9–48. The patient is placed in the right lateral decubitus position with the right buttock and scapula at the edge of the table. The abdominal incision is marked.

Table 9–2. PELVIC RECURRENCES AFTER 553 CURATIVE RESECTIONS FOR RECTAL CANCER (1966 TO 1981)

Operation	Dukes Classification	No. of Patients	Pelvic Recurrences	Percentage of Pelvic Recurrences
Anterior resection	A	82	2	2.4
	B	108	12	11.1
	C	71	14	19.7
	All	261	28	10.7
Abdominosacral resection	A	49	3	6.1
	B	56	4	7.1
	C	51	13	25.4
	All	156	20	12.8
Abdominoperineal resection	A	35	1	2.9
	B	48	4	8.3
	C	53	12	22.6
	All	136	17	12.5

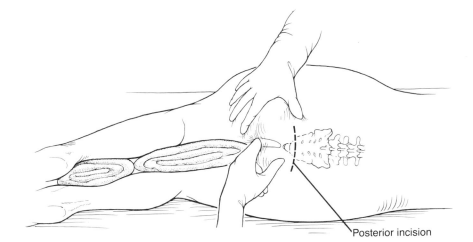

Figure 9–49. The posterior incision is marked at the sacrococcygeal joint.

Posterior incision

and redraping the patient. The surgeon can return to the abdomen to mobilize the proximal colon further to avoid tension on the colorectal anastomosis, or to perform a protective colostomy. The advantages of abdominosacral resection in the lateral position are analogous to the advantages of synchronous abdominoperineal resection in the Lloyd-Davies position.

Abdominal Phase

The abdomen is opened through an oblique incision starting between the left costal margin and the iliac crest, running parallel to the inguinal ligament, and curving across the rectus abdominis muscles above the pubis. The incision is carried through all layers of the abdominal wall. The oblique incision affords excellent exposure of the splenic flexure and the pelvic organs. After the abdomen is thoroughly explored, the small bowel is excluded from the operative field by laparotomy pads. Exposure is facilitated by means of a mechanical retractor with multiple adjustable arms.

The splenic flexure is mobilized by sharp division of its lateral peritoneal attachments. Gerota's fascia is identified, because the dissection will be carried distally in this plane between the retroperitoneum and the mesocolon. Injury to the spleen is avoided by maintaining upward traction on omentum as the colon is freed by sharp dissection in the avascular embryonic fusion plane. Freeing of the omentum is carried far enough to the right to allow the transverse colon to rotate on the middle colic artery.

The left colon is drawn downward to the patient's right, and its lateral peritoneal attachments are divided. The peritoneal incision is carried down the lumbar gutter into the pelvis. Mobilization of the colon continues in the retroperitoneal plane established on Gerota's fascia. The left gonadal vessels and ureter are identified. As the superior hemorrhoidal vessels come into

view, the sympathetic nerve plexus is identified. These nerves lie outside the fascia propria of the rectum and bear no relationship to the lymphovascular pedicle. Preservation of these nerves maintains normal ejaculation. More important, it leads to the proper plane for posterior mobilization of the rectum without troublesome bleeding from presacral veins.

The colon is drawn upward to the patient's left, and the right leaf of the sigmoid mesentery is incised at its base. The right ureter is identified and swept laterally.

The sigmoid mesentery containing the superior hemorrhoidal vessels and lymphatics is now easily swept upward from the aorta. This lymphovascular pedicle is isolated, clamped, divided, and suture-ligated, usually at the level of the origin of the left colic artery (Fig. 9–50).

Mobilization of the proximal colon should be sufficient to allow it to lie loosely in the pelvis, conforming to the curve of the sacrum after colorectal anastomosis. The left colic artery may be divided at its origin when additional length is necessary, because the left colon is often tethered by this vessel. In that case, the marginal artery must be preserved, because the blood supply to the colon stump is now based on the middle colic artery. The mesosigmoid colon is divided to the site selected for the proximal margin. Cope-DeMartel clamps are applied at this site, and the colon is divided.

The rectum is mobilized from the hollow of the sacrum by blunt dissection in the loose areolar plane on the fascia propria of the rectum to the tip of the coccyx. This virtually bloodless plane preserves the previously identified sympathetic nerves (see Fig. 9–50). A deeper plane may be entered if the tumor is adherent, but the risk of presacral vein bleeding is thereby incurred.

The peritoneal incisions at the base of the mesosigmoid colon are continued anteriorly to meet in the cul-de-sac, and the anterior wall of the rectum is freed on Denonvilliers' fascia to the level of the seminal vesicles

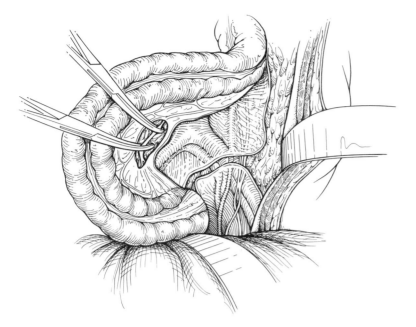

Figure 9–50. The colon is mobilized, and the superior hemorrhoidal vessels are divided and ligated. The avascular plane on fascia propria of rectum is entered.

or upper vagina. This dissection can be continued bluntly on the posterior wall of the prostate or vagina.

When the anterior and posterior dissections are completed, the lateral ligaments of the rectum containing the middle hemorrhoidal vessels are identified. The left lateral ligament is divided first (Fig. 9–51). The broad band of tissue that is the lateral ligament is dissected as far distally as possible, encircled, clamped near the pelvic sidewall, divided, and ligated. Upward displacement of the rectum now exposes the right lateral ligament, which is also encircled, divided, and ligated.

The rectum has now been mobilized as completely as possible. The seminal vesicles or upper vagina is visible. The tip of the coccyx, the levator ani muscle diaphragm, and the puborectalis sling are palpable. If mobilization provides sufficient length to permit anterior resection, the operation is completed through the abdomen. For many midrectal cancers, the posterior exposure is necessary. Before the posterior incision is made, the pelvis is irrigated with saline and meticulous hemostasis is achieved. Oozing may be controlled by a pelvic pack. Complete hemostasis is facilitated after the rectum is delivered from the pelvis through the posterior wound.

Posterior Phase

A transverse incision is made over the sacrococcygeal joint and deepened to the gluteus maximus muscles and the sacrum (Fig. 9–52). Depression of the tip of the coccyx facilitates its disarticulation and excision.

Waldeyer's fascia is incised, and the retrorectal space is entered (Fig. 9–53). Brisk bleeding from presacral vessels is controlled by electrocautery.

The posterior wound is enlarged to admit four fingers by splitting the levators in the direction of their fibers (Fig. 9–54). A transverse incision is suitable, because it may be lengthened without limitation by the sacrum or the anus. If necessary, the gluteal muscles may be split for further exposure. Part of the sacrum may be excised with a rongeur. The sacrotuberous ligament serves as a craniad limit protecting the sciatic nerve.

The rectosigmoid stump is now delivered through the posterior wound by using the DeMartel clamp as a handle (Fig. 9–55). The rectosigmoid stump is most safely delivered by pushing through the abdomen and applying gentle traction from the posterior wound. Firm traction on the levator ani muscles enhances exposure of the pelvis. The lower rectum can now be further mobilized for wide lateral and distal clearance.

The lowermost portions of the lateral ligaments that remain are divided at the pelvic sidewalls (Fig. 9–56). The anterior surface of the rectum can be freed from the prostate or the lower vaginal wall. The posterior surface of the rectum is dissected to the puborectalis sling.

The extent of the tumor is determined, and the distal margin of at least 3 cm is measured with a ruler (see Fig. 9–56). The precise limits of small tumors may be determined by means of sigmoidoscopy through the rectosigmoid stump.

The distal margin is cleared of fat circumferentially to bare the longitudinal muscle. A right-angle renal pedicle clamp is applied at this site.

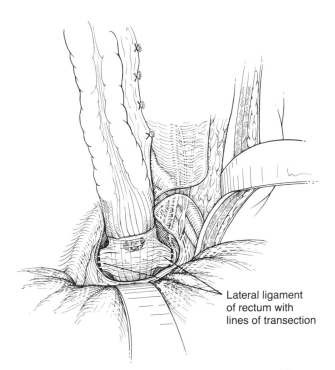

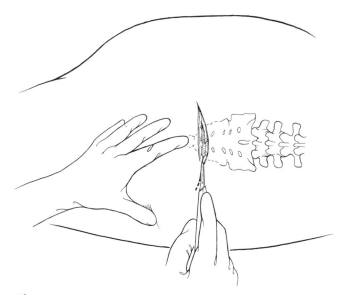

Figure 9–51. The left lateral ligament containing the middle hemorrhoidal vessels is encircled, clamped, divided, and ligated.

Lateral ligament of rectum with lines of transection

Figure 9–52. A posterior transverse incision is made at the sacrococcygeal joint.

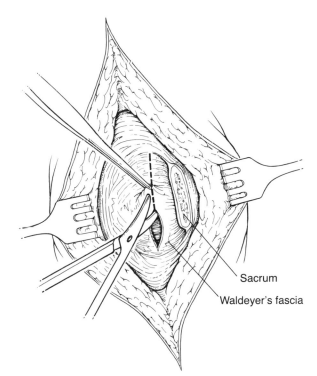

Sacrum

Waldeyer's fascia

Figure 9–53. The coccyx has been disarticulated with a knife and excised. Waldeyer's fascia is incised, and the retrorectal space is entered.

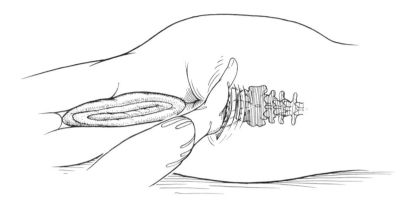

Figure 9–54. The wound is enlarged by blunt dissection, splitting the levators in the direction of their fibers.

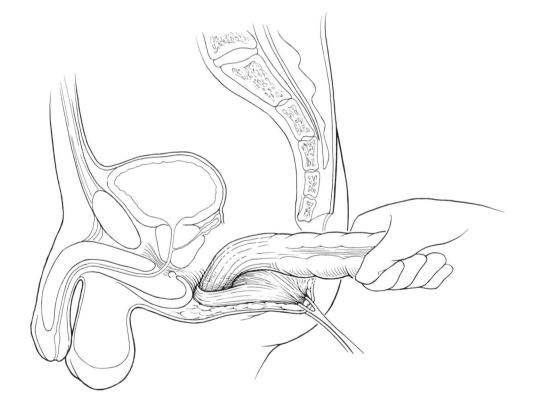

Figure 9–55. The specimen is delivered posteriorly.

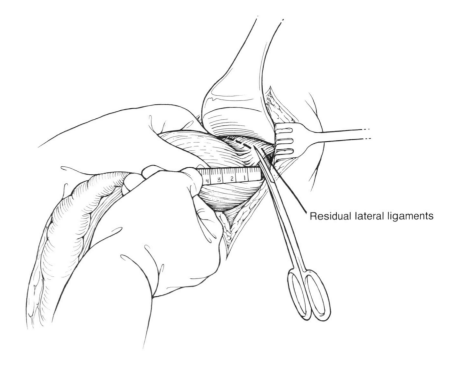

Residual lateral ligaments

Figure 9–56. Additional dissection is done to clear the pelvis completely to the levators. The lowermost portions of the lateral ligaments are divided. The extent of the tumor is determined, and a distal margin of at least 3 cm is measured without tension. The rectum is cleared at this site and a right-angle bowel clamp is applied.

Stapled Anastomosis

The end-to-end coloanal anastomosis may be facilitated by the use of a circular stapler. One of the technical difficulties associated with a stapled coloanal anastomosis is a size discrepancy between the rectal stump and the proximal colon. The rectum is usually larger in diameter than the proximal colon, making inclusion of the entire circumference of the rectum in the pursestring suture difficult. This problem may be obviated by routinely extending the distal resection to the puborectalis muscle. The rectum narrows at this point to pass through the puborectalis muscle, and the chance for an incomplete doughnut is minimized. This contributes to the safety of the anastomosis and enhances the distal margin. The largest-diameter stapler should be used in every case. If the proximal colon is narrow and thick-walled, further resection may allow use of a larger stapler head.

As the rectum is incised, a full-thickness suture of 0-0 polypropylene is inserted (Fig. 9–57). The incision is enlarged and the suturing continued circumferentially until the specimen is amputated and the pursestring is completed. The suturing may be an over-and-over whipstitch, as shown, which permits close spacing of stitches. An alternative method is to employ a true pursestring suture, which is somewhat easier to tie snugly around the shaft of the stapler.

A pursestring is placed in the proximal colon and tied over the anvil. The patient is in the lateral position, and the stapler is easily inserted through the anus,

thereby allowing the surgeon to pass the instrument and to observe its appearance at the anorectal stump. The anorectal pursestring suture is tied around the shaft of the stapler (Fig. 9–58). The distal suture may be inspected easily for inclusion of the entire circumference of rectum. The proximal bowel is guided down to the pelvis by the abdominal route. The stapled anastomosis is completed under direct vision through the posterior wound.

Sutured Anastomosis

The proximal colonic stump is delivered, care being taken to avoid axial rotation of the bowel. The latch of the DeMartel clamp or the marking stitch is a convenient guide for maintaining proper orientation of the colon. An extra 3 to 4 cm of proximal colon is pulled through posteriorly as illustrated. This allows the suturing to be done without hindrance by the DeMartel clamp.

A series of interrupted Cushing stitches of 4-0 silk are placed. After all the sutures have been placed, they are tied and cut; the first and last are retained to mark the corners of the anastomosis.

The adjoining walls of the colon and rectum are incised. The cut edges should show brisk bleeding that indicates a good blood supply. The inner row of sutures is started at the center of the anastomosis by using a double-armed 4-0 chromic catgut or Dexon suture. This suture is tied and run in both directions as a full-

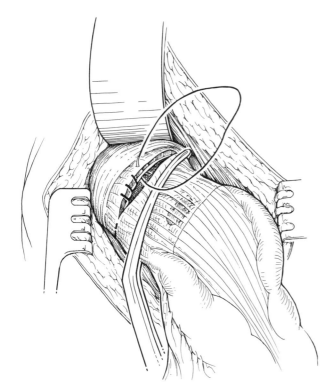

Figure 9–57. A distal pursestring polypropylene suture is inserted for the stapled anastomosis.

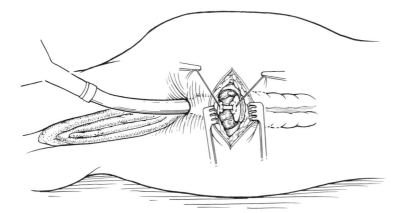

Figure 9–58. The distal pursestring suture is tied around the shaft of the stapler. The anvil in the proximal bowel is guided down to the pelvis for completion of the stapled anastomosis.

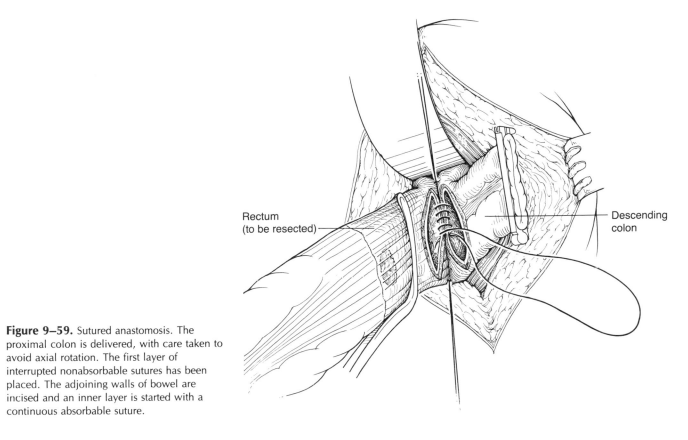

Rectum
(to be resected)

Descending
colon

Figure 9–59. Sutured anastomosis. The proximal colon is delivered, with care taken to avoid axial rotation. The first layer of interrupted nonabsorbable sutures has been placed. The adjoining walls of bowel are incised and an inner layer is started with a continuous absorbable suture.

thickness, loosely locked stitch (Fig. 9–59). The remaining wall of the rectum is divided and the specimen is removed. Excess proximal colon contained within the DeMartel clamp is excised.

The catgut suture is brought out at the corners of the anastomosis, and the inner layer is completed as a continuous Connell suture. The outer layer is completed using interrupted Cushing sutures of 4-0 silk.

COMPLICATIONS

The most significant complications associated with abdominosacral resection are massive presacral venous hemorrhage, ureteral injury, and anastomotic leakage. The first two complications are avoidable, and the third should be infrequent. These complications are by no means limited to abdominosacral resection but are common to all radical sphincter-saving operations for cancer of the rectum. Abdominosacral resection in the lateral position requires reorientation in the surgeon's view of anatomic structures, but dissection in well-defined anatomic planes minimizes these problems. A mechanical retractor with multiple arms avoids the problem of placing assistants and frees both of the surgeon's and assistants' hands. Mobilization of the left colon and rectum in the proper plane lifts these

structures and their lymphovascular pedicles from the retroperitoneum and leaves the gonadal vessels, ureters, sympathetic nerves, and presacral veins undisturbed.

Ureteral Injury

Ureteral injury may occur proximally during division of the superior hemorrhoidal lymphovascular pedicle or distally during mobilization of the rectum and division of the lateral ligaments. If dissection is started at the splenic flexure, identification of Gerota's fascia establishes the proper retroperitoneal plane superficial to the left gonadal vessels and left ureter. Following this same plane displaces the ureter laterally throughout its length. At the pelvic brim, identification of the ureter may be confirmed medial to the gonadal vessels and across the iliac artery at its bifurcation. After incision of the peritoneum at the pelvic brim, the ureters may be swept laterally by blunt dissection. Anterior mobilization of the rectum should begin in the midline to avoid injury of the distal ureter. After the anterior and posterior dissection of the rectum is completed, lateral ligaments of the rectum are encircled and divided deep within the pelvis, because the ureters lie at a higher level. Position of both ureters should be reconfirmed before the superior hemorrhoidal pedicle or the lateral ligaments are clamped and divided.

If the ureter is injured, direct repair by using fine interrupted absorbable sutures over a temporary stent is the simplest approach. If the ureter is transected distally, it may be reimplanted via an oblique tunnel through the bladder wall and sutured to the bladder mucosa from within. Finally, if a long segment is missing, replacement by ileal interposition is more complex but equally effective.

Massive Pelvic Bleeding

Troublesome hemorrhage may occur from injury to presacral veins or hypogastric veins in the pelvic sidewalls. To mobilize the rectum, dissection should be done on the fascia propria, which envelops the lymphovascular pedicle. Preservation of the sympathetic nerve plexus on the aortic bifurcation and the two hypogastric nerves that run on either side of the rectum will lead to this bloodless plane. A deeper plane may be entered if the tumor is adherent. Bleeding from presacral veins should be controllable by suture ligature or temporary packing. Electrocautery is usually ineffective for control of these veins and may result in increased bleeding.

Bleeding from the pelvic sidewalls from the hypogastric vessels is less common, but it may occur during isolation and division of the lateral ligaments. Whenever possible, the lateral ligaments should be clamped and divided and the middle hemorrhoidal vessels ligated under direct vision. When exposure is limited by obesity or a narrow pelvis, the lateral ligaments may be divided blindly or avulsed by sweeping the hand along the pelvic sidewall. Bleeding from such injury to the hypogastric vessels may be massive, and exposure limited. The best policy is temporary control by packing and definitive hemostasis after posterior delivery of the rectum permits visualization of the pelvis.

Anastomotic Leak

The precautions observed to minimize the incidence of anastomotic leakage have been described in the discussion of operative technique, but certain points should be emphasized. Careful dissection to minimize tissue damage, adequate mobilization to avoid tension, adequate blood supply, and precise stapled or sutured anastomosis are essential.

The pelvic and sacral wounds are thoroughly irrigated with saline, and hemostasis is secured. The omentum is delivered through the posterior incision and wrapped around the anastomosis when possible.

The position of the omentum may be maintained by attaching it to the levator ani with several sutures.

No attempt is made to close the defect in the pelvic peritoneum. Loops of small bowel will fill the pelvic dead space, and fluid accumulating in the pelvis can drain into the peritoneal cavity. As a precaution, a soft closed suction drain of silicone rubber may be left in the pelvis. Drainage volumes of 100 to 250 ml are not unusual in the first 48 hours. The drain is removed as soon as possible.

Protective Colostomy

A proximal colostomy is constructed if there is any doubt about the integrity of the anastomosis. Current practice is a lateral transverse colostomy brought through a wide defect in the abdominal wall and a small skin aperture.[2] This practice allows the colon to rise to the skin level, where a small lateral opening is sutured to the skin only. Adequate mechanical bowel preparation and a satisfactory anastomosis make complete diversion unnecessary. For the first 5 to 9 days, intraluminal contents consist of only liquid and gas. A lateral opening, which bleeds off liquid and gas, prevents distention and offers sufficient protection. In fact, when bowel function returns, almost all stool is discharged through this lateral stoma. If the anastomosis is sound, the colostomy may easily be closed in several weeks.

Treatment of Anastomotic Leak

Anastomotic leaks may be clinically undetectable or may produce peritonitis and sepsis. Early in the series, four patients with significant leaks in unprotected anastomoses required emergency diverting colostomy for peritonitis. More commonly, the leaks (19 of 23) after abdominosacral resection resulted in well-controlled posterior fistulas. The posterior wound in abdominosacral resection undoubtedly increased the detection rate for small leaks because of the easy egress of fecal matter by this route. Nonetheless, the anastomosis constructed after abdominosacral resection is lower than that established after anterior resection and is therefore inherently more tenuous. Moreover, the close proximity of the posterior wound to the anastomotic suture line may actually predispose to leakage. For this reason, the omentum is interposed between the anastomosis and the posterior wound whenever possible.

All fistulas healed after temporary diversion of the fecal stream. In two instances, small fistulas that were detected after hospital discharge (2 weeks or more postoperatively) healed spontaneously without colostomy. These late fistulas can be safely managed by bowel rest with parenteral nutrition or low-residue enteral diets.

SUMMARY

Abdominosacral resection is the most reliable radical sphincter-saving operation for midrectal cancers that are too low for anterior resection. The posterior incision provides maximum exposure for wide resection of the tumor, a measured distal margin, and an accurate anastomosis. The procedure can be carried out consistently to the pelvic floor without disrupting the anal sphincters and their innervation. Sphincter function is consistently preserved. The mortality rate is no higher than for other radical rectal resections. Morbidity can be limited by the selective use of protective colostomy. The recent use of the end-to-end circular stapler and mechanical retractors have improved the ease and safety of the operation. The combined abdominal and posterior approach allows mobilization of the rectum to the levators in every case, and resection is limited only by distance of the tumor from the sphincter, not by poor exposure due to obesity or a narrow pelvis. In the treatment of 926 consecutive patients with rectal cancer, sphincter-saving resection was possible in 78%. In our experience, abdominosacral resection extends the range of sphincter-saving resection beyond that which is possible by the abdominal approach alone with no compromise in safety and no increased risk of local recurrence or death from cancer.

REFERENCES

1. Beart RW Jr, Kelly KA. Randomized prospective evaluation of the EEA stapler for colorectal anastomoses. Am J Surg 1981;141:143–147.
2. Eng K, Localio SA. Simplified complementary transverse colostomy for low colorectal anastomosis. Surg Gynecol Obstet 1981;153:734–735.
3. Goligher JC. Recent trends in the practice of sphincter-saving excision for carcinoma of the rectum. In: Jordan GL Jr, ed. Advances in Surgery. Chicago: Year Book, 1979, pp 15–22.
4. Goligher JC. Use of circular stapling gun with perianal insertion of anorectal purse-string suture for construction of very low colorectal or colo-anal anastomoses. Br J Surg 1979;66:501–504.
5. Knight CD, Griffen FD. An improved technique for low anterior resection of the rectum using the EEA stapler. Surgery 1980;88:710–714.
6. Localio SA, Eng K, Coppa GF. Abdominosacral resection for midrectal cancer: A fifteen year experience. Ann Surg 1983;198:320–324.
7. Mason AY. Transsphincteric approach to rectal lesions. Surg Ann 1977;9:171–174.
8. Parks AG. Transanal technique in low rectal anastomosis. Proc R Soc Med 1972;65:975–976.

Tumors of the Anal Canal

Jerome J. DeCosse

Although operations for anal canal tumors and perianal tumors are the primary subject matter of this chapter, the proximity of the anus to other structures justifies consideration of approaches to tumors behind the anus and rectum in the precoccygeal and distal presacral space and to some small tumors in the distal rectum.

Understanding the anatomy of the anal canal is the key to understanding and obtaining operative access to the kinds of tumors that arise on, within, and deep into the structures of the anal area.

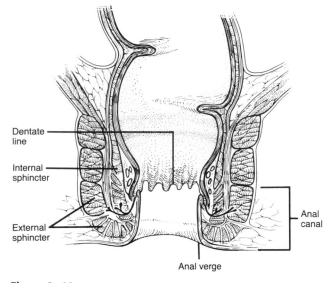

Figure 9–60. Anatomic points of reference for localization of and access to anal and perianal tumors.

ANATOMIC LANDMARKS

Several anatomic points provide a background for localization and access (Fig. 9–60). The dentate line is readily identified by viewing the crypts and columns of Morgagni. The mucosa at the dentate line is a transitional epithelium extending about 5 mm distally and up to 20 mm proximally. This narrow band, the site of embryologic fusion of the proctodeum with the hindgut, may be the site of cloacogenic cancers. Above, or cephalad, is the columnar epithelium of the rectum, and below, or caudad, is hairless, modified squamous epithelium that extends distally for several centimeters to the anal verge. This surface constitutes the anal margin. Beyond the anal verge resides the hair-bearing skin of the perineum and the buttock. Definitions of the distal or caudad boundary of the perianal area, also called the pecten, vary; some definitions include the skin of the adjacent buttock beyond the anal verge.

The anal canal is conical and, on average, about 3 cm long; this length is worth remembering during proctosigmoidoscopy, because it must be subtracted in calculation of the distance of a rectal mass from the dentate line. The anal canal may be longer in muscular men, whereas the dentate line may be visible in a senescent person with a patulous anus. Small external skin tags, which might be labeled external hemorrhoids, are so frequent in older people as to merit being considered normal.

PREOPERATIVE PREPARATION

Before anal and distal rectal tumors other than retrorectal tumors are operated on, a biopsy specimen

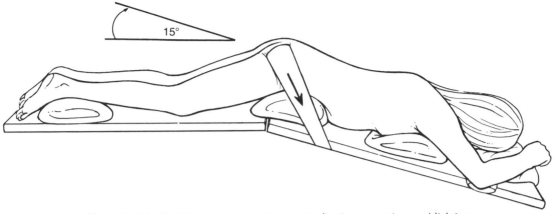

Figure 9–61. The Kraske position optimizes visualization, retraction, and lighting.

should always be obtained and histopathology confirmed.

The patient merits a thorough mechanical bowel preparation and, in my opinion, both oral preoperative antibiotics and perioperative intravenous, broad-spectrum, antibiotic coverage. In addition, intraluminal rectal povidone-iodine may be useful. Rare instances of devastating necrotizing infection might have been avoided by more intensive preparation.

This chapter does not address office surgery other than biopsy. The procedures described are best performed in an ambulatory surgery setting or hospital environment with regional or general anesthesia and with excellent lighting. Headlamps are often useful.

PATIENT POSITIONING AND ANESTHESIA

Flexibility in positioning the patient and in choosing anesthesia are important elements of safe and successful anal surgery. For anterior and many lateral lesions of the anus and distal rectum and for retrorectal surgery, the prone, hip-flexed, knee-chest (Kraske) position optimizes visualization, retraction, and lighting (Fig. 9–61). Hip flexion need not exceed 15 to 20 degrees. Padding should be placed below the pelvis to support hip flexion, below the chest to ease breathing, and below the feet to reduce pressure. The buttocks should be retracted laterally by taping to the operative table.

Posterior anal and distal rectal tumors may require the lithotomy position, whereas the left lateral Sims' position may be appropriate for left-sided or anterior lesions. Although the prone-flexed position has notable advantages, positioning and anesthesia should be appropriate for the patient and the lesion.

The prone position lends itself to regional anesthesia.

If general anesthesia is used, endotracheal intubation is essential. Spinal or caudal block, supplemented by mild sedation, provides a comfortable setting to both patient and surgeon for most anal surgery.

Given meticulous preparation, anal and rectal incisions can be closed primarily with absorbable sutures, and oral nutrition can promptly be resumed. Prolonged postoperative restriction of defecation by starvation and constipating agents is cruel and unnecessary. Primary closure of vertical incisions in the anal canal prevents development of a guttering defect that may lead to partial anal incontinence.

OVERVIEW OF OPERATIVE MANAGEMENT

The aim of modern anal and rectal tumor surgery is to achieve a cure while preserving gut integrity and function. As a result, the initial (and usually only) operation may be a conservative one for which prediction of success depends on both operative findings and subsequent histopathologic scrutiny. Patients who may need a second, more extensive operation must be informed that subsequent radical surgery may be necessary and must participate in and accept the surgeon's recommendations before the initial intervention takes place.

The anal sphincters can be divided, preferably posteriorly; the surgeon can mark individual components during the course of division and then approximate them, preserving continence. However, in patients with distal rectal tumors who may later require an abdominoperineal resection, presacral tissue planes may be divided to expose the presacral space posterior to the investing fascia of the rectum. A few patients have experienced perineal recurrence after local rectal surgery was followed by radical resection. Although there is no proof of harm, it is worthwhile to anticipate a possibility of more extensive secondary surgery and avoid violation of these critical tissue planes. Thus, for cases in which it is possible, intraluminal rectal surgery may be preferable.

TUMORS OF THE ANAL AREA

We now address tumors that occur in the anal margin, the perianal skin from just below the dentate line to the anal verge.

By far the most frequent malignant tumor of this area is epidermoid carcinoma.[1] This tumor may appear as a small, hard, perianal nodule or as an ulcerated or exophytic mass. Frequently, an unsuspected epidermoid carcinoma may be found in an external hemorrhoid, venereal wart, or biopsy specimen from an anal fissure or fistula; hence, tissues from these operative procedures should be submitted for microscopic examination. The differential diagnosis includes leukoplakia, condyloma acuminata, and chronic skin disorders.

Epidermoid carcinoma of the anal margin commonly occurs against a background of anal inflammatory disease. The incidence of epidermoid carcinoma at this site may be increasing in persons at risk for acquired immunodeficiency syndrome (AIDS). Patients with this tumor should be asked about other risk factors for AIDS, and a request for a human immunodeficiency virus (HIV) test may be in order. Anal epidermoid cancer also has a strong association with the human papillomavirus (HPV).[2]

Most epidermoid tumors of the anal margin are small. Their superficiality is highlighted by free mobility and lack of infiltration into underlying surrounding structures.

Operative excision with a margin and with primary closure can be performed easily for most small, mobile anal margin tumors, and a cure rate in excess of 90% can be anticipated. Primary closure with absorbable sutures should be accomplished in the vertical plane of the anal canal. Small tumors can probably be handled with equal effectiveness by radiotherapy, but the simplicity and ease of surgery favor operation.

Several rare tumors may be found within the perianal area.[3, 4] Basal cell carcinomas have a typical "rodent ulcer" configuration with a raised, pearly edge and central ulceration. Because histologic findings show compact sheets of basophilic cells, this tumor must be differentiated from basaloid cancer of the anal canal. Basal cell carcinoma rarely invades or metastasizes. The mobile tumors can almost always be managed effectively by wide local excision.

Bowen's disease is an intraepithelial carcinoma with distinctive, vacuolated, hyperchromatic nuclei called Bowenoid cells. The tumor appears as a discrete, reddish, plaquelike area with scaly eczematoid features. Ulceration suggests invasive cancer. Bowen's disease is often associated with internal cancer and may be found more frequently among patients who are HIV-positive. Treatment of perianal Bowen's disease is by wide local excision with frozen section of margins. Closure of the wound may require a skin graft or rotation flaps.

Like Paget's disease of the breast, perianal Paget's disease appears as a pale, gray, rusty, plaquelike lesion that seems inflamed and indurated. Pruritus may be severe. An underlying mass may or may not be palpable. Skin biopsy shows characteristic mucin-containing intraepithelial cells that stain positively with aldehyde-fuchsin and with Alcian blue. In the absence of an underlying mass, local excision suffices. An underlying mass indicates the presence of infiltrating cancer: If the tumor is more than 2 cm in diameter, an abdominoperineal resection should be considered.

Malignant melanoma also may occur in the anal canal or even in the last few centimeters of the rectum. The tumor may appear as a small, brownish-black, grapelike growth or as a large ulcerated mass. Only about one half of anorectal melanomas have visible pigmentation, and some are amelanotic on electron microscopy. Malignant melanoma of the perianal area, no matter how superficial, requires an abdominoperineal resection in a potentially curable patient.

Soft tissue tumors, particularly leiomyoma and leiomyosarcoma, also can be found in the perianal and perirectal tissues. These smooth muscle tumors may be small, superficial, rubbery, and mobile, or they may be large, deep, poorly outlined, and obviously infiltrating. Assessment of life-threatening potential depends more on clinical features than on histopathologic findings. Smooth muscle tumors cannot be treated effectively by superficial enucleation; they require more aggressive management.

Operative Management of Superficial Tumors of the Perianal Area

Small superficial tumors in the perianal area that demonstrate easy mobility may be excised with a 1-cm margin and closed primarily with absorbable suture. The superficial portion of the external sphincter is exceptionally close, and it is virtually impossible to perform a full-thickness excision without removing part of the external sphincter. No harm is done. However, vertical strips of anoderm must be preserved to ensure healing. Circumferential excision or destruction of the anoderm results in anal stenosis.

Larger, mobile, cutaneous tumors may require interposition of skin. In general, a skin graft should be avoided because it entails substantial problems of postoperative care. If a skin graft is necessary, the patient, purged preoperatively, should be maintained postoperatively on a no-residue intake and constipating agents, such as codeine derivatives, to prevent bowel movements for 4 to 6 days.

A rotation flap, sliding advancement flap, or V-Y triangular flap is preferred (Fig. 9–62). Rotation flaps should originate from the buttock and should not be lifted from the thin, midline intergluteal skin. The advancement flap and the V-Y triangular flap gain mobility by being detached from surrounding skin. Preservation of the bulk of subcutaneous attachment maintains both vascularity and sensation, the latter being important in the anal canal for continence. If necessary, flaps can be approximated to the dentate line with absorbable sutures.

Histopathologic findings must always be obtained and adequate lateral and deep margins ensured. The postoperative patient can promptly resume functional activity.

Initial conservative treatment is probably inappropriate if the diameter of the anal margin tumor exceeds 5 cm or if tethering to the sphincteric musculature is evident. Prognosis correlates with depth of invasion. Larger or fixed tumors, or the presence of positive microscopic margins after conservative management, warrant additional treatment. Although conventional secondary management is an abdominal perineal resection, combined radiotherapy and chemotherapy are assuming an increasingly prominent role.

In the absence of skin grafts, limited surgery in the anal margin is seldom associated with postoperative complications. Skin necrosis or wound dehiscence may require a prolonged period of Sitz baths before secondary healing is achieved. Secondary healing can result in a guttering defect and minor anal incontinence.

Operative Management of Deep Tumors of the Perianal Area

Localized smooth muscle tumors are typically embedded in the sphincteric musculature. Such tumors call for an extensive local excision, which may require removal of portions of the sphincteric apparatus. The surgeon must decide whether the circumstances warrant a limited local effort or require an abdominal perineal resection for cure. If a rectal or perianal leiomyosarcoma is small and histologically low-grade, a wide, local excision with supplemental radiotherapy may be appropriate.[5]

Depending on location and size, a sphincterotomy can provide access to the tumor and allow excision with a margin. Excision also can be accomplished through a transanal cutaneous approach. A sphincterotomy is best performed in the posterior midline, but local excision may be accomplished in any part of the circumference of the anal canal if the musculature is accurately identified and reconstructed. The basic procedure consists of accurate identification of the sphincteric musculature by means of sutures or clamps, excision of the mass with a margin, and accurate reconstruction of the sphincters with overlapping nonabsorbable sutures and primary closure of the skin. In anal repair, the conical form of the anal canal should be reconstructed, because the anal epithelium adjacent to the dentate line is necessary for control of continence.

If postoperative infection results in dehiscence of a sphincterotomy, the severity of ensuing fecal incontinence may require a sigmoid colostomy. Prolonged secondary healing and subsequent anal repair may be necessary before the colostomy can be closed.

If tumor margins are involved after deeper anal surgery is performed, an abdominoperineal resection is necessary. Although abdominoperineal resection is described in detail, special aspects related to anal tumors are considered here.

EPIDERMOID CANCER OF THE ANAL CANAL

Malignant tumors that occur in the narrow band of transitional epithelium at and adjacent to the dentate line are variously called epidermoid or squamous cancer, mucoepidermoid cancer, cloacogenic cancer, transitional cell cancer, and basaloid cancer. These histopathologic terms carry similar therapeutic and prognostic implications: All are variants of epidermoid cancer. Rare anal gland adenocarcinomas also occur in this area. These can be difficult to distinguish from poorly differentiated epidermoid cancer of the anal canal and from bulky, very distal rectal cancer.

The presenting symptoms are pain and/or bleeding. Examination in the office can be unreliable. A palpable, distal, submucosal, rectal mass can be confused with rectal cancer. Careful scrutiny, which often requires a regional or general anesthesia, shows a mucosal defect at or near the dentate line.

Staging is also difficult to accomplish in the office. Pain may preclude testing the mobility of the tumor. Tethering or fixation indicates invasion of the anal musculature and levator mechanism. Computed tomography and magnetic resonance imaging are helpful.

The treatment of epidermoid cancer of the anal canal has changed considerably during the past 10 to 15 years. At this time, the initial treatment of anal

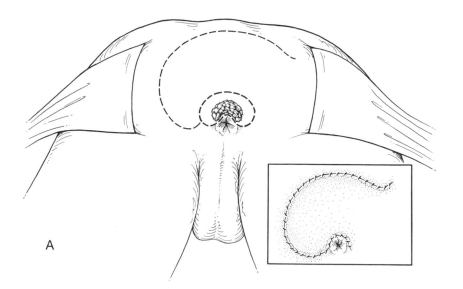

A

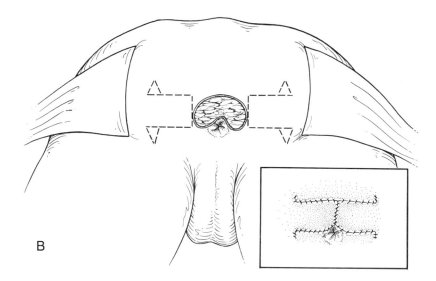

B

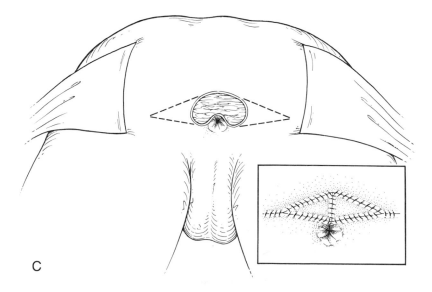

C

Figure 9–62. *A,* Rotation flap. *B,* Advancement flap. *C,* V-Y triangular flap.

canal cancer ought to be combined chemotherapy and radiotherapy while operative intervention shifts to a secondary role of staging and rescue.[6, 7]

The conventional combined treatment consists of the following: mitomycin C, 15 mg/m², as a single intravenous bolus on day one; 5-fluorouracil (5FU), 750 mg/m² per day, as a continuous intravenous infusion for 5 days; and radiotherapy as 3,000 rad divided into fractions of 200 rad overlapping the 5FU and finishing in about 3 weeks. The 5FU infusion may be repeated at that time. The 5FU is thought to have a radiosensitizing effect. Unlike chemotherapy of other tumors, the current treatment strategy is primarily induction, without a consolidation or maintenance program. Future developments in this area may well include additional chemotherapy as well as more radiotherapy.

About 4 to 6 weeks after the induction treatment is completed, the patient should be operatively staged. Although persistent tumor may be evident at outpatient examination, in general the anal canal is too irritated and tender to permit thorough outpatient examination.

Hence, patients with no apparent persistent disease are best treated by the surgeon in an ambulatory surgical setting while they are under regional or general anesthesia. It is necessary to obtain a biopsy specimen from the site of the cancer, to excise any suspicious area, and to perform one or two needle biopsies of the deeper muscular tissues. Examination provides both staging and recovery mechanisms. If examination is negative, no further treatment is needed.

Tumors that fail to respond to chemotherapy and radiotherapy conventionally require an abdominoperineal resection. If the anal canal cancer was less than 5 cm in initial diameter, the likelihood of cure with combined treatment exceeds 80%. If the tumor was more than 5 cm in diameter at initial presentation, or if there is evident persistent disease at the staging examination, an abdominoperineal resection should be considered. If biopsy at the staging examination shows only residual microscopic disease, the patient should probably have an abdominoperineal resection. However, in the setting of persistent or recurrent tumor, some oncologists now provide additional radiotherapy and chemotherapy in an effort to destroy residual disease; thus, abdominoperineal resection is becoming a backup system in case of failure of supplementary treatment. Anal canal cancer tends to recur locally before distant dissemination is found.

Operative Management of Anal Canal Cancer

In the presence of a bulky anal canal cancer, recurrence or persistence of disease following chemotherapy and radiotherapy, or complications of radiotherapy, an abdominoperineal resection may be necessary.

Although the basic technique of an abdominoperineal resection is described elsewhere, several technical points of particular utility during radical operations for anal cancer merit description. The tissues within the ischiorectal space must be widely excised. The structures of the levator ani muscles should be divided at their lateral boundaries. It should be impossible to approximate the levator musculature during closure of the perineal floor. If the tumor involves the anterior anal wall in a woman, excision of the posterior vaginal wall is appropriate. In curable patients, pelvic lymph node involvement, if any, is almost always confined to the distal sigmoid and rectum; hence, ligation of the mesenteric vessels at the aortic bifurcation is appropriate.

In principle, one should approximate primarily the skin and subcutaneous tissues of the perineal floor with nonabsorbable mattress sutures, which should remain in place for almost 2 weeks. Before closure, sump drains should be inserted into the presacral space through separate perineal stab wounds, and these should remain until drainage virtually ceases, about 8 days after operation.

One reason for primary closure is that most patients have had extensive radiotherapy. In those who have had such therapy, perineal wounds heal very slowly. An irradiated perineal wound that is packed may take many months to heal.

If subsequent radiotherapy is anticipated, the pelvic peritoneum should be reperitonealized. The uterus should be retroflexed. It also is helpful to isolate the omentum on the left gastrocolic artery for placement in the pelvis as a buffer between the site of proposed irradiation and small bowel. The omentum can be tunneled through the transverse mesocolon and brought down the left gutter.

During primary radiotherapy of anal canal cancer, both inguinal and femoral areas are included in the radiation port. The result of prophylactic groin dissection in patients with clinically positive findings for inguinal or femoral lymph nodes is exceptionally poor, and given previous therapeutic levels of radiotherapy, the value of prophylactic excision is doubtful.

The most threatening complication of abdominoperineal resection is operative or early postoperative bleeding, which usually arises from the middle hemorrhoidal veins, other branches of the hypogastric venous plexus, or the middle sacral venous plexus. These risks can be lessened by a two-team approach to abdominoperineal resection and by deliberate clamping and ligating of the middle rectal vessels.

Dissection of the presacral space ought to be performed under direct vision immediately posterior to the fascia propria of the rectum. For bleeding from the middle sacral vessels that cannot be controlled by other measures, a sterilized thumbtack has been found useful.[8]

Except perhaps in neurosurgery and cardiac surgery, there is no venous bleeding that cannot be controlled by a pack. When major pelvic bleeding occurs during the operation, the area should be packed and pressure maintained while hypovolemia is corrected and appropriate resources for lighting, exposure, and repair are marshaled. Doing otherwise is futile and dangerous. The hypogastric vein can be ligated or repaired by vascular suture. As a last resort, it may be necessary to pack the pelvis through the open perineal wound.

EDITORIAL COMMENT

Large, invasive epidermoid carcinomas of the anal canal and tumors that persist after chemotherapy and radiotherapy require abdominoperineal resection. Before one embarks on an abdominoperineal resection or while one is staging the patient, a gallium scan is useful to demonstrate occult metastases.

The editors propose that attempts at conservatism while performing an abdominoperineal resection are inappropriate. The patient is subjected to a mutilating procedure requiring a permanent stoma and may suffer sexual and bladder dysfunction. Therefore, given the price that the patient must pay, every attempt should be made to excise all potential sites of regional metastases. The lymphatic drainage of the anal canal is extensive; not only is there drainage superiorly via the rectal mesentery along the superior rectal artery and laterally along the midrectal vessels, but there is inferior drainage via the inferior rectal nodes that potentially may involve the inguinal, external iliac, and obturator nodes. Although we do not advocate "prophylactic" or elective dissections of Scarpa's triangle, involvement of these nodes requires a dissection of the femoral region. Irrespective of the status of the femoral nodes, we advocate clearance of the external iliac and obturator lymph nodes as part of the operation when an abdominoperineal resection for anal canal carcinoma is performed. As in operations for rectal cancer, we also perform a dissection of the hypogastric and common iliac nodes in addition to total excision of the rectal mesentery and midrectal nodes. We have salvaged patients with metastases in the obturator and/or iliac nodes by this dissection.

RETRORECTAL TUMORS

The retrorectal space is defined as the space anterior to the sacrum and coccyx, posterior to the fascia propria of the rectum, cephalic to the levator ani and coccygeal muscles, and caudal to the pelvic peritoneal reflection. Within this space, a variety of rare benign and malignant tumors may develop.[9] The most frequent are dermoid cysts in women and sacrococcygeal teratomas in infants and men. Sacrococcygeal teratomas are considered in Chapter 25. Middle-aged men are likely to have solid malignant tumors, whereas women and children tend to have congenital and cystic lesions. The symptom is ordinarily pain on sitting. A congenital cyst may present with a perirectal abscess.

Virtually all retrorectal tumors can be palpated by rectal digital examination. Hence, it is necessary to examine the posterior distal aspect of the rectum routinely with the examining finger. Palpation may be enhanced by a thumb on the perianal skin.

A sacral radiograph should be obtained for all patients in whom a presacral mass is suspected. If there is a sacral bone defect or bone destruction, the tumor is probably malignant. Suspicion of a chordoma calls for myelography. Two thirds of patients with a sacrococcygeal teratoma have calcifications in a soft tissue mass seen on sacral radiographs.

Computed tomography (CT) and magnetic resonance imaging (MRI) are the definitive preoperative studies. MRI may be superior. Nearly all solid tumors are chordomas. Cystic tumors include sacrococcygeal teratomas.

In general, preoperative biopsy is not indicated, because aspiration of an anterior sacral meningocele may initiate a lethal meningitis. The mass must be removed. Biopsy is warranted only if the mass is solid and deemed incurable.

Operative Management of Retrorectal Tumors

Posterior access with the patient in a prone, flexed position provides optimal exposure for operating on a benign tumor. A mechanical bowel preparation and perioperative antibiotics are used. The Kraske approach is widely used (Fig. 9–63). The incision may be vertical or transverse. The coccyx is readily identified and removed, the retrorectal space entered, and the fascia propria of the rectum recognized. A benign cyst can then be excised. For a malignant tumor such as a sacrococcygeal chordoma, a combined abdominal and sacral approach is necessary.

In this approach, the coccyx and fourth and fifth sacral segments with their corresponding nerve roots can be dissected bilaterally and removed with maintenance of normal bowel and bladder control. Higher dissection leads to increasing sensory and motor loss. Any bone resection requires ligation of the middle sacral artery. Both third sacral nerve roots and the pudendal nerves on one side must be preserved.

The Yorke-Mason incision provides an alternative

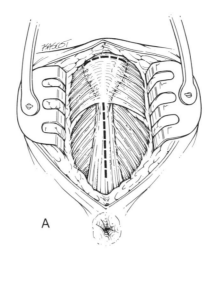
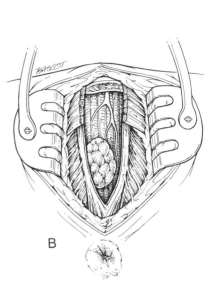

Figure 9–63. *A* and *B,* The Kraske approach to management of retrorectal tumors.

access to the retrorectal space (Fig. 9–64).[10] Patients should have a mechanical bowel preparation and perioperative antibiotics. A parasacral, oblique incision is made adjacent to the border of the sacrum, and the retrorectal space is entered after the levator muscles are divided. The components of the levator musculature are carefully identified with stay sutures for subsequent approximation. Access to retrorectal benign tumors may be obtained without division of the anal sphincteric musculature. The Yorke-Mason incision is also drained with a presacral drain, although the operation is usually performed without entering the rectum.

DISTAL RECTAL TUMORS

Small, mobile, distal rectal cancers and malignant colorectal adenomas can be removed transanally with a high level of clinical success.[11] Local excision of a distal rectal cancer constitutes a total biopsy with a margin. The criteria for conservative management after local excision include the following: excision is complete with a margin; the tumor is well or moderately well differentiated; mucinous components are absent; there is no vascular or lymphatic invasion; and, tumor does not invade through the muscularis propria. In the presence of adverse prognostic factors, the patient merits a low anterior resection or an abdominoperineal resection. Invasion through the muscularis propria is associated with about a 12% incidence of lymphatic metastasis. In our experience, ulceration of a small

mobile tumor alone does not constitute an adverse factor.

We have had experience with patients who had adverse prognostic factors and who refused abdominoperineal resection, had subsequent radiotherapy, and remained free of evidence of recurrence for longer than 5 years. Hence, adjuvant radiotherapy is a useful adjunct to local excision.

Rectal carcinoids are generally found in the distal rectum. Most are within reach of the examining finger, and they are usually small, hard, submucosal, and mobile; on endoscopic inspection, the mucosal surface is yellow. Rectal carcinoids are not associated with the carcinoid syndrome, but they are associated with visceral cancer elsewhere, and systemic evaluation is necessary. Rectal carcinoids of up to two cm in diameter are regarded as benign. Depending on their size and location, they can be managed by endoscopic excision, transanal excision, or posterior sphincterotomy. Rectal carcinoids larger than 2 cm in diameter behave more aggressively and require anterior resection or abdominoperineal resection.

Operative Management of Small Distal Rectal Tumors

In principle, a rectal tumor that can be reached with the examining finger and is mobile can be removed transanally. If the tumor is tethered or fixed to the examining finger, local excision should not be performed. A mechanical and antibiotic bowel preparation and perioperative antibiotics are administered. The

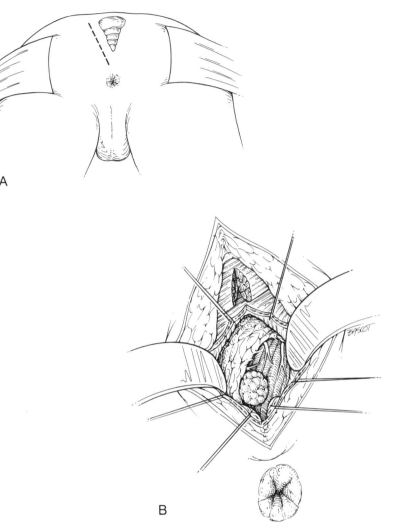

Figure 9–64. *A* and *B,* The Yorke-Mason incision, an alternative means of access to the retrorectal space.

patient should be positioned on the operating table to provide the greatest access to the growth. The operating headlight is useful.

When adequate exposure is attained, a full-thickness excision with a margin is performed (Fig. 9–65). Successive figure-eight chromic stay sutures and Allis clamps help bring the tumor distally to the anal outlet. Improper use of retractors can impede mobilization of the tumor.

Once stay sutures are applied above and below the tumor and the mucosa adjacent to the tumor is grasped with an Allis clamp, a full-thickness diathermy excision is performed from cephalad to caudad as an ellipse, to achieve a lateral mucosal margin of at least 5 mm from the tumor. As the tumor is excised, a running, locking, 0-0 chromic suture approximates the adjacent, full-thickness rectal wall and achieves hemostasis. Any arterial bleeders are clamped and individually ligated or oversewn.

At completion of the excision, one must orient the specimen with pins on a small plastic frame so that the mucosal side faces outward. This orientation permits proper fixation and sectioning by the pathologist.

Instead of a full-thickness excision into perirectal fat by intent, a submucous resection (Fig. 9–66) may be warranted in cases of large mobile villous adenomas in the distal rectum where many biopsies have not demonstrated cancer. The preparation for operation is the same. Here infiltration of the submucosa with 1 to 400,000 epinephrine in saline lifts the mucosa off the muscularis and permits a careful submucous resection with ophthalmic scissors or diathermy. It is not possible to approximate the mucosa; bleeding points are carefully coagulated, and the wound heals surprisingly well by secondary intention. The fresh specimen should be carefully oriented for subsequent microscopic examination.

EDITORIAL COMMENT

A common and often perplexing problem is the operative management of large or circumferential villous adenomas at or adjacent to the dentate line. Excision of these circumferential tumors without mucosal repair results in stenosis of the anorectum. For this entity we advocate a submucosal excision of the tumor. This procedure is also attributed to Yorke-Mason and is described by Dr. Dozois in Chapter 13 on prolapse of the rectum.

For this operation the patient is positioned in the prone position, and the hips are flexed 45 degrees. The use of a Wilson frame is advantageous. The anal canal is exposed by two Gelpi retractors and the mucosa beneath the tumor infiltrated with a dilute (1:100,000) epinephrine solution. The tumor-bearing mucosa is excised submucosally; this procedure is akin to the mucosectomy employed for an endorectal pull-through operation. A margin of normal mucosa should be obtained both superior and inferior.

After the submucosal incision, the circular muscle of the rectum is visible throughout the area of excision. Several rows of stout, absorbable sutures are placed in an axial fashion in the muscular layers. When these sutures are drawn together and tied, an accordionlike shortening of the rectum is obtained, which approximates the superior and inferior margins of mucosa. The mucosal defect is then repaired by interrupted absorbable sutures.

The operative specimen is pinned on a board and submitted to the pathologist for whole-mount examination and serial sectioning. If a benign villous adenoma is confirmed, or if there is only carcinoma in situ or superficial invasion, nothing other than surveillance need be done. If an invasive carcinoma is detected, an appropriate cancer operation is performed as a secondary procedure.

We have utilized this procedure with excellent results for villous adenomas exceeding 6 cm in length.

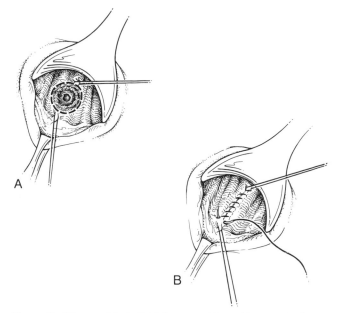

Figure 9–65. *A* and *B*, Full-thickness excision with a margin for management of small distal rectal tumors.

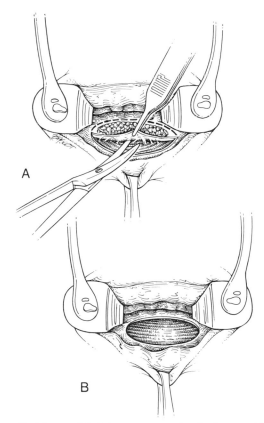

Figure 9–66. *A* and *B*, Submucous resection for large mobile villous adenomas in the distal rectum.

REFERENCES

1. Greenall MJ, Quan SHQ, Stearns MW, Urmacher C, DeCosse JJ. Epidermoid cancer of the anal margin. Am J Surg 1985;149:95–101.
2. Scholefield JH, Talbot IC, Whatrup C, et al. Anal and cervical intraepithelial neoplasia: Possible parallel. Lancet 1989;2:765–769.
3. Quan SHQ. Rare tumors of the anus and rectum. In: DeCosse JJ, Todd IP, eds. Anorectal Surgery Clinical Surgery International. Vol 15. New York: Churchill Livingstone, 1988, pp 171–177.
4. Gordon PH. Current status: Perianal and anal canal neoplasms. Dis Colon Rectum 1990;33:799–808.
5. Minsky BD, Cohen AM, Hajdu SI, Nori D. Sphincter preservation in rectal sarcoma. Dis Colon Rectum 1990;33:319–322.
6. Greenall MJ, Quan SHQ, Urmacher C, DeCosse JJ. Treatment of epidermoid carcinoma of the anal canal. Surg Gynecol Obstet 1985;161:509–517.
7. Vokes EE, Weichselbaum RR. Concomitant chemotherapy: Rationale and clinical experience in patients with solid tumors. J Clin Oncol 1990;8:911–934.
8. Khan FA, Fang DT, Nivatvongs S. Management of presacral bleeding during rectal resection. Surg Gynecol Obstet 1987;165:274–276.
9. Rosen CB, Beart RW. Presacral tumors. In DeCosse JJ, Todd IP, eds. Anorectal Surgery Clinical Surgery International. Vol 15. New York: Churchill Livingstone, 1988, pp 178–192.
10. Yorke-Mason A. Trans-sphincteric exposure of the rectum. Ann Roy Coll Surg Engl 1972;51:320–331.
11. DeCosse JJ, Wong RR, Quan SHQ, et al. Conservative treatment of distal rectal cancer by local excision. Cancer 1989;63:219–223.

Radiotherapy of Colorectal and Anal Carcinomas

David G. Brachman
Daniel J. Haraf
Ralph R. Weichselbaum

Radiotherapy for colorectal cancer is not new. The first published report was written by Symonds in 1914, only 6 years after Miles described the abdominoperineal resection and 2 decades before Dixon Mayo's popularization of the low anterior resection.[1] Despite the long history of radiotherapy, a clear delineation of its role in the management of colon, rectal, and anal cancer has only recently begun to emerge. This subchapter focuses on the use of curative and adjuvant radiotherapy to decrease the often-devastating morbidity of local recurrence and increase the overall survival rate from these cancers.

RECTAL CANCER

Sphincter-Preserving Radiotherapy for Early Lesions

For selected early-stage (Dukes A) rectal cancers, sphincter-saving endocavitary irradiation can be performed with little morbidity and an excellent chance for cure.[2, 3] The ultimate success of this approach lies in the careful selection of suitable patients based on specific criteria that include stage, size, location within the rectum, and degree of differentiation. Suitable cases are mobile lesions confined to the mucosa that are less than 5×3 cm and located below the peritoneal reflection but above the dentate line in patients with moderately or well-differentiated histologic findings without palpable perirectal lymph nodes on digital examination.[2] Transrectal ultrasonography is helpful in determining not only the status of these lymph nodes but also the extent of the primary tumor. The incidence of local lymph node metastases is in the range of 10% in the lesions described, but it increases with poorly differentiated histologic findings.[4] Encroachment on the anal canal is a relative contraindication to endocavitary irradiation.

Treatment is given through a specially designed proctoscope with a maximum diameter of 3 cm; lesions up to 5 cm in maximum dimension are encompassed by overlapping two adjacent treatment fields. An enema is administered before treatment is given, but no special diet is required, and the therapy is done on an outpatient basis. If local anesthesia is desired, a perianal block may be used. The procedure is performed on a proctologic tilt table by using a 50-kV hand-held fiberoptic-equipped treatment scope, and patients receive a total of 100 to 120 Gy in three to four treatments at 2- to 3-week intervals over 6 to 8 weeks. Each treatment takes less than 4 minutes, and patients may resume normal activities immediately thereafter. The fraction size and total dose given are nonstandard and are probably tolerated because of the relatively short depth of penetration of 50-kV x-rays.

The importance of follow-up at regular intervals is emphasized. Digital examination and direct visualization should be performed every 3 to 6 months for the first 5 years and laboratory and imaging studies utilized when appropriate. After therapy is completed, the site of treatment is typically atrophic, and biopsy of an otherwise benign-appearing site to confirm a complete response should not be done. As an alternative to biopsy, Papillon advocates cytologic examination of scrapings from the treatment area. In Sischy's series, 22% of treated patients exhibited some superficial necrosis in the treated area with healing occurring in all cases either spontaneously or with the use of steroid enemas.[3] Occasionally, patients experience telangiectasias and minor bleeding. This complication can be minimized by avoiding excessive roughage and platelet inhibitors (especially aspirin).

In his experience at the University of Rochester, Sischy achieved local control in 95% of patients (183 of 192) treated with curative intent.[3] Nine patients had local recurrence, and five of these patients were salvaged by surgery. Ninety-three percent of patients (74 of 80) followed for more than 5 years were free of disease, and 45 patients have died of intercurrent disease. In Papillon's series from Lyon, 245 patients have been followed for a minimum of 5 years.[2] Local failure has occurred in 5.3%, and nodal failure is 4.9%. Although only 8.9% of patients died from cancer, an additional 13.3% patients died of intercurrent disease for an overall survival rate of 76.3%. The treatment policy as practiced at Lyon dictates that polypoid lesions less than 12 cm from the anal canal are treated with contact therapy through the proctoscope, as noted. Ulcerated lesions of the lower half of the rectum (2 to 9 cm above the anal canal) are first treated with contact therapy followed 1 month after the last treatment by an iridium-192 implant for an additional 20 to 40 Gy to the tumor bed. On occasion, larger, more locally advanced lesions not initially suitable for this program can be downstaged with external-beam pelvic radiotherapy before being managed by endocavitary irradiation.

Papillon reports on 33 elderly patients (mean age 77 years) given 3,000 rad external-beam radiation via arc fields in 10 fractions before endocavitary irradiation.[2] Eighty-five percent (28 of 33) were locally controlled at 2 to 7 years; three of five patients with failed radiotherapy underwent successful surgical salvage. It is generally agreed that injudicious application of this technique to more advanced or higher-grade lesions would likely jeopardize the survival of patients who may be cured by other types of therapy that can more effectively manage the regional lymphatics. Nevertheless, in our experience, this highly valuable technique is underutilized in the treatment of this large subset of patients for whom it is wholly appropriate and should constitute at least an alternative to surgical resection.

Adjuvant Radiotherapy of Rectal Carcinoma

When potentially curative surgery is used as the sole method of treatment in locally advanced rectal cancer, local recurrence is both the most common site of failure and the leading cause of morbidity and mortality.[5] The incidence of local failure is usually 10% or less in early-stage disease (modified Astler-Coller A or B1), but it increases rapidly if the tumor penetrates the bowel wall and/or spreads to regional lymph nodes, with local recurrence rates that range from 20% to 50% or higher.[5] The higher incidence of local recurrence as a first or only site of failure in locally advanced rectal cancer contrasts sharply with the pattern of failure seen in colon cancer of a similar stage.

The principal reason for the higher rate of local failure seen in rectal cancer is anatomic constraints imposed by the pelvis on obtaining adequate margins of surgical resection. This is especially true for radial margins; they are often measured in millimeters, in contrast to the 3- to 15-cm (or wider) margins obtainable proximally or distally after an abdominoperineal resection or low anterior resection. In addition, the lymphatic drainage of the middle and lower rectum is not only to the inferior mesenteric lymph nodes, but also to the internal iliac and obturator chains, regions not easily reached by standard surgical approaches. Finally, an anastomotic recurrence is most likely to be seen when the distal margin is minimal after a low anterior resection for a relatively low-lying tumor. In all three instances, local recurrence would be expected to be higher for advanced tumors in the middle and lower rectal segments as a result of anatomic factors not encountered during colonic resections.[6]

Although definitions of the segments vary, the literature points to a relationship between the likelihood of local failure and the location of the tumor with respect to the peritoneal reflection (Table 9–3).[4, 7–10]

Table 9–3. LOCAL RECURRENCE RATE BY
LOCATION IN RECTUM

Author	Lower	Middle	Upper	Reference No.
Morson et al.	15%	8%	5%	4
McDermott et al.	26%	21%	14%	7
Philipshen et al.	31%	30%	10%	8
Moossa et al.	32%	10%	4%*	9
Adloff et al.	38%	33%	11%	10

*Includes rectosigmoid.

Lesions above the peritoneal reflection are more likely to entail a complete surgical removal of the primary and draining lymphatics and so are less likely to show any benefit from even the most effective local adjuvant treatment.

Numerous randomized and nonrandomized studies have been done to assess the impact of adjuvant radiotherapy on the rates of local failure and overall survival in patients with rectal cancer.[11–22] These investigations include reports of radiotherapy administered preoperatively, postoperatively, both pre- and postoperatively, and, more recently, with concomitant single or multidrug chemotherapy regimens. Representative randomized trials are summarized in Tables 9–4 to 9–7. Discussion focuses on local control, disease-free and overall survival rates, and therapy-related complications as they pertain to radiotherapy as an adjuvant to surgery in rectal cancer.

Preoperative Radiotherapy

Potential benefits from the use of preoperative radiotherapy include the following: (1) possible pathologic downstaging of a lesion, with an improvement in resectability of advanced lesions and the possibility of more conservative (i.e., sphincter-sparing) surgery; (2) a potential decrease in the viability of tumor cells dislodged at surgery, thereby lowering the incidence of operative seeding and distant metastases; and (3) the chance to irradiate tumor cells and normal tissues before their blood supply is compromised. This latter point is important, because tumor hypoxia appears to lessen the effectiveness of radiotherapy in controlling some tumor types and may therefore decrease the therapeutic ratio.

For most histologic types, it has generally been found that the minimum dose of radiation needed to sterilize well-oxygenated clinically occult micrometastases with a probability of greater than 90% control is approximately 45 to 50 Gy delivered over 4 to 5 weeks. The relationship of increasing dose to increased tumor control for rectal cancer was demonstrated in nonrandomized studies by Stevens et al. as well as by Fortier et al., in which patients received varying doses of preoperative radiation.[23, 24] An increased probability of local control was seen over the dose range from 40 to 60 Gy at 1.8 to 2.0 Gy/day over 4 to 6 weeks. In the Fortier report, local recurrence was 33% at 40 Gy and 9% at 50 Gy, and no local failures occurred at 60 Gy.

Because of concern about operative delay and the possible adverse effects on wound healing, many surgeons have been reluctant to use relatively high-dose (45 to 50 Gy) standard-fraction (1.8 to 2.0 Gy/day) preoperative radiotherapy. Therefore, most preoperative studies have used "hypofractionation," in which a lower total dose is delivered in a shorter time in the hope of achieving the same tumoricidal effect seen with the conventional fractionation studies already noted. Despite extensive mathematical models attempting to delineate "bioequivalent" treatments, it is unlikely that these compressed treatment schedules and larger doses per fraction at a lower total dose have a tumor-control potential equal to that of the more usual total dose and fractionation programs.

Low-dose or hypofractionated preoperative radiotherapy has been investigated in randomized trials (Table 9–4). In the largest such study, 849 patients were enrolled in the Stockholm Rectal Cancer Group trial, which compared 25 Gy over 5 to 7 days 1 week before surgery to surgery alone.[11] The incidence of pelvic failure in the radiotherapy group was 10.8% (46 of 424) versus 22.8% (97 of 425) (p < .01) for surgery alone at a median follow-up of 4.5 years. Of patients undergoing radiotherapy, 14% versus 9% of controls had postoperative wound infections. The rates of small bowel obstruction and anastomotic leaks were 2% each in the treatment arm and 3% each in the control group. The postoperative mortality rate at 30 days was 8% in the treated group but 2% in the surgery-alone group; however, this excess mortality was confined to the patient population older than 75 years of age (16% radiotherapy versus 2% surgery). The two therapies differed in neither disease-free survival nor overall survival.

Two large randomized studies using radiation doses of more than 30 Gy have been published, each with a surgery-only control arm. The Veterans Administration Surgical Oncology Group Trial II used 31.5 Gy in 1.75 Gy/day fractions; at 5 years, the survival rate in both treated and control groups for patients undergoing potentially curative resection was 50%, and no difference in local control or operative complications was observed.[12] Because the relationship of total radiation dose, fraction size, and overall time of delivery to tumor control is a probability function, it is not surprising that no impact on local control was noted in this study, in which a relatively low dose and fraction size were employed.

The European Organization on Research and Treatment of Cancer (EORTC) randomized 466 patients to

Table 9–4. SELECTED RANDOMIZED PREOPERATIVE ADJUVANT RADIOTHERAPY TRIALS IN RECTAL CANCER PATIENTS

Study	No. of Patients	Treatment Arms	Local Failure (%)	Overall Survival	Reference No.
Stockholm Rectal Cancer Study Group (1990)	425	Control	22.8 (p <0.1)*	—	11
	424	Radiotherapy (25 Gy in 2.5 Gy/fx)	10.8	—	
Veterans Administration Surgical Oncology Group Trial II (1986)	180	Control	—	49.6	12
	181	Radiotherapy (31.5 Gy in 1.75 Gy/fx)	—	50.3	
European Organization on Research and Treatment of Cancer (1988)	233	Control	30	59.1 (p = n.s.)	13
	233	Radiotherapy (34.5 Gy in 2.3 Gy/fx)	15	69.1	

— = not stated; fx = fraction; n.s. = not statistically significant.

*p values, where cited, are from the original texts; comparison is made between treatment in rows immediately above and below value.

preoperative radiotherapy with 34.5 Gy in 2.3 Gy fractions followed by surgery in an average of 11 days versus surgery alone.[13] For patients undergoing curative resection, local recurrence rates were 15% for radiotherapy plus surgery and 30% for surgery alone (p = .003). A trend toward increased survival was seen at 5 years; 69% of patients were alive in the radiotherapy plus surgery group and 59% alive in the surgery-only arm. Thirty-two percent of control and 21.6% of adjuvant radiotherapy plus surgery patients died of rectal cancer. Of the tumors in this study, 90% were within the last 10 cm of the rectum. Although no definite survival benefit was observed in these trials, it does appear that the incidence of local recurrence can be cut roughly in half by well-tolerated moderate-dose preoperative irradiation.

Postoperative Radiotherapy

A major advantage of a postoperative approach to adjuvant radiotherapy is that it allows exclusion from treatment those patients found at surgery to have either modified Astler-Coller Stage A or B1 disease or distant metastases. Approximately 25% to 50% of patients in preoperative radiotherapy series are unlikely to derive any demonstrable benefit, because these series contain patients found to have early-stage lesions (11% to 37%) and metastases (11% to 13%) at the time of operation. Two randomized trials of postoperative radiotherapy have been reported (Table 9–5).

A Danish study of 494 patients who received either no further therapy or postoperative radiotherapy to 50 Gy demonstrated no survival advantage with radiotherapy; however, patients with Stage C disease had a decrease in local failure rates.[14] This study was somewhat unusual in that 20% of patients randomized to receive postoperative treatment received none or an incomplete course, and more than 50% of patients had upper rectal or rectosigmoid lesions. As can be seen from Table 9–3, these patients appear less likely to benefit from local adjuvant therapy.

In a more recent EORTC trial, 172 patients with locally advanced (B2 to C3, modified Astler-Coller staging) disease were randomized to either surgery

Table 9–5. SELECTED RANDOMIZED POSTOPERATIVE ADJUVANT RADIOTHERAPY TRIALS IN RECTAL CANCER PATIENTS

Study	No. of Patients	Treatment Arms	Local Failure (%)	Overall Survival (%)	Reference No.
Danish Multicenter Study (1986)	250	Control	Stage B 12	B/C 67*	14
	244	Radiotherapy (50 Gy split course in 2 Gy/fx)	Stage C 25	B/C 82*	
European Organization on Research and Treatment of Cancer	87	Control	Stage B 2–C 25	B 63 C 39	(B. Nordlinger: unpublished communication)
	84	Radiotherapy (46 Gy in 2 Gy/fx)	Stage B 2–C 19	B 65 C 43	

*Local recurrence-free survival.

fx = fraction.

Table 9–6. RANDOMIZED TRIALS OF PREOPERATIVE VERSUS POSTOPERATIVE ADJUVANT RADIOTHERAPY IN RECTAL CANCER

Study	No. of Patients	Treatment Arms	Local Failure (%)	Overall Survival (%)	Reference No.
Radiation Therapy Oncology Group (1990)	148	5 Gy in 1 fx preoperatively + surgery + postoperative radiation (if B2–C) to 45 Gy in 1.8 Gy/fx	21 (p = n.s.)*	75 (p = n.s.)	15
	156	Surgery + postoperative radiation (if B2–C) to 45 Gy in 1.8 Gy/fx	31	68	
Stockholm Rectal Cancer Group (1990)	236	Preoperative radiation (25.5 Gy in 5.1 Gy/fx)	12 (p = .02)	~46†	16
	235	Postoperative radiation (60 Gy split course in 2 Gy/fx)	21	~40†	

*p values, where cited, are from the original texts; comparison is made between treatments in rows immediately above and below the value.
†Local recurrence-free survival.
fx = fraction; n.s. = not statistically significant.

alone or surgery followed by postoperative radiotherapy to a total of 46 Gy in 23 fractions, given 4 to 8 weeks after surgery. At a mean follow-up of over 4 years, no significant difference was seen in overall survival rates; local failure was 25% in the surgery group and 19% in the adjuvant radiotherapy arm (B. Nordlinger: unpublished communication).

Two reports attempted to settle the issue of the optimum timing of adjuvant radiotherapy relative to surgery (Table 9–6). The Radiation Therapy Oncology Group (RTOG) sought to test the value of adding preoperative to postoperative radiotherapy plus surgery ("sandwich therapy"). Patients were randomized to either no therapy or 5 Gy in one fraction 24 hours before surgery.[15] Following surgical resection, patients with Stage A or B1 disease received no further treatment, whereas patients with Stage B2, B3, or C disease underwent postoperative radiotherapy to 45 Gy. At 36 months, there are no significant differences between the two arms of the study in the rates of distant metastases, local control, and survival.

In the Stockholm Rectal Cancer Study Group trial, a total of 471 patients with resectable cancer were randomized to either 25.1 Gy in five daily fractions followed in 1 week by surgery, or postoperative treatment to directly compare pre- and postoperative radiotherapy.[16] Radiation consisted of 50 Gy in 2 Gy/day fractions to a pelvic field followed by a reduced treatment volume for an additional 10 Gy to a total dose of 60 Gy. The postoperative treatment was limited to patients with Astler-Coller B2, C1, or C2 lesions found at the time of surgery. At a mean follow-up of 6 years, the local failure rate is 21% in the postoperative versus 12% in the preoperative group (p = .02), with no difference seen in the rate of distant metastases, disease-free or overall survival. Perineal wound sepsis occurred in 33% of preoperative patients versus 18%

of postoperative patients (p < .001); all other surgical complications were equally distributed between the two groups. All but one patient randomized to preoperative radiotherapy received treatment, whereas 16% of postoperative treatment patients received no radiotherapy.

Of radiobiologic concern is the "split-course" technique used to deliver the postoperative radiotherapy; after 40 Gy was administered, a 2-week break was taken before treatment was resumed. There is evidence that the percentage of clonogenic cells can increase during interruptions in radiotherapy as a result of tumor cell proliferation and that a prolonged break from treatment can make tumor cell eradication more difficult. This relationship between decreased control from split-course treatment regimens and accelerated repopulation during breaks has been demonstrated for various disease sites.

Despite the general effectiveness of adjuvant radiotherapy in lessening the incidence of local failure, compared with surgery alone, this result has not led to an increase in overall survival rates. The optimum dose and timing of adjuvant radiotherapy have yet to be determined. Although it is possible that further refinements in radiotherapy alone may result in a much-desired increase in cure rates, distant failure occurs in 20% to 40% of patients who are candidates for local adjuvant therapy. Therefore, for any adjuvant therapy to be truly effective, it needs to address the dual problem of distant and local failure.

Radiotherapy With or Without Chemotherapy

Several trials have addressed the issue of distant and local failure by administering 5-fluorouracil (5FU) or 5FU-based chemotherapy with or without concomitant

Table 9–7. RANDOMIZED TRIALS OF ADJUVANT RADIOTHERAPY AND/OR CHEMOTHERAPY IN RECTAL CANCER

	No. of Patients	Treatment Arms	Local Failure (%)	Overall Survival (%)	Disease-Free Survival (%)	Reference No.
Preoperative						
European Organization on Research and Treatment of Cancer (1984)	121	Preoperative radiotherapy (34.5 Gy in 2.3 Gy/fx)	—	59 (p = .06)*	—	17
	126	Preoperative radiotherapy (34.5 Gy in 2.3 Gy/fx) + 5FU	—	46	—	
Postoperative						
National Surgical Adjuvant Bowel and Breast Project RO1 (1988)	184	Surgery alone	25 (p = .06)	43	30	
	184	Postoperative radiotherapy (46 Gy in 2 Gy/fx ± boost to 53 Gy)	16	41	34	
	187	Postoperative chemotherapy (MOF)	21	53	42	
Gastrointestinal Tumor Study Group (1985, 1986)	48	Postoperative chemotherapy (MF)	18.8	54†	~43†	19,20
	50	Postoperative radiotherapy (40–48 Gy in 2 Gy/fx)	18	~52	~43	
	58	Surgery alone	20.6	~45 (p = .005)	~28 (p = .05)	
	46	Postoperative radiotherapy + 5FU, followed by MF chemotherapy	6.5	~67	~57	
Gastrointestinal Tumor Study Group (1990)	104	Postoperative radiotherapy + 5FU, then 5FU × 5 mo	—	76	69 (p = n.s.)	
	95	Postoperative radiotherapy + 5FU, then MF × 12 mo	—	66	54	22
North Central Cancer Treatment Group–Mayo Clinic (1991)	100	Postoperative radiotherapy alone (50.4 Gy in 1.8 Gy/fx)	25 (p = .036)	38 (p = 0.43)	38 (p = .0025)	21
	104	Postoperative MF chemotherapy, then radiotherapy + 5FU followed by additional MF chemotherapy × 2 mo	13.5	53	58	

*p values, where cited, are from the original texts; comparison is made between treatments in rows immediately above and below the value.
†Survivals are estimates from most recent published graphic data available.
MOF = methyl-CCNU + 5FU; MF = methyl-CCNU + 5FU; 5FU = 5-fluorouracil; fx = fraction; — = not stated; n.s. = not statistically significant.

radiotherapy as an adjuvant treatment in locally advanced rectal cancer (Table 9–7). In an early study, the EORTC compared preoperative radiotherapy of 34.5 Gy in 2.3 Gy fractions with and without concomitant 5FU.[17] In the combined treatment group, a trend toward decreased distant metastases was seen, primarily in the liver (p = .07), but no change in the rate of local failure or disease-free survival was noted. Overall, an increased incidence of death from intercurrent disease occurred in the combined treatment group and resulted in a lower overall survival for patients in this arm.

In protocol RO-1, the National Surgical Adjuvant Bowel and Breast Project randomized patients to surgery alone, postoperative radiotherapy, or a postoperative adjuvant chemotherapy regimen consisting of 5FU, methyl-N-C2-chloroethyl-N'-cyclohexyl-N-nitrosourea (CCNU), and vincristine (Oncovin).[18] Com-

pared with the group receiving surgery alone, the postoperative radiotherapy patients showed a reduction in local-regional failure from 25% to 16% without a significant benefit in overall survival. For the chemotherapy arm, subset analysis revealed a disease-free survival advantage with Dukes B and C disease, limited to male patients, and an overall survival rate increase with Dukes B (but not Dukes C) disease, also limited to male patients. The survival of females was adversely affected by the administration of this chemotherapy regimen. Although this study did not contain a concomitant chemotherapy-radiotherapy arm, three large studies have been published that employed a postoperative combined modality therapy.

In the first Gastrointestinal Tumor Study Group (GITSG) trial, 202 patients with perirectal fat extension and/or positive lymph nodes were randomized to one of four arms: (1) surgery alone, (2) combination chemotherapy with methyl-CCNU and 5FU, (3) pelvic radiotherapy (44 or 48 Gy), or (4) pelvic radiotherapy with methyl-CCNU and 5FU.[19] In the most recent update with a minimum follow-up of 6.3 years, overall survival was 58% in the combination radiotherapy plus chemotherapy arm, 44% in both chemotherapy-only and radiotherapy-only arms, and 28% in the surgery-only arm (p = .005 for combination therapy versus surgery alone).[20] The major effect of combination therapy is to enhance local control; local regional relapse occurred in 20.6% of surgery-alone patients, 18.8% of chemotherapy-alone patients, 18% of radiotherapy-alone patients, and only 6.5% of combination therapy patients. Distant metastases occurred in 34%, 27%, 30%, and 26% of these same patient groups, respectively. This study is interesting in that the large decrease in local failure is a major reason for a reduction in disease-specific and overall mortality rates seen in the combined modality group, relative to surgery alone.

A trial of radiotherapy alone versus radiotherapy plus 5FU and methyl-CCNU chemotherapy by the North Central Cancer Treatment Group–Mayo Clinic produced similar results.[21] A group of 207 patients with modified Astler-Coller B2 to C3 disease were randomized to either postoperative radiotherapy with boost to a reduced field and no further treatment or two cycles of postoperative 5FU with methyl-CCNU followed by pelvic radiotherapy with 5FU given for 3 days during week 1 and week 5 of radiotherapy. Radiation doses were identical in each arm, and after radiotherapy was completed, an additional cycle of 5FU with methyl-CCNU was administered to the patients in the combined modality arm.

At a median follow-up of over 7 years, local recurrence, disease-free and overall survival rates were all significantly higher in the combination therapy arm. Local failure was 25% in the control and 13.5% in the combination treatment arm, and distant metastasis rates were 46% and 29% in these same groups. Disease-free survival was 38% versus 58% (p = .0025), favoring the combination therapy arm. No deaths from toxicity were seen, and only two patients (one in each treatment arm) had severe diarrhea requiring hospitalization; the major side effects were hematologic and generally mild. Severe delayed reactions were seen in 13 patients (6.7%); 10 of these were small bowel complications (9 obstructions and hemorrhage). Six of these patients received combined therapy and four had radiotherapy alone; one death attributed to sepsis occurred in each group. A second study by the GITSG that randomized patients to radiotherapy and 5FU with or without methyl-CCNU showed no advantage in disease-free survival or in local recurrence rates for methyl-CCNU, compared with 5FU alone.[22]

Randomized trials in Stages B and C colon cancer have shown a decreased recurrence rate and increased overall survival for patients who received adjuvant 5FU and levamisole.[25, 26] Therapy was well tolerated, and the results reached statistical significance for patients with Dukes C disease. On the basis of these encouraging results, a National Cancer Institute–sponsored cooperative group randomized study has been opened to extend this regimen to manage rectal cancer as well; patient accrual has just begun.

Incompletely Resected and Unresectable Carcinomas

Cytotoxic therapies are generally more effective when the tumor cell burden is small, and resection should attempt to achieve appropriate tumor-free margins, including resection of portions of adjacent organs when tumor invasion or adherence is present. Areas suspicious for or known to harbor residual tumor should be noted, and the placement of titanium clips to define areas of concern helps greatly to localize these sites on radiotherapy planning films postoperatively. Table 9–8 summarizes the results of several nonrandomized series of radiation for known residual disease.[27–32] Although the radiation doses used and criteria for local failure were not uniform, the overall survival rate of patients with microscopic residual disease is greater than that of patients with gross residual disease at the time of completion of surgery. Furthermore, interstudy comparison suggests that there is an increasing likelihood of local failure over time.

Given the need for improvement in this class of patients and the encouraging local control rates achieved with the combination of radiation and chemotherapy in the adjuvant trials noted, we are now utilizing such an approach in these cases. Radiotherapy for 45–50 Gy to the pelvis and a reduced-field dose of 15 Gy for a total of 60–66 Gy to areas of known residual disease is given in conjunction with 5FU chemotherapy. Early results are encouraging, but further patient accrual and follow-up are needed. Another strategy in this difficult group of patients is the use of preoperative radiation; in contrast to the moderate doses used in an adjuvant setting, high doses (55 to 60 Gy or more) are usually delivered by standard fractionation techniques (2 Gy/fraction). Surgery is delayed until 4 to 6 weeks after radiation is completed, in order to obtain the maximum benefit of any radiotherapy-induced downstaging.

A report from Jefferson University, Philadelphia, details their experience on 85 patients with complete extrarectal fixation, 92% of whom had tumors within the distal 6 cm of the rectum.[33] A dose of 55 Gy was given in 25 fractions, followed by surgery in 4 to 6 weeks. In 70% of cases, sphincter-sparing surgery was

Table 9–8. EXTERNAL-BEAM RADIOTHERAPY FOR POSTOPERATIVE RESIDUAL DISEASE

Author	Dose Range (Gy)	Microscopic Residual		Gross Residual		Minimum Follow-up	Reference No.
		Local Control	*Survival*	*Local Control*	*Survival*		
Brizel and Tepperman	9–64	68%	*	71%	*	6 mo	27
Wang and Schulz	20–50	†		*	22%	<12 mo	28
Ghossein et al.	31–60	85%	77%	50%	39%	12 mo	29
Allee et al.	45–70	74%	59%	48%	68%	*; survival given at 3 yr	30
Rominger et al.	50–70	72%	58%	50%	28%	15 mo	31
Schild et al.	40–60	30%	30%	14%	14%	5 yr	32

* = not stated; † = only cases of gross residual reported.

possible, and at 5 years, local control was 84% with a disease-free survival of 42%. Complications requiring reoperation occurred in 6% of patients, and there were no treatment-related deaths.

For patients with ulcerated lesions larger than 5 cm in diameter and found to be only marginally resectable on the basis of fixation and/or bulk, Sischy employed preoperative radiotherapy with 5FU and mitomycin C, based on his protocol for the treatment of anal carcinoma.[34] Surgery in all cases was an abdominoperineal resection, and 33 patients treated in this manner have been followed for a minimum of 5 years. Local control has been sustained in 85% of patients; 64% are alive with no evidence of disease; distant failure is 12%, and 9% died of intercurrent disease without recurrence.

In an attempt to gain the downstaging advantages of preoperative radiotherapy and restrict the highest-dose areas as much as possible, some centers have used a combination of preoperative and intraoperative radiotherapy. Doses of 45 to 55 Gy delivered by external-beam radiation are followed in 4 weeks by surgery and intraoperative radiotherapy for an additional 15 to 20 Gy in a single fraction. Used after tumor resection but before reanastomosis, this technique allows delivery of radiotherapy under surgical guidance and direct visualization. Small bowel can be excluded from the high-dose area, and the rapid depth-dose fall-off of the electron beam ensures that a minimum of normal tissue is included in the field.

Both the Mayo Clinic and the Massachusetts General Hospital have updated their series.[35, 36] For patients with nonrecurrent locally advanced disease, survivals of 55% to 58% at greater than 3 years are reported, and local control is achieved in 77% to 83% of cases. Complication rates are only slightly higher than in patients treated with surgery alone (21% versus 16%, respectively, in the Massachusetts General Hospital series). This compares favorably with the 35% rate of complications from the same hospital seen with high-dose preoperative external-beam radiotherapy and re-

section. Intraoperative radiotherapy finds its greatest utility when only suspicious or microscopically positive surgical margins remain after resection. As with external-beam radiotherapy alone, local control is higher in patients with microscopic residual, as opposed to gross residual, disease at the time of intraoperative radiotherapy administration. The results obtained in the treatment of recurrent disease are less favorable, although 20% to 25% of patients are free of disease at 5 years.[35, 36] The Mayo Clinic is currently evaluating the addition of chemotherapy to the preoperative external-beam portion of this regimen; an analysis is not yet available.

Occasionally, a patient in need of local therapy is, for medical reasons, inoperable or refuses potentially curative surgery. External-beam radiotherapy used alone in these settings was initially reported by Rider and updated by Cummings from the Princess Margaret Hospital.[37] A group of 144 patients with lesions staged as either "mobile" or "fixed" were treated with a usual dose of 50 Gy in 2.5-Gy fractions. For patients with mobile tumors, the 5-year local control rate was 39% with an overall survival rate of 36%, whereas those with fixed lesions had local control and 5-year survival rates of 11%, respectively. Of long-term survivors, 76% maintained anal function, and 70% did not require a colostomy at any point (before or after radiotherapy) in their illness. The prolonged time to a maximum regression is interesting. In patients with mobile lesions, it was not seen until over 3 months after radiotherapy was completed. Two fatal cases of acute radiation enteritis were seen, as was one late death from complications of pelvic fibrosis. Although the overall radiation dose was not greater than that used in most postoperative adjuvant studies, the high daily dose per fraction and the lack of multiple treatment fields per day are likely to have contributed to these complications. These results give hope in cases of medical inoperability or patient refusal to accept colostomy at any cost.

We believe that future strategies for rectal cancer treatments should explore the issues of optimum combinations and timing of surgery, chemotherapy, and radiation for each stage of disease. We concur with the philosophy of the National Institutes of Health Consensus Statement on Adjuvant Therapy for patients with colon and rectal cancer that at the current time, postoperative combined chemoradiotherapy appears to offer the best chance to attain improved local control and overall survival and should be considered the standard of care for patients with locally advanced rectal cancer.[38]

COLON CARCINOMA

General Considerations

The role of radiotherapy for the treatment of colon cancer is less clearly defined than for that of rectal carcinoma. Whereas radiotherapy has been shown to be beneficial in preventing local recurrence in rectal carcinoma, the indications for radiotherapy in cases of colon carcinoma require further investigation. Although there is a high rate of local failure in rectal carcinoma, the number of local failures is much less pronounced for colon carcinoma, as described in the discussion of rectal carcinoma. Fewer nodal groups, which are easier to evaluate and excise at the time of surgery, drain the colon, compared with rectal lesions. These factors increase the likelihood of complete removal of the primary lesion and the draining lymphatics, resulting in a lower risk of local recurrence. Therefore, it is more difficult to show any benefit from adjuvant local therapy.

However, a number of series suggest that in certain circumstances, locoregional failure is a significant problem after selected colon cancers are resected.[39–43] The risk of locoregional recurrence may vary for different segments of the colon for anatomic reasons. The ascending and descending colon lack a true mesentery, whereas the cecum has a variable mesentery and limited mobility. These features make it difficult to obtain an adequate surgical margin in circumferential lesions or those with posterior penetration through the bowel wall. Thus, carcinoma of the colon tends to be a heterogeneous group of neoplasms that require that anatomic and pathologic factors be taken into account in considering patients for adjuvant radiotherapy.

Adjuvant Radiotherapy

Adjuvant radiotherapy for treatment of colon carcinoma has not been widely studied. The information available thus far seems to indicate that adjuvant radiotherapy may be beneficial for selected patients with colon carcinoma. In general, adjuvant radiotherapy appears to be indicated for the same stages of colon carcinoma as of rectal carcinoma. Data from the Massachusetts General Hospital indicate that patients with Stages A and B1 disease have a few local failures after curative resection and would benefit little from adjuvant radiotherapy.[41] However, patients with lesions in the cecum, ascending colon, and descending colon who have penetration through the bowel wall (modified Astler-Coller Stages B3, C2, and C3) have a relatively high risk of local failure (20% to 50%) and should be considered for additional treatment.[41] In a subsequent study, Duttenhaver et al. gave 4,500 to 5,040 cGy to the tumor bed in 80 patients with Stage B2 to C disease and found a decrease in the local recurrence rates.[44] Other authors have reported an increase in the local control rates after adjuvant radiotherapy, compared with historical controls.[45–47]

Although it has been difficult to demonstrate that an increase in local control results in an increase in survival, local failure can result in significant morbidity, and postoperative radiotherapy to the tumor bed in doses of 4,500 to 5,400 cGy has not been reported to result in significant toxicity. Patients at increased risk of local failure include those with Stage B2 to C disease in the ascending colon, descending colon, or cecum and should be considered candidates for adjuvant irradiation. Other patients who should be referred for postoperative radiotherapy include those with positive or close margins of resection and those with gross involvement of neighboring structures.

Inoperable or Unresectable Colon Carcinoma

Unlike rectal carcinoma, most colon carcinomas are resectable, and information about the use of preoperative radiotherapy to influence resectability is limited. In one small series, five patients with unresectable lesions of the sigmoid or transverse colon were given 4,500 to 5,000 cGy preoperative radiotherapy and re-evaluated 4 to 6 weeks after radiation was given. All five patients were able to undergo complete resection of their tumors.[48] Radiotherapy as the sole treatment modality for carcinoma of the colon is not recommended, because over 6,500 cGy would be required in an attempt to sterilize gross disease and could result in significant small bowel toxicity. Although doses of 5,000 to 5,400 cGy may provide significant palliation, the increased risk of toxicity with curative doses of radiation can be justified in patients who cannot be operated on for medical reasons.

Conclusions

The role of radiotherapy in the treatment of colon and rectal cancer varies with disease site, stage, and individual patient factors. In colon cancer, treatment decisions depend heavily on operative findings, including location and adherence. With early-stage rectal cancer, endocavitary irradiation is a highly successful and cost-effective sphincter-sparing approach for a select group of patients. For modified Astler-Coller Stage B2 to C rectal cancer, we believe that postoperative adjuvant combined chemotherapy and radiotherapy should be considered for all patients able to undergo such therapy. Decreased local recurrence rates as well as emerging evidence for increased disease-free and overall survival rates as a result of combined radiotherapy and 5FU or 5FU-based regimens make these combinations the standard against which all other treatments should be compared. Definitive external-beam radiotherapy and intraoperative radiotherapy have a place in the management of patients who are unsuitable for operation as well as patients with lesions that cannot be completely removed surgically.

ANAL CANCER

General Considerations

Anal carcinoma is much less common than colon and rectal cancer and accounts for only 1% to 2% of all large bowel cancer in the United States. Many different cell types are present in the anal region, and each can give rise to malignancy. Over 80% of neoplasms in this area are epidermoid carcinomas; most are squamous cell or basaloid (cloacogenic) carcinomas.[49] Basaloid or cloacogenic carcinomas arise from the transitional epithelium and, stage for stage, have a prognosis similar to that for squamous cell carcinoma.[50] Other rare histologic types may give rise to malignancy such as small cell carcinoma, melanoma, and lymphoma.

The treatment of anal carcinomas has changed over the past decade. Until relatively recently, the most common treatment was operative and employed abdominoperineal resection. Other therapeutic options have been explored in an attempt to preserve anal function. Limited local excision has been used with some success in well-selected patients.[51, 52] The ability of radiotherapy to cure epidermoid anal carcinoma and preserve anal function without producing serious morbidity has not been widely accepted until recently. However, radiotherapy alone for the treatment of anal carcinomas has been widely used in Europe with good results.[53, 54] Programs have combined radiotherapy with chemotherapy and conservative resection in the treatment of these uncommon cancers.

Radiation as the Sole Method of Treatment

Radiotherapy has been hampered by concerns about the risk of painful anal stenosis and doubts about the ability of orthovoltage or interstitial implants to control regional lymph node metastases. For these reasons, radical surgery was preferred over radiotherapy in many centers.[55] Nevertheless, a number of centers have reported their results with megavoltage external-beam radiation or interstitial implant, or a combination of these two techniques. These studies showed that radiotherapy alone can produce 5-year survival rates similar to those achieved by radical surgery while preserving anal function, as shown in Table 9–9.

Table 9–9. RESULTS OF RADIOTHERAPY ALONE FOR ANAL CANCER

Series	Technique	No. of Patients	Five Year Survival	Local Control*	Retain Anal Function
Eschwege et al.[53]	EB alone	64	46%	52(81%)	47(74%)
Cummings et al.[59]	EB I	51	59%	29(57%)	39(76%)
Cantril et al.[56]	EB†	33	NS	26(79%)	26(79%)
James et al.[60]	I alone	68	49%	33(49%)	27(40%)
Salmon et al.[61]	EB I‡	195	58%	132(68%)	126(65%)
Doggett et al.[57]	EB alone	35	92%	27(77%)	28(80%)
Papillon[58]	I and EB	154	68%	124(80%)	131(85%)
Schlienger et al.[63]	EB alone	193	68%	128(66%)	106(55%)

*Local control with radiation alone excluding surgical salvage.
†Three patients received a portion of radiotherapy by implant.
‡Twelve patients received a portion of radiotherapy by implant.
EB = external beam; I = implant; NS = not stated.

In 1983 Cantril et al. reported their experience of utilizing radiotherapy alone in the treatment of anal carcinoma.[56] Of the 35 patients treated with radiation, 28 (80%) remained locally controlled without further therapy, and all retained anal continence. Only one local failure was recorded in the 24 patients with lesions smaller than 5 cm. Four of the seven patients who developed local failure were salvaged by surgery. A subsequent report with longer follow-up reports continued good results in patients with lesions smaller than 5 cm.[57] Local control was 77% (28 of 35) with radiation alone. Seven of the eight failures were able to be salvaged surgically: five by abdominoperineal resection and two by local excision, for an overall local control of 97%. The actuarial 5-year disease-free survival rate was 92%, and anal continence was maintained in 80% (28 of 35). Similar results have been obtained at the Institut Gustav-Roussy in 64 patients treated with external-beam radiotherapy alone. These authors report an 81% local control rate with 74% of patients retaining anal function.[53]

Other centers have combined external-beam radiotherapy with an interstitial implant in the treatment of anal carcinoma with equally good results. Papillon initially employed an interstitial implant alone in the treatment of epidermoid anal carcinoma. He later modified the treatment technique to include external-beam radiation and the implant when he encountered painful local reactions and difficulty encompassing larger tumors with the implant alone.[58]

The results of radiotherapy alone have been encouraging. However, a number of reports have suggested that a subgroup of patients have large tumors and may be at a higher risk of local failure when radiotherapy is the sole treatment modality. For example, some radiotherapy series examined tumor size before the beginning of treatment and reported a correlation between the size of the lesion and the local control rate following radiotherapy. Results of these series are shown in Table 9–10. Although a number of retrospective series present evidence indicating that radiotherapy alone can cure a sizable number of epidermoid carcinomas of the anal canal and preserve sphincter function, these results also indicate that radiotherapy alone has difficulty controlling lesions larger than 3 to 5 cm.

The role of surgical salvage following radical radiotherapy has not been systematically studied. The limited data available on surgical salvage after radiation is administered are presented in Table 9–11. However, the data must be interpreted with caution. As noted in Table 9–11, surgery was not attempted on all local failures. The literature does not clarify whether surgery was not technically possible or not considered an option because of medical reasons or the presence of metastatic disease. In the series by Salmon et al.,[61] abdominoperineal resection was part of the therapeutic plan for all patients who did not achieve a complete clinical response within 6 months of radiotherapy. In this series, 27 patients who did not achieve a complete response with radiotherapy underwent operation, and the salvage rate was 85%. No mention was made of the number of histologically sterile operative specimens obtained. This same series reports 42 patients whose disease recurred locally more than 6 months after therapy. Resection was attempted only on 24 (57%) and was successful in 12. Thus, it appears that abdominoperineal resection can salvage 20% to 85% of all local failures after radiotherapy. However, the salvage

Table 9–10. EFFECT OF TUMOR SIZE ON LOCAL CONTROL FOLLOWING RADIOTHERAPY

Series	Lesion Size	No. of Patients	Five Year Survival	Local Control*
James et al.[60]	<5 cm	42	60%†	27(64%)
	>5 cm	26	30%†	6(23%)
Cantril et al.[56]	<5 cm	26	96%†	23(88%)
	>5 cm	7	79%†	3(43%)
Salmon et al.[62]	25%‡	49	70%	31(63%)
	50%	101	61%	47(47%)
	75%	16	19%	0(0%)
	100%	17	19%	0(0%)
Schlienger et al.[63]	T1, T2§	63	NS	45(71%)
	T3a	38	NS	28(74%)
	T3b	57	NS	35(61%)
	T4	35	NS	20(57%)
Papillon[58]	≤4 cm	39	NS	35(90%)
	>4 cm	58	NS	44(76%)

*Local control with radiation alone excluding surgical salvage.
†Actuarial survival calculation.
‡Reported as percentage circumference of anal canal involvement.
§1987 UICC staging criteria.
NS = not stated.

Table 9–11. RESULTS OF SALVAGE SURGERY FOLLOWING RADIOTHERAPY

Series	No. of Patients	No. Local Failure after Radiation	No. Surgery Attempted	No. Salvaged*	Ultimate Local Control
James et al.[60]	68	35	18	7(20%)	59%
Cummings et al.[59]	51	22	10	8(36%)	73%
Cantril et al.[56]	33	7	NS	4(57%)	91%
Salmon et al.[61]	195	27† 42‡	27 24	23(85%) 12(29%)	86%
Schlienger et al.[63]	193	65	41	19(29%)	76%

*Reported as number salvaged/number local failures after radiation.
†This group did not have a complete response and underwent abdominoperineal resection within 6 months.
‡This group developed a local recurrence more than 6 months after radiation.
NS = not stated.

rate ranges from 38% to 85% for patients undergoing operation. The data from one series suggest that surgical salvage may be more successful when performed within 6 months of radiotherapy.[61]

Although there has been much concern about the potential for complications following curative radiotherapy, the actual number of complications requiring surgery have been few. As can be seen in Table 9–9, 40% to 80% of patients retain anal function after radiotherapy; surgery is reserved for radiotherapy failures. The number of complications following radiotherapy has been acceptable and is shown in Table 9–12. If patients who develop local recurrence are excluded, the rate of major complications that require surgery ranges from 4% to 18%, with most modern series reporting less than 10% major complications. The major complication rate does not change, regardless of whether external-beam radiation or implant, or a combination of both techniques is used. The definition of moderate complications varies from series to series and occurs in 7% to 20% of patients. Generally mild or moderate complications consist of occasional incontinence or anal bleeding, anal stricture, fibrosis, pain, and edema, which can be treated medically or do not require treatment.

Radiotherapy and Chemotherapy

In an effort to improve the results of radiotherapy, investigators have begun to employ chemotherapy as a biologic response modifier to sensitize cells and potentiate the curative effects of radiation, permitting the eradication of larger tumors with radiation doses tolerated by normal tissues. Investigators at Wayne State University were one of the first to report the results with a protocol consisting of preoperative radiotherapy (3,000 cGy) and chemotherapy (5FU and mitomycin C) as adjuvant therapy, given to reduce the bulk of disease to a more localized form for more effective removal by radical surgery.[64]

When no tumor could be found in the operative specimens of five of the first six patients treated, the protocol was changed and the requirement for radical resection was eliminated. Patients with gross disappearance of tumor underwent an excisional biopsy of the scar to determine if microscopic disease was present. Additional reports by the same investigators with more patients and additional follow-up demonstrated that a low dose of radiation given concomitantly with chemotherapy resulted in histologically complete disappearance of tumor in over 85% of patients.[65, 66]

Since the report by Nigro et al. was published, other investigators have published results with combined modality therapy which are summarized in Table 9–13. All of the larger series have followed a chemotherapy protocol similar to that pioneered by Nigro with mitomycin C given as a bolus injection, 24-hour continuous infusion 5FU and concurrent or sequential radiotherapy. The concurrent regimens begin chemotherapy and radiotherapy on the same day while the sequential regimens administer chemotherapy before

Table 9–12. MAJOR COMPLICATIONS FOLLOWING RADIOTHERAPY

Series	Total Dose	Major Complications*
James et al.[60]	≈55 Gy	6%
Cantril et al.[56]	58–80 Gy	12%
Salmon et al.[62]	60–65 Gy	4%
Schlienger et al.[63]	60–65 Gy	5%
Cummings et al.[59]	45–50 Gy	6%
Doggett et al.[57]	45–75 Gy	6%
Papillon[58]	62–68 Gy	5%

*Complications following radiotherapy alone. Patients who underwent surgery for local recurrence are excluded.

Table 9–13. COMBINED MODALITY THERAPY IN EPIDERMOID CARCINOMA OF THE ANAL CANAL

	Wayne State University[67]	Memorial Hospital[68]	Highland Hospital[34]	Princess Margaret Hospital[69]	Fresno Community Hospital[70]	Radiation Therapy Oncology Group[71]
Mitomycin C	15 mg/m²	15 mg/m²	10 mg/m²	10 mg/m²	15 mg/m²	10 mg/m²
5-Fluorouracil	1,000 mg/m² × 4 d × 2 cycles	750 mg/m² × 4 d	1,000 mg/m² × 4 d × 2 cycles	1,000 mg/m² × 4 d	1,000 mg/m² × 4 d × 2 cycles	1,000 mg/m² × 4 d × 2 cycles
Radiation	30 Gy	30 Gy	50–57 Gy	50 Gy	40–50 Gy	40 Gy
RT/Chemotherapy	Concurrent	Sequential	Concurrent	Concurrent	Concurrent	Concurrent
No. patients	45	30	33	30	30	79
No. APR/LE/Bx*	45	30	4	0	22	65
Histologic CR	38 (84%)	16 (53%)	4 (100%)		22 (100%)	57 (88%)
Clinical CR			30 (91%)	28 (93%)		
Local recurrence	7%	47%	9%	7%	3%†	20%‡
Major complications	0%	NS	0%	16%	0%	NS
Retain anal function	60%	NS	88%	83%	97%	NS
Follow-up (months)	24–132	5–74	12–108	8–50	9–76	NS

*The number of patients undergoing APR, local excision (LE) or biopsy (Bx) as part of the protocol prior and excluding patients who later underwent surgery for local failure.
†Three of four local failures salvaged with additional chemotherapy and radiotherapy.
‡Estimated from data presented.
APR = abdominoperineal resection; RT = radiation; NS = not stated.

radiotherapy. In addition to differences in the timing of administration, these centers have varied the total dose of radiation given and the daily dose of radiation.

In the Wayne State University and Memorial Hospital series, chemotherapy was given before a planned surgical procedure was performed. Early in these studies, the surgical procedure was an abdominoperineal resection, which later was modified to local excision when histologically sterile specimens were obtained in the first patients. Other series have not incorporated surgery into the original treatment plan. Instead, these studies have employed higher doses of radiation as definitive treatment and reserved surgery for treatment failures or those with palpable residual tumor after combined chemotherapy and radiotherapy.

In spite of the differences among these trials, there is little evidence to suggest one schedule is markedly superior to another. All trials were conducted on relatively small numbers of patients, and all have similar response and survival rates. None of the trials was randomized, and results are compared to historical controls. Nevertheless, these investigations do suggest that the majority of patients with early and moderately advanced epidermoid carcinoma of the anal canal can be cured with combined radiotherapy and chemotherapy while preserving anal sphincter competence.[34, 67–70]

Analysis of the combined modality trials to date results in a number of interesting observations. The studies from Wayne State University and Memorial Hospital employed a relatively low dose (3,000 cGy) of radiation followed by abdominoperineal resection or excisional biopsy of the scar in all patients, and residual carcinoma was found in 16% (Wayne State) and 47% (Memorial) of patients. The Memorial Hospital series used a lower dose of 5FU, compared with the Wayne State University study, and administered the chemotherapy and radiotherapy sequentially, instead of concomitantly, which may explain the higher incidence of positive surgical specimens. These data suggest that concomitant chemotherapy and radiotherapy may be superior, at least when combined with lower doses of radiation than traditionally used for gross disease.

The dose of radiation required for optimum local control with a minimum of major complications has not been defined when combined with chemotherapy. Series reporting the results of radiotherapy alone indicate that doses in excess of 60 Gy are needed for local control and that even these doses have difficulty controlling the larger lesions. Therefore, one might hypothesize that the number of local failures would be higher if local excision were not part of the Wayne State University and Memorial Hospital protocols. The series from Princess Margaret Hospital employed a higher dose of radiation and reserved surgery (abdominoperineal resection and local excision) for patients with residual disease on clinical examination.[69] Although only 2 of 30 patients developed a local failure, the number of major complications that required surgery was higher than that seen in other studies. The greater number of major complications in the Princess Margaret Hospital series has been attributed to the fraction size (250 cGy) used to treat these patients. Other series have employed higher doses of radiotherapy (40 to 57 Gy) utilizing fraction sizes of 180 to 200 cGy and have obtained local control rates of over 90% without local excision or major complication.[34]

Although the dose of radiation combined with chemotherapy required to control local disease has not been defined, studies suggest that higher doses are needed for larger tumors. Studies that have looked at the size or stage of the lesion before beginning therapy report higher numbers of local failures, residual disease on biopsy, and the requirement for surgical salvage in patients with larger or later-stage lesions.[67, 70] Preliminary results from the RTOG report a local control rate of 84% and 66% at 1 year for lesions smaller than 3 cm and 3 cm or larger, respectively, following radiotherapy and chemotherapy.[71] Thus, it appears that local excision may be necessary in patients with larger lesions receiving low-dose (30 Gy) radiotherapy and concomitant chemotherapy. Also, the need for local excision can be eliminated with higher radiation doses without increasing the risk of major complications.

Technique

Many techniques employing external-beam and interstitial radiation have been described. Interstitial techniques alone have limited applicability, because it is difficult to encompass the larger lesions adequately. In addition, interstitial implants do not manage disease that may be present in the inguinal or pelvic nodes. Thus, interstitial therapy alone should be reserved for patients with well-differentiated squamous cell carcinomas of the distal canal and anal verge that are less than 3 cm in diameter and who are considered to be at low risk of having regional node metastases. In most cases, interstitial therapy may be valuable as a "boost" following external-beam treatment.

Except for the small well-differentiated lesions already described, treatment of the primary tumor and regional nodes with external-beam radiation is recommended. A minimum of two fields should be employed with all fields treated each day; this minimizes the chances of a major complication. The initial fields used should encompass the primary tumor, inguinal nodes, and pelvic nodes with an adequate margin and custom blocking should be employed to exclude tissues not at risk of containing disease from the treatment volume. Great care should be taken to ensure that the inferior border of the field extends below the lower limit of the tumor. Bolus may be necessary with megavoltage equipment to ensure that the tumor receives an adequate dose. A boost field, which is reduced in size, should be considered in the situations described next; this consists of two to four ports encompassing the original gross disease.

When external-beam radiation without chemotherapy is used, a dose of 60 to 65 Gy is recommended for the primary tumor. Fraction sizes should not exceed 180 to 200 cGy, because the data suggest larger fraction sizes result in a greater number of major complications.[69] The primary tumor and regional nodes are encompassed in the fields described earlier for the initial 45 Gy. A reduced volume is treated to spare the pelvic small bowel and rectosigmoid colon while gross disease is included for an additional 15 to 20 Gy. If concomitant chemotherapy and radiation are given, a modification in the dosage is often used; however, the optimal dose of radiation required, when combined with chemotherapy, has not yet been defined. Investigators at Wayne State University obtained good results after 30 Gy combined with abdominoperineal resection or local excision.[67] Patients with larger lesions had a higher incidence of residual tumor in the operative specimen, suggesting that 30 Gy may not be sufficient without local excision in the larger and/or higher-stage lesions. Papillon reports a local failure rate of 26% in 77 patients with T3 lesions treated with radiation alone to a dose of 63 to 68 Gy. When chemotherapy was added to the same radiation scheme in a second group of 70 patients with T3 lesions, the local failure rate decreased to 13%.[54] Other studies showed that doses of 50 to over 60 Gy combined with chemotherapy resulted in excellent local control without excision or excessive complications.[34, 69] Therefore, we currently recommend that the primary tumor receive a minimum of 50 Gy when concomitant therapy is employed. Higher doses (54 to 60 Gy) may be necessary for cure and should be considered for patients who have larger (over 4 cm) lesions at the time of diagnosis or residual disease after receiving the initial 50 Gy, before proceeding to abdominoperineal resection.

Conclusions

Substantial progress has been made in the treatment of anal canal carcinoma toward the goals of uncomplicated cure and preservation of anal function. However, many unresolved issues remain. The basic question of whether surgery alone, radiation alone, or combined modality therapy is superior treatment is unlikely to be answered in a randomized trial, because patients will be unlikely to participate in studies in which one or more options offer a chance to avoid colostomy. A comparison of the published series suggests that for small and moderately sized lesions, modern radiotherapy alone or combined modality therapy (chemoradiotherapy) can result in survival rates similar to those reported following radical surgery. Furthermore, it appears that local control, survival, and complication rates are similar in patients treated with radiation alone versus radiation combined with 5FU and mitomycin C. The series from the Princess Margaret Hospital does provide a historical comparison of radiotherapy to combined modality therapy from within a single institution.[69] Although survival rates, cause-specific survival rates, and complications for the two groups were similar, the colostomy-free survival rate was superior in the combined modality group. Again, the limitations of a nonrandomized trial prevent definitive conclusions.

Even though formal clinical trials are lacking, the available data support the use of radiotherapy alone or in combination with chemotherapy as the initial treatment of epidermoid cancer of the anus, which would preserve anal function in the majority of patients. Radical surgery should be held in reserve for patients with residual or recurrent carcinoma. However, a number of questions still need to be addressed. For example, some investigators advocate combined modality therapy as the only standard of care. However, there is no compelling evidence to support the superiority of this treatment to radiotherapy alone. This is particularly true in patients with early anal cancers for whom radiotherapy alone results in excellent local control. Perhaps radiotherapy alone is sufficient for small, early-stage lesions, whereas combined modality therapy should be reserved for the more advanced lesions. This question needs to be addressed

in a randomized trial. Other questions that need to be addressed include the optimal radiation techniques and the radiation doses, alone and in combination with chemotherapy, that are sufficient to control disease. The number of chemotherapeutic drugs and the dose necessary in combined modality therapy need to be studied, along with the related toxicities. Currently the RTOG is conducting a randomized prospective trial to determine whether mitomycin C represents an important component of the combined modality program. Clinical trials are under way in Europe to answer the question of whether radiotherapy or combined modality therapy is superior. All these trials are made difficult by the relative rarity of this tumor.

EDITORIAL COMMENT

The value of radiotherapy combined with chemotherapy is well established for epidermoid carcinoma of the anal canal. Radiotherapy is effective, at least for palliation, for the treatment of recurrent or residual disease, particularly in the pelvis and perineum. The effectiveness of multidrug chemotherapy as an adjuvant treatment for rectal carcinoma is as yet unclear and is disappointing in the treatment of recurrent and/or metastatic disease. The role of radiotherapy to the pelvis as adjuvant therapy has not been precisely determined, but the evidence presented in this chapter suggests that it is beneficial in lowering recurrence rates and may even affect long-term survival. There is debate as to the timing of radiotherapy: Should it be given preoperatively or after operation, or both? The long-term complications from modern radiotherapy have not yet been well evaluated.

In view of the data available and the many unanswered questions regarding radiotherapy, we have empirically adopted a protocol of utilizing postoperative radiotherapy. We can, therefore, eliminate patients with superficial lesions who are at low risk and restrict our treatment to those who have a high probability of recurrence: patients with many lymph nodes involved by tumor, microinvasion of nerves, lymph channels and capillaries; and patients with mucinous tumors. By this selection, only patients at high risk are subjected to the possible hazards of radiation enteritis or cystitis. The risk of radiation enteritis may also be reduced by elevating the small bowel from the pelvis by an omental flap or synthetic mesh.

REFERENCES

1. Symonds CJ. Cancer of rectum: Excision after application of radium. Proc R Soc Med 1914;7,(part 1):152.
2. Papillon J. New prospects in the conservative treatment of rectal cancer. Dis Colon Rectum 1984;127(11):695–700.
3. Sischy B, Hinson EJ, Wilkinson DR. Definitive radiation therapy for selected cancers of the rectum. Br J Surg 1988;75:901–903.
4. Morson BC, Path MC, Bussey HJR. Surgical pathology of rectal cancer in relation to adjuvant radiotherapy. Br J Radiol 1967;40:161–165.
5. Rich T, Gunderson LL, Lew R, et al. Patterns of recurrence of rectal cancer after potentially curative surgery. Cancer 1983;52:1317–1329.
6. Tepper JE. Reflections in rectosigmoid: Retro-peritoneal vs. intra-peritoneal. Int J Radiat Oncol Biol Phys 1988;14:1043–1046.
7. McDermott FT, Hughes ES, Pihl E, et al. Local recurrence after potentially curative resection for rectal cancer in a series of 1008 patients. Br J Surg 1985;72:34–37.
8. Philipshen SJ, Heilweil M, Quan SH, et al. Patterns of pelvic recurrence following definitive resections of rectal cancer. Cancer 1984;53:1354–1362.
9. Moossa AR, Ree PC, Marks JE, et al. Factors influencing local recurrence after abdominoperineal resection for cancer of the rectum and rectosigmoid. Br J Surg 1975;62:727–730.
10. Adloff M, Arnaud JP, Schloegel M, Thibaud D, et al. Factors influencing local recurrence after abdominoperineal resection of cancer of the rectum. Dis Colon Rectum 1985;28:413–415.
11. Stockholm Rectal Cancer Study Group. Preoperative short-term radiation therapy in operable rectal carcinoma. Cancer 1990;66:49–55.
12. Higgins GA, Humphrey EW, Dwight RW, et al. Preoperative radiation and surgery for cancer of the rectum. Veterans Administration Surgical Oncology Group Trial II. Cancer 1986;58:352–359.
13. Gerard A, Buyse M, Nordlinger B, et al. Preoperative radiotherapy as adjuvant treatment in rectal cancer. Ann Surg 1988;208:606–614.
14. Balslev JB, Pedersen M, Teglbjaerg PS, et al. Postoperative radiotherapy in Dukes' B and C carcinoma of the rectum and rectosigmoid. A randomized multicenter study. Cancer 1986;58:22–28.
15. Sause WT, Martz KL, Noyes D, et al. RTOG-81-15 ECOG-83-23 evaluation of preoperative radiation therapy in operable rectal carcinoma. Int J Radiat Oncol Biol Phys 1990;19(Suppl 1):179.
16. Pahlman L, Glimelius B. Pre- or postoperative radiotherapy in rectal and rectosigmoid carcinoma. Report from a randomized multicenter trial. Ann Surg 1990;211:187–194.
17. Boulis-Wassif S, Gerard A, Loygue J, et al. Final results of a randomized trial on the treatment of rectal cancer with preoperative radiotherapy alone or in combination with 5-fluorouracil,

followed by radical surgery. Trial of the European Organization on Research and Treatment of Cancer Gastrointestinal Tract Cancer Cooperative Group. Cancer 1984;53:1811–1818.

18. Fisher B, Wolmark N, Rockette H, et al. Postoperative adjuvant chemotherapy or radiation therapy for rectal cancer: Results from NSABP protocol R-01. J Natl Cancer Inst 1988;80:21–29.

19. Gastrointestinal Tumor Study Group. Prolongation of the disease-free interval in surgically treated rectal carcinoma. N Engl J Med 1985;312(23):1294–1295.

20. Gastrointestinal Tumor Study Group. Survival after postoperative combination treatment of rectal cancer. N Engl J Med 1986;315:294–295.

21. Krook JE, Moertel CG, Gunderson LL, et al. Effective surgical adjuvant therapy for high-risk rectal carcinoma. N Engl J Med 1991;324:709–713.

22. Gastrointestinal Tumor Study Group (GITSG). Radiation therapy and 5-fluorouracil (5-FU) with or without MeCCNU for the treatment of patients with surgically adjuvant adenocarcinoma of the rectum. Proc ASCO 1990;9:106.

23. Stevens KR, Allen CV, Fletcher WS. Preoperative radiotherapy for adenocarcinoma of the rectosigmoid. Cancer 1976;37:2866–2874.

24. Fortier GA, Krochak RJ, Kim JA, Constable WC. Dose response to preoperative irradiation in rectal cancer: Implications for local control and complications associated with sphincter-sparing surgery and abdominoperineal resection. Int J Radiat Oncol Biol Phys 1986;12:1559–1563.

25. Laurie JA, Moertel CG, Fleming TR, et al. Surgical adjuvant therapy of large-bowel carcinoma: An evaluation of levamisole and the combination of levamisole and fluorouracil. J Clin Oncol 1989;7(10):1447–1456.

26. Moertel CG, Fleming TR, MacDonald JS, et al. Levamisole and fluorouracil for adjuvant therapy of resected colon carcinoma. N Engl J Med 1990;322:352–358.

27. Brizel HE, Tepperman BS. Postoperative adjuvant irradiation for adenocarcinoma of the rectum and sigmoid. Am J Clin Oncol 1984;7:679–685.

28. Wang CC, Schulz MD. The role of radiation therapy in the management of carcinoma of the sigmoid, rectosigmoid, and rectum. Radiology 1962;79:1–5.

29. Ghossein NA, Samala EC, Alpert S, et al. Elective postoperative radiotherapy after incomplete resection of colorectal cancer. Dis Colon Rectum 1981;24:252–256.

30. Allee PE, Gunderson LL, Munzenrider JE. Postoperative radiation therapy for residual colorectal carcinoma. Int J Radiat Oncol Biol Phys 1981;7:1208.

31. Rominger CJ, Gelber RD, Gunderson LL, Conner N. Radiation therapy alone or in combination with chemotherapy in the treatment of residual or inoperable carcinoma of the rectum and rectosigmoid or pelvic recurrence following colorectal surgery. Am J Clin Oncol 1985;8:118–127.

32. Schild SE, Martenson JA, Gunderson LL, et al. Long-term survival and patterns of failure after postoperative radiation therapy for subtotally resected rectal adenocarcinoma. Int J Radiat Oncol Biol Phys 1989;16:459–463.

33. Tobin RL, Mohiuddin M. Preoperative radiation for cancer of the rectum with extrarectal fixation. Int J Radiat Oncol Biol Phys 1990;19(Suppl 1):180.

34. Sischy B. The use of radiation therapy combined with chemotherapy for the management of squamous cell carcinoma of the anus and marginally resectable adenocarcinoma of the rectum. Int J Radiat Oncol Biol Phys 1985;11:1587–1593.

35. Gunderson LL, Martin JK, Beart RW, et al. Intraoperative and external beam irradiation for locally advanced colorectal cancer. Ann Surg 1988;207(1):52.

36. Willet CG, Shellito PC, Wood WC. Intraoperative electron beam radiation therapy for locally advanced rectal and rectosigmoid carcinoma. Int J Radiat Oncol Biol Phys 1990;19(Suppl 1):214.

37. Cummings BJ. Radiation therapy and rectal carcinoma: The Princess Margaret Hospital experience. Br J Surg 1985;72(Suppl):64–66.

38. National Institutes of Health Consensus Statement. Adjuvant therapy for patients with colon and rectum cancer. NIH Consensus Development Conference 1990;8(4):179.

39. Gunderson LL, Sosin H, Levitt S. Adenocarcinoma of the colon: Areas of failure in a reoperation series (second or symptomatic looks). Int J Radiat Oncol Biol Phys 1985;11:731.

40. Russell AH, Pelton J, Reheis CE, et al. Adenocarcinoma of the proximal colon: An autopsy study with implications for new therapeutic strategies. Cancer 1985;56:1446.

41. Willett CG, Tepper JE, Cohen AM, et al. Local failure following curative resection of colonic adenocarcinoma. Int J Radiat Oncol Biol Phys 1984;10:645.

42. Cass AW, Million RR, Pfaff WW. Patterns of recurrence following surgery alone for adenocarcinoma of the colon and rectum. Cancer 1976;37:2861–2865.

43. Willett CG, Tepper JE, Cohen AM, et al. Failure patterns following curative resection of colonic carcinoma. Ann Surg 1984;200:685–690.

44. Duttenhaver JR, Hoskins RB, Gunderson LL, et al. Adjuvant postoperative radiation therapy in the management of adenocarcinoma of the colon. Cancer 1986;57:955–963.

45. Shehata WM, Meyer RL, Jazy FK, et al. Regional adjuvant irradiation for adenocarcinoma of the cecum. Int J Radiat Oncol Biol Phys 1987;13:843–846.

46. Wong CS, Harwood AR, Cummings BJ, et al. Postoperative local abdominal irradiation for cancer of the colon above the peritoneal reflection. Int J Radiat Oncol Biol Phys 1985;11:2067–2071.

47. Kopelson G. Adjuvant postoperative radiation therapy for colorectal carcinoma above the peritoneal reflection: I. Sigmoid colon. Cancer 1983;51:1593–1598.

48. Emami B, Pilepich M, Willett C, et al. Effect of preoperative irradiation on resectability of colorectal carcinomas. Int J Radiat Oncol Biol Phys 1982;8:1295–1299.

49. Peters RK, Mack TM. Patterns of anal carcinoma by gender and marital status in Los Angeles County. Br J Cancer 1983;48:629.

50. Bowman BM, Moertel CG, O'Connell MJ, et al. Carcinoma of the anal canal. A clinical and pathologic study of 188 cases. Cancer 1984;54:114.

51. Hardcastle JD, Bussey HJR. Results of surgical treatment of squamous cell carcinoma of the anal canal and anal margin seen at St. Mark's Hospital 1928–1966. Proc R Soc Med 1968;61:629.

52. Greenall MJ, Quan SHQ, Sterns MW, et al. Epidermoid cancer of the anal margin: Pathologic features, treatment and clinical results. Am J Surg 1985;149:95.

53. Eschwege F, Lasser P, Charry A, et al. Squamous cell carcinoma of the anal canal: Treatment by external beam irradiation. Radiother Oncol 1985;3:145.

54. Papillon J, Montbarbon JF. Epidermoid carcinoma of the anal canal: A series of 276 cases. Dis Colon Rectum 1987;30:324.

55. Cummings BJ. The place of radiation therapy in the treatment of carcinoma of the anal canal. Cancer Treat Rev 1982;9:125.

56. Cantril ST, Green JP, Schall GL, Schaup WC. Primary radiation in the treatment of anal carcinoma. Int J Radiat Oncol Biol Phys 1983;9:1271.

57. Doggett SW, Green JP, Cantril ST. Efficacy of radiation therapy alone for limited squamous cell carcinoma of the anal canal. Int J Radiat Oncol Biol Phys 1988;15:1069.

58. Papillon J. Rectal and Anal Cancers. Conservative Treatment by Irradiation—An Alternative to Radical Surgery. Berlin: Springer-Verlag, 1982.

59. Cummings BJ, Thomas GM, Keane TJ, et al. Primary radiation therapy in the treatment of anal canal carcinoma. Dis Colon Rectum 1982;25:778.

60. James RD, Pointon RS, Martin S. Local radiotherapy in the management of squamous carcinoma of the anus. Br J Surg 1985;72:282.

61. Salmon RJ, Zafrani B, Labib A, et al. Prognosis of cloacogenic and squamous cancers of the anal canal. Dis Colon Rectum 1986;29:336.

62. Salmon RJ, Fenton J, Asselain B, et al. Treatment of epidermoid and canal cancer. Am J Surg 1984;147:43.

63. Schlienger M, Krzisch C, Pene F, et al. Epidermoid carcinoma

of the anal canal treatment results and prognostic variables in a series of 242 cases. Int J Radiat Oncol Biol Phys 1989;17:1141.

64. Nigro ND, Vaitkevicius VK, Considine B. Combined therapy for cancer of the anal canal: A preliminary report. Dis Colon Rectum 1974;17:354.

65. Nigro ND, Seydel HG, Considine B, et al. Combined preoperative radiation and chemotherapy for squamous cell carcinoma of the anal canal. Cancer 1983;51:1826.

66. Nigro ND. An evaluation of combined therapy for squamous cell cancer of the anal canal. Dis Colon Rectum 1984;27:763.

67. Leichman L, Nigro N, Vaitkevicius VK, et al. Cancer of the anal canal. A model for preoperative adjuvant combined modality therapy. Am J Med 1985;78:211.

68. Michaelson RA, Magill GB, Quan SHQ, et al. Preoperative chemotherapy and radiation therapy in the management of anal epidermoid carcinoma. Cancer 1983;51:390.

69. Cummings B, Keane T, Thomas G, et al. Results and toxicity of the treatment of anal canal carcinoma by radiation therapy or radiation therapy and chemotherapy. Cancer 1984;54:2062.

70. Flam MS, John MJ, Mowry PA, et al. Definitive combined modality therapy of carcinoma of the anus: A report of 30 cases including the results of salvage therapy in patients with residual disease. Dis Colon Rectum 1987;30:495.

71. Sischy B, Doggett RLS, Krall JM, et al. Definitive irradiation and chemotherapy for radiosensitization in management of anal carcinoma: Interim report on radiation therapy oncology group study #8314. J Natl Cancer Inst 1989;81:850.

Vascular Diseases of the Colon

C H A P T E R 1 0

Ronald N. Kaleya
Scott J. Boley

During the past 3 decades, vascular diseases of the colon have been recognized as a major cause of morbidity, especially in the geriatric patient population. These diseases commonly become manifest either as ischemic insults or as bleeding. Diagnosis and treatment require an understanding of the differences in the pathology, physiology, and etiology as well as the natural history of the various forms of these diseases.

Ischemic disorders of the colon can result from interference with blood flow to the colon only, as in colonic ischemia, or from more global interruption of mesenteric blood flow, as in acute mesenteric ischemia. Colonic bleeding can be caused by an array of pathologic vascular diseases, such as colonic ectasias and hemangiomas (Fig. 10–1).

ISCHEMIC DISEASES OF THE COLON

Colonic ischemia (CI) is recognized as one of the most common colonic disorders of the elderly population. Although it was described more than a century ago, CI continues to be a difficult clinical problem because of the diverse outcomes associated with ischemic injury to the colon. Inadequate blood flow to all or part of the colon can produce a heterogeneous spectrum of clinical syndromes and pathologic findings, ranging from completely reversible intramural and submucosal hemorrhage to transmural colonic gangrene. Although some patients develop the severe complications of gangrene, perforation, ischemic stricture, and persistent colitis, most episodes of CI are noncatastrophic with transient symptoms and pathologic changes. CI isolated to the right colon is often a manifestation of acute mesenteric ischemia (AMI), which has a more fulminant course, and therefore is discussed separately.

Colonic Circulation

Reduction in blood flow to the colon may be a reflection of diverse pathologic conditions, ranging from inadequate systemic perfusion during cardiogenic shock to local morphologic or functional changes in the colonic vasculature. Atherosclerotic or thrombotic occlusion of the superior or inferior mesenteric artery, focal cholesterol or blood clot emboli, and vasculitides or spontaneous or drug-induced vasoconstriction can lead to insufficient blood flow and cellular ischemia. Regardless of the cause of the ischemic insult, the results are the same—a spectrum of bowel damage ranging from completely reversible functional alterations to total hemorrhagic necrosis of portions or all of the colon and/or small intestine.

The colon is normally protected from ischemia by its abundant collateral circulation. Communications among the celiac artery (CA), superior mesenteric artery (SMA), inferior mesenteric artery (IMA), and iliac arterial beds are numerous. Collateral flow around small arterial branches is made possible by the multiple arcades within the colonic mesentery, and SMA or IMA occlusions are bypassed via the arch of Riolan (meandering artery), the central anastomotic artery, and the marginal artery of Drummond. Additionally, within the bowel wall there is a network of communi-

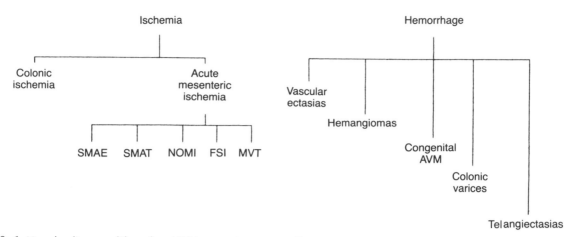

Figure 10–1. Vascular diseases of the colon. (AVM = arteriovenous malformation; SMAE = superior mesenteric artery embolism; SMAT = superior mesenteric artery thrombus; NOMI = nonocclusive mesenteric ischemia; FSI = focal segmental ischemia; MVT = mesenteric venous thrombus.)

cating submucosal vessels that can maintain viability of short segments of the colon where the extramural arterial supply has been compromised.

The colon has an inherently lower blood flow than the small intestine, and is therefore more sensitive to injury during acute reductions in blood flow. More importantly, experimental studies have shown that functional motor activity of the colon is accompanied by decreased blood flow. In addition, the pronounced effect of "straining" on systemic arterial and venous pressures in constipated patients, compared with normal individuals, provides indirect evidence that constipation may accentuate the adverse circulatory effects of defecation. Geber has postulated that "the combination of normally low blood flow and decreased blood flow during functional activity would seem to make the colon (1) rather unique among all areas of the body where increased motor activity is usually accompanied by an increased blood flow and (2) more susceptible to pathology."[1]

Colonic Ischemia

Before 1950 CI was considered to be synonymous with colonic infarction. However, during the 1950s, there were many reports of different forms of iatrogenic ischemic injury of the colon resulting from high ligation of the IMA in the course of aneurysmectomy or colectomy for colon carcinoma.[2, 3] In 1963, Bernstein and Bernstein termed the persistent colitis following iatrogenic ischemic injuries "ischemic ulcerative colitis."[4]

Also in 1963, on the basis of retrospective and experimental studies, Boley, Schwartz, and coworkers described the clinical, radiographic, and pathologic features of the previously unrecognized noniatrogenic,

noncatastrophic reversible forms of ischemic colonic injury.[5, 6] Later animal research by Boley and others, reported in 1965, confirmed that spontaneous CI could also result in irreversible pathologic colonic injury, specifically, stricture, gangrene, and chronic colitis. Subsequently in 1966, Marston and associates applied the term ischemic colitis to a group of 16 patients; 1 had colonic gangrene, 12 had ischemic strictures, and 3 suffered from reversible colitis.[8]

The term colonic ischemia is currently used to describe a general pathophysiologic process that causes a variety of clinical conditions. These conditions are classified as reversible or nonreversible and then further categorized as (1) reversible ischemic colopathy (submucosal or intramural hemorrhage), (2) reversible or transient ischemic colitis, (3) chronic ulcerative ischemic colitis, (4) ischemic colonic stricture, (5) colonic gangrene, or (6) fulminant universal colitis (Fig. 10–2).

Clinical Manifestations

Although for most patients colonic ischemic episodes have no identifiable cause, features of the clinical history that suggest CI include previous episodes of either CI or small bowel ischemia, or a precipitating cardiovascular event leading to a transient low-flow state. Up to 20% of the patients have an associated lesion, such as a partially obstructing colonic stricture, carcinoma, or diverticulitis, which not only obscures the diagnosis but may complicate treatment.

Patients with CI usually present with the sudden onset of mild abdominal pain, which is usually localized to the left lower quadrant and crampy in character. Less commonly, the pain is severe or can be described only retrospectively, if at all. An urgent desire to defecate frequently accompanies the pain and is fol-

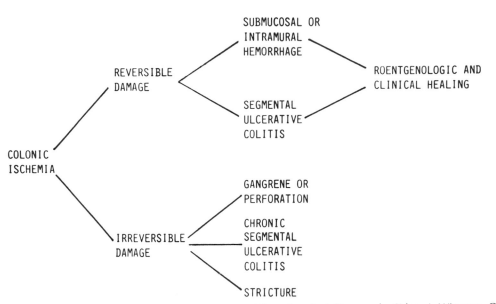

Figure 10–2. End results of colonic ischemia. (From Management of Gastrointestinal Diseases, by Sidney J. Winawer, Gower Medical Publishing, New York, NY, 1992.)

lowed within 24 hours by the passage of either bright red or maroon blood in the stool. The bleeding is usually not vigorous, and blood loss requiring transfusion is so rare that it should suggest an alternative diagnosis. Physical examination may reveal mild to severe abdominal tenderness elicited over the site of the involved segment of bowel.

Any part of the bowel may be affected, but the splenic flexure and descending and sigmoid colons are the most common sites (Fig. 10–3). Although specific etiologies, when identified, tend to affect defined areas of the colon, no prognostic implications can be derived from the distribution of the disease. Nonocclusive ischemic injuries usually involve the "watershed" areas of the colon—the splenic flexure and the junction of the sigmoid colon and rectum—whereas ligation of the inferior mesenteric artery produces changes in the sigmoid colon. Similarly, the length of bowel affected varies with the cause. For example, atheromatous emboli result in short-segment changes, and nonocclusive injuries usually involve much longer portions of the colon. Depending on the severity and duration of the ischemic insult, the patient may develop fever or leukocytosis. There is usually no acidemia, hypotension, or septic shock. In more severe ischemia, signs of peritonitis may develop.

The diagnosis of CI is usually made after the period of ischemia has passed and blood flow to the affected segment of colon has returned to normal. Many cases of transient or reversible ischemia are probably missed because a barium enema or colonoscopy is not performed early in the course of the disease. No study has provided an accurate determination of the incidence of CI.

In addition, several retrospective reviews of older clinical material have revealed many cases of CI that were either undiagnosed or misdiagnosed because the various clinical manifestations of this disorder were not recognized. Using the modern clinical radiologic and pathologic criteria for the diagnosis of CI, two retrospective reviews of 154 patients in whom colitis was identified after the age of 50 years revealed that 72% to 74% of the patients had CI.[9, 10] One half of these patients had previously been diagnosed as having inflammatory bowel disease.

Our experience with more than 250 cases of CI shows no significant sex predilection. Approximately 90% of patients with this disease are older than 60 years of age and have other evidence of systemic atherosclerotic disease. Oral contraceptives and cocaine, however, are responsible for an increasing number of cases in the younger population.[11, 12] Other associated causes are listed in Table 10–1. What finally triggers an ischemic episode remains conjectural in most instances; whether increased demand by colonic tissues is superimposed on an already marginal flow or whether flow itself is acutely diminished has yet to be ascertained.

Natural History

Despite similarities in the initial presentation of most episodes of CI, the outcome cannot be predicted at its onset unless the initial physical findings indicate an unequivocal intra-abdominal catastrophe. The ultimate course of an ischemic insult depends on many factors including (1) the cause, that is, occlusive or nonocclusive; (2) the caliber of an occluded vessel; (3) the

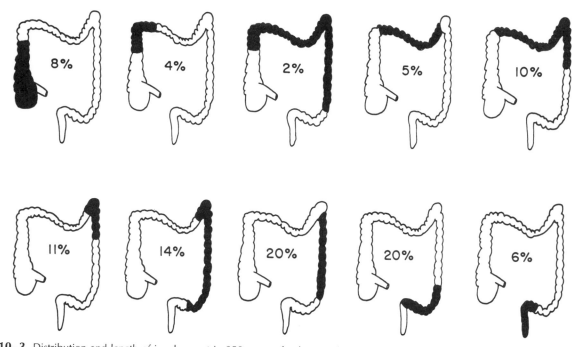

Figure 10–3. Distribution and length of involvement in 250 cases of colonic ischemia. (From Kaleya RN et al. Mesenteric ischemic disorders. In: Maingot R, ed. Abdominal Operations. 9th ed. East Norwalk, CT: Appleton & Lange, 1990.)

duration and degree of ischemia; (4) the rapidity of onset of the ischemia; (5) the condition of the collateral circulation; (6) the metabolic requirements of the affected bowel; (7) the presence and virulence of the bowel flora; and (8) the presence of associated conditions, such as colonic distention.

Most commonly, symptoms subside within 24 to 48 hours, and clinical, radiographic, and endoscopic evidence of healing is seen within 2 weeks. More severe, but still reversible, ischemic damage may take 1 to 6 months to resolve. In about one half of patients with CI the ischemic damage is too severe to heal, and the patients ultimately develop irreversible disease. Approximately two thirds of these patients follow a more protracted course, developing either chronic segmental ulcerative colitis or ischemic stricture. The remaining one third of patients develop signs and symptoms of an intra-abdominal catastrophe, such as gangrene with or without perforation, which becomes obvious within hours of the initial presentation.

Because the outcome of an episode of CI usually cannot be predicted, patients must be examined serially for evidence of peritonitis, rising temperature, elevation of the white blood count, or increasing severity of symptoms. Patients with diarrhea or bleeding persisting beyond the first 10 to 14 days usually progress to perforation or, less frequently, a protein-wasting enteropathy. Strictures may develop over weeks to months, and they may be asymptomatic or may produce progressive bowel obstruction. Some of the asymptomatic strictures resolve spontaneously over many months.

Diagnosis

Early and appropriate diagnosis of CI depends on serial radiographic and/or colonoscopic evaluation of the colon in addition to repeated clinical evaluations of the patient. The more severe cases of CI may be difficult to distinguish from AMI, whereas the less severe cases may have the same clinical signs that accompany acute and chronic idiopathic ulcerative colitis, Crohn's colitis, infectious colitis, and diverticulitis. A combination of radiographic, colonoscopic, and clinical findings may be necessary to establish the diagnosis of CI.

In patients with suspected CI, if abdominal radiographs are nonspecific, sigmoidoscopy is unrevealing, and no signs of peritonitis are observed, a gentle barium enema or colonoscopy should be performed in the unprepared bowel within 48 hours of the onset of symptoms. The most characteristic finding is "thumbprinting" or "pseudotumors" on the barium enema (Fig. 10–4), or hemorrhagic nodules or bullae during colonoscopy. Segmental distribution of these findings, with or without ulceration, suggests CI; however this diagnosis cannot be made conclusively on the basis of a single study. In fact, persistence of the thumbprints suggests a diagnosis other than CI, for example, lymphoma or amyloidosis.

Table 10–1. CAUSES OF COLONIC ISCHEMIA

Hemodynamic causes
    Cardiogenic shock
    Hemorrhagic shock
    Arrhythmia
Occlusive causes
    Inferior or superior mesenteric artery emboli, minor
      or major
    Cholesterol emboli syndrome, especially following
      angiography or angioplasty
    Inferior mesenteric artery thrombosis
Traumatic causes
    Blunt or penetrating trauma
    Ruptured ectopic pregnancy
    Aneurysmectomy
    Aortoiliac reconstruction
    Gynecologic operations
    Colonic bypass procedures
    Lumbar aortography
    Colectomy with high ligation of the inferior
      mesenteric artery
    Strangulated hernia
Drug-induced causes
    Digitalis
    Oral contraceptives
    Cocaine
Systemic causes
    Periarteritis nodosa
    Systemic lupus erythematosus
    Rheumatoid arthritis
    Necrotizing arteritis
    Thromboangiitis obliterans
    Polycythemia vera
    Parasitic infestation

Repeated radiographic or endoscopic examinations of the colon together with observation of the clinical course are necessary to confirm the diagnosis. Segmental colitis associated with a tumor or other potentially or partially obstructing lesions is also characteristic of ischemic disease. The radiographic findings of universal colonic involvement, loss of haustrations, or pseudopolyposis are more typical of chronic idiopathic ulcerative colitis, whereas skip lesions, linear ulcerations, or fistulas suggest Crohn's colitis.

It is imperative to obtain the diagnostic study early in the course of the disease, because the thumbprinting disappears within days, as the submucosal hemorrhages resorb or evacuate into the colon lumen when the overlying mucosa ulcerates and sloughs. A barium enema or colonoscopy performed 1 week after the initial study should reflect the evolution of the disease, either by the return to normal or by the replacement of the thumbprints with a segmental ulcerative colitis pattern. If colonoscopy is chosen as the initial study, caution is indicated. Distention of the bowel with air to pressures above 30 mm Hg diminishes colonic blood flow, shunts blood from the mucosa to the serosa, and causes a progressive decrease in arteriovenous oxygen extraction. Kozarek and colleagues showed that, during routine colonoscopy, intraluminal pressures exceed 30 mm Hg. Therefore, this modality can potentially induce or exacerbate CI.[13] This risk can be minimized by insufflation with carbon dioxide, which increases colonic blood flow at similar pressures.[14]

Biopsy specimens of nodules or bullae identified endoscopically early in the course of CI reveal submucosal hemorrhage, whereas biopsy specimens of the surrounding mucosa usually reveal nonspecific inflammatory changes.[15] Histologic evidence of mucosal infarction, although rare, is pathognomonic for ischemic injury. Angiography seldom shows significant vascular occlusion or other abnormalities and is not indicated in patients suspected of having CI, except for those in whom the disease is isolated to the right colon.

When the clinical presentation does not allow a clear distinction between CI and AMI, and plain films of the abdomen do not show the characteristic thumbprinting pattern of colonic ischemia, an "air enema" is performed by gently insufflating air into the colon under fluoroscopic observation. The submucosal edema and hemorrhages that produce the thumbprinting pattern of CI can be accentuated and identified in this manner (Fig. 10–5).

Once the provisional diagnosis of CI is made, a gentle barium enema is performed to determine the site and distribution of the disease and any associated lesion that predisposed the patient to the episode of ischemia, that is, carcinoma, stricture, or diverticulitis. If, however, thumbprinting is not observed and the air enema does not suggest the diagnosis of CI, a selective mesenteric angiogram is immediately performed to exclude the diagnosis of AMI. Because AMI progresses rapidly to an irreversible outcome and optimal diagnosis and treatment of this condition require angiography, the diagnosis of AMI must be established or excluded before a barium study is performed. Residual barium from a contrast study of the colon may obscure the mesenteric vessels and therefore preclude an adequate angiographic examination and intervention.

Management

GENERAL PRINCIPLES

Once the diagnosis of colonic ischemia has been established and if the physical examination does not suggest intestinal gangrene or perforation, the patient is treated expectantly. Parenteral fluids are administered, and the bowel is allowed to rest. Broad-spectrum antibiotics including therapy for gram-negative rods, enterococcus, and anaerobic organisms is prescribed, because antibiotic therapy reduces the length of bowel damaged by ischemia, although it does not prevent colonic infarction. Cardiac function is optimized to ensure adequate systemic perfusion. Medications that cause mesenteric vasoconstriction, for example, digitalis and vasopressors, should be withdrawn if possible. The

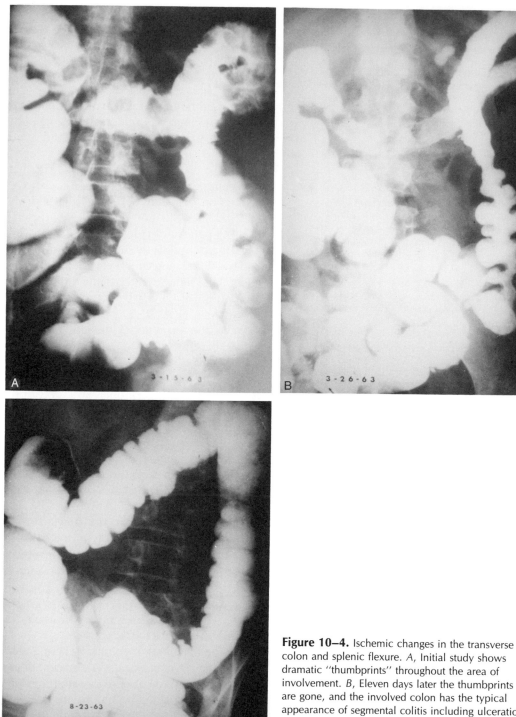

Figure 10–4. Ischemic changes in the transverse colon and splenic flexure. *A*, Initial study shows dramatic "thumbprints" throughout the area of involvement. *B*, Eleven days later the thumbprints are gone, and the involved colon has the typical appearance of segmental colitis including ulceration *(arrow)*. *C*, Five months after onset there is complete return to normal. The patient was asymptomatic 3 weeks after the onset of her illness. (From Boley SJ et al. Colonic ischemia: Reversible ischemic lesion. In: Vascular Disorders of the Intestines. New York: Appleton-Century-Crofts, 1971.)

urine output is monitored. Patients whose output is inadequate are rescuscitated with parenteral isotonic fluids. The clinically or radiographically distended colon is decompressed with a rectal tube, with or without gentle saline irrigations. In spite of their efficacy in ulcerative colitis, parenteral corticosteroids are contraindicated because they increase the possibility of perforation and secondary infection. Appropriate management of patients seen during or soon after the ischemic episode requires serial radiographic or endoscopic evaluations of the colon and continued clinical monitoring.

The white blood cell count, hemoglobin, and hematocrit values should be measured frequently during the acute episode. Although they are rarely needed, blood products should be administered when required. Potassium and magnesium must be monitored, as the levels of these electrolytes may be disturbed by the associated diarrhea and tissue necrosis. Serum levels of lactate dehydrogenase, creatine phosphokinase, serum glutamic-oxaloacetic transaminase, and serum glutamate-pyruvate transaminase may reflect the degree of bowel necrosis, but they are nonspecific. Parenteral nutrition is initiated early for patients having significant diarrhea. Narcotics should be withheld until it is clearly established that an intra-abdominal catastrophe is not present and that the patient is clinically improving. Cathartics are contraindicated. No attempt should be made to prepare the bowel for surgery in the acute phase, because this may precipitate perforation.

Increasing abdominal tenderness, guarding, rebound tenderness, rising temperature, and paralytic ileus during the period of observation are indicative of colonic infarction. Although not specific for CI, these signs dictate the need for expedient laparotomy for resection of the affected segment of colon. The serosal appearance of infarcted colon ranges from that of wet tissue paper to mottled, thickened, aperistaltic bowel. The resected specimen should be opened in the operating suite and examined for mucosal injury. If the margins are involved, additional colon should be removed until the margins appear grossly normal.

COURSE OF DISEASE

Despite similarities in the initial presentation of most episodes of CI, the outcome cannot be predicted at its onset unless the initial physical findings indicate an unequivocal intra-abdominal catastrophe. Most commonly, symptoms subside within 24 to 48 hours, and clinical, radiographic, and endoscopic evidence of healing is seen within 2 weeks (Table 10–2). More severe, but still reversible, ischemic damage may take 1 to 6 months to resolve. In approximately 50% of patients with CI, the ischemic damage is too severe to heal, and the patient ultimately develops irreversible disease.

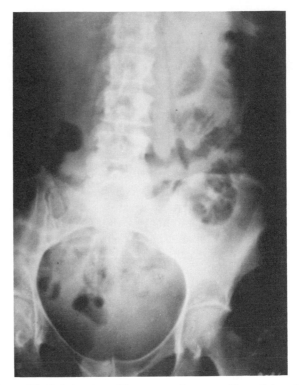

Figure 10–5. Ischemic colitis seen on air enema. (From Kaleya RN et al. Colonic ischemia. In: Perspectives in Colon and Rectal Surgery. St Louis: Quality Medical Publishing, 1990.)

Table 10–2. OUTCOME OF COLONIC ISCHEMIA AT MONTEFIORE MEDICAL CENTER

Reversible ischemia	44%
Persistent colitis	19%
Ischemic stricture	13%
Gangrene or perforation	19%
Undetermined outcome	5%

In approximately two thirds of these patients, CI follows a more protracted course, developing into either chronic segmental ulcerative colitis or ischemic stricture. In the remaining one third, signs and symptoms of an intra-abdominal catastrophe, such as gangrene with or without perforation, become obvious within hours of the initial presentation.

MANAGEMENT OF REVERSIBLE LESIONS

In patients with the mildest cases of CI, signs and symptoms of illness disappear within 24 to 48 hours, submucosal and intramural hemorrhages resorb, and complete clinical and radiographic resolution occurs within 1 to 2 weeks (Fig. 10–6). No further therapy is indicated for these patients. More severe ischemic insults result in necrosis of the overlying mucosa with ulceration and inflammation and the subsequent development of segmental ulcerative colitis. Varying amounts of mucosa may slough, and healing may ultimately occur over several months. Patients with such protracted healing may be clinically asymptomatic, even in the presence of persistent radiographic or endoscopic evidence of disease. These asymptomatic patients are placed on a high-residue diet and are followed frequently to confirm complete healing or the development of a stricture or persistent colitis. Recurrent episodes of bacteremia or sepsis in asymptomatic patients with segmental ulcerative colitis are usually caused by the diseased segment of bowel and are an indication for elective resection.

MANAGEMENT OF IRREVERSIBLE LESIONS

Patients with persistent diarrhea, rectal bleeding, protein-losing enteropathy, or recurrent sepsis for more than 10 to 14 days usually experience infarction with perforation. Hence, resection is indicated to prevent this complication. A GoLytely bowel preparation is administered along with oral and intravenous antibiotics prior to operation. At no time, however, should enemas be used to prepare the bowel.

Despite a normal serosal appearance, extensive mucosal injury may be present. The extent of resection should be guided by the distribution of disease as demonstrated on the preoperative studies, rather than by the serosal appearance at the time of operation. As in all resections for CI, the specimen must be opened immediately to ensure that the mucosa at the margins is viable. If the segmental ulcerative colitis involves the rectum at the time of operation, a mucous fistula or Hartmann procedure with an end-colostomy should be performed. The mucous fistula can be fashioned through diseased bowel, and in some cases, this segment heals sufficiently to allow subsequent restoration of bowel continuity. Local steroid enemas may be helpful in this setting; however parenteral steroids are again contraindicated. A simultaneous proctocolectomy is rarely indicated.

In patients with concurrent or recent myocardial infarctions or in patients with major medical contraindications to surgery, a trial of prolonged parenteral nutrition with concomitant intravenous antibiotic therapy may be considered as an alternative, albeit less than optimal, method of management.

MANAGEMENT OF THE LATE MANIFESTATIONS

CI may not become symptomatic during the acute episode but may nonetheless produce chronic segmental ulcerative colitis. Patients with this form of CI are frequently misdiagnosed if not seen during the acute episode. Barium enema studies may show a segmental colitis pattern, a stricture simulating a carcinoma, or even an area of pseudopolyposis (Fig. 10–7). At this stage of disease the clinical course is often indistinguishable from other causes of colitis or stenosis, unless the patient has been followed from the time of the acute episode. Crypt abscesses and pseudopolyposis, usually considered histologically diagnostic of chronic idiopathic ulcerative colitis, can be found with ischemic colitis. Regardless, the de novo occurrence of segmental ulcerative colitis or stricture in an elderly patient should be considered ischemic in origin and treated accordingly.

The natural history of segmental ulcerative colitis in the elderly patient is that of ischemic colitis: the involvement remains localized, the resection is not followed by recurrence, and the response to steroid therapy is usually poor. Patients with chronic segmental ulcerative colitis are initially managed symptomatically. Local steroid enemas may be helpful, but parenteral steroids should be avoided. In patients whose symptoms cannot be controlled by medication, segmental resection of the diseased bowel should be performed.

MANAGEMENT OF ISCHEMIC STRICTURES

Patients with asymptomatic segmental ulcerative colitis may develop a stenosis or stricture of the colon. Strictures that produce no symptoms should be observed. Some return to normal over 12 to 24 months

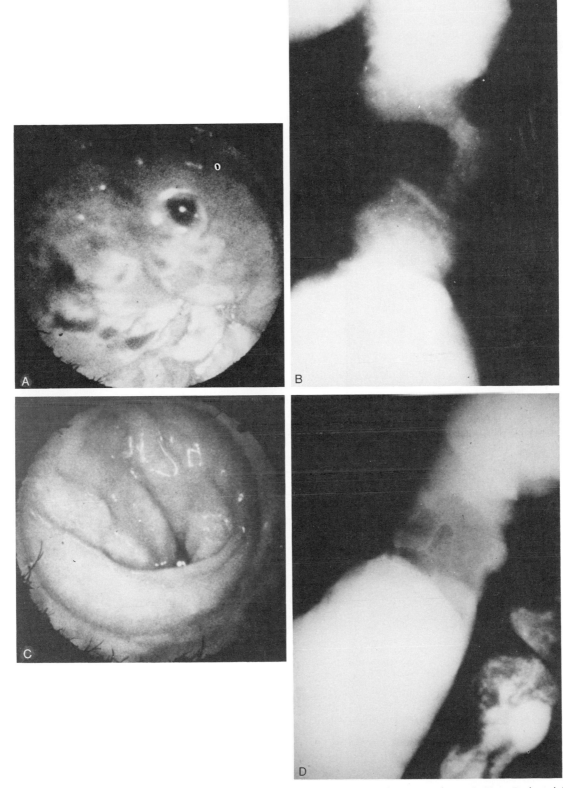

Figure 10–6. Ischemic lesion of the rectosigmoid. *A,* Sigmoidoscopic appearance of the colon at initial examination. Dark nodular mass is a submucosal hemorrhage, below which are ulcerations where other areas of hemorrhage have broken down. *B,* Initial barium enema showing typical thumbprints corresponding to submucosal hemorrhages seen at sigmoidoscopy. *C,* Three weeks later, there is complete healing of the rectal mucosa. *D,* Barium enema has returned to normal. (From Littman L, et al. Sigmoidoscopic diagnosis of reversible vascular occlusion of the colon. Dis Colon Rectum 1963;6:142.)

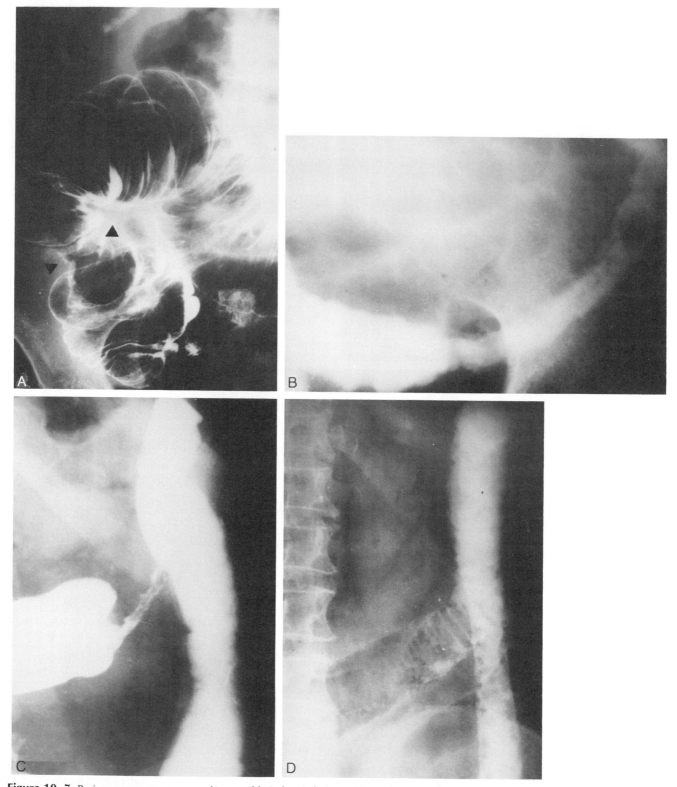

Figure 10–7. Barium enema appearance of irreversible ischemic lesions of the colon. *A,* Ischemic stricture *(between arrowheads)* with characteristics of carcinoma. *B,* Chronic segmental ulcerative colitis. *C,* Stricture. *D,* Pseudopolyposis. (*A,* From Brandt LJ et al. Simulation of colonic carcinoma by ischemia. Gastroenterology 1985;88:1137. *D,* From Boley SJ et al. Ischemic disorders of the intestines. In: Ravitch MM, ed. Current Problems in Surgery. Chicago: Year Book Medical Publishers, 1978.)

with no further therapy. If symptoms of obstruction develop, however, a segmental resection should be undertaken.

MANAGEMENT OF SPECIFIC CLINICAL PROBLEMS

Colonic Ischemia Complicating Abdominal Aortic Surgery. Mesenteric vascular reconstruction is not indicated in most cases of CI, but it may be required to prevent CI during and after aortic reconstruction. A small percentage of patients develop clinically symptomatic CI, but a higher incidence—up to 10%—is noted when routine colonoscopy is performed after abdominal aortic surgery.[16] The 1% to 2% of patients that develop clinical signs of CI following aortic replacement account for approximately 10% of the postoperative deaths.[17] Factors that contribute to the development of postoperative CI include rupture of the aneurysm, hypotension, operative trauma to the colon, hypoxemia, arrhythmias, prolonged aortic cross-clamp time, and improper management of the IMA during aneurysmectomy.

The most important aspect of management of CI following aortic surgery is its prevention. Collateral blood flow to the left colon after occlusion of the IMA comes from the SMA via the arch of Riolan (the meandering artery) or the marginal artery of Drummond and from the internal iliac arteries via the middle and inferior hemorrhoidal arteries (Fig. 10–8A). If these collateral pathways are intact, postoperative CI rarely occurs. Therefore, aortography to determine the patency of the celiac axis, SMA, IMA, and internal iliac artery, is advised prior to aneurysmectomy. The presence of a meandering artery does not itself allow safe ligation of the IMA, because the blood flow in the meandering artery frequently originates from the IMA and reconstitutes an obstructed SMA. Ligation of the IMA in the latter circumstance can be catastrophic, leading to infarction of the small and large bowels. Ligation of the IMA is safe only when angiography confirms that the blood flows in the meandering artery from the SMA to the IMA. Therefore, reimplantation of the IMA and revascularization of the SMA are required when the SMA is occluded or tightly stenosed and the IMA provides inflow to the meandering artery (Fig. 10–8B).

Occlusion of both hypogastric arteries on the preoperative arteriogram indicates that the rectal blood flow is dependent on collateral flow from the IMA or from the SMA via the meandering artery (Fig. 10–8C). In this circumstance, reconstitution of flow to one or both hypogastric arteries as well as to the IMA is desirable at the time of aneursymectomy.

The IMA can be excised with a small cuff of the aneurysm wall (a Carrell patch). At the conclusion of the aneurysmectomy and prosthetic graft placement, a partially occluding vascular clamp is provided across the anterior wall of the graft in a convenient position for reimplantation of the IMA. The patch is sewn in place with running polypropylene vascular sutures. The SMA can be revascularized, either by reimplanting it in the graft wall in a similar manner or by fashioning a lateral extension of the aortic graft with prosthetic material or reversed saphenous vein in an end-to-side fashion.

During the operation cross-clamp time should be minimized, and hypotension must be avoided. If a meandering artery is identified, it should be carefully preserved. Because the serosal appearance of the colon is not a reliable indicator of collateral blood flow, several methods have been suggested to determine the need for IMA reimplantation. Stump pressure in the transected IMA greater than 40 mm Hg or a ratio of mean IMA stump pressure to mean systemic blood pressure that is greater than 0.40 indicates adequate collateral circulation and reliably obviates the need to revascularize the IMA. Pulsatile Doppler ultrasound flow signals at the base of the mesentery and at the serosal surface of the colon with temporary IMA inflow occlusion also suggest that the IMA can be ligated safely without reimplantation.

Tonometric determination of intraluminal pH of the sigmoid colon has been used to identify inadequate collateral colonic blood flow during aneurysmectomy.[18, 19] A tonometric balloon is passed into the sigmoid colon per rectum before the aorta is cross-clamped. After the aorta is occluded, the intraluminal pH is determined. The intraluminal pH is a metabolic marker of tissue acidosis and reflects clinically significant ischemia, thus indicating the need for reimplantation of the IMA or revascularization of the SMA while the abdomen is open.

The difficulty of accurately assessing CI postoperatively and the significant mortality associated with it mandate that postoperative colonoscopy be performed in high-risk patients. Patients at high risk of developing postoperative CI following aortic reconstruction are those with ruptured abdominal aortic aneurysms, prolonged cross-clamping times, patent IMA on preoperative aortographies, nonpulsatile flows in the hypogastric arteries at operation, and postoperative diarrhea. In these patients colonoscopy is routinely performed within 2 to 3 days of the operation, and if CI is identified, therapy is begun before major complications develop.

Fulminating Universal Colitis. A rare fulminating form of CI involving all or most of the colon and rectum has been identified in a few patients. They have the sudden onset of toxic universal colitis evidenced by bleeding, fever, severe diarrhea, abdominal pain and tenderness, and often signs of peritonitis. The clinical course is rapidly progressive. The management

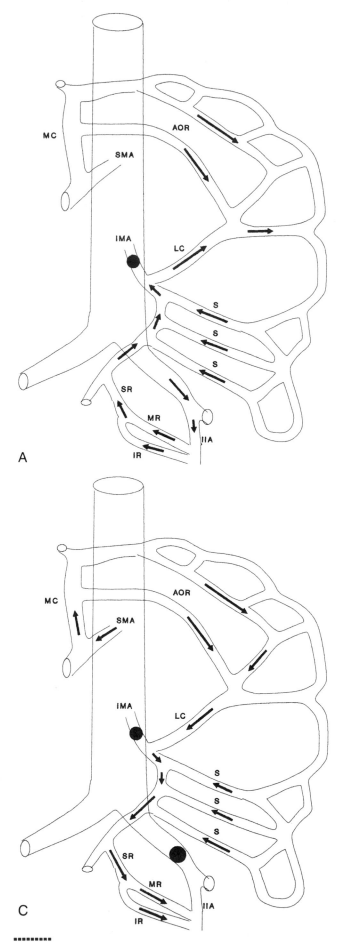

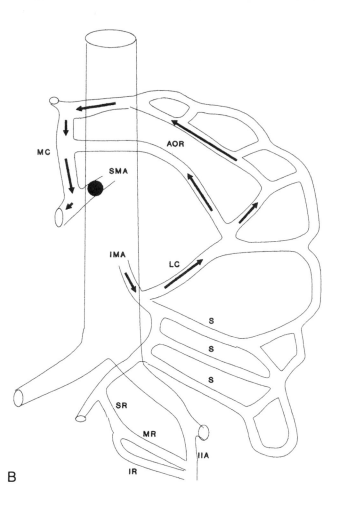

Figure 10–8. Collateral blood flow to the colon. *A,* Collateral blood flow from the marginal artery, arch of Riolan, and internal iliac artery via the inferior and middle rectal arteries to an occluded inferior mesenteric artery (IMA). *B,* Collateral blood flow from the IMA via the marginal artery and arch of Riolan to an occluded superior mesentery artery (SMA). *C,* The entire rectal blood flow dependent on collateral flow due to occlusion of both internal iliac arteries. The IMA is also occluded leaving the rectal flow dependent on collateral flow from the SMA via the arch of Riolan and marginal artery and then via the superior rectal vessel to the middle and inferior rectal arteries. (MC = middle colic artery; AOR = arch of Riolan; LC = left colic artery; S = sigmoid arteries; SR = superior rectal artery; MR = middle rectal artery; IR = inferior rectal artery; and IIA = internal iliac artery.)

of this condition is similar to that of other forms of fulminating colitis, and total abdominal colectomy with an ileostomy is usually required. A second-stage proctectomy has been necessary in some patients within 1 month of the original operation. The histologic appearance is a combination of ischemic changes and severe colitis.

Lesions Mimicking Colon Carcinoma. Patients with ischemic colitis can present with lesions that appear, on barium enema and colonoscopy, to be colon carcinoma. Colonoscopy may be able to distinguish the malignant lesions from those resulting from ischemic cicatrization, and it is advisable when an annular lesion is identified on barium enema. The treatment is local resection with immediate restoration of bowel continuity.

Colitis Associated with Colon Carcinoma. Acute colitis in patients with carcinoma of the colon has been recognized for many years.[20] The colitis is usually, but not always, proximal to the tumor and occurs with or without clinical obstruction. It is ischemic in origin and has the radiologic and endoscopic appearance of ischemic colitis. Clinically, patients may have symptoms of CI or symptoms related to the primary cancer, that is, chronic, crampy abdominal pain, bleeding, and acute colonic obstruction. In most cases, however, the predominant complaints relate to the ischemic insult—sudden onset of mild to moderate abdominal pain, fever, bloody diarrhea, and abdominal tenderness.

It is imperative that both the radiologist and the surgeon be aware of the frequent association of CI and colon cancer. The radiologist must exclude cancer in every case of CI, and the surgeon should examine any colon resected for cancer to exclude the presence of an ischemic process in the area of the anastomosis, because ischemia at the anastomosis may lead to a stricture or a leak.

Colonic Ischemia as a Manifestation of Acute Mesenteric Ischemia

CI localized to the right side of the colon may be the initial manifestation of interference with the SMA circulation. If a thumbprinting pattern or colonoscopy reveals CI isolated to the right colon, we consider this an indication for selective mesenteric angiography before the patient's discharge from the hospital in order to exclude the diagnosis of some form of AMI. AMI is a spectrum of disorders affecting the SMA blood flow, including superior mesenteric arterial embolus (SMAE), nonocclusive mesenteric ischemia (NOMI), superior mesenteric arterial thrombosis (SMAT), and mesenteric venous thrombosis (MVT). We have seen three patients who presented with right-sided CI and developed small bowel ischemia within 1 month. All

had advanced atherosclerotic disease involving the SMA.

In part because of an absolute rise in the incidence of this family of diseases but also because of a familiarity with the syndromes produced by vascular insufficiency of the intestines, AMI has been diagnosed increasingly in the past 30 years. The higher incidence has been attributed to the aging of the population, as AMI occurs predominantly—although not exclusively—in geriatric patients, especially those with significant cardiovascular and systemic disorders. Similarly, the widespread use of coronary and surgical intensive care units and other extraordinary means of cardiopulmonary support has salvaged patients who otherwise would have died rapidly of cardiovascular conditions, only to permit them to develop AMI as a later consequence of the primary disease.

The exact incidence of AMI is difficult to determine, but as the number of elderly individuals in the population grows, disorders affecting the mesenteric circulation will continue to grow. In our large metropolitan medical center, AMI is responsible for approximately 0.1% of all admissions.

There has been a changing distribution of causes of AMI over the past 50 years (Fig. 10–9). Acute MVT was believed to be the major cause of AMI in the early studies; for example, in 1926 Cokkinis reported that 60% of his patients presenting with AMI had MVT.[21] However, after Ende described the nonocclusive form of AMI in 1958, it was recognized that many patients considered to have MVT before Ende's report were, in actuality, suffering from NOMI.[22] This observation was reflected in Jackson's report in 1963, in which MVT accounted for only 25% of the cases of AMI.[23] As the diagnosis of NOMI by angiography became standard, the incidence of MVT fell to under 10% by 1973,[24] and to under 5% at our institution by 1983.

In most of the more recent series, SMAE and NOMI were responsible for 70% to 80% of cases of AMI. We have noted a decline in the incidence of nonocclusive ischemia, possibly a result of the increase of systemic vasodilators, such as the calcium channel blocking agents and nitrates, in coronary intensive care units. In addition, the more common employment of left ventricular assist devices in the treatment of cardiogenic shock has decreased the period of profound hypotension associated with left ventricular failure and has presumably attenuated its effect on the mesenteric circulation.

Acute Mesenteric Ischemia

Emboli to the SMA are responsible for 40% to 50% of episodes of AMI. The emboli usually originate from

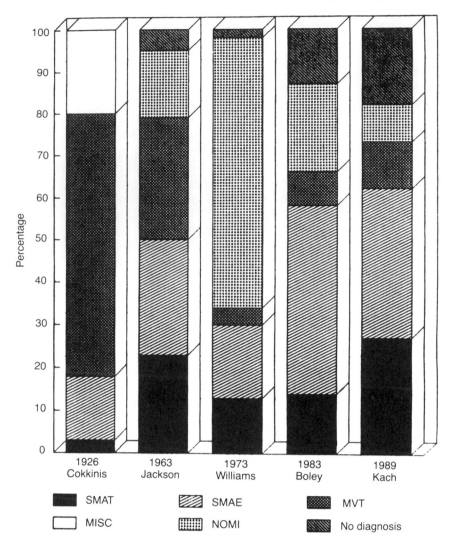

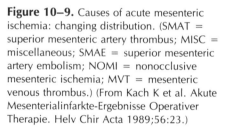

Figure 10–9. Causes of acute mesenteric ischemia: changing distribution. (SMAT = superior mesenteric artery thrombus; MISC = miscellaneous; SMAE = superior mesenteric artery embolism; NOMI = nonocclusive mesenteric ischemia; MVT = mesenteric venous thrombus.) (From Kach K et al. Akute Mesenterialinfarkte-Ergebnisse Operativer Therapie. Helv Chir Acta 1989;56:23.)

a left atrial or ventricular mural thrombus. The thrombus embolizes after being dislodged or fragmented during a period of arrhythmia. Many patients with SMAE have a history of previous peripheral artery embolism, and approximately 20% have synchronous emboli in other arteries. Emboli to the SMA tend to lodge at points of normal anatomic narrowings, usually immediately distal to the origin of a major branch (Fig. 10–10). In 10% to 15% of patients the emboli lodge peripherally in branches of the SMA or in the SMA distal to the origin of the ileocolic artery. The embolus may completely occlude the arterial lumen, but more commonly it only partially occludes the vessel. After a period of partial occlusion and diminution of blood flow distal to the embolus, vasoconstriction develops in arteries both proximal and distal to the embolus (Fig. 10–11), and this vasoconstriction can impair collateral blood flow to the SMA and its branches distal to the embolus, exacerbating the ischemic insult.

Nonocclusive mesenteric ischemia causes 20% to 30% of episodes of AMI and is thought to result from splanchnic vasoconstriction initiated by a period of decreased cardiac output associated with hypotension caused by arrhythmias, cardiogenic shock, hypovolemic shock, or vasoactive medications. The vasoconstriction may persist even after the precipitating cause has been eliminated or corrected. Predisposing factors for NOMI include acute myocardial infarction, congestive heart failure, aortic insufficiency, hepatic diseases, renal diseases—especially in patients requiring hemodialysis—and major cardiac or intra-abdominal operations. In addition, a more immediate precipitating cause, such as acute pulmonary edema, cardiac arrhythmia, or shock, is usually present, although the consequent intestinal ischemia may not become manifest until hours or days later.

SMAT occurs at areas of severe atherosclerotic narrowing, most often at the origin of the SMA (see Fig. 10–10). The acute ischemic episode is commonly superimposed on chronic mesenteric ischemia; hence

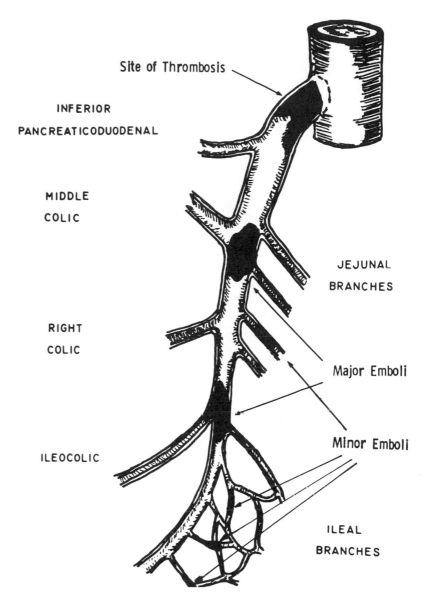

Site of Thrombosis

INFERIOR
PANCREATICODUODENAL

MIDDLE
COLIC

RIGHT
COLIC

ILEOCOLIC

JEJUNAL
BRANCHES

Major Emboli

Minor Emboli

ILEAL
BRANCHES

Figure 10–10. Common sites of superior mesenteric artery (SMA) emboli. Emboli distal to the iliocolic branch or in segmental branches are considered minor emboli. All others are major emboli. Thrombosis usually occurs near the origin of the SMA. (From Kaleya RN et al. Mesenteric ischemic disorders. In: Maingot R, ed. Abdominal Operations. 9th ed. East Norwalk: Appleton & Lange, 1990.)

approximately 20% to 50% of these patients have a history of abdominal pain with or without evidence of malabsorption and weight loss during the weeks to months preceding the acute episode. Additionally, most patients with SMAT have severe and diffuse atherosclerosis with a prior history of coronary, cerebrovascular, or peripheral arterial insufficiency.

Pathophysiology of Mesenteric Vasoconstriction

Collateral pathways open immediately on occlusion of a major vessel in response to arterial hypotension distal to the obstruction. Increased blood flow through the collateral pathways continues as long as the pressure in the vascular bed distal to the obstruction remains below systemic pressure. If, however, vasoconstriction develops in the distal arterial bed, the arterial pressure rises owing to increased resistance, which ultimately impairs collateral flow to the dependent segment.

Despite the adequate collateral vasculature in most patients, acute interruption or diminution of blood flow in the mesenteric circulation caused by emboli or hypotension results in intestinal ischemia secondary to persistent vasospasm. A decrease in SMA flow initially produces local mesenteric vascular responses that tend to maintain intestinal blood flow, but if the diminished flow is prolonged, active vasoconstriction develops, which may persist even after the primary cause of decreased flow is corrected. Boley and associates have shown that following an acute 50% reduction in SMA blood flow in anesthetized dogs, the mesenteric arterial pressure (MesAP) in the peripheral mesenteric arteries fell to 49% of mean control values.[25] When the SMA

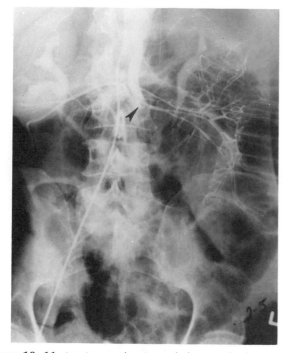

Figure 10–11. Arteriogram showing embolus completely occluding the SMA *(large arrowhead)* with associated vasospasm *(small arrowheads)* occluding blood flow. (From Brandt LJ et al. Ischemic intestinal syndromes. In: McLean LD, ed. Advances in Surgery. Chicago: Year Book Medical Publishers, 1981.)

flow was maintained at 50% of normal, the MesAP returned to control values in 1 to 6 hours while the celiac flow, which had initially increased, fell to control levels. The increased vascular resistance caused by vasoconstriction ultimately resulted in decreased collateral perfusion from the celiac and inferior mesenteric systems. If the flow restrictor was removed from the SMA as soon as the MesAP rose to control values, the flow through the SMA also returned to normal. However, if the SMA occlusion was maintained for 30 to 240 minutes after the MesAP had returned to control levels, the flow in the SMA never returned to normal. It remained at 30% to 50% of the control value because of persistent arterial vasoconstriction, despite the removal of the SMA flow restrictor. This decreased flow continued for up to 5 hours of observation but could be corrected by direct infusion of papaverine into the SMA. In this manner, mesenteric vasoconstriction plays a significant role in the development of ischemia, in both the acute occlusive and the nonocclusive arterial forms of mesenteric ischemia.

When papaverine was infused during the 50% flow restriction, the MesAP remained low throughout 4 hours of observation, and the SMA flow returned to normal on release of the obstruction. On the basis of these observations, intra-arterial papaverine infusions are recommended for the management of both the occlusive and the nonocclusive forms of AMI. Intra-arterial papaverine is also recommended for some patients with the venous forms of mesenteric vascular diseases because venous thrombosis has experimentally been shown to cause arterial spasm.[26]

It had been presumed that in NOMI the bowel injury occurs during the period of diminished cardiac output, or hypotension, and that with correction of these cardiovascular problems the mesenteric blood flow returns to normal. This simplistic concept is contradicted by operative findings of persistent bowel ischemia when no arterial or venous obstruction is found and cardiac function has been optimized. In patients with NOMI the onset of abdominal signs and symptoms caused by intestinal ischemia may actually begin after the correction of the primary systemic problem. This paradox can be explained by the experimental observations that an episode of low mesenteric flow, as short as 2 hours in duration, can produce mesenteric ischemia as a result of vasoconstriction and that the vasoconstriction and ischemia may continue after correction of the initiating problem.

The end result of an ischemic episode depends on many factors. Thus the extent of intestinal injury is a function of (1) the state of the systemic circulation, (2) the degree of functional or anatomic compromise, (3) the number and caliber of vessels affected, (4) the response of the vascular bed to diminished perfusion, (5) the nature and capacity of the collateral circulation to supply the needs of the dependent segment of bowel, (6) the duration of the insult, and (7) the metabolic needs of the dependent segment as dictated by its function and bacterial population.

Clinical Manifestations

Early identification of AMI requires a high index of suspicion by the clinician in patients who have significant risk factors associated with this disease. AMI occurs most frequently in patients over 50 years of age who have chronic heart disease and long-standing congestive heart failure, especially those poorly controlled with diuretics or digitalis. Cardiac arrhythmias, commonly atrial fibrillation, recent myocardial infarction, and hypotension due to burns, pancreatitis, or hemorrhage all predispose patients to AMI. Previous or synchronous arterial emboli increase the likelihood of an acute SMAE. The development of sudden abdominal pain in a patient with any or all of these risk factors should suggest the diagnosis of AMI.

A history of abdominal pain, often after meals, for weeks to months before the onset of an acute episode has been considered a frequent finding in patients with AMI. This misconception was based on reports by Dunphy in 1936[27] and again by Mavor and colleagues in 1962,[28] who found that 50% of patients with AMI had antecedent abdominal symptoms. The prodromal abdominal pain occurred, however, only in patients with acute SMAT superimposed on chronic mesenteric ischemia—the cause of AMI in less than 25% of patients. Thus postprandial abdominal pain in the weeks to months preceding the acute onset of severe abdominal pain occurs in only a small percentage of patients with AMI.

Acute abdominal pain varying in severity, nature, and location occurs in 75% to 98% of patients with intestinal ischemia. Characteristically, in early AMI the pain experienced by the patient is markedly out of proportion to the physical findings. Therefore sudden, severe abdominal pain accompanied by rapid and often forceful bowel evacuation, especially with minimal or no abdominal signs, strongly suggests an acute arterial occlusion in the mesenteric circulation.

Unexplained abdominal distention and gastrointestinal bleeding may be the only indications of acute intestinal ischemia, especially in nonocclusive disease, because pain is absent in up to 25% of these patients. Patients surviving cardiopulmonary resuscitation who develop culture-proven bacteremia and diarrhea without abdominal pain should be evaluated for NOMI.[29] Distention, although absent early in the course of mesenteric ischemia, is often the first sign of impending intestinal infarction. The stool contains occult blood in 75% of patients, and this bleeding may precede any other symptom of ischemia. Right-sided abdominal pain associated with the passage of bright red or maroon blood in the stool, although characteristic of CI, strongly suggests the diagnosis of AMI.

Although there are no abdominal findings early in the course of intestinal ischemia, as infarction develops, increasing tenderness, rebound tenderness, and muscle guarding reflect the progressive loss of intestinal viability and the presence of transmural gangrene. Significant abdominal findings strongly indicate infarcted bowel. Nausea, vomiting, hematochezia, hematemesis, massive abdominal distention, back pain, and shock are other late signs.

Diagnosis

Leukocytosis exceeding 15,000 cells/mm^3 occurs in approximately 75% of patients with AMI, whereas about 50% present with a metabolic acidemia. Elevations of serum amylase and phosphate as well as peritoneal fluid intestinal alkaline phosphatase and inorganic phosphate have been described, but the sensitivity and specificity of these markers of intestinal ischemia have not been established. Leukocytosis out of proportion to the clinical findings, elevated hemoglobin and hematocrit values, and blood-tinged peritoneal fluid, often with an elevated amylase content, are not specific for AMI but suggest advanced intestinal necrosis and sepsis.

Plain abdominal radiographs are usually normal in early mesenteric ischemia before infarction occurs. Late in the course of the disease, formless loops of small intestine or small intestinal "thumbprinting" can suggest the diagnosis of AMI. Isolated thumbprinting of the right colon may be the only indication of AMI. Even if colonoscopy reveals the hemorrhagic bullae characteristic of CI, the finding of CI confined to the right colon may be the result of decreased perfusion of the SMA rather than simple CI and should be treated as such.

Laparoscopy may be useful in patients whose clinical status precludes angiography.[30] However SMA blood flow decreases profoundly with intraperitoneal pressures exceeding 20 mm Hg, making laparoscopy potentially dangerous in the setting of suspected AMI.[31] Lower intraperitoneal pressures for brief periods, though, produce only minimal alterations in mesenteric perfusion. Laparoscopic examination of the bowel is limited to the serosal surface, making it unreliable for diagnosing early mucosal necrosis at a time when the serosa still appears relatively normal.

Duplex scanning has been of some value in identifying portal and superior MVT and, in a few patients, SMA occlusion. The flow in the SMA can be reproducibly determined by this method, but the wide range of normal SMA blood flow from 300 to 600 ml/min limits the value of this test in diagnosing ischemia.[32]

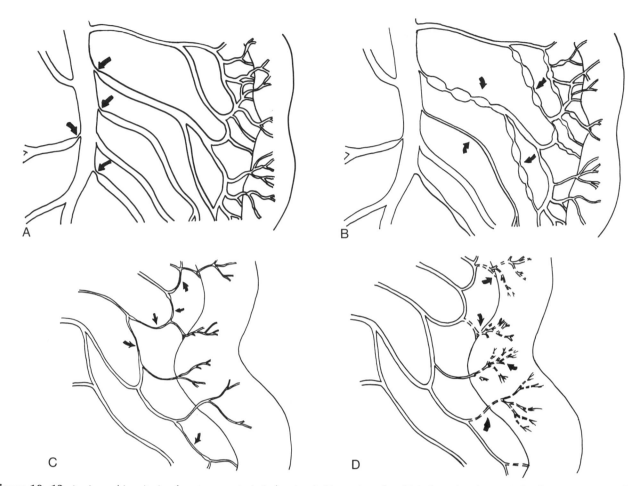

Figure 10–12. Angiographic criteria of acute mesenteric ischemia: *A,* Narrowing of multiple branches *(arrows),* *B,* Alternate spasm and dilatation of intestinal branches ("string of sausages" sign) *(arrows),* *C,* Spasm of arcades *(arrows),* *D,* Impaired filling of intramural vessels *(arrows).* (From Kaleya RN et al. Mesenteric vascular diseases. In: Maingot R, ed. Abdominal Operations. 9th ed. East Norwalk: Appleton & Lange, 1990.)

As the capabilities of this modality improve and clinical trials determine its sensitivity and specificity, it may become a reliable screening method for the detection of the occlusive forms of AMI. Computed tomography (CT) has also been utilized to identify arterial and venous thromboses as well as ischemic bowel but only in the late stages of the disease.

Historically, angiography was limited to identifying arterial occlusions by embolus or thrombosis. Currently, selective angiography is the mainstay of both the diagnosis and initial treatment of AMI.[33] On the basis of experimental and retrospective studies of patients undergoing abdominal angiography, Siegelman, Sprayregen, and Boley identified four reliable angiographic criteria for the diagnosis of mesenteric vasoconstriction: (1) narrowing of the origins of multiple branches of the SMA, (2) irregularity in the intestinal branches, (3) spasm of the arcades, and (4) impaired filling of intramural vessels (Fig. 10–12).[34]

Although mesenteric vasoconstriction occurs in hy-

potensive patients and in those with pancreatitis, its presence in patients with suspected intestinal ischemia who are not in shock, do not have pancreatitis, and are not receiving vasopressors is diagnostic of NOMI. Therefore, if angiography is performed sufficiently early in the disease, patients with occlusive and non-occlusive AMI can be identified before bowel infarction develops and before clinical and radiologic signs of infarction make the diagnosis of intestinal ischemia evident.

Management

GENERAL PRINCIPLES

Patients over 50 years of age who have any of the previously enumerated risk factors for AMI and who develop a sudden onset of abdominal pain that is severe enough to contact a physician and lasts for more than 2 hours should be suspected of having AMI. These patients should be managed according to an aggressive radiologic and surgical algorithm (Figs. 10–13 and 10–14). Less absolute indications for inclusion within this protocol include unexplained abdominal distention, colonoscopic evidence of isolated right-sided CI, or acidosis without an identifiable cause. Because diagnostic clinical or radiologic signs usually indicate irreversible intestinal injury, broad selection criteria are essential if early diagnosis and successful treatment are to be achieved. Some negative studies must be accepted in order to identify and salvage patients who do have AMI.

PREOPERATIVE MANAGEMENT

Initial treatment is directed toward resuscitation and correction of the predisposing or precipitating causes of the ischemia. Relief of acute congestive heart failure and correction of hypotension, hypovolemia, and cardiac arrhythmias must precede any diagnostic evaluation. Efforts to improve mesenteric blood flow will be futile if low cardiac output, hypovolemia, or hypotension persists. Frequently patients with AMI are septic with low systemic vascular resistance and sequestration of fluid into the "third space." Optimal cardiac performance can best be achieved under these circumstances with the aid of a Swan-Ganz catheter by using serial cardiac profiles to ensure maximal systemic perfusion. After resuscitation is accomplished, plain films of the abdomen are obtained. These films are taken not to establish the diagnosis of AMI but rather to exclude other identifiable causes of abdominal pain, for example, a perforated viscus with free intraperitoneal air. A normal plain film does not exclude AMI; ideally patients are studied before radiologic signs are present, as such findings indicate infarcted bowel. If no alternative diagnosis is made on the basis of the plain abdominal films, selective SMA angiography is performed immediately. On the basis of angiographic findings and the presence or absence of peritoneal signs, patients are treated according to the algorithms in Figures 10–13 and 10–14.

Even when the decision to operate has been made on clinical grounds, a preoperative angiogram should be obtained in order to manage the patient properly at celiotomy. Moreover, relief of mesenteric vasoconstriction is essential to correctly treating emboli and thromboses as well as the nonocclusive low-flow states. Intra-arterial infusion of papaverine through an angiography catheter placed percutaneously in the origin of the SMA is the recommended method of relieving mesenteric vasoconstriction before and after the operation. It is infused at a constant rate of 30 to 60 mg/hr by means of an infusion pump. Although almost all the papaverine infused into the mesenteric circulation is cleared during one passage through the liver, in some cases this dose may have systemic effects. Therefore the systemic arterial pressure and cardiac rate and rhythm must be monitored constantly during the papaverine infusion. The clinical and angiographic responses of the patient to the vasodilator therapy determine the duration of the papaverine infusion.

MANAGEMENT AT CELIOTOMY

Celiotomy is indicated in AMI to restore intestinal arterial flow after an embolus or thrombosis and/or to resect irreparably damaged bowel. Revascularization should precede evaluation of intestinal viability, because bowel that initially appears infarcted may show surprising recovery after adequate blood flow is restored.

After revascularization, intestinal viability can be assessed by several methods. Traditionally, the bowel is placed in warm, saline-soaked laparotomy pads and observed over a period of 10 to 20 minutes for return of normal color, peristalsis, and presence or absence of pulsations in the intestinal arteries. This clinical assessment is of limited accuracy, however, and a more sensitive and specific evaluation depends on technologic aids. Techniques that have been proposed include surface fluorescence,[35] perfusion fluorometry,[36] Doppler measurements of arterial flow,[37] electromyography,[38] surface temperature, serosal pH, surface oxygen consumption, and radioisotope uptake determinations. Only Doppler pulse determinations, fluorescence using an ultraviolet light after an intravenous injection of fluorescein, and perfusion fluorometry have gained wide clinical acceptance. Surface fluorescence increases the accuracy of differentiating viable from nonviable bowel; the equipment is inexpensive and the dye is safe, but the technique remains subjective. Perfusion fluorometry is more objective, allows repeated estimations, and is more accurate in general than surface fluorescence. However the equipment is expensive, and only small areas of the bowel can be evaluated at one time. Although Doppler probes are available in most operating rooms, this modality is again limited to examining small areas of the intestine. A practical solution is initial surface fluorescence, with perfusion fluorometry or Doppler examination being reserved for evaluating the equivocal areas when diffuse patchy involvement is seen or for evaluating the margins of unresected bowel.

Short segments of bowel that are nonviable or questionably viable after revascularization occurs are resected, and a primary anastomosis is performed. If extensive portions of the bowel are involved, only the clearly necrotic bowel is resected, and a planned reexploration (second look) is performed within 12 to 24 hours. The ends of the questionable bowel can simply be closed or a double ostomy performed. One decides to perform a second-look operation during the initial celiotomy if major portions or multiple segments of intestine are of questionable viability, and the second-

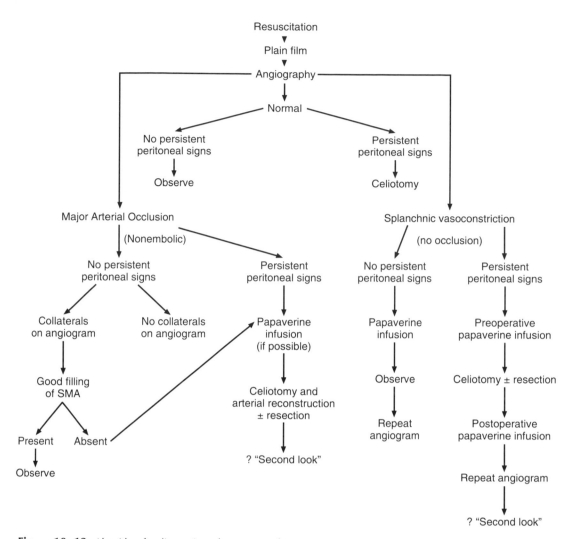

Figure 10–13. Algorithm for diagnosis and treatment of acute mesenteric ischemia (continues in Fig. 10–14).

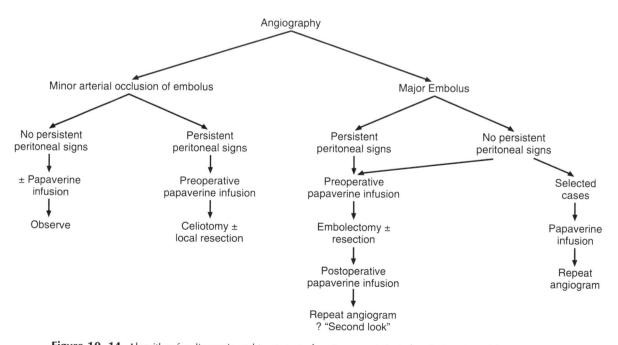

Figure 10–14. Algorithm for diagnosis and treatment of acute mesenteric ischemia (continued from Fig. 10–13).

look celiotomy must be done irrespective of the patient's subsequent clinical course. The purpose of the second-look celiotomy, as proposed by Shaw, is "not just to allow a clear definition between dead and live bowel to take place, but also to allow time for the institution of supportive measures which may render more of the bowel viable."[39] Such measures may include, among others, optimizing cardiac output, SMA infusion of papaverine, antibiotic therapy, and anticoagulant therapy.

If at celiotomy there is obvious infarction of all or most of the small bowel with or without a portion of the right colon, then the surgeon confronts a philosophical decision: whether to do anything at all. Resecting all of the involved bowel inevitably produces a patient with short-bowel syndrome with its attendant problems, and almost certainly in an older patient a commitment to life-long parenteral nutrition. A preoperative discussion with the patient and the patient's family concerning this problem is warranted so that an acceptable decision can be reached if this situation is encountered at surgery.

POSTOPERATIVE MANAGEMENT

The use of anticoagulants for management of AMI remains controversial. Heparin anticoagulation may cause intestinal, submucosal, or intraperitoneal hemorrhage, and except in the case of mesenteric venous thrombosis, we have not used it in the immediate postoperative period. However late thrombosis following embolectomy of arterial reconstruction occurs frequently enough that anticoagulation 48 hours postoperatively seems advisable. Some authors have advocated immediate anticoagulation in all patients, especially when a second look is required.

Both systemic and locally administered antibiotics have been shown to improve the survival of ischemic bowel.[40] For this reason, and because of the high incidence of positive blood cultures in patients with AMI, broad-spectrum systemic antibiotics are begun as soon as the diagnosis is entertained and are continued throughout the postoperative period as dictated by the findings at celiotomy.

MANAGEMENT OF SPECIFIC TYPES

Superior Mesenteric Artery Embolus. Upon identification of an SMAE at angiography, a papaverine infusion is begun through the catheter placed selectively in the origin of the SMA, proximal to the occlusion. The patient is then managed according to the algorithm in Figure 10–14, on the basis of the site of the embolus, the presence or absence of peritoneal signs, the extent of the collateral blood flow, and the degree of vasospasm in the vascular beds both proximal and distal to the embolus, as determined by an angiogram obtained after a selective intra-arterial bolus injection of 25 mg of tolazoline.

Minor emboli are those limited to the branches of the SMA or to the SMA distal to the origin of the ileocolic artery (see Fig. 10–10). Patients who have minor emboli and whose pain is relieved by the vasodilator therapy can be managed expectantly. However, patients with major emboli selected for nonoperative therapy must fulfill these criteria: They must have (1) significant contraindications to surgery, (2) no peritoneal signs, and (3) adequate perfusion of the vascular beds distal to the embolus following administration of a bolus of vasodilator into the SMA. Direct infusion of thrombolytic agents through selectively placed catheters has been employed successfully by others in a few patients, but this approach must still be considered experimental.

Embolectomy is always performed before assessing intestinal viability. The embolus is approached directly, or less optimally through a proximal arteriotomy (Fig. 10–15). The proximal SMA is exposed by drawing the transverse colon cephalad and anteriorly, as the small intestine is retracted inferiorly. The inferior leaf of the transverse mesocolon is incised, and the proximal SMA is dissected free between the pancreas and the fourth portion of the duodenum. The SMA is exposed for 2 to 3 cm proximal and distal to the origin of the middle colic artery. The SMA is palpated gently to determine the most distal extent of arterial pulsation, or the artery may be examined directly with a Doppler probe to identify the site of the embolus. Once the site of the embolus is found, the SMA and its branches are controlled proximally and distally with vessel loops or gentle vascular clamps. A longitudinal arteriotomy is made over the embolus or just proximal to it, and the embolus is removed; residual clots are flushed out of the artery by briefly releasing the vessel loops. A Fogarty balloon catheter is then passed proximally and distally to remove all remaining clots. The arteriotomy is closed with or without a vein patch.

Following embolectomy, bowel viability is determined. If no second look is planned, the papaverine infusion is continued for an additional 12 to 24 hours. An arteriogram is then obtained to exclude persistent vasospasm before the arterial catheter is removed. If a second look is performed, the infusion is continued through the second procedure and until no vasoconstriction is present on a follow-up angiogram.

Nonocclusive Mesenteric Ischemia. NOMI is diagnosed when the angiographic signs of mesenteric vasoconstriction are seen in a patient who has the clinical picture of mesenteric ischemia and is neither in shock nor receiving vasopressors. The angiographic findings may vary from the previously described local signs to a pruned appearance of the entire mesenteric vascu-

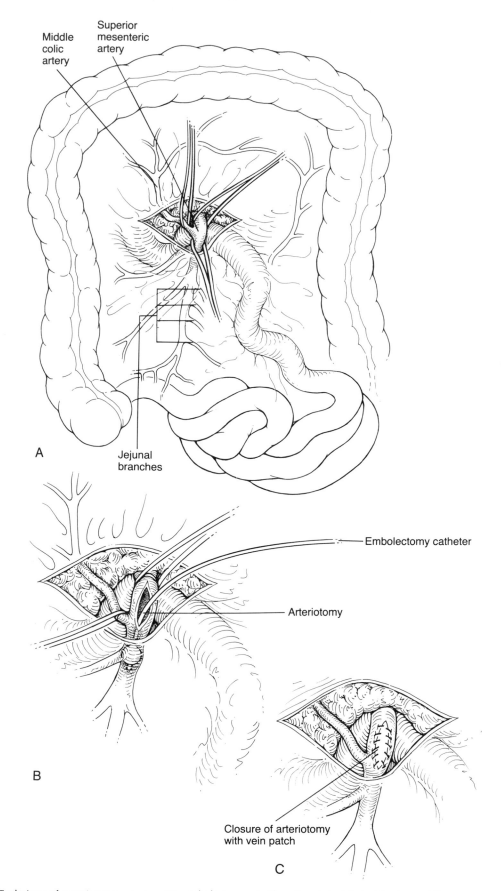

Figure 10–15. Technique of superior mesenteric artery embolectomy. *A*, The artery is isolated at the base of the mesentery over the site of the embolus. *B*, Longitudinal arteriotomy is made, and the vessel is cleared of debris. *C*, The arteriotomy is closed primarily or with a vein patch (shown). (From Boley SJ et al. An aggressive roentgenologic and surgical approach to acute mesenteric ischemia. In: Nyhus LM, ed. Surgery Annual. New York: Appleton-Century-Crofts, 1973.)

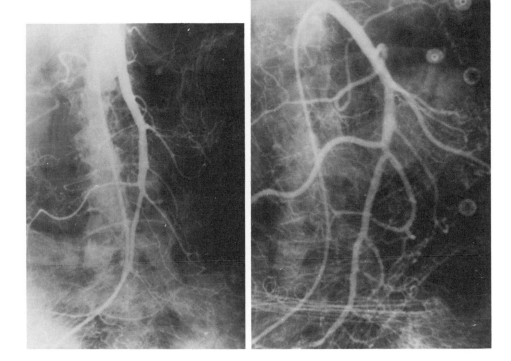

Figure 10–16. Patient with nonocclusive mesenteric ischemia managed with papaverine infusion for 3 days. *A*, Initial angiogram showing spasm of the main superior mesenteric artery, origins of branches, and intestinal arcades. *B*, Angiogram repeated after 36 hours of papaverine infusion. Study was obtained 30 minutes after papaverine was replaced with saline. At this time the patient's abdominal symptoms and signs were gone. (From Boley SJ et al. Acute mesenteric ischemia. In: Ravitch MM, ed. Current Problems in Surgery. Chicago: Year Book Medical Publishers, 1978.)

lature (Fig. 10–16). A selective SMA infusion of papaverine is begun in all patients with NOMI as soon as the diagnosis is made. In patients with persistent peritoneal signs, the infusion is continued during and after exploration. At operation, manipulation of the SMA is minimized. Overtly necrotic bowel is resected, and a primary anastomosis is performed only if no second look is planned. We believe it is preferable to leave bowel of questionable viability rather than to perform a massive enterectomy, because frequently the bowel improves with supportive measures or is demarcated more clearly by the time of the second look.

When a papaverine infusion is the primary treatment for NOMI, it is continued for approximately 24 hours, after which the infusion is changed to normal saline for 30 minutes prior to a repeat angiogram. On the basis of the clinical course of the patient and the presence or absence of vasoconstriction on the repeat angiogram, the infusion is either discontinued or maintained for an additional 24 hours. Angiography is repeated daily until there is no radiographic evidence of vasoconstriction (see Fig. 10–16) and the patient's clinical symptoms and signs are gone. Infusions have usually been discontinued after 24 hours but have been maintained for as long as 5 days.

When papaverine is used in conjunction with surgery for nonocclusive disease, a second-look operation is frequently necessary. In such cases the infusion is continued as previously described for second-look operations following embolectomy. The arterial catheter

is removed when no angiographic signs of vasoconstriction are seen 30 minutes after cessation of vasodilator therapy.

Acute Superior Mesenteric Artery Thrombosis. SMAT is most often identified on a flush aortogram showing complete occlusion of the SMA within 1 to 2 cm of its origin. Some filling of the SMA distal to the obstruction via collateral pathways is almost always present. Branches both proximal and distal to the obstruction may show local spasm or diffuse vasoconstriction. Differentiation between thrombosis and an embolus can be difficult, and in such cases the patients are treated initially for SMAE. A more difficult problem arises in patients with abdominal pain and without abdominal signs and complete occlusion of the SMA on aortogram. In these patients one must differentiate between an acute and a long-standing occlusion, as the latter may be coincidental to an unrelated presenting illness. Prominent collateral vessels between the superior mesenteric and the celiac or inferior mesenteric circulations are characteristic of chronic SMA occlusion. If large collaterals are present and there is good filling of the SMA on the late films during the angiogram, the occlusion can be considered chronic and the abdominal pain is probably unrelated to mesenteric vascular disease. In the absence of peritoneal signs, such patients are treated expectantly. The absence of collateral vessels or the presence of collaterals with inadequate filling of the SMA indicates an acute occlusion. In the latter instance the middle colic artery is probably occluded, which interrupts the collateral cir-

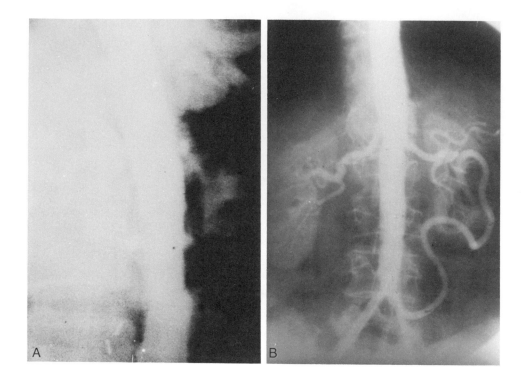

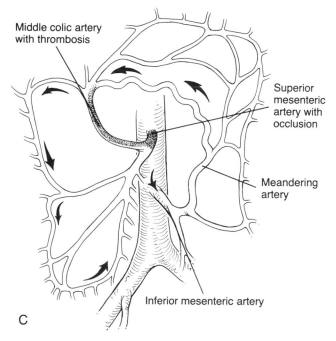

Middle colic artery
with thrombosis

Superior
mesenteric
artery with
occlusion

Meandering
artery

Inferior mesenteric artery

C

Figure 10–17. Chronic versus acute superior mesenteric artery (SMA) occlusion. *A,* Lateral projection showing occlusion of major vessels. *B,* Chronic occlusion with a large meandering artery providing collateral flow to the SMA via the middle colic artery. *C,* Diagrammatic depiction of chronic SMA occlusion and collateral flow through the meandering artery. Acute thrombosis of the middle colic branch interrupts flow to the right colon and the entire SMA vascular bed. Arrows indicate the direction of flow. (*B,* From Boley SJ et al. Ischemic disorders of the intestines. In: Ravitch MM, ed. Current Problems in Surgery. Chicago: Year Book Medical Publishers, 1978.)

culation from the IMA via the meandering artery to an already marginal system (Fig. 10–17). Prompt intervention is indicated, irrespective of the abdominal findings in these patients.

An angiographic catheter is placed in the proximal SMA, and a papaverine infusion is begun. If the origin of the SMA cannot be identified or cannulated at angiography, a small Silastic catheter should be advanced proximally into the SMA through a jejunal artery at the time of operative revascularization to treat the associated vasospasm. This catheter is brought out through a separate incision in the abdominal wall and is used for postoperative papaverine infusion (Fig. 10–18).

Revascularization procedures for SMAT are similar to those for chronic mesenteric ischemia, in which thrombectomy and endarterectomy, or some form of bypass graft to the SMA distal to the obstruction is employed. Although a short graft from the aorta to the SMA is the simplest procedure, extensive aortic atherosclerotic disease often precludes this option. The internal or external iliac artery may be the most successful source of inflow in these cases. Although autologous reversed saphenous vein is the preferred conduit, polytetrafluoroethylene (PTFE) has been used successfully, even in the presence of peritoneal contamination. Percutaneous balloon and laser angioplasty of the SMA also have been reported.[41] Because currently there is no good method of monitoring end-organ injury and because of the danger of rethrombosis with irreparable bowel loss, as was the case with one of our patients, we do not recommend these techniques for acute SMA occlusions.

Reimplantation. Reimplantation is performed by transecting the artery distal to the occlusion and performing an anastomosis directly to the aorta. This procedure is technically difficult owing to the short length of available vessel and the presence of severe aortic atherosclerotic disease in the region of the origins of the celiac and SMA trunks. This procedure should be reserved solely for situations in which the aorta is being replaced and the revascularization done prophylactically.

Endarterectomy. Endarterectomy has been attempted both through the diseased vessel and through the aorta itself (Fig. 10–19). Both approaches are technically difficult and can result in embolization of atheromatous fragments into the distal visceral and systemic circulation. The transarterial approach is usually unsuccessful, because the most proximal extent of the occlusion is difficult to remove safely. The transaortic "trapdoor" endarterectomy requires cross-clamping the aorta in the supraceliac position, which increases the possibility of ischemic injury to the kidneys and distal circulation.[42] Although this approach offers the theoretical advantage of clearing both the

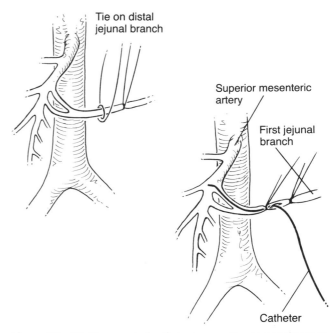

Figure 10–18. Placement of catheter in superior mesenteric artery (SMA) via a small jejunal branch at the time of laparotomy. A small distal jejunal branch is identified and dissected. A distal tie is placed on the branch and a small arteriotomy is made. A catheter is threaded into the main SMA and secured in place with either a silk or an elastic thread tie. The end of the catheter is brought through a separate incision in the abdominal wall and attached to an infusion pump. Placement of this catheter can be confirmed either by an intraoperative angiogram or by the injection of fluorescein at the time of surgery.

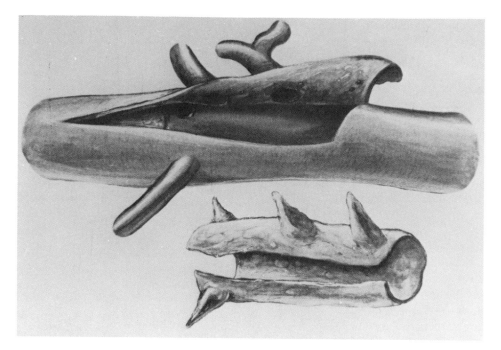

Figure 10–19. Combined visceral and renal endarterectomy with sleeve aortic endarterectomy. (From Wylie EJ et al. Manual of Vascular Surgery. Vol 1. New York: Springer Verlag, 1980.)

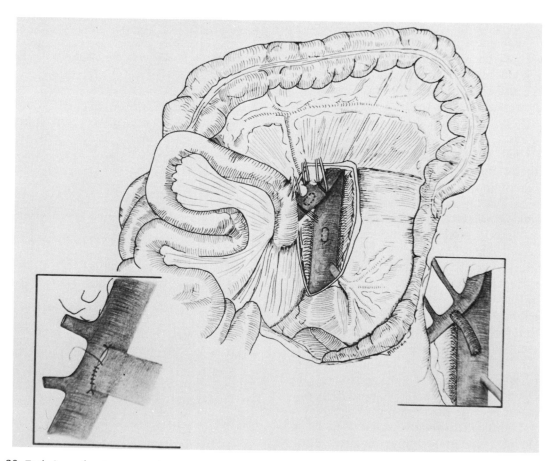

Figure 10–20. Technique of aorta–to–superior mesenteric artery (SMA) bypass. An incision in the retroperitoneum has been made over the aorta and carried superiorly to divide the ligament of Treitz. This provides exposure of the aorta and the SMA in the region of the middle colic artery. Sites of the anastomosis are shown. Inset left shows the fine suture technique of anastomosis. Inset right shows the completed anastomosis.

visceral and renal vessels and is completely autogenous, it is a much more major operation than a bypass operation.

Bypass. Mesenteric bypass from the aorta or the iliac artery to the side of the SMA distal to the occlusion is the procedure of choice (Fig. 10–20). Reversed autologous saphenous vein, after gentle distention, is at least 5 mm in its smallest diameter and is the preferred graft material. PTFE or knitted Dacron is a suitable substitute if the saphenous vein is unavailable or inadequate.

The optimal site of origin of the graft has been disputed. Because of the mobility of the SMA, grafts originating from the infrarenal aorta may be occluded with the movement of the mesentery of the small intestine. In addition, late failure due to progressive atherosclerotic disease of the infrarenal aorta has led some surgeons to use the supraceliac aorta as the inflow for the graft. Most infrequently the common, external, and internal iliac arteries are the only non-calcified vessels, and we have successfully used these as the source of inflow.

RESULTS OF THERAPY FOR ACUTE MESENTERIC ISCHEMIA

Traditional methods of managing AMI have resulted in mortality rates between 70% and 90%.[43, 44] Using the aggressive approach previously outlined, this catastrophic mortality rate has been substantially reduced. Overall, 50% or more of the patients presenting with AMI and treated according to the present algorithm survive, and approximately 70% to 90% lose less than 1 meter of intestine.[32, 34]

VASCULAR LESIONS CAUSING COLONIC BLEEDING

Vascular lesions of the lower gastrointestinal tract, considered uncommon 15 years ago, are now recognized as a major cause of colonic blood loss, particularly in elderly patients. Confusion and controversy remain concerning the pathogenesis, natural history, appropriate therapy, and proper names for these vascular abnormalities of the colon. Although many reports have grouped them together, several distinct entities (Table 10–3), all having the passage of blood per rectum as a common presentation, can be identified.

Vascular Ectasias

Vascular ectasias of the colon are by far the most common vascular lesions found in the colon and are

EDITORIAL COMMENT

Few clinical entities present to the surgeon such a vast array of distressing problems as does intestinal ischemia. The diagnosis is often obscure, the treatment options may be limited because of the extent of nonviable bowel, and attempts at treatment often fail or result in a disabling short-gut syndrome. The authors have presented a rational classification of ischemic disease and an algorithmic approach to its problems, which, taken together, are a thoughtful alternative to the traditional therapeutic nihilism with its inevitable catastrophes.

The editors endorse the concept of a "second look" (or even a third look) and rarely, if ever, perform a primary anastomosis in these circumstances. We prefer to employ multiple stomas until the patient is well stabilized and then to re-establish intestinal continuity as an elective procedure. A perforation or an anastomotic leak in these tenuous patients may well be the coup de grâce.

We recognize the inevitable problems of continued vascular access and the physiologic sequelae of lifelong total parenteral nutrition, but we have been successful in sustaining a large number of patients with continuous partial or total parenteral nutrition for many years of life of good quality. If there is a "common denominator" of relative success or failure in these patients, it appears to be the presence of a significant amount of colon and the eventual re-establishment of intestinal continuity. These patients fare far better than their counterparts with an end-ileostomy and its attendant restrictions on oral intake and the practical difficulties of huge stomal outputs.

probably the most frequent cause of recurrent lower intestinal bleeding in patients beyond 60 years of age.[45] They are distinct pathologic and clinical entities,[46, 47] and in our concept of their pathogenesis, they arise from age-related degeneration of previously normal colonic blood vessels. Vascular ectasias almost always occur in the cecum or the proximal ascending colon; are usually multiple and less than 5 mm in diameter;

EDITORIAL COMMENT

The automatic assumption that a patient presenting with significant bleeding per rectum suffers from diverticulitis is well challenged by the authors. The authors' logical and well-reasoned diagnostic and therapeutic algorithms will avoid unnecessary, ill-timed, and inappropriate operations.

If operation for vascular ectasia is necessary, it is important to resect all of the ectatic lesions to avoid recurrent hemorrhage. Immediate injection of the vascular pedicle by the pathologist for a contrast specimen radiograph may reveal ectatic vessels at the margins of the specimen, requiring further resection.

If, following the suggested diagnostic algorithms, diverticulitis is indeed found to be the cause of hemorrhage, the various options and treatments presented in Chapter 8 apply.

Table 10–3. VASCULAR LESIONS OF THE COLON

Vascular ectasias
Hemangiomas
Congenital arteriovenous malformations
Colonic varices
Telangiectasias
Klippel-Trénaunay-Weber syndrome
Others
    Vascular spiders and venous stars of liver
      disease
    Degenerative phlebectasia of the elderly
    Vasculitic lesions
    Focal hypervascularity of ulcerative, Crohn's,
      and ischemic colitis
    Neovascularity of radiation colitis
    Kaposi's sarcoma of the colon and anus

are rarely identified by gross inspection or routine pathologic examination; are diagnosed by colonoscopy or angiography; and, unlike many congenital or neoplastic vascular abnormalities, are not associated with synchronous angiomatous lesions of the skin, mucous membranes, or other viscera.

Incidence and Pathophysiology

There is no sex predilection for the development of vascular ectasias. Most patients are over 50 years of age, and two thirds are over 70 years. Mucosal vascular ectasias of the right colon can be found in more than 25% of asymptomatic patients over the age of 60 years who undergo routine colonoscopy.[48]

Any hypothesis concerning the formation of colonic vascular ectasias must account for their prevalence in elderly patients, their small size and multiplicity, and their preponderance in the cecum and right colon. Although the cause of these lesions has not been definitively established, injection and clearing studies led us to postulate that vascular ectasias are degenerative lesions associated with aging and represent a unique entity distinct from previously described intestinal vascular abnormalities. We believe that over time, normal contraction and distention of the colon causes repeated, partial, intermittent, low-grade obstruction of submucosal veins, especially where they pierce the muscular layers of the colon. These repeated episodes of transiently elevated venous pressures initially cause dilatation and tortuosity of the submucosal veins, and then, in a retrograde manner, of the venules and the arteriolar-capillary-venular units draining into them. Ultimately, the capillary rings surrounding the crypts dilate and the competency of the precapillary sphincters is lost, producing a small arteriovenous communication (Fig. 10–21). The latter represents the "early-filling vein," which was the original angiographic criterion for diagnosis of this lesion. These abnormal submucosal veins found in the absence of a mucosal lesion, or underlying a minute mucosal ectasia supplied by a normal artery, suggested that submucosal vein dilatation was the primary pathologic change rather than a result of "arterialization" from an arteriovenous communication. The theory that intramural veins are partially obstructed by functional colonic activity is supported by several earlier studies. Venous flow in the bowel is diminished by colonic motility, increased wall tension, and increased intraluminal pressure.[49–51] Rhythmic alterations in venous blood flow and venous pressure related to colonic contractions also have been demonstrated.[52] The presence of these degenerative lesions in the cecum and right colon may be explained by Laplace's law, because during periods of colonic distention the wall tension will be greatest in the portion of the bowel with the widest diameter (cecum and right colon).

Approximately 25% of patients with bleeding ectasias have a diagnosis of aortic stenosis. Some investigators ascribe a causative role for ectasias to aortic valvular disease. We do not believe that there is an etiologic relationship between aortic stenosis and colonic ectasias. Rather, some feature of aortic stenosis, perhaps the low pulse pressure or decreased systemic perfusion characteristic of this disorder, may increase the chance of bleeding in individuals who have vascular ectasias. For instance, a low-flow state may lead to ischemic necrosis of the single endothelial layer that separates the ectatic vessels from the colonic lumen. Alternately, a roughened or stenotic aortic valve could produce a mild consumptive coagulopathy or a subtle alteration in platelet function; these defects, combined with a thin-walled, dilated, mucosal vascular lesion, may cause an ectasia to bleed.[53]

In view of these factors and of contradictory evidence concerning the beneficial effect of aortic valve replacement in the treatment of bleeding ectasias, it seems prudent to consider cardiac disease and colonic lesions as separate and only potentially related entities. A rational approach appears to be initial therapy directed to the colonic lesion if the patient's cardiac status does not require surgical correction. However if valvular replacement is indicated, this should be done first, and treatment of the colonic ectasia deferred unless or until there is continuing or recurrent postoperative bleeding.

Microscopically, vascular ectasias consist of dilated, distorted, thin-walled vessels, mostly lined by only endothelium and less frequently by a small amount of smooth muscle. Structurally, they appear to be ectatic veins, venules, and capillaries. The degree of distortion of the normal vascular architecture varies among different lesions, but the most consistent, and apparently the earliest, abnormality noted in all lesions we have studied is the presence of dilated, often huge, submucosal veins (Fig. 10–22A). Progressively more exten-

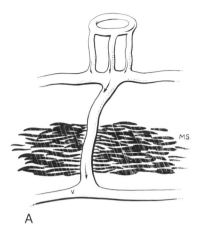
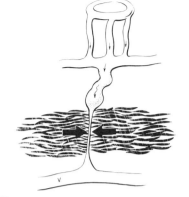
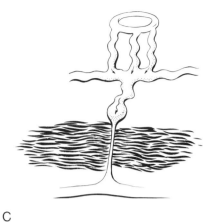

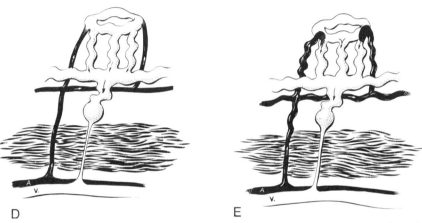

A   B   C

D   E

Figure 10–21. Diagrammatic illustration of proposed concept of the development of cecal vascular ectasias. *A,* Normal state of vein (V) perforating muscular layers. *B,* With muscular contraction or increased intraluminal pressure, the vein is partially obstructed. *C,* After repeated episodes over many years, the submucosal vein becomes dilated and tortuous. *D,* Later the veins and venules draining into the abnormal submucosal vein become similarly involved (A = artery). *E,* Ultimately the capillary ring becomes dilated, the precapillary sphincter becomes incompetent, and a small arteriovenous communication is present through the ectasia. (*A* to *E,* From Boley SJ et al. On the nature and etiology of vascular ectasias of the colon: Degenerative lesion of aging. Gastroenterology 1977;72:650.)

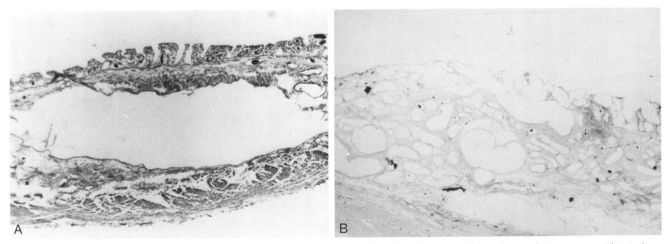

A   B

Figure 10–22. *A,* A large distended vein completely filling the submucosa with a few dilated venules in the overlying mucosa. This is the hallmark of an early ectasia. Hematoxylin & eosin × 50. *B,* Advanced lesion showing total disruption of the mucosa with replacement by ectatic vessels. Only one layer of endothelium separates the lumen of the cecum from those dilated vessels. Hematoxylin & eosin × 50. (*A,* From Boley SJ et al. Vascular ectasias of the colon. Surg Gyn Obstet 1979;149:353. *B,* From Boley SJ et al. Vascular lesions of the colon. Adv Intern Med 1984;29:301.)

sive lesions show increasing numbers of dilated and deformed vessels traversing the muscularis mucosa and involving the mucosa until, in the most severe lesions, the mucosa is replaced by a maze of distorted, dilated vascular channels (Fig. 10–22*B*).

Clinical Aspects

Except for gastrointestinal bleeding, vascular ectasias of the colon are asymptomatic. Bleeding from ectasias is usually recurrent and low-grade. Approximately 15% of patients, however, present with massive hemorrhage, and a smaller percentage present in hemorrhagic shock. During repeated episodes, bleeding in an individual patient may range from gross hematochezia to maroon-colored stools, melena, or occult blood in the stool. Tarry stools are passed in 20% to 25% of episodes, and blood loss is manifested by iron-deficiency anemia and stools that intermittently contain occult blood in 10% to 15% of patients. This spectrum reflects the varied rate of bleeding from the ectatic capillaries, venules, and in advanced lesions, arteriovenous communications. In more than 90% of patients, the bleeding stops spontaneously.

In the early series as many as 30% of patients with colonic vascular ectasias had undergone prior operations for other suspected sources of intestinal bleeding, including partial gastrectomy, vagotomy with antrectomy or pyloroplasty, and left colon resection for purported diverticular bleeding. None of the patients in our series who had left colectomy had angiographic or histologic documentation of a bleeding site at the time of the prior operations. More recently the proportion of patients who have had previous operations has decreased as the diagnosis is established earlier. Physicians have been more willing to refer patients for endoscopic ablation or operation before repeated episodes of bleeding occur.

The problem of differentiating blood loss from vascular ectasias or diverticulosis when bleeding is not demonstrated endoscopically or angiographically is compounded by the frequent occurrence of these lesions without bleeding in people over 60 years of age. Diverticulosis occurs in up to 50% of people older than 60 years, and nonbleeding mucosal vascular ectasias of the right colon have been found in more than one quarter of people the same age. Therefore, in the absence of a demonstrated site of hemorrhage, bleeding can be attributed to an ectasia or diverticulosis only indirectly by observing the course of the patient after resection of the suspected lesion. Furthermore, in some patients with angiographically confirmed vascular ectasias, another unrelated and undetected nondiverticular lesion may be responsible for the blood loss.[54, 55] The prevalence of a second type of lesion in patients with vascular ectasias is not known. However recurrent

lower intestinal bleeding occurs in 15% to 20% of patients who have undergone right hemicolectomy for angiographically proven vascular ectasias, which suggests that a second source may have been present.[56, 57]

Diagnosis

The diagnostic approach we use in patients with lower gastrointestinal (LGI) bleeding (Table 10–4) varies with their age, the presence or absence of active bleeding, and the severity of hemodynamic compromise caused by the blood loss. All patients with LGI bleeding should have a coagulation profile performed, including a platelet count, prothrombin time, and partial thromboplastin time, to identify clotting abnormalities. Further evaluation of patients with LGI bleeding depends on the rate of blood loss.

MAJOR BLEEDING

Major bleeding is defined as (a) acute blood loss causing hemodynamic signs of hypovolemia or (b) the sudden passage of large amounts of bloody, maroon, burgundy, or melenic stools in the absence of hemodynamic compromise.

Because 10% to 15% of major LGI bleeding begins in the upper gastrointestinal (UGI) tract,[58] nasogastric lavage follows assessment of the coagulation status and

Table 10–4. DIAGNOSTIC SCHEMA FOR LOWER INTESTINAL BLEEDING

Digital rectal examination coagulation studies	

Major bleeding	*Nonmajor bleeding*
Nasogastric aspiration	Colonoscopy
UGI endoscopy	UGI endoscopy
Rigid sigmoidoscopy	Barium studies
99-Tc scintigraphy	UGI series
	Small bowel
	? Colon
	Selective angiography
	Small bowel enteroscopy
	111-In scintigraphy

Bleeding, active	*Bleeding, ceased*
Colonoscopy	Colonoscopy
Selective angiography	Barium studies
	Colon
	UGI series
	Small bowel
	Selective angiography
	Ancillary tests
	Small bowel enteroscopy
	Long tube aspiration
	String test

digital rectal examination. A bloody aspirate indicates UGI bleeding in most cases, whereas the absence of blood and the presence of bile in the aspirate virtually excludes bleeding proximal to the ligament of Treitz. A clear, nonbilious aspirate, however, is an indication for UGI endoscopy in actively bleeding patients, because there may be a lesion distal to a closed pylorus. A blood urea nitrogen level greater than 30 mg/dl occurs in approximately two thirds of patients with major bleeding proximal to the colon and may help guide the clinician toward a putative bleeding site. Standard proctosigmoidoscopic examination is done to exclude anorectal and distal sigmoid pathology.

Rigid sigmoidoscopy is followed by abdominal scintigraphy in actively bleeding patients, because the latter may localize the bleeding site or may confirm the cessation of bleeding, enabling clinicians to choose colonoscopy or angiography as the next diagnostic modality. Scintigraphy is noninvasive, safer than angiography and colonoscopy, more sensitive in detecting active bleeding than angiography, and capable of identifying bleeding over a 24-hour period—not just during the brief period of a colonoscopic examination or an angiographic contrast injection.[59, 60]

Two radionuclides commonly used to detect intestinal bleeding are technetium-99m–labeled sulfur colloid and technetium-99m–labeled red blood cells. Previously, technetium-99m sulfur colloid scanning was considered the more sensitive of these two techniques, and because it is rapidly cleared from the circulation (plasma half-life of only 2 to 3 minutes), the most effective agent for detecting active bleeding. Although it was thought to be less sensitive than sulfur colloid scanning, technetium-99m red blood cell scanning was considered valuable for detecting intermittent bleeding, primarily because of the 24-hour half-life of technetium-99m–labeled red blood cells. It now appears that only technetium-99m red blood cell labeling is necessary, as both clinical and experimental studies have found it as sensitive as sulfur colloid, reliably detecting active bleeding even at rates below 0.1 ml/min.[61, 62] Unlike sulfur colloid scanning, with red cell scintigraphy, serial studies can be obtained for up to 36 hours following a single injection of the radionuclide, detecting lesions that bleed intermittently. Furthermore, technetium-99m red blood cells are not cleared by the liver and spleen, as is sulfur colloid, so that bleeding in the area of these organs, which is often obscured with sulfur colloid, can be visualized.

Active Major Bleeding. If scintigraphy demonstrates a bleeding site in the colon and the patient is hemodynamically stable, colonoscopy is performed. Under this circumstance, clotted blood within the colon often obscures visibility and increases the risks of the procedure. Because of these increased dangers, if the bleeding site is shown by the scan to be proximal to

the mid–transverse colon, colonoscopy should be abandoned if technical difficulties are encountered. If a site of hemorrhage is identified distal to the mid–transverse colon, extra efforts to cleanse the bowel and proceed cautiously are usually rewarding.

Although colonoscopy is playing an increasingly larger role in the diagnosis of colonic vascular lesions, the endoscopist's ability to diagnose the specific lesion is limited by the similar appearances of many vascular, inflammatory, neoplastic, and iatrogenic abnormalities. Indeed, vascular ectasias can be mimicked by any of the lesions listed in Table 10–3. Thus, vascular lesions should be evaluated preferably on entering the colon rather than on withdrawing from it, thereby avoiding traumatic and suction artifacts that limit the endoscopist's ability to identify and differentiate these lesions.[63]

Angiography is performed if neither scintigraphy nor colonoscopy reveals the bleeding site, if colonoscopy is not technically feasible, if scintigraphy demonstrates bleeding within the small bowel, or if the patient continues to bleed actively. A selective superior mesenteric arteriogram is the initial study performed because 50% to 80% of all LGI bleeding occurs in the vascular bed fed by the SMA. Selective inferior mesenteric artery and celiac axis studies are performed in that order if the initial SMA arteriogram does not identify the lesion. Flush aortography is of no use in identifying bleeding lesions and is not done.

Mesenteric arteriography may be productive both in patients with active bleeding and in those who have stopped bleeding. Extravasation of contrast material is the angiographic hallmark of active hemorrhage and can be seen with bleeding rates as low as 0.5 ml/min.[64] Angiographic signs of tumor neovascularization or vascular ectasias may identify a presumed cause and location of the hemorrhage.

Angiography can both be diagnostic and provide access for treatment. In 80% of cases active bleeding can be at least temporarily stopped by the transcatheter infusion of vasopressin. Transcatheter embolization of ectasias has been reported, but it should be employed only in extreme situations because it may result in bowel infarction.

Angiography successfully identifies the source of lower intestinal bleeding in approximately two thirds of patients. Pooling of extravasated contrast material in a diverticulum is the angiographic sign of diverticular bleeding and was present in 75% of patients with diverticular bleeding in the series reported by Welch and colleagues.[65] In contradistinction, extravasation has been shown in only 10% to 20% of patients bleeding from vascular ectasias of the colon, because the bleeding is usually episodic. However, other angiographic signs make possible the diagnosis of colonic ectasias or other vascular lesions of the small and large bowel, even in the absence of active bleeding. There

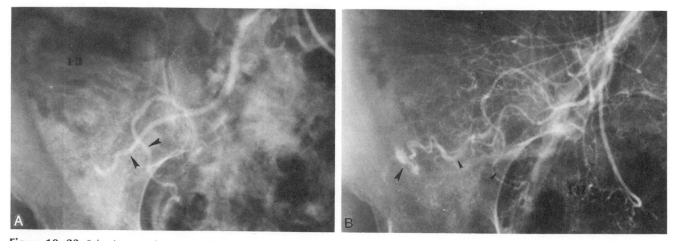

Figure 10–23. Selective superior mesenteric arteriogram in a patient with cecal vascular ectasias showing *A*, two densely opacified, slowly emptying, dilated, tortuous cecal veins *(arrowheads)* 14 seconds after the arterial injection. Note the late visualization of the ileocolic vein after the nearby veins have cleared of contrast material. *B*, Arterial phase of the same arteriogram showing vascular tuft *(large arrowhead)* and two early-filling veins *(small arrowheads)* at 6 seconds. (From Boley SJ et al. The pathophysiologic basis for the angiographic signs of vascular ectasias of the colon. Radiology 1977;125:615.)

are three major angiographic signs of ectasias (Fig. 10–23). The earliest sign to develop in the evolution of an ectasia, and hence the one most frequently seen, is a densely opacified, dilated, tortuous, slowly emptying intramural vein that reflects ectatic changes in the submucosal veins. This sign is found in more than 90% of patients with ectasias. A vascular tuft, seen in 70% to 80% of patients, represents a more advanced lesion and corresponds to extension of the degenerative process to mucosal venules. An early-filling vein is a sign of even more advanced changes and reflects an arteriovenous communication through a dilated arteriolar-capillary-venular unit. It is a late sign, present in only 60% to 70% of the patients. All three angiographic signs are found in more than one half of patients with bleeding ectasias. Intraluminal extravasation of contrast material alone is inadequate to diagnose an ectasia, but when seen in conjunction with at least one of the three signs of ectasias is indicative of a ruptured mucosal lesion.

On rare occasions vigorous resuscitation with intravenous fluids and blood products may fail to stabilize the patient with major bleeding. Colonoscopy is best avoided in hemodynamically unstable patients, and thus emergent angiography is the procedure of choice. Transcatheter or intravenous vasopressin usually controls such bleeding and converts an emergency situation into an elective one, thus saving the patient from unnecessary and potentially debilitating surgery.

Major Bleeding That Has Ceased. In patients with major LGI bleeding in whom proctosigmoidoscopy and nasogastric aspiration are negative and bleeding has ceased, scintigraphy is not performed and colonoscopy

is the initial diagnostic procedure. The presence of blood clots may severely limit visualization, obscure lesions, and make passage of the colonoscope technically difficult and hazardous. In these instances, enemas delivered through the colonoscope can be used to clean the lumen and bowel wall. If these efforts fail, the examination is postponed to prepare the patient with a polyethylene glycol-based agent (GoLytely, Colyte).

If a complete and satisfactory colonoscopic examination reveals no explanation for the bleeding other than diverticulosis, then double-contrast barium studies of the colon, the UGI tract, and the small bowel are indicated. If both colonoscopy and barium opacification studies are normal or show only the presence of diverticula, selective mesenteric angiography has been the most informative study in our experience. Other techniques such as sequential long-tube aspiration of the intestine and small bowel enteroscopy may also be of value. During angiography, the SMA, IMA, and CA are injected in that order. Arteriography, when performed in patients whose bleeding has stopped, is utilized primarily to diagnose tumor neovascularity or vascular lesions, many of which have characteristic angiographic findings permitting them to be identified in the absence of extravasation.

Occasionally, an initially negative technetium-99m red blood cell study, performed because it was not clinically apparent whether bleeding had stopped, may reveal extravasation during serial scanning and localize a lesion that bleeds intermittently. Patients with recurrent or persistent major bleeding for which no site of hemorrhage is found may require exploratory laparotomy with attempts at intraoperative localization (e.g., intraoperative enterocolonoscopy) in order to avoid "blind" resection of part or all of the colon.

NONMAJOR BLEEDING

Nonmajor bleeding is identified by (a) a chemical test for blood in the stool (occult LGI bleeding) or (b) the passage of hemodynamically insignificant amounts of either gross blood per rectum or melena. Although bleeding of this type has been identified in 25% to 30% of patients with ectasias, it is probably less common. Until more recently, evaluation of patients with minor bleeding consisted of rigid proctosigmoidoscopy followed by single-contrast barium enema. However, this approach is inadequate because (1) even flexible fiberoptic sigmoidoscopy cannot visualize the right colon and therefore misses 40% of mass lesions and all vascular ectasias, and (2) double- or air-contrast barium enema shows equivocal results in 20% of cases and regularly misses 40% of polyps, one third of cancers, 60% of discrete ulcerations and colitides, and all mucosal or submucosal vascular lesions.[66-68] Conversely, colonoscopy can reliably visualize the entire mucosal surface of the colon and should be the initial diagnostic study in patients with nonmajor bleeding. Retroflexion of the colonoscope in the rectal vault combined with meticulous examination of the anus during withdrawal of the instrument provides sufficient examination of the anorectum, thereby eliminating the need for rigid proctosigmoidoscopy. Barium enema is necessary only when the entire colon cannot be visualized endoscopically.

If colonoscopy findings are negative, esophagogastroduodenoscopy (EGD) is performed, preferably on the same day, in order to examine the UGI tract. Negative EGD findings are followed by double-contrast radiography of the UGI tract and small bowel. On rare occasions, repeat endoscopic studies or barium enema may be contributory. If these studies are repeatedly normal but occult or "slow" bleeding continues, small bowel enteroscopy,[69] indium-111 platelet scintigraphy,[70] or mesenteric angiography may at times be helpful. Less commonly, exploratory laparotomy with attempts at intraoperative localization may be the only alternative.[71]

Treatment

Once a colonic vascular ectasia has been identified, management consists of controlling the acute hemorrhage and definitive treatment of the lesion itself. Major changes in management have occurred since the original descriptions of vascular ectasias and include the increasing roles of radionuclide scanning and colonoscopy in identifying the cause and site of bleeding and transcolonoscopic ablation of focal lesions.

CONTROL OF ACUTE HEMORRHAGE

In most patients, the acute hemorrhage can be controlled by nonoperative means, and an emergency operation, with its increased morbidity and mortality, avoided. In patients in whom colonoscopy has been successful, and an actively bleeding ectasia or fresh mucosal thrombus (i.e., a sentinel clot) identified, endoscopic ablation of the lesion is an effective mode of therapy. In patients who undergo angiography because colonoscopy was unsuccessful or technically not feasible, vasopressin infusions, either intravenously or intra-arterially through the angiographic catheter, successfully arrest hemorrhage in more than 80% of patients in whom extravasation is demonstrated. The intravenous route appears as effective as the intra-arterial route when the bleeding is in the left colon, but intra-arterial administration has been more successful when the bleeding is from the right colon or small bowel.

DEFINITIVE TREATMENT

During the first 15 years after vascular ectasias were described, definitive treatment was some type of colonic resection. Endoscopic electrocoagulation was a therapeutic option mainly reserved for the elderly with complicated medical illnesses. Today, treatment with the argon laser, neodymium yttrium aluminum garnet (Nd-YAG) laser, endoscopic sclerosis, monopolar electrocoagulation, bipolar electrocoagulation, and the heater probe for miscellaneous vascular lesions throughout the gastrointestinal tract is well described. In institutions where physicians experienced in endoscopic surgery are available, a greater number of patients can be managed endoscopically, and resection is often reserved for patients whose bleeding cannot be stopped or in whom endoscopic treatment is unsuccessful.

Asymptomatic vascular ectasias are frequently noted incidentally during colonoscopy in many elderly patients. Most surgeons do not recommend treating asymptomatic cecal vascular lesions, but if increasing experience with some of the newer modes of therapy, for example, bipolar electrocoagulation and heater probe, prove to be safe, a more aggressive approach to these lesions may be warranted.

Right hemicolectomy remains the treatment of choice in patients who have bled and in whom an ectasia of the right colon has been identified either by colonoscopy or by angiography if (1) the bleeding cannot be stopped; (2) an endoscopist experienced in transcolonoscopic ablation is not available; and (3) endoscopic ablation has been unsuccessful or is not feasible for technical reasons, for example, in large or multiple lesions. In the latter two situations, the right hemicolectomy is done as an elective procedure once active bleeding is controlled. The extent of colonic resection is not altered by the presence or absence of diverticulosis in the left colon; only the right half of the colon is removed. The entire right half of the colon must be removed to ensure that no ectasias remain. Because up to 80% of bleeding diverticula are located in the right side of the colon, the risks of leaving the left colon are far outweighed by the increased morbidity and mortality of subtotal colectomy. Recurrent bleeding can be expected in up to 20% of patients so treated and was observed in 4 of our 27 patients with angiographically proven ectasias. Subtotal colectomy should be performed only in patients who have persistent colonic bleeding and normal colonoscopic findings and selective angiograms.

Other Vascular Lesions

As shown in Table 10–2, many vascular lesions other than ectasias can affect the LGI tract, some as part of a syndrome or systemic disease and others as single or multiple lesions unrelated to disease elsewhere in the body.

Hemangiomas

The second most common vascular lesion of the colon is the hemangioma. Although hemangiomas are considered by some to be true neoplasms, they are generally thought to be hamartomas because of their presence at birth in most cases. Colonic hemangiomas may occur as solitary lesions, as multiple growths limited to the colon, or as part of diffuse gastrointestinal or multisystem angiomatoses. Individual hemangiomas may be broadly classified as cavernous, capillary, or mixed. Most hemangiomas are small, ranging from a few millimeters to 2 cm. Larger lesions do occur, however, especially in the rectum.

Clinically, bleeding from colonic hemangiomas is usually slow, producing occult blood loss with anemia or melena. Hematochezia is less common, except in the case of large cavernous hemangiomas of the rectum, which can cause massive hemorrhage. The diagnosis is best established by colonoscopy; radiographic studies, including angiography, may be normal. In the presence of gastrointestinal bleeding, hemangiomas of the skin or mucous membranes should suggest the possibility of associated bowel lesions.

Pathologically, hemangiomas are well circumscribed but not encapsulated. Grossly, cavernous hemangiomas appear as polypoid or moundlike, reddish-purple lesions of the mucosa. Sectioning of the lesion reveals numerous dilated, irregular blood-filled spaces within the mucosa and submucosa, sometimes extending through the muscular wall to the serosal surface. The vascular channels are lined by flat endothelial cells with flat or plump nuclei. Their walls do not contain smooth muscle fibers but are composed of fibrous tissue of varying thickness. Capillary hemangiomas are plaquelike or moundlike, reddish-purple lesions composed of a proliferation of fine, closely packed, newly formed capillaries separated by very little edematous stroma. The endothelial lining cells are large, usually hypertrophic, and in some areas may form solid cords or nodules with ill-defined capillary spaces. There is little or no pleomorphism or hyperchromasia.

Small hemangiomas that are either solitary or few in number can be treated by colonoscopic laser coagulation. Large or multiple lesions usually require resection of either the hemangioma alone or the involved segment of colon. The hemangioma can either be palpated directly or revealed by transilluminating the bowel wall with an operative endoscope. The affected area can be resected as shown in Figure 10–24. Often this can be accomplished without opening the bowel, as shown.

CAVERNOUS HEMANGIOMAS OF THE RECTUM

A distinct form of colonic hemangioma is the cavernous hemangioma of the rectum. These lesions are usually not associated with other gastrointestinal hemangiomas and are extensive, involving the entire rectum, portions of the rectosigmoid, and the perirectal tissues. They cause massive and sometimes uncontrollable hemorrhage, which often begins in infancy. The diagnosis can usually be suggested on plain films of the abdomen by the presence of phleboliths and by displacement or distortion of the rectal air column.[72] A barium enema study showing narrowing and rigidity of the rectal lumen, scalloping of the rectal wall, and an increase in the size of the presacral space further supports the diagnosis. Endoscopically, elevated nodules or vascular congestion causing a plum-red coloration is seen. Ulcers and signs of proctitis may be evident. Angiograms can demonstrate these lesions but are rarely necessary to establish the diagnosis.

The massive bleeding resulting from these rectal hemangiomas often necessitates excision of the rectum by either abdominal perineal or low anterior resection, but because lesions occasionally involve the perirectal tissues, attempts at maintaining continence via "pull-through" procedures may fail. Ligation and embolization of major feeding vessels have been employed with varying degrees of success, and although local measures (e.g., electrocoagulation, sclerotherapy) are usually only temporarily effective, they have been of value in some instances.

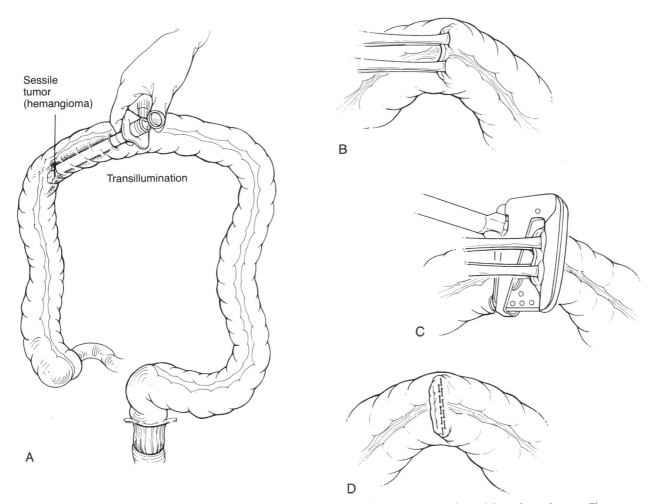

Figure 10–24. Resection of a hemangioma of the colon. *A,* Intraoperative rigid endoscopy is performed through a colotomy. The hemangioma is transilluminated. *B,* The affected area of colon is distracted with Allis forceps. *C,* The affected area of colon is resected with a linear stapling device. *D,* The closure of the colotomy after the resection of the hemangioma is shown.

DIFFUSE INTESTINAL HEMANGIOMATOSIS

Diffuse intestinal hemangiomatosis denotes numerous, as many as 50 to 100, lesions involving the stomach, small bowel, and colon.[73] Bleeding or anemia usually leads to the diagnosis in childhood. Hemangiomas of the skin or soft tissues of the head and neck are frequently present. Continuous slow but pernicious bleeding requiring transfusions, or an intussusception led by one of the lesions, may necessitate surgical intervention. The diagnosis may be made by endoscopy and barium studies; angiography may be normal in spite of numerous lesions. The hemangiomas are similar in appearance to solitary lesions and are usually cavernous, although some have the histologic appearance of hemangioendotheliomas (benign lesions in children). At operation all identifiable lesions should be excised either through enterotomies or limited bowel resections. Transillumination and compression of the bowel wall are helpful in finding small lesions.

When multiple lesions are present, the colon can be opened along a tenia and then intussuscepted upon itself. Each hemangioma can be ligated with a surgical clip or with polyglycolic acid sutures (Fig. 10–25). Unfortunately, repeated operations may be necessary to control blood loss.

Universally miliary hemangiomatosis is usually fatal in infancy. Fortunately, it is a rare condition in which hundreds of hemangiomas involve the skin, brain, lung, and abdominal viscera. Death results from congestive heart failure due to large arteriovenous shunts or may result from the local effects of the lesions. Colonic lesions are rarely significant.

BLUE-RUBBER-BLEB NEVUS SYNDROME (CUTANEOUS AND INTESTINAL CAVERNOUS HEMANGIOMAS)

In 1860, Gascoyen reported an association among cutaneous vascular nevi, intestinal lesions, and GI

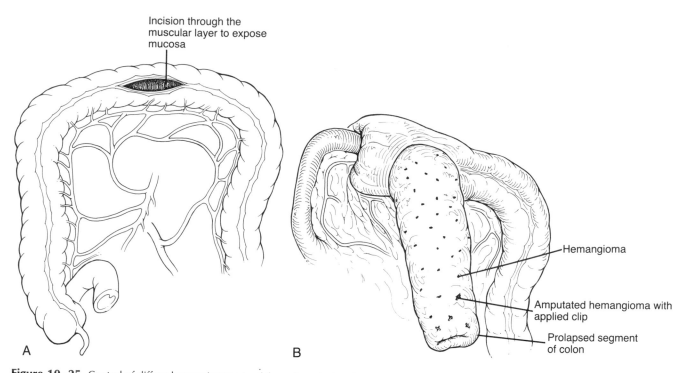

Figure 10–25. Control of diffuse hemangiomatosis of the colon. *A*, A colotomy is made along a tenia. *B*, The right colon (or left) can be inverted upon itself through the colotomy, and each of the hemangiomas can either be oversewn or ligated with a surgical clip. This is an extraordinarily tedious approach to treatment for this disease.

bleeding. Bean later coined the name "blue-rubber-bleb syndrome" and distinguished it from other cutaneous vascular lesions.[74] A familial history is infrequent, although a few cases of transmission in an autosomal-dominant pattern have been reported.

The lesions in this syndrome are distinctive. They vary in size from 0.1 to 5.0 cm, are blue and raised, and have a wrinkled surface. Characteristically the contained blood can be emptied by direct pressure, leaving a wrinkled sac. The hemangiomas may be single or innumerable and are usually found on the trunk, extremities, and face but not on mucous membranes. They increase in size and number with advancing age and do not undergo malignant transformation.[75] They may be present in any portion of the gastrointestinal tract, but they are most common in the small bowel. In the colon they occur more commonly on the left side and in the rectum. They are infrequently seen by barium opacification or angiographic studies and are detected most successfully by endoscopy if they are proximal to the ligament of Treitz or in the colon. Microscopically, they are cavernous hemangiomas composed of clusters of dilated capillary spaces lined by cuboidal or flattened endothelium with connective tissue stroma. In the bowel, they are located in the submucosa. Resection of the involved segment of bowel is recommended for recurrent hemorrhage, although endoscopic laser coagulation is an attractive therapeutic option.

Congenital Arteriovenous Malformations

Congenital arteriovenous malformations (AVMs) are embryonic growth defects and are considered to be developmental anomalies. Although they are found mainly in the extremities, they can occur anywhere in the vascular tree. In the colon they may be small, similar to ectasias, or they may involve a long segment of bowel. The more extensive lesions are seen most often in the rectum and sigmoid colon.

Histologically, AVMs are persistent communications between arteries and veins located primarily in the submucosa. Characteristically there is "arterialization" of the veins, that is, tortuosity, dilatation, and thick walls with smooth muscle hypertrophy and intimal thickening and sclerosis. In long-standing AVMs, the arteries are dilated with atrophic and sclerotic degeneration.

Angiography is the primary means of diagnosis. Early-filling veins in small lesions and extensive dilatation of arteries and veins in large lesions are pathognomonic of arteriovenous malformations (Fig. 10–26). Patients with significant bleeding should have resection of the involved segment of colon.

Colonic Varices

Varices of the colon are very rare, but they may be a cause of hematochezia or melena. In most cases the

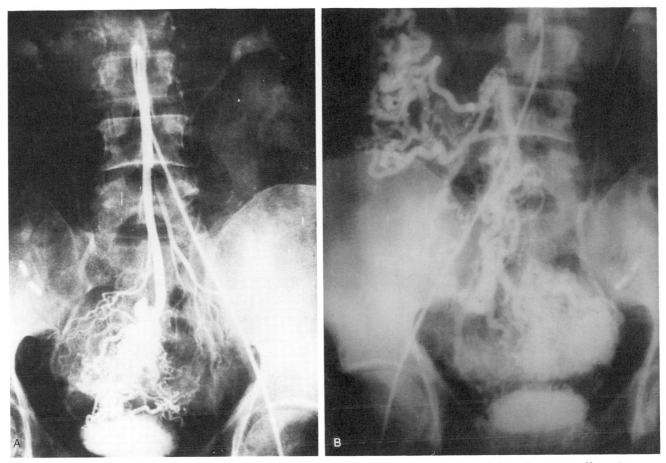

Figure 10–26. *A,* Arterial phase of selective inferior mesenteric arteriogram from a patient with congenital arteriovenous malformation showing multiple dilated arteries going into a large segment of the rectosigmoid. *B,* Venous phase of the same arteriogram showing dilated tortuous vessels to the same segment as well as other more proximal areas. (From Boley SJ et al. In: Stollerman GH, ed. Advances in Internal Medicine. Vol. 29. Chicago: Year Book Medical Publishers, 1984.)

varices are located in the rectosigmoid and are found progressively less often in the more proximal colon. The most common cause of colonic varices is portal hypertension; congenital anomalies, mesenteric venous obstruction, congestive heart failure, and pancreatitis account for the others.[76] Why varices form so rarely in the colon and why they bleed are unclear. Varices are easily diagnosed by proctosigmoidoscopy, colonoscopy, or angiography and may even be seen on conventional barium studies of the colon. Therapy consists of segmental colonic resection, protocaval shunting, or local ligation or sclerosis.

Telangiectasias

Telangiectasias are small vascular lesions found on cutaneous, mucocutaneous, and mucosal surfaces throughout the body. On gross examination and at endoscopy they are millet seed–sized and appear as cherry-red spots, vascular spiders, smooth hillocks, or lesions resembling ectasias. They may be hereditary or

acquired and have been described in association with many disorders (e.g., chronic renal failure, progressive systemic sclerosis, von Willebrand's disease, CRST [*C*alcinosis cutis, *R*aynaud's phenomenon, *S*cleroderma, *T*elangiectasis] syndrome),[77–79] but are most commonly known as part of the Osler-Weber-Rendu disease, or hereditary hemorrhagic telangiectasis.

Hereditary hemorrhagic telangiectasis is a familial disorder characterized by telangiectasias of the skin and mucous membranes and recurrent gastrointestinal bleeding. Lesions are noticed frequently in the first few years of life, and recurrent epistaxis in childhood is characteristic of the disease. By age 10 years, about one half of patients will have had some bleeding, but severe hemorrhage is unusual before the fourth decade of life and occurs with a peak incidence in the sixth decade. In almost all patients, bleeding presents as melena, whereas epistaxis and hematemesis are less frequent. Bleeding may be severe, and patients not uncommonly receive more than 50 transfusions in a lifetime. A family history of disease has been reported in 80% of patients with the disorder, but less commonly in those with bleeding, especially when the bleeding occurs later in life.

Telangiectasias are almost always present on the lips, oral and nasopharyngeal membranes, tongue, or hand, and lack of involvement of these sites casts suspicion on the diagnosis. Lesions on the lips are more common in patients with gastrointestinal bleeding than in those without it. Telangiectasias occur in the colon but are far more common in the stomach and small bowel. UGI lesions are more apt to cause significant bleeding.

The telangiectasias are not demonstrable on barium enema examination but are easily seen on endoscopy. Occasionally, in the presence of severe anemia and blood loss, they transiently become less visible, but with blood replacement they again increase in prominence. Angiography is usually normal but may demonstrate arteriovenous communications or small clusters of abnormal vessels.

Pathologically, the major changes involve the capillaries and venules, but arterioles may also be affected. The lesions consist of irregular, ectatic, tortuous blood-filled spaces lined by a delicate single layer of endothelial cells and supported by a fine layer of fibrous connective tissue. No elastic lamina or muscular tissue is present in these vessels. The arterioles show some intimal proliferation and often have thrombi in them, suggesting vascular stasis, but the most conspicuous findings are in the venules. In contrast to those in vascular ectasias, these venules are abnormally thick and have very prominent, well-developed longitudinal muscles. Apparently these abnormal venules play the major role in regulating blood flow to the telangiectasia. Many treatments have been recommended, including oral and parenteral estrogen therapy and multiple resections of involved bowel. At present, endoscopic electrosurgery and laser coagulation appear to be the most promising techniques, and they may be performed during active bleeding or before any bleeding episodes occur. Although endoscopic therapy has diminished the need for resecting bowel in some cases, long-term follow-up studies are needed to evaluate the ultimate course of patients so treated.

Klippel-Trenaunay-Weber Syndrome

Originally described by Klippel and Trenaunay in 1900, this syndrome is characterized by unilateral congenital lesions of the lower extremities, including (1) cutaneous hemangiomas, usually of the flat, diffuse capillary type, (2) varicose veins dating from childhood, and (3) soft tissue hypertrophy and bony elongation. Involvement of the colon is uncommon and poorly defined, usually involving the rectum or rectosigmoid when it occurs.[80]

The cause of the syndrome has been variably ascribed to congenital arteriovenous fistulas and to aplasia, hypoplasia, dysplasia, atresia, and obstruction of the deep venous system. Rectal lesions usually cause bleeding during childhood and have been described by some as cavernous hemangiomas or as varicosities of the rectal veins.[81] CT scanning and ultrasonography have been found helpful in determining the extent of colonic and other visceral disease.[82]

Major rectal or bladder bleeding has occurred in a few children, with one reported mortality. Ligation of bleeding hemorrhoids or sclerosis of rectal veins is often temporarily effective, but proctectomy may be necessary in some patients.

REFERENCES

1. Geber WF. Quantitative measurements of blood flow in various areas of the small and large bowel. Am J Physiol 1960;198:985.
2. Shaw RS, Green TH. Massive mesenteric infarction following inferior mesenteric artery ligation in resection of the colon for carcinoma. N Engl J Med 1953;248:890.
3. Smith RF, Szilagyi DE. Ischemia of the colon as a complication in the surgery of the abdominal aorta. Arch Surg 1960;80:806.
4. Bernstein WC, Bernstein EF. Ischemic ulcerative colitis following inferior mesenteric artery ligation. Dis Colon Rectum 1963;6:54.
5. Boley SJ, Schwartz S, Lash J, Sternhill V. Reversible vascular occlusion of the colon. Surg Gynecol Obstet 1963;116:53.
6. Schwartz S, Boley SJ, Lash J. Roentgenological aspects of reversible vascular occlusions of the colon and its relationship to ulcerative colitis. Radiology 1963;122:533.
7. Boley SJ, Krieger H, Schultz L, et al. Experimental aspects of peripheral vascular occlusion of the intestine. Surg Gynecol Obstet 1965;121:789.
8. Marston A, Phiels MT, Thomas ML, Morson BC. Ischemic colitis. Gut 1966;7:1.
9. Brandt LJ, Boley SJ, Goldberg L, et al. Colitis in the elderly. Am J Gastroenterol 1981;76:239.
10. Wright HG. Ulcerating Colitis in the Elderly. Epidemiological and Clinical Study of an Inpatient Hospital Population. [Thesis]. New Haven, CT: Yale University, 1970.
11. Barcewicz PA, Welch JP. Ischemic colitis in young adult patients. Dis Colon Rectum 1980;23:109.
12. Fishel R, Hamamoto G, Barbul A, et al. Cocaine colitis. Is this a new syndrome? Dis Colon Rectum 1985;28:264.
13. Kozarek RA, Ernest DL, Silverman ME. Air pressure induced colon injury during diagnostic colonoscopy. Gastroenterology 1980;78:7.
14. Brandt LJ, Boley SJ, Sammartano RJ. Carbon dioxide and room air insufflation of the colon. Gastrointest Endosc 1986;32:324.
15. Boley SJ, Brandt LJ, Veith FJ. Ischemic disorders of the intestine. Curr Prob Surg 1978;15:1.
16. Ernst CB, Hagihara PF, Daugherty ME, et al. Ischemic colitis incidence following abdominal aortic reconstruction: A prospective study. Surgery, 1976;80:417.
17. Kim MW, Hundahl SA, Dang CR, et al. Ischemic colitis following aortic aneurysmectomy. Am J Surg 1983;145:392.
18. Fiddian-Green RG, Amelin PM, Herrmann JB. Prediction of the development of sigmoid ischemia on the day of aortic surgery. Arch Surg 1986;121:654.
19. Poole JW, Sammartano RJ, Boley SJ, et al. The use of tonometry to detect sigmoid ischemia during aneurysmectomy. Presented at the New York Surgical Society, November, 1987.
20. Teitjen GW, Markowitz AM. Colitis proximal to obstructing colonic carcinoma. Arch Surg 1975;110:1133.

21. Cokkinis AJ. Mesenteric Venous Occlusion. London: Bailliére Tindall, 1926.
22. Ende N. Infarction of the bowel in cardiac failure. N Engl J Med 1958;258:879.
23. Jackson BB. Occlusion of the Superior Mesenteric Artery [Monograph]. In: American Lectures in Surgery. Springfield, IL, Charles C Thomas, 1963.
24. Wittenberg J, Athanasoulis CA, Shapiro JH, Williams LF. A radiological approach to the patient with acute extensive bowel ischemia. Radiology 1973;106:13.
25. Boley SJ, Regan JA, Tunick PA, et al. Persistent vasoconstriction—a major factor in nonocclusive mesenteric ischemia. Curr Top Surg Res 1971;3:425.
26. Laufman H. Significance of vasospasm in vascular occlusion [Thesis]. Chicago: Northwestern University Medical School, 1948.
27. Dunphy JE. Abdominal pain of vascular origin. Am J Med Sci 1936;192:109.
28. Mavor GE, Lyall AD, Chrystal KMR, Tsapogasi M. Mesenteric infarction as a vascular emergency: The clinical problems. Br J Surg 1962;50:219.
29. Gaussorgues P, Guerugniand PY, Vedrinne JM, et al. Bacteremia following cardiac arrest and cardiopulmonary resuscitation. Intensive Care Med 1988;14:575.
30. Serreyn RF, Schoofs PR, Baetens PR, Vandekerckhove D. Laparoscopic diagnosis of mesenteric venous thrombosis. Endoscopy 1986;18:249.
31. Kleinhaus S, Sammartano RJ, Boley SJ. Variations in blood flow during laparoscopy. Physiologist 1976;19:255.
32. Qamar MI, Read AE, Skidmore R, et al. Transcutaneous Doppler ultrasound measurements of superior mesenteric artery blood flow in man. Gut 1986;27:100.
33. Boley SJ, Sprayregen S, Siegelman SS, Veith FJ. Initial results from an aggressive roentgenological and surgical approach to acute mesenteric ischemia. Surgery 1977;82:898.
34. Siegelman SS, Sprayregen S, Boley SJ. Angiographic diagnosis of mesenteric arterial vasoconstriction. Radiology 1974;122:533.
35. Stolar CJ, Randolph JG. Evaluation of ischemic bowel viability with a fluorescent technique. J Pediatr Surg 1978;13:221.
36. Carter M, Fantini G, Sammartano RJ, et al. Qualitative and quantitative fluorescein fluorescence for determining intestinal viability. Am J Surg 1984;147:117.
37. Shah S, Andersen C. Prediction of small bowel viability using Doppler ultrasound. Ann Surg 1981;194:97.
38. Brolin RE, Semmelow JL, Koch RA. Myoelectric assessment of bowel viability. Surgery 1987;102:32–38.
39. Shaw RS. The "second look" after superior mesenteric arterial embolectomy or reconstruction for mesenteric infarction. In: Ellison EH, Frieser SR, Mulholland JH, eds. Current Surgical Management. Philadelphia: WB Saunders, 1965, p 509.
40. Cohn I, Floyd CE, Dresden CF, Bornside GH. Strangulation obstruction in germ-free animals. Ann Surg 1962;156:692.
41. Becker GJ, Katzen BT, Dake MD. Noncoronary angioplasty. Radiology 1989;170:921.
42. Wylie EJ, Stoney RJ, Ehrenfeld WK. Manual of Vascular Surgery. Vol I. New York: Springer-Verlag, 1980, p 210.
43. Hibbard JS, Swenson JC, Levin AG. Roentgenology of mesenteric vascular occlusion. Arch Surg 1933;26:20.
44. Koveker G, Reichow W, Becker HD. Ergebnisse der Therapie des akuten Mesenterialgefassverschlusses. Langenbecks Arch Chir 1985;366:536.
45. Boley SJ, Sammartano RJ, Adams A, et al. On the nature and etiology of vascular ectasias of the colon: Degenerative lesions of aging. Gastroenterology 1977;72:650.
46. Mitsudo S, Boley SJ, Brandt LJ, et al. Vascular ectasias of the right colon in the elderly: A distinct pathological entity. Hum Pathol 1979;10:585.
47. Boley SJ, Dibiase A, Brandt LJ, et al. Lower intestinal bleeding in the elderly. Am J Surg 1979;137:57.
48. Hamoniere G, Grenner A, Lalloue C, et al. Recherchessur Pangiectasie du colon droit. Ext Lyon Chir 1982;78:125.
49. Semba T, Fujii Y. Relationship between venous flow and colonic peristalsis. Jpn J Physiol 1976;20:408.
50. Chou CC, Dabney JM. Interrelation of ileal wall compliance and vascular resistance. Am J Dig Dis 1967;12:1198.
51. Noer RJ, Derr JW. Effect of distension on intestinal revascularization. Arch Surg 1949;59:542.
52. Sidky M, Bean JW. Influence of rhythmic and tonic contraction of intestinal muscle on blood flow and blood reservoir capacity in dog intestine. Am J Physiol 1958;193:386.
53. Love JW. The syndrome of calcific aortic stenosis and gastrointestinal bleeding. Resolution following aortic valve replacement. J Thorac Cardiovasc Surg 1982;83:779.
54. Steger AC, Galland RB, Hemingway A. Gastrointestinal haemorrhage from a second source in patients with colonic angiodysplasias. Br J Surg 1987;74:726.
55. Riley JM, Wilson PC, Grant AK. Double pathology as a cause of occult gastrointestinal blood loss. Br Med J 1981;282:686.
56. Boley SJ, Sammartano R, Brandt LJ, et al. Vascular ectasias of the colon. Surg Gynecol Obstet 1979;149:353.
57. Salem RR, Thompson JN, Rees HC, et al. Outcome of surgery in colonic angiodysplasia. Gut 1985;26:1155.
58. Cello JP. Diagnosis and management of lower gastrointestinal hemorrhage: Medical staff conference. West J Med 1985;143:80.
59. Alavi A. Scintigraphic demonstration of acute gastrointestinal bleeding. Gastrointest Radiol 1980;5:205.
60. Winzelberg GG, Froelich JW, McKusick KA, et al. Scintigraphic detection of gastrointestinal bleeding: A review of current methods. Am J Gastroenterol 1983;78:324.
61. Smith R, Copely DJ, Bolen FH. ^{99m}Tc RBC scintigraphy: Correlation of gastrointestinal bleeding rates with scintigraphic findings. Am J Radiol 1987;148:869.
62. Thorne DA, Datz FL, Remley K, et al. Bleeding rates necessary for detecting acute gastrointestinal bleeding with ^{99m}Tc labeled red blood cells in an experimental model. J Nucl Med 1987;28:514.
63. Frank MS, Brandt LJ, Boley SJ, et al. Iatric submucosal hemorrhage. Am J Gastroenterol 1981;75:209.
64. Nusbaum M, Baum S. Radiographic demonstration of unknown sites of gastrointestinal bleeding. Surg Forum 1963;14:374.
65. Welch CE, Athanasoulis CA, Galdabini JJ. Hemorrhage from the large bowel with special reference to angiodysplasia and diverticular disease. World J Surg 1978;2:73.
66. Gilberstein V. Colon cancer screening: The Minnesota experience. Gastrointest Endosc 1980;26:315–319.
67. Tedesco FJ, Gottfried EB, Corless JK, et al. Prospective evaluation of hospital patients with nonactive lower intestinal bleeding—timing and role of barium enema and colonoscopy. Gastrointest Endosc 1984;30:281–286.
68. Tedesco FJ, Waye JD, Raskin JB, et al. Colonoscopic evaluation of rectal bleeding—a study of 304 patients. Ann Intern Med 1978;89:907–911.
69. Lewis B, Waye J. Gastrointestinal bleeding of obscure origin: The role of small bowel enteroscopy. Gastroenterology 1988;94:1117–1121.
70. Schmidt KS, Rasmussen JW, Grove D, et al. The use of indium 111 labelled platelets for scintigraphic localization of gastrointestinal bleeding with special reference to occult bleeding. Scand J Gastroenterol 1986;21:407–409.
71. Lau WY, Fan ST, Wong SH, et al. Preoperative and intraoperative localization of gastrointestinal bleeding of obscure origin. Gut 1977;28:869–873.
72. Hellstrom J, Hultborn KA, Engstedt L. Diffuse cavernous hemangioma of the rectum. Acta Chir Scand 1955;109:277.
73. Mellish RWP. Multiple hemangiomas of the gastrointestinal tract in children. Am J Surg 1971;121:412.
74. Bean WB. Vascular Spiders and Other Related Lesions of the Skin. Springfield IL: Charles C Thomas, 1958, pp 178–185.
75. Wong SH, Lau WY. Blue rubber bleb nevus syndrome. Dis Colon Rectum 1982;25:371–376.
76. Izsak EM, Finlay JM. Colonic varices. Three case reports and review of the literature. Am J Gastroenterol 1980;73:131.
77. Zuckerman GR, Cornette GL, Clouse RE, et al. Upper gastrointestinal bleeding in patients with chronic renal failure. Ann Intern Med 1985;102:588–590.
78. Marshall JB, Settles RH. Colonic telangiectasias in scleroderma. Arch Intern Med 1980;140:1121–1124.

79. Durray PH, Marcal JM, LiVolsi VA, et al. Gastrointestinal angiodysplasia: A possible component of von Willebrand's disease. Hum Pathol 1984;15:539–544.

80. Ghahremani CG, Kangarloo H, Volberg F, et al. Diffuse cavernous hemangioma of the colon in Klippel-Trenaunay syndrome. Radiology 1976;118:673.

81. Servelle M, Bastin R, Loygue J, et al. Hematuria and rectal bleeding in the child with Klippel and Trenaunay syndrome. Ann Surg 1976;183:418.

82. Jafri SZH, Bree RL, Glazer GM. Computed tomography and ultrasound findings in Klippel-Trenaunay syndrome. J Comput Assist Tomogr 1983;7:457–461.

Large Bowel Obstruction

C H A P T E R   1 1

A. R. Moossa
Ralph Crum

The incidence of large bowel obstruction varies with age and predisposing factors. Neonates and newborn infants are a group with an increased incidence of the disorder, which is influenced by the stress of prematurity and developmental conditions. They require rapid diagnosis and specialized care. Hirschsprung's disease, necrotizing enterocolitis, meconium ileus, congenital atresia, volvulus neonatorum, and imperforate anus represent the most common causes.[1-3] Infants and children may rarely present with a strangulated hernia, intussusception, complication of Meckel's diverticulum, or Hirschsprung's disease diagnosed beyond the newborn period, which occurs in 10% of patients.[1, 4] Young adults rarely present with colonic obstruction but may develop a complication of Crohn's disease, a strangulated hernia, or volvulus.[1] Adhesions following previous abdominal operations are virtually never a direct cause of large bowel obstruction. The majority of colonic obstruction cases occur in adults secondary to cancer, diverticular disease, volvulus, strangulated hernia, fecal impaction, or intestinal ischemia.[1, 5-8]

PATHOLOGY

The distended gut proximal to an obstructed segment contains both gas and fluid. Gas accumulation was demonstrated by Wangensteen to be secondary to swallowed air.[9] Measurements of regional blood flow in nonstrangulated obstruction reveal a temporary decrease in blood flow just proximal to the obstruction. This is followed by a significant and sustained 85% increase in blood flow just proximal to the obstruction and a 45% increase in the bowel just distal to the obstructed segment.[10] Progressive bowel distention impairs venous outflow and increases capillary hydrostatic pressure. This leads to increased intracellular edema and iso-osmolar fluid loss into the gut lumen.[1] Hypoalbuminemia may contribute to osmotic flow of fluid into the interstitial space and to losses into the intestinal lumen.[1] Increases in bacterial organisms above the obstruction, especially *Bacteroides* spp., contribute to local bowel edema and aggravate the inflammatory response.[10] Strangulation may result in hemorrhage into the bowel and, in addition to ischemic and toxic bacterial effects, results in further iso-osmolar intravascular volume depletion.

Obstruction leads to dramatic changes in intestinal muscular activity. Initial hypermotility of the colon resulting from obstruction is short-lived, a state of hypomotility proximal to the obstruction supervenes within 5 hours, and chronic obstruction results in a dramatic loss of contractile power.[11] Studies of myoelectric activity in mechanical obstruction lasting more than 24 hours demonstrate a significant delay in myoelectric recovery time, whereas early intervention results in a shorter period for bowel recovery.[12]

DIAGNOSIS

History

Diagnosis of large bowel obstruction is straightforward in most patients. The usual presenting feature is an insidious onset of abdominal discomfort or pain (81%) with progressive abdominal distention (80%).[7, 13] Severe spasmodic pain with vomiting is a common feature of right-sided lesions that may decompress into the small bowel because of an incompetent ileocecal valve, which occurs in 20% to 40% of patients.[5] Shock and dehydration are late features in the course of the syndrome.

Intussusception of a tumor mass or sudden impaction of a fecal mass is the probable cause of acute obstruction in a previously asymptomatic cancer patient. More often there is a history of weeks or months of increasing bowel disturbance. A few of the usual prodromal symptoms are progressive constipation requiring purgatives; blood or slime in the stools; and transient abdominal distention with colicky, central abdominal pain relieved by the passage of flatus.[1] Weight loss and decreased appetite may also occur.

The patient with pseudo-obstruction is in a different clinical category and usually is already in the hospital after undergoing trauma, cesarean section, or laparotomy. On examination, the patient does not appear unusually ill, but this finding is largely influenced by the concurrent disease.[1] The most consistent (100%) and dramatic finding is massive abdominal distention, occurring acutely and progressing.[1, 14] Although constipation is common, 41% of patients continue to have flatus and/or diarrhea.[14] The patient complains of colicky abdominal pain; on auscultation, bowel sounds may be normal or obstructive in quality with splashing, rushing, and tinkling sounds.[1] Although grossly distended, the abdomen is often soft and nontender, except during episodes of colic. Persistent tenderness is common when perforation or ischemia is present (87%).[14, 15] The rectum is usually empty and nontender to digital examination.

Physical Examination

Observation of the patient as a whole, and the abdomen in particular, aids in establishing the appropriate working diagnosis. Small clues including posture, activity, apprehension, observation of the distribution of abdominal distention, visible peristalsis, and association of peristalsis with colicky pain at once suggest the presence of an obstructing bowel lesion.[1] The hernia orifices and abdomen must be palpated for signs of localized tenderness, muscle spasm, rebound tenderness, and masses. Auscultation usually reveals increased bowel sounds with splashing, rushing, tinkling, and borborygmi, all indicative of mechanical obstruction. Digital rectal examination may reveal ballooning of the rectum, a palpable mass or swelling at the pelvic brim, and blood or slime on the examining finger.

Resuscitation

Many patients with acute large bowel obstruction are in relatively good general condition, because vomiting with its attendant dehydration and electrolyte imbalance occurs late. Some are frail, and a great percentage are elderly with concomitant systemic disorders involving the cardiovascular, pulmonary, and renal systems. A proper period of resuscitation is essential to correct extracellular volume depletion and electrolyte imbalance. Baseline values for biochemical and hematologic parameters must be measured and monitored as deemed appropriate in the individual patient. During resuscitation the vital signs are closely monitored. Urinary output is usually a reliable guide to the adequacy of rehydration. In elderly patients, monitoring of the central venous pressure and, occasionally, insertion of a Swan-Ganz catheter may be required.

A sump nasogastric tube should always be passed and connected to low continuous suction. This is especially important if vomiting is a symptom or if x-ray films reveal small bowel distention. Long intestinal tubes are probably unsuitable in this emergency setting, owing to the time and manipulation that are often required to induce them to negotiate past the pylorus and duodenum. Decompression of the small bowel rarely affects the condition of a large bowel obstruction. Parenteral antibiotics effective against colonic flora should be administered, because contamination at operation is seldom avoidable. We prefer the use of ampicillin or a cephalosporin combined with metronidazole or an aminoglycoside.

Whether routine anaerobic coverage with clindamycin or metronidazole is essential remains a debatable issue. Intravenous antibiotics should be started preoperatively and continued for at least 24 to 48 hours postoperatively.

Diabetic patients should have their blood glucose monitored and appropriately controlled with small intravenous doses of regular insulin. Patients with clinical or electrocardiographic evidence of cardiovascular disease should be managed with the close cooperation of a cardiologist.

Diagnostic Tests

Radiology

Routine examinations should include a posteroanterior chest radiograph and supine and erect or right lateral decubitus abdominal films. Upright films must include both diaphragms and symphysis pubis and should be taken after the patient has been in position for at least 5 minutes. Plain abdominal radiographs are still the most useful diagnostic measure in cases of colonic obstruction. Eisenberg and Heineken, in a review of 1,780 examinations, developed criteria for predicting positive findings in cases of abdominal pain.[16] Three clinical factors with high positive likelihood ratios proved to have value in predicting radiographic evidence of bowel obstruction: (1) distention, (2) history of abdominal operation, and (3) increase in high-pitched bowel sounds. Of the 49 patients with generalized abdominal pain, 27 had radiographic evidence of bowel obstruction. Positive findings include dilated colon proximal to the obstruction and absence of air-filled bowel distally. The large bowel can be distinguished from the small bowel by its size, peripheral location, and presence of haustrations in the ascending and transverse portions. When the ileocecal valve is incompetent, air and fluid are decompressed into the small bowel, which occurs more often with proximal colonic lesions.

Sigmoidoscopy or Colonoscopy

Proctosigmoidoscopy is usually indicated and is especially helpful for lesions (cancer) of the distal sigmoid and rectosigmoid, for reduction of sigmoid volvulus, and for rectal biopsy in ulcerative colitis and Hirschsprung's disease. In addition to a therapeutic role in volvulus, proctosigmoidoscopy may also be used to convert obstructing cancers in the rectosigmoid to partially obstructing lesions by means of a guide wire and a lubricated tube.[1, 5, 17] Provided decompression is achieved, further preparation of the colon for primary resection and anastomosis under elective conditions may be carried out.[5, 17]

Colonoscopy is the most accurate method for evaluation of the entire colon.[18, 19] Because of the obstruction and inadequate bowel preparation it is rarely useful preoperatively in obstruction caused by cancer.[5] However, postoperative evaluation of the entire colon and rectum is mandatory to detect the 6% to 7% synchronous carcinomas and the 29% to 36% synchronous neoplastic polyps.[18, 19] Colonoscopy can play important diagnostic and therapeutic roles in pseudo-obstruction of the colon and is discussed in the following section.

ACUTE PSEUDO-OBSTRUCTION OF THE COLON (OGILVIE'S SYNDROME)

Acute pseudo-obstruction of the colon, named after Sir Heenage Ogilvie who first described this syndrome in 1948, is characterized by acute massive dilatation of the right colon and cecum without any organic cause being found by contrast radiology, colonoscopy, laparotomy, or autopsy.[15, 20–26] If untreated, distention may cause perforation, peritonitis, and death.[1, 14]

The fundamental cause of, or "common denominator" for, the development of Ogilvie's syndrome is unknown. Review of the literature from 1948 to 1987

documented 427 cases, with 88% of the patients having extracolonic conditions.[14, 15, 22, 24, 25, 27] The most commonly associated disorders are nonoperative trauma and some surgical procedures, such as cesarean section and hip surgery (replacement and pinning).[14] Medical conditions are present in 45% of cases; infections, cardiac disorders, neurologic problems, and respiratory disease are the most likely associated conditions.[14]

Etiology

The pathophysiologic mechanism accounting for acute colonic distention is unknown. The most common theory for the development of this condition is disruption in autonomic control of the colon.[23] A direct or reflux disturbance in sacral parasympathetic outflow to the left colon results in a condition similar to Hirschsprung's disease in children.[14, 23, 25] The proximal normal part of the colon becomes dilated and terminates at the splenic flexure, where the abnormal and collapsed left colon causes a functional obstruction.[23]

Radiographic Findings

The most useful diagnostic measure is a plain radiograph of the abdomen, which is suggestive of a distal colonic obstruction with segmental proximal colonic dilatation.[1, 14, 15, 22, 25, 26] The dilated colon has well-defined septa, preserved haustration, smooth inner colonic contour, and minimal fluid, making air-fluid levels uncommon.[14, 25, 26, 29] A contrast radiographic examination is a diagnostic procedure that requires expertise to rule out mechanical obstruction in the unprepared bowel and to avoid perforation.[14] A barium contrast radiograph gives higher resolution than meglumine diatrizoate (Gastrografin), but it must be done carefully and the procedure terminated as soon as barium reaches the dilated bowel.[1]

Treatment

Acute pseudo-obstruction of the colon is usually self-limiting.[23] By stopping oral intake and decompressing the stomach with a nasogastric tube, one prevents air swallowing from contributing to the bowel distention.[22, 23] Correction of volume deficits and electrolyte abnormalities, as well as discontinuation of narcotics, usually results in resolution within 3 to 6 days.[14, 15, 23] Supine and dependent abdominal radiographs should be taken every 12 hours to measure cecal diameter and to check for free air.[14] Re-examination at frequent intervals by a single examiner is essential because free air may be absent on x-ray films

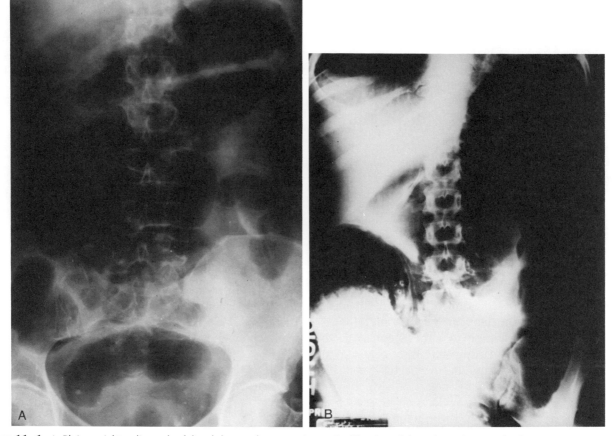

Figure 11–1. *A,* Plain upright radiograph of the abdomen demonstrating toxic dilatation of the colon. This was the first episode of colitis that the patient suffered. Note the sawtooth margins of the transverse colon indicating ulcerative colitis and the increased space between the loops of bowel coincident to bowel wall edema. *B,* Patient with gross perforation of a toxic megacolon with pneumoperitoneum. The patient underwent a successful abdominal colectomy with mucous fistula and end-ileostomy and survived.

in one half of the cases of perforation.[30] Colonoscopic decompression is indicated for all patients whose cecal diameter is greater than 12 cm and who have no clinical peritonitis or localized pain, and for all patients without clinical or radiographic improvement following 12 hours of conservative therapy.[20, 24] This procedure can be both therapeutic and diagnostic, and an 80% to 90% initial success rate with 15% to 20% recurrence can be expected.[14, 20, 21, 24, 28] Recurrence tends to occur in cases in which the small bowel is also dilated with air.[22] A second colonoscopy usually achieves equally good success, but a much higher (40%) recurrence rate can be expected.[14]

Surgical Intervention

Surgical intervention is mandatory when mechanical obstruction cannot be ruled out, when nonsurgical therapy fails to control cecal diameter (>9 cm), when perforation is suspected or present, and when evidence of ischemia (bloody discharge or purple, friable he-

morrhagic mucosa) is identified during colonoscopy.[1, 14, 15, 22, 25] Without perforation or with a single perforation and absence of serosal tears or splitting of the teniae, a cecostomy is the procedure of choice because of the high success rate (95% to 100%) and the relatively low rates of morbidity (3% to 9%) and mortality (15% to 21%).[14, 22] Diverting ileostomies, transverse colostomies, and intraoperative decompression are not recommended because of their limited success and associated high mortality rates.[14] Resection by right hemicolectomy, ileostomy, and mucus fistula is the procedure of choice for extensive disruption of the serosa and teniae coli, for perforation, and for an ischemic right colon.[14, 15, 22]

TOXIC MEGACOLON

Toxic megacolon, more appropriately named toxic dilatation of the colon, is a variant of colonic pseudo-obstruction (Fig. 11–1).[31] It may occur in any patient who develops a severe attack of colitis, whether ulcerative, Crohn's, or amebic colitis. It occurs primarily in the younger age group of patients, particularly in those who present with an initial severe attack of colitis or those who have had inflammatory bowel disease of recent onset. Fazio reports 26% of his series as having colitis for less than 3 months prior to colonic dilatation.[32]

Colonic Features

Toxic dilatation of the colon is not usually a sudden event, but it is frequently preceded by symptoms and signs of acute colitis. Pain may not be a prominent feature, because it is often masked by steroids and/or analgesics. Abdominal examination may reveal the contour of the dilated transverse colon, with or without localized or diffuse tenderness and guarding. A rectal examination invariably reveals the presence of blood and/or mucus in the stool. Some irregularity or nodularity of the rectal mucosa may be palpated. The most important features of toxic megacolon are the systemic manifestations of the disorder. Fever, signs of dehydration, and mental confusion are often prominent.

Diagnosis

A plain radiograph of the abdomen is diagnostic. In the past, definition of toxic megacolon as a clinical entity was based on a fixed figure for transverse diameter of the colon, and 5.5 cm was taken as the upper limit of normal for the mean diameter of the transverse colon. The current approach is to base the diagnosis on serial changes seen on repeated radiographs, along with any other relevant radiologic indices as well as with the overall clinical picture. At the Cleveland Clinic, the mean diameter at the point of maximal dilatation was 9.2 cm, and this was the same for patients with or without colon perforation.[32] It is therefore impossible to set a lower limit in toxic dilatation beneath which perforation is unlikely to occur.

Radiographically, although the entire colon is usually affected, the transverse colon and splenic flexure are the structures most commonly involved with the dilatation. The rectum is usually spared. Additional clues on the plain radiograph are the loss of haustral pattern and a linear strip of gas in proximity to the colon wall representing, respectively, a large submucosal ulcer and a free perforation locally sealed by omentum. The bowel wall may appear nodular in parts, representing thickened and inflamed mucosa.

Etiology

The precise mechanism responsible for toxic dilatation remains unclear. Opiates, anticholinergic drugs, and purgatives are often precipitating factors. The dilatation may also be precipitated by unnecessary investigation during an acute colitis episode. Barium enema studies, colonoscopy, sigmoidoscopy, and all investigations requiring air insufflation or biopsies have been known to precipitate an attack.

Hypocalcemia and hypoalbuminemia are usually associated with severe disease and are probably a consequence of the toxicity itself rather than a factor directly predisposing to dilatation. A linear relationship between alkalosis in colitis and an increasing amount of intestinal gas has been demonstrated. Toxic megacolon is seen with increasing frequency in patients with severe colitis when the blood pH reaches or exceeds 7.50. Any patient with an acute attack of colitis with a pH of 7.50, gaseous distention of several ileal and jejunal loops, and severe plasma protein and electrolyte depletion, must be suspected of developing an impending megacolon that warrants intensive medical treatment.[33] This can be detected only by careful biomedical and radiographic monitoring of the patient with acute colitis.

Treatment

Toxic megacolon is a potential surgical emergency, and all medical treatment must be regarded as resuscitative in nature and preparatory to operation. The operative mortality increases from about 5% to 50% once gross perforation of the colon has occurred. As expected, after adequate resuscitation, including steroid and antibiotic administration, the patient's general condition often improves, but the surgeon must not be lured into a false sense of security because the diseased colon may perforate at any time. Thus, a general response to medical treatment does not necessarily imply that an operation can be avoided. Even before perforation occurs, peritoneal sepsis is likely to be present owing to transmigration of bacteria across the diseased, thinned colonic wall. It is common at the time of laparotomy to find turbid peritoneal fluid loaded with organisms in the absence of gross perforation. This intermediate state makes the signs of perforation difficult to assess, and for this reason operative intervention is indicated for *established* toxic megacolon as soon as resuscitation is complete.

Accurate preoperative replacement of fluids and electrolytes is essential. Large-bore intravenous catheters, including a central venous line, should be inserted for fluid administration and monitoring of the right atrial pressure. A nasogastric tube is inserted and connected to continuous low-grade suction. A urinary catheter must also be placed to monitor urinary output. Significant extracellular fluid volume depletion together with hypoalbuminemia invariably exists in these patients and requires correction with electrolyte and salt-free albumin solutions. Potassium supplementation and blood transfusion should be given as required. Any metabolic acidosis that does not respond to rehydration is corrected with intravenous sodium bicarbonate. Corticosteroids are administered to support those patients whose adrenal function has been suppressed by the chronic use of exogenous steroids. An initial dose of 100 mg of hydrocortisone given intravenously is recommended, followed by at least 50 mg given intravenously every 4 hours. A broad-spectrum antibiotic cover is started after blood cultures are obtained. If amebic colitis is suspected, treatment with metronidazole is mandatory. Resuscitation is considered adequate when a urine output of 40 ml/hr is achieved with a sustained central venous pressure between 5 and 10 cm of water.

Surgical Management

Cecostomy, decompressing ileostomy, and colostomy have no place in the management of the patient with toxic megacolon. Turnbull originally proposed that a diverting ileostomy and a decompressive colostomy at one or two sites ("blow-hole" operation) should be performed as an initial procedure to prevent fecal spillage during colectomy. According to his thesis, once the acute crisis is over the patient can have an elective colectomy with a much lower risk. The modern concept is that emergency abdominal colectomy is essential and represents the treatment of choice. The rectal stump can be preserved as a Hartmann pouch. Once the patient has recovered from the fulminant episode of colitis, a second procedure can electively be considered, depending on the state of the rectal stump and the histologic diagnosis obtained from the colectomy specimen. Ileorectal anastomosis can be considered in Crohn's colitis if the rectum is relatively spared. This can also be achieved in many cases of pseudomembranous colitis or amebic colitis. If the patient has ulcerative colitis, a second-stage proctectomy and restorative proctocolectomy, consisting of a mucosal proctectomy and ileoanal anastomosis with a proximal ileal reservoir, are the two options.[34]

ACUTE VOLVULUS OF THE COLON

Intestinal obstruction secondary to twisting and kinking of the large bowel is rare in the United States, representing only 2% to 6% of all cases of mechanical obstruction.[1, 31, 32] The worldwide variation in the incidence of colonic volvulus is well known, and volvulus represents the major cause of mechanical bowel obstruction in some areas of eastern Europe, India, and Africa.[1, 32, 33] Volvulus occurs most frequently in the sigmoid colon, less often in the right colon, and rarely in the transverse colon and splenic flexure.[1, 9, 31, 34]

The geographic and anatomic differences in the incidence of volvulus result from multiple etiologic factors. Congenital abnormalities of faulty rotation or inadequate attachment of the colon to the posterior abdominal wall can create a loop of bowel with a long mobile mesentery or mesocolon.[1] Congenital colonic redundancy and increased mobility combined with a

---

EDITORIAL COMMENT

There is general agreement that the severely ill patient suffering from either fulminant colitis or toxic megacolon is best treated by an initial abdominal colectomy and ileostomy and should *not* be subjected to a one-stage proctocolectomy or endorectal pull-through as an emergency procedure. The method of managing the retained rectosigmoid colon, however, engenders some debate. In practice, the setting in which the operation is performed is often the determining factor.

If the patient is known to suffer from ulcerative colitis, the rectosigmoid may be exteriorized as a mucous fistula if the bowel lends itself to this manipulation. This is the safest alternative. If inflammation is severe or if perforation is likely, a Hartmann pouch closure is the other alternative. In this situation I prefer to close the rectum as a "low pouch" that is extraperitoneal and well below the sacral promontory. This maneuver has several advantages: it avoids the dangerous closure of diseased bowel within the peritoneal cavity; if proctectomy is later elected, it can be performed via a perineal approach without laparotomy; and if endorectal pull-through is chosen, the procedure is simplified by the previous resection. In this last instance, I prefer an interval of at least 3 months between the two procedures so that the dense inflammation subsides allowing an easier dissection.

If, at the time of abdominal colectomy, the diagnosis is known to be Crohn's colitis or is in doubt, the status of the rectum is the determining factor. If the patient is known to suffer from Crohn's disease and there is rectal sparing, as much rectosigmoid and terminal ileum as possible should be spared. An anastomosis between a shortened small bowel and a rectal pouch of less than 10 to 14 cm from the anal verge may result in poor function with frequent and often uncontrolled stools. At the initial procedure the disease-free rectum may be safely closed or exteriorized. In these instances I usually opt for closure.

If the diagnosis as to the type of colitis is not known, conservatism should prevail, preserving as much rectosigmoid as possible, usually via a mucous fistula. The type of secondary procedure to be performed will be determined by the eventual diagnosis.

narrow mesenteric base increase the likelihood of twisting.[1, 32]

Acquired factors include colonic distention associated with dietary factors, distal obstruction, and a manifestation of one of the various forms of megacolon.[33] Intraoperative manipulation and postoperative adhesions may fix a loop of bowel at its apex or narrow the mesenteric base, contributing to the incidence of volvulus. At the Mayo Clinic between 1960 and 1980, 53% cases of sigmoid volvulus and 68% of cecal volvulus followed laparotomy, and in the latter group 27% of patients developed volvulus within 2 weeks of a previous surgical procedure.[31]

RIGHT COLON VOLVULUS

Acute volvulus of the right colon is an uncommon surgical emergency accounting for less than 2% of all cases of adult intestinal obstruction.[35] Within the control population of the Mayo Clinic, 41% of volvulus cases involved the right colon.[31] Necropsy examination has shown that 20% of the general population have a cecum sufficiently mobile to allow the development of volvulus.[35] Contributing factors include previous abdominal operation, congenital bands, malrotation, pregnancy, and cyst or pelvic tumor that displaces the cecum upward, and any obstructing lesion of the left colon.[1, 35]

Torsion of the ileocecal segment most often occurs in a clockwise direction with cecum passing upward and then to the left.[1] A sufficiently mobile cecum may also twist along the axis of the right colon or may simply fold anteriorly and superiorly over a fixed ascending colon, resulting in the "cecal bascule," which occurs in 10% of cases.[31, 36]

Clinical Features

Three series by O'Mara, Ballantyne, and Anderson and Welch were combined for a total of 190 cases of cecal volvulus; the majority (59% to 74%) of patients were women with mean ages of 51 to 60 years.[35, 36, 40] Variation in the frequencies of previous laparotomies (17% to 38%) were noted. A temporal relation with another acute medical problem was observed in 28% of each series.

The patients' symptoms began, on average, 2 days before presentation, with pain (84% to 97%) and distention (76% to 96%) being the most common features. Nausea and vomiting (52% to 87%) and constipation (50% to 60%) occurred less frequently, and obstructive bowel sounds or peritoneal signs were poor indicators of bowel injury. A tympanic abdominal mass in the hypogastrium or on the right side was present in 33% of Anderson's 69 patients and represented the distended cecum 87% of the time.

Radiographic Diagnosis

Plain abdominal radiographs can be diagnostic in up to 50% of cases; most commonly, the displacement of the cecum is into the epigastrium or left upper quadrant.[37] The presence of a single fluid level and visualization of the ileocecal valve are the most helpful radiologic signs.[1] Usually there are distended loops of small intestine located to the right of the cecal gas shadow. In patients with complete obstruction, no gas can be seen beyond the point of obstruction (Fig. 11–2).

Barium enema examination shows the opaque medium being cut off at the transverse colon or the hepatic flexure, beyond which is seen the gas-filled right colon.[1] When barium enema is done, special consideration should be given to the possibility of distal obstructive lesions associated with cecal volvulus.[40]

Colonoscopic reduction of cecal volvulus was attempted in four patients at the Mayo Clinic, and reduction was accomplished in one.[31]

Treatment

Operative treatment is mandatory. The abdomen is explored through a generous midline incision. When the bowel is viable and detorsion successful, acute cases should be treated with cecopexy and tube cecostomy.[35] Anchoring the acutely distended and thin-walled cecum to the parietal peritoneum may occasionally be difficult, and although O'Mara and coworkers[40] and Bellantyne[42] report no recurrence with cecopexy alone, Anderson and Welch[39] report a 20% recurrence rate. An incidental appendectomy should be performed whenever it is safely possible, in order to avoid later diagnostic confusion. Mortality rates associated with operation on viable bowel range from 7% to 12%.[31, 35, 36] Gangrene of the involved ileocolic segment requires resection with ileostomy and mucous fistula. Primary anastomosis may be considered in highly selected cases. Nonviable bowel is present in 20% to 29% of acute cases, and expected mortality rates range from 33% to 40%.[31, 35, 36] Mortality is related to age, associated medical illnesses, delay in diagnosis, and delay in surgical therapy.

SIGMOID COLON VOLVULUS

Volvulus of the sigmoid colon is a fascinating condition with wide geographic variation as well as a peculiar

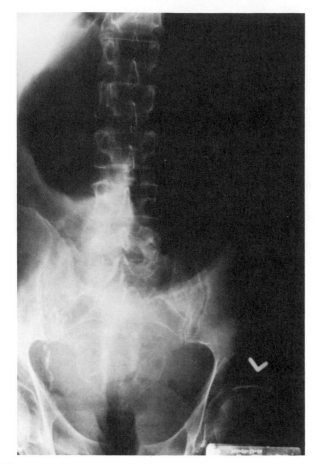

Figure 11–2. Flat plate of the abdomen showing a typical cecal volvulus. Note that the cecum and right colon are grossly distended and are located in the left upper quadrant of the abdomen. The right iliac fossa is devoid of any bowel gas.

association with mental deficiency and old age. Unlike cecal volvulus, in the majority of cases of sigmoid volvulus there is a possibility of treating for the immediate emergency by nonoperative means.[1] The natural history of sigmoid volvulus has been known since ancient times.[38] Detorsion was recognized even in ancient Egypt as the fundamental requirement for treatment and for averting what is otherwise a fatal intra-abdominal catastrophe.[38] By the early twentieth century, modalities for both operative and nonoperative therapy have been developed. Unfortunately, an additional half century was needed for a union between acute nonoperative emergency management followed by definitive elective surgical therapy. With this combination treatment, the successful outcome achieved in the management of sigmoid volvulus is dependent on prompt recognition, urgent decompression, and elective resection of viable but redundant bowel.

In the United States, volvulus of the colon represents 2% to 6% of all cases of intestinal obstruction.[1, 31, 32, 37, 39] It accounts for approximately 10% to 13% of all large bowel obstruction.[39] Most cases of colonic volvulus occur in the sigmoid colon.[1, 34, 37, 39, 40] Among English-speaking countries, affected patients tend to be elderly, with a slight predominance of males and a well-documented association with institutionalized patients.[1, 31, 32, 39] In pregnant American women, sigmoid volvulus is the most common cause of intestinal obstruction.[31] Factors that predispose adults to sigmoid volvulus are largely acquired. A long, redundant sigmoid colon is an important etiologic factor. Coarse vegetable fiber diets, chronic constipation, colonic mobilization as part of a previous procedure, and ethnic (black) and gender (male) differences may be contributing factors.[31, 40] Abnormal bowel mobility and megacolon secondary to Hirschsprung's disease, Chagas' disease, ischemic colitis, and myenteric damage caused by anthraquinone laxatives, anticholinergics, and other drugs have been implicated. A narrow mesosigmoid parietal attachment secondary to mesosigmoiditis, either surgically created or the result of adhesions, contributes to an anatomic situation predisposing to a volvulus. Finally, adhesion with fixation of the apex of a long redundant loop creates the second stationary pivot point and the axis for rotation.

Clinical Features

Four series published between 1978 and 1987 have been reviewed to illustrate the clinical features of acute sigmoid volvulus.[31, 32, 39, 41] Patients are in general elderly (mean ages 61 to 72 years) with a slight male predominance (48% to 57%). The most common symptom was the presenting complaint of abdominal pain (74% to 85%). Even more common was the

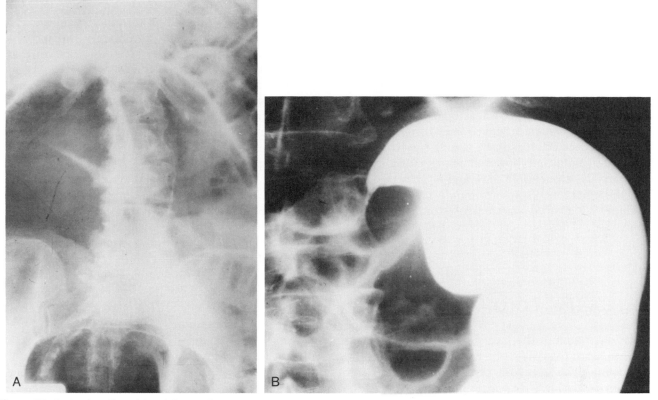

Figure 11–3. *A,* Plain film of the abdomen showing a sigmoid volvulus. Note the grossly dilated loop of sigmoid colon coming out of the pelvis, resembling a thin-walled "pregnant uterus" filled with air. *B,* Barium contrast radiograph showing a typical bird's beak appearance of the obstruction in the lower sigmoid colon. This is pathognomonic of sigmoid volvulus.

finding of abdominal distention (88% to 94%). Abnormal bowel sounds, usually obstructive in quality; constipation; and occasionally nausea and vomiting, were reported in that order. The least common symptom was diarrhea. The least common findings were absence of bowel sounds and evidence of peritonitis; when present, these were associated with gangrenous bowel.

Acute medical problems and recent abdominal operations were associated with sigmoid volvulus and contributed to morbidity and mortality.[31, 32, 39, 41]

Radiographic Diagnosis

Signs considered diagnostic of sigmoid volvulus without requiring barium enema include a distended haustral sigmoid loop ("bent inner tube") with overlap, apex below the left diaphragm and above the tenth dorsal vertebral body, inferior convergence to the left, and a fulcrum below the lumbosacral angle.[42] It is predicted that one third of plain abdominal films will be nondiagnostic; however, a wide range (37% to 83%) of patients' x-ray findings are actually positive.[31, 32, 39, 41] A distended proximal or descending colon, a low sigmoid loop apex, and occasionally a low-lying transverse colon are the most common causes of interpretive errors.[42] A barium enema usually demonstrates a "bird's beak" appearance or "mucosal spiral" pattern (Fig. 11–3).[42]

Management

Proctosigmoidoscopy, preferably using a flexible scope, followed by placement of a rectal tube into the sigmoid colon, is successful in 79% to 89% of patients.[31, 32, 39, 41] The incidence of recurrence without surgical therapy is high, 40% to 50%, and operation should follow decompression during the same hospitalization in most cases.[31, 39] In patients undergoing elective procedures, primary anastomosis following adequate bowel preparation is clearly desirable. When a volvulus is identified and reduced at laparotomy, the distended colon can be decompressed by gentle "milking" down into a rectal tube (placed prior to laparotomy) connected to gentle suction. If the colon is viable, resection is *still mandatory*. Primary anastomosis must be avoided, even when protected by a diverting colostomy. A Hartmann procedure or mucous fistula and end-colostomy are preferable in most instances. If gangrenous bowel is identified, resection of all nonviable bowel is mandatory with creation of an end-colostomy. A sigmoid mucous fistula or a Hartmann procedure should be performed with the distal bowel. Exteriorization-resection of the Paul-Mikulicz type results in inadequate resection, retraction of distal limb, and a higher recurrence rate.[32, 41] Primary anastomosis without proximal diversion results in suture line disruption and a 30% occurrence of fecal fistula among survivors.[44] The presence of nonviable bowel increases mortality from less than 10% to between 38% and 80%.[39]

In the emergency setting, operative detorsion, sigmoidopexy, and tube sigmoid colostomy are *not* recommended. They subject the patient to additional surgical risks and to increased risk of recurrence.

OBSTRUCTING COLON CANCER

Adenocarcinoma of the large intestine is the etiologic factor in more than 60% of patients with acute colonic obstruction. The prognosis of patients with this complication is considerably poorer than the overall prognosis of patients with cancer of the colon.[43–46] The poor outlook for these patients results from the increased incidence of locally unresectable cancer, metastatic disease, sepsis, advanced age, and associated medical conditions.[43, 46–48] The influence of surgical therapy on reducing the morbidity and mortality rates in these gravely ill patients is directly reflected in the immediate and long-term disease-free survival rates.

Data accumulated from the Large Bowel Cancer Project (1986) analyze 4,292 patients and indicate that the highest risk of obstruction (49%), postoperative cardiopulmonary complication (36%), and in-hospital mortality (18%) and the lowest age-adjusted 5-year survival (28%), even after curative resection (38%), occur with carcinoma at the splenic flexure.[49] The high incidence of obstruction appears to be the main associated risk for in-hospital mortality at this site. These data confirm the findings of Schein, Umpleby, and Fitchett in their previous reviews of 4,583 patients in 1985.[5, 48–51] Taken together, these reports indicate that 19% of colon cancer patients present with obstruction; that there is a higher frequency of obstructed left colon cancers over right-sided lesions; and that there is an increased incidence among Dukes' Stage B cases and among women.[5, 49–55] The lowest risk of obstruction was in the rectum (6%) and with Duke's Stage A cases.[48, 49]

Ohman, in a review of 1,071 cancers of the large bowel, found that 148 of these (14%) presented with complete obstruction and that the overall 5-year survival rate was 16%, less than one half the rate for nonobstructed patients (34%).[50] An additional 23,000 cases were reviewed with an overall 15% incidence of obstruction. The risk for obstruction with cancers located in the right colon was 12%, the transverse and left colon 25%, and the rectum 4% to 5%. Age and sex did not differ between obstructed and nonobstructed patients.

In contrast to these findings, Waldron and colleagues found that age correlated with the risk of perioperative death in emergency colorectal operations.[56] In a review of 1,033 patients, 527 (51%) were over 70 years old. Of these "elderly" patients, 301 (58%) constituted emergency admissions, compared with 222 (43%) emergency admissions in a second, younger group. No differences in the duration of symptoms or indications for emergency admissions were observed, and obstruction (46% Group I, 48% Group II) was the leading cause. Emergency perioperative mortality was 38% in Group I and differed significantly from the 18% mortality in the group under 70 years of age. No difference in stage at presentation (66% Stages B and C; 28% Stage D) was identified. The perioperative mortality in the group over 70 years of age was significantly higher in both elective (18% versus 11%) and emergency (38% versus 19%) cases, but it was following emergency operation that the older patients fared particularly poorly.[56]

The National Surgical Adjuvant Bowel Project (NSABP) clinical trials have studied the significance of tumor location and bowel obstruction in colorectal cancer in Duke's Stages B and C.[57] Tumor location proved to be a strong prognostic discriminant, and the effects of bowel obstruction were influenced by the location of the tumor. Bowel obstruction in the right colon was associated with a significantly diminished disease-free survival and an estimated risk of treatment failure three times greater than that in the nonobstructed patient, whereas obstruction in the left colon demonstrated no such effect. This phenomenon was independent of nodal status and tumor encirclement; the latter two factors proved to be of prognostic significance independent of tumor obstruction.[57]

An analysis of prognostic indicators performed by the Gastrointestinal Tumor Study Group (GITSG) in 1986 in 572 patients with Duke's Stages B2 and C colon cancers revealed that obstruction, perforation, and rectal bleeding were prognostic factors. Tumor location was of little prognostic importance and did not affect disease-free survival. Whereas NSABP reported a 14% difference at 3 years between disease-free curves for left versus right colon involvement, the difference shown in the GITSG data is approximately 2%. Colonic obstruction and perforation in the NSABP and GITSG studies were significant prognostic indicators and, independent of stage, were associated with decreased 5-year and disease-free survivals. Two studies at the Massachusetts General Hospital and the Lahey Clinic confirm the poorer 8-year survival rates associated with obstruction.[43, 44, 53, 54, 58]

Etiology

Malignant tumors of the colon begin in polyps.[18] About 5% of tubular adenomas and 30% to 40% of villous adenomas eventually exhibit malignant changes in one or several polyps.[49] The tumor may grow above mucosal level into the bowel lumen or may ulcerate the mucosa and invade the muscular wall encircling the bowel.[5] As the colonic lumen narrows, the proximal colon dilates and becomes loaded with liquid and solid feces.[1] Work hypertrophy leads to thickening of the bowel wall, and eventually the proximal bowel margin tends to become flattened and the distal margin more elevated, producing a liplike structure that overhangs the mucosa.[1, 5] Partial obstruction may appear on retrograde barium study as complete obstruction because of the valve action at the tumor margin.[5] Complete obstruction is rarely the result of total occlusion of the bowel by the cancerous growth but is the result of edema, impaction of feces, or intussusception.[1] In selected cases, careful management may allow bowel preparation for elective colonic excision.[5]

Diagnosis

History and Physical Examination

Chapuis and Dent, in a review of 709 patients using multivariate analysis of clinical and pathologic variables, found that the only symptom with an independent effect on survival was obstruction.[59] Improved survival was associated with rectal bleeding. A longer duration of symptoms was associated with a higher survival rate. Abdominal pain, intestinal obstruction, abnormal findings on abdominal examination, and symptoms of less than 4 weeks' duration were all associated with lower survival rates. Anemia, altered bowel habits, and tumor location were of no statistical predictive value.[59] A similar review of Vanek and Whitt confirms these findings in an additional 315 cases of adenocarcinoma of the colon.[60]

Contrast Radiographs

When there is question regarding the site of mechanical obstruction, a dilute barium or water-soluble contrast radiograph may be performed. In unprepared bowel using dilute contrast material, confirmation of obstruction and its site can be accurately determined; however, no analysis of mucosal detail is possible or desirable in the completely obstructed colon. Stewart and Finan, in a prospective study of 99 patients whose plain films suggested mechanical obstruction, found that by means of a single Diodone enema, complete obstruction was identified in 52 patients and its site relocated in 11.[61] There was a free flow of contrast material to the cecum in the remaining 35, 11 of whom had pseudo-obstruction; 6 patients were later proved to have carcinomatosis and in 3 patients partially obstructing cancers were missed. There was no false-positive result in this series. Confirmation of the diagnosis and its site has many advantages. When the obstruction results from malignant disease and the surgeon's policy is to manage the carcinoma in a staged fashion, then the first stage (i.e., a defunctioning colostomy) can be performed "blindly" through a small incision. The second stage may then be performed through a new vertical incision rather than one that is a few weeks old and perhaps inappropriately situated. Alternatively, where the policy is to perform a primary resection with or without a primary anastomosis, then the laparotomy can be performed through an appropriate abdominal incision.[61, 62]

Sigmoidoscopy

Sigmoidoscopy has a long history as an excellent tool for establishing the diagnosis of obstruction in the rectosigmoid. Flexible sigmoidoscopy for decompression of the obstructed bowel by using a guide wire and lubricated tube appears to be safe and effective.[17] This can be supplemented by the appropriate use of saline enemas. Further clinical trials will establish the risks and usefulness of this procedure.

Treatment

Emergency Right Colectomy

Resection and primary anastomosis without diversion is the usual therapeutic procedure for obstructing cancers of the right colon. Removal of the edematous and friable bowel, including the cancer and its lymphatic and vascular supply, and anastomosis of nondilated ileum and distal colon complete the operation. When the ileocecal valve is incompetent and the small bowel dilated, no anastomosis should be performed; the ends of the ileum and colon should be exteriorized because of the edematous and friable bowel wall and the prospect of performing the anastomosis in a heavily contaminated field.[7, 63] Preoperative shock, advanced age, associated injuries, or illnesses may influence the latter decision. If a preliminary diversion is considered, the performance of a loop ileostomy is the procedure of choice.[64] Perforation is an absolute indication for resection. Drainage should be performed only when indicated, and no anastomosis should be attempted following resection of a perforated cancerous lesion or, more commonly, a cecal perforation in the dilated segment proximal to the obstruction.

Opponents of Left Colon Resection and/or Anastomosis

In two major reviews of obstructing carcinoma, Welch and Donaldson and Dutton et al presented five cases each of left-sided lesions primarily resected with 60% mortality.[13, 51] These results compared poorly to obstructing left-sided cancers treated by staged resection. With diversion followed by resection, the reported mortality was 2% (1 of 51 patients) and 5.5% of (3 of 54 patients), respectively. Welch and Donaldson found a high rate (55%) of large and small bowel dilatation secondary to obstructing cancers and concluded that among this series of patients, loop transverse colostomy is the diverting procedure of choice.[13]

Ohman, in a review of 148 obstructing carcinomas of the colon, found that the mortality was higher (14% versus 5%) and 5-year survival lower (19% versus 35%) when patients were treated by primary resection compared with staged treatment.[50] These results are not comparable, however, even if the two groups of patients had similarly staged disease, because the methods of treatment were not randomly allocated and variability among surgeons could not be evaluated.

Emergency Left Colectomy

The theory that primary resection for obstructing cancer, especially on the left side, carries a higher operative mortality rate than the staged procedure has been challenged during the 1980s. Reasons for attempting primary resection include higher long-term survival rates and resectability, prevention of progression of the cancer between decompression and primary resection, and one or two fewer operations than staged tumor removal.

Clark et al recommend that no primary anastomosis should be performed following left or right colon resection for obstructing carcinoma.[65] Instead, both cut ends of bowel should be exteriorized as a colostomy/ileostomy and mucous fistula. Anastomotic leakage and disruption are cited as the major causes of 27% (left colon) and 35% (right colon) of mortalities among these patients. Restoration of bowel continuity may be attempted a few months later and provides a chance for a "second-look" laparotomy. Their series studied patients who were operated on during the 1960s and earlier largely by residents in training with varying degrees of supervision.

Carson et al, in a review of 129 cases of colonic obstruction from left-sided cancers, found that primary resection resulted in decreased operative mortality, decreased incidence of postoperative sepsis, and increased long-term survival, compared with colostomy alone or colostomy as part of a staged procedure.[66] All primary resections were protected by a proximal diverting colostomy.

Valerio and Jones developed a policy of resection in large bowel emergencies and achieved resection in 65% with a 15% operative mortality.[6] Anastomosis of proximal and distal segments usually followed resection, and the anastomosis was protected by a proximal diverting colostomy. Fielding et al, in a prospective study of outcome following staged or primary resection, found that although the mortality of primary tumor resection was high (25%), it was no higher than that of staged tumor resection. Of patients with distal tumors in whom a staged resection was planned, 35% died after a loop colostomy. However primary resection was more desirable insofar as the duration of hospital stay for patients was one half that of the former group.[67] The most striking result was that the ratio of postoperative deaths for trainee surgeons compared with fully trained surgeons was 3 to 1.[67]

Koruth and Hunter reviewed 104 cases of emergency laparotomy, and 82 (79%) had a primary resection with a mortality of 12.2%, an intraperitoneal sepsis rate of 2.4%, and a wound sepsis rate of 8.7%.[62] One half of the patients who had resections involving obstructing cancers of the left colon underwent primary anastomosis, and 13.3% died. Intraoperative antegrade colonic irrigation was performed prior to all primary anastomoses. Two other series by White and Macfie (35 patients) and Amsterdam and Mayer (25 patients) performed primary resection and colostomy as the procedure of choice in obstructing cancers of the left colon.[68, 69]

Operative mortalities were 8.5% and 12% respectively, with complication rates of 29% and 62%. In both groups the distended remaining proximal bowel was emptied by a mixture of aspiration, irrigation, and "milking" maneuvers.[68, 69] The largest series comparing primary resection and staged resection for obstructing carcinomas is drawn from the Large Bowel Cancer Project, which demonstrates high in-hospital mortality rates (19% versus 22%) and equivalent 5-year survival rates (25%) for both procedures.[49, 52, 57] Completed staged resection was reported with a 6% mortality rate; however 25% (36 of 157 patients) died before the second stage could be completed. The major disadvantage of primary anastomosis was the high clinical leak rate (18%) reported following left-sided resection and anastomosis. This compares to rates of 10% in right-sided obstruction and 6% in elective resection. The major advantage for primary resection was the shorter hospital stay (20 + 1.7 compared with 40 + 4.6 days) and fewer wound infections.[49, 52, 57]

Total Abdominal Colectomy and Anastomosis

Primary resection has been carried one step further to include subtotal or total colectomy with reported complication rates of 26.6% to 40%, operative mortality rates of 7% to 20%, and average hospital stays of 8.4 to 18 days.[70–73] Advocates include Klatt et al[70] (5 patients) Deutch et al[71] (14 patients), Hughes et al[72] (52 patients), and Feng et al[73] (9 patients). The procedure is performed without proximal diversion. If intraperitoneal contamination occurs during mobilization or resection, exteriorization should replace primary anastomosis. The results are good, with a com-

bined mortality rate of less than 10%, and are strongly influenced by patient selection and experience in performing the larger operation. In addition to the benefits cited for primary resection, subtotal colectomy removes additional synchronous tumors and a possible septic focus, which is the distended and contaminated colon. Feng et al report that 3 months after operation, the average number of bowel movements was 1.8 per day in their subtotal or total colectomy patients.[73]

INTUSSUSCEPTION

Intussusception is the invagination of proximal bowel (intussusceptum) into the distal lumen (intussuscipiens). About 90% to 95% of intussusceptions occur in infancy or early childhood, and 85% to 95% of these are ileocolic and idiopathic.[74–76] In adults, intussusception is rare, accounting for 5% to 15% of cases, most patients being over 50 years of age.[74–77] Felix et al, in a review of 1,214 reported cases, estimated that 63% (759 of 1,214) of all intussusceptions in adults are tumor-related.[78] Among the colonic intussusceptions (45%, or 546 of 1,214 patients), 48% resulted from malignant tumors and 21% from benign tumors. Of the small bowel intussusceptions (55%, or 668 of 1,214 patients), 17% were attributable to malignant tumors and 40% to benign tumors.

In a review of the world literature including 1,593 patients, Nichter and Busuttil noted an even distribution of cases throughout the gastrointestinal tract.[74] In adults, approximately 85% of instances were secondary to a specific intramural lesion, and, in general, older patients had a greater chance of having a malignant tumor. Overall, 39% of cases were secondary to malignancy; there is a 55% risk with colonic intussusception and a 24% risk with the small bowel.[74]

History

The duration of symptoms is variable, and most patients suffer from chronic, intermittent, partial obstruction[74, 77, 79]; less than 20% have complete obstruction.[77, 80] Pain is present in 71% to 96% of patients and is usually crampy and intermittent.[74, 77, 79, 81–83] Nausea and vomiting are present in 68% to 82% of patients and occur with greater frequency with increasingly more proximal obstructions.[74, 77, 79, 81] Passage of bloody bowel movements may occur, and melena is observed in 38% to 47% of patients.[74, 79] Tenderness (60%) and distention (45%) are the most common findings on examination.[80, 81] A palpable abdominal mass (20% to 50%) is sometimes present only during the attacks.[74, 77, 78, 79]

Diagnostic Studies

Plain abdominal radiographs sometimes reveal, aside from the typical hydrogaseous formations, a soft mass protruding into the lumen of the dilated bowel.[80] Barium enema studies may show "crescent-edge," "coiled spring," "pitchfork," or "bird's beak" signs.[74] No attempt should be made at hydrostatic reduction in adults.[74, 80, 81, 84]

Ultrasonography usually shows a dense, echogenic core corresponding to the lumen of the gas and mucus-filled intussusception and presenting a series of interfaces, while it is surrounded by a peripheral sonolucent zone corresponding to the edematous bowel wall.[80] Ultrasonography is the preferred method of diagnosis in the 4% to 6% of intestinal obstructions caused by intussusception during pregnancy.[83]

Computed tomographic scanning also enables a diagnosis to be made. It has the additional advantage of helping to determine the nature of the tumor and thus to decide, to some extent, on the possibility of malignancy.[83]

In rare cases, the diagnosis is made after pathologic examination of sloughed or autoamputated portions of bowel wall.[82, 85] Thirty total cases of spontaneous expulsion of an amputation portion of bowel with healing and restoration of bowel continuity have been reported.[85]

Treatment

Surgical management of adult intussusception is the procedure of choice.[74, 77, 80] No attempt at reduction prior to resection should be performed for fear of intraluminal seeding and/or venous embolization of tumor cells, and also the possibility of peritoneal soiling if strangulation is present.[77] The operation should include wide resection of the colon and its associated mesentery.[74, 77] Primary anastomosis following small intestine or right colon resection is usually possible. Staged reanastomosis should follow left colon resection. For patients with sigmoidorectal intussusception, abdominoperineal amputation should not be performed unless histologic evidence of malignancy has first been obtained.[80]

DIVERTICULITIS CAUSING COLONIC OBSTRUCTION

The most common acute complication of diverticular disease is perforation with spreading peritonitis.[6, 86–90] However about 60% to 70% of diverticulitis patients have some degree of large bowel obstruction, and 10% develop acute large bowel obstruction.[7] This constitutes the second most common cause of acute colonic obstruction in adults.[7] For a stable population of almost 400,000 people in northeast Scotland, Kyle and Davidson reported a combined hospital incidence of six patients per year being admitted to three Aberdeen Hospitals over two 5-year periods.[91] Rodkey and Welch, in a review of 338 cases of diverticular disease, present several theories about why the sigmoid colon is prone to develop pulsion diverticula.[92] Circular muscle thickening and hypertrophy result in segmentation of the colon and markedly increased intraluminal pressures within these closed compartments. Because the sigmoid is the narrowest portion of the colon, it develops the highest intraluminal pressure per unit of muscular wall tension (Laplace's law). Increased irritability of the sigmoid has also been identified in patients with diverticular disease, compared with normal controls. Therefore, not only is the sigmoid colon capable of developing high intraluminal pressure, but it also has the propensity to do so more often than other areas of the colon.[92] Acute obstruction is the result of fibrous stenosis from previous inflammation and acute inflammatory processes with resultant edema and spasm.[87]

Diagnosis

History and Physical Examination

Letwin was able to elicit a history of diverticulitis in 74% of 46 patients proved to have acute sequelae of diverticular disease.[87] Abdominal pain, tenderness, and some variation in bowel function were present in most patients. Abdominal distention and nausea were usually present with obstruction (14 patients). A palpable abdominal mass was present in nine patients. In their evaluation of patients for colonic diverticular disease, Kyle and Davidson use the following as diagnostic clinical features: (1) left-sided or lower abdominal pain, (2) deep tenderness in the left iliac foss, (3) altered bowel habit, (4) rectal bleeding, (5) pyrexia over 37.5%, and (6) leukocytosis of $10,000/mm^3$ or more.[91]

Diagnostic Studies

Radiographic studies, including plain and upright films of the abdomen and barium enema, aid in confirming the suspicion of obstruction and in elucidating the cause. Findings on barium study that help differentiate obstruction due to diverticular disease from that caused by cancer include the following: (1) diverticular disease usually affects a long segment of bowel, whereas in carcinoma the lesion is often short (although there are many exceptions to this rule); (2) in carcinoma, the transition from normal to diseased bowel is usually abrupt, whereas in diverticular disease it is more gradual; (3) a bizarre fringed contour is more often associated with diverticulitis; (4) in the benign lesion, the mucosa is intact, whereas in carcinoma it is destroyed; (5) the presence of diverticula in the bowel above or below the area of narrowing is rather in favor of a diagnosis of diverticulitis, although both conditions may coexist, and having diverticula does not render a patient immune from carcinoma of the colon; (6) spasm of the colon is more constant in diverticular disease than in carcinoma.[1]

Treatment

Krukowski and Matheson, in a review of the literature from 1957 to 1984, cited 57 publications totaling 1,282 patients.[89] During a period of review, the majority of patients (64%) have been treated by a conservative operation (i.e., diverting colostomy with or without drainage of any pericolic abscess) with a combined mortality of 25%. This is in contrast to the results for any form of primary resection in which the combined mortality is 11%. Although a wide range of differences in operative technique and perioperative management must be taken for granted in this collected series, it is clear that the mortality for extirpative surgery is less than one half that for more conservative procedures.[89]

In a second article, Krukowski et al state that emergency resection of the sigmoid colon is the preferred treatment for patients with generalized or fecal peritonitis, but most patients present with less florid disease, in which case aggressive surgery is inappropriate.[86] Among their 57 patients admitted with "acute diverticulitis," 37 were managed conservatively without operation. Even among four patients who had pericolic and/or pelvic abscesses at operation, no resection was performed. Lambert et al agree with Krukowski that the Hartmann procedure is the procedure of choice in cases of communicating perforation; however, defunctioning colostomy and drainage has an acceptably low mortality under "favorable" conditions.[82] Classen et al, in a 10-year retrospective study using the three-stage procedure, reported a combined operative mortality of 11% with over 200 patients.[93] However, over one quarter of these patients did not have the diseased colon resected.

Problems with staged resection or colostomy and drainage as primary therapy for these acute cases of diverticulitis include (1) recurrence of symptoms in 50% to 70% of patients,[86] (2) retained carcinoma with sigmoid colon and upper rectal lesions in up to 25% of patients,[90] (3) continued sepsis and death,[94–96] (4) progressive fibrosis and overt colon obstruction. Less

severe problems include the prolonged disability and prolonged hospitalization with similar postoperative complications.[94–96] Fistula formation with or without repair of unrecognized small perforation can be expected in 20% of patients.

Auguste and Wise[95] and Liebert and DeWeese[94] reported favorable results with resection and the Hartmann procedure for the treatment of perforated diverticulitis, sometimes with abscess and obstruction. In both reports 100% of their 43 patients left the hospital cured. Eisenstat et al,[97] Underwood and Marks,[96] and Nagorney et al[98] agree that their results with resection and the Hartmann procedure make it the recommended alternative approach for the acute complications of diverticulitis: perforation, obstruction, abscess, and fistula formation. Killingback further clarifies the objectives of surgical therapy in his review of 248 cases in 1983.[88] The aim of the operation is to excise a relatively small segment of the bowel with its perforation. This removes the affected segment and prevents further contamination. An end-colostomy with a Hartmann closure of the rectal stump is mandatory. It is not the time to perform a formal or definitive resection of diverticular disease of the left part of the colon.

EDITORIAL COMMENT

In keeping with our preference for primary resection for obstructing cancers, we also recommend primary resection *without* anastomosis as the treatment of choice for diverticulitis complicated by obstruction or perforation. We agree with the authors that a definitive resection of all diverticular disease is not the purpose of the emergency procedure. The site of obstruction or fecal contamination is removed, the proximal colon brought out as an end-colostomy, and the distal segment closed as a Hartmann pouch. In rare instances the rectum is so inflamed that safe closure is impossible. In this situation a controlled fistula may be established by a large-bore tube placed in the end of the tenuously closed rectum. The drainage tube is brought to the abdominal wall extraperitoneally. The rectum is then irrigated free of feces after completion of the procedure, and a Foley catheter is inserted through the anus into the rectum. The catheters are then irrigated frequently or continuously, and after a few days both catheters can be removed with safety. In the few cases in which we have resorted to this technique, we have been rewarded by spontaneous closure without a pelvic abscess.

A diverting colostomy is reserved for patients in whom there is a large pericolic or pelvic abscess complicating the diverticulitis. For these patients, extraperitoneal drainage of the abscess and complete fecal diversion, usually by a right transverse colostomy, are accomplished as the initial operative procedure. Percutaneous drainage by a small-bore catheter will usually fail, so open drainage via an extraperitoneal route is our recommended treatment.

REFERENCES

1. Ellis H. Intestinal Obstruction. New York: Appleton-Century-Crofts, 1982.
2. Ricketts RR. Workup of neonatal obstruction. Am Surg 1984;50:517–521.
3. Ghory MJ, Sheldon CA. Newborn surgical emergencies of the gastrointestinal tract. Surg Clin North Am 1985;65:1083–1098.
4. Starling JR, Croom RD, Thomas CG. Hirschsprung's disease in young adults. Am J Surg 1986;151:104–109.
5. Fitchett CW, Hoffman GC. Obstructing malignant lesions of the colon. Surg Clin North Am 1986;66:807–820.
6. Valerio D, Jones PF. Immediate resection in the treatment of large bowel emergencies. Br J Surg 1978;65:712–716.
7. Moossa AR, Altorki N. Large bowel obstruction. In: Cameron J, ed. Current Surgical Therapy. Burlington, Ontario: BC Decker, 1985–1986, 103–104.
8. Irvin GL III, Horsley J, Caruana JA. The morbidity and mortality of emergent operations for colorectal disease. Ann Surg 1984;199:598–603.
9. Wangensteen OH, Rea CE. The distention factor in simple intestinal obstruction; experimental study with exclusion of swallowed air by cervical esophagotomy. Surgery 1939;5:327.
10. Papanicolaou G, Nikas D, Ahn Y, Condos S, Fielding P. Regional blood flow and water content of the obstructed small intestine. Arch Surg 1985;120:926–932.
11. Coxon JE, Dickson C, Taylor I. Changes in colonic motility during the development of chronic large bowel obstruction. Br J Surg 1985;72:690–693.
12. Brolin RE, Reddell MT. Gastrointestinal myoelectric activity in mechanical intestinal obstruction. J Surg Res 1985;38:515–523.
13. Welch JP, Donaldson GA. Management of severe obstruction of the large bowel due to malignant disease. Am J Surg 1974;127:492–499.
14. Vanek VW, Al-Salti M. Acute pseudo-obstruction of the colon (Ogilvie's syndrome): An analysis of 400 cases. Dis Colon Rectum 1986;29:203–210.
15. Soreide O, Bjerkeset T, Fossidal JE. Pseudo-obstruction of the colon (Ogilvie's syndrome), a genuine clinical condition? Dis Colon Rectum 1977;20:487–491.
16. Eisenberg RL, Heineken P, Hedgcock HW, et al. Evaluation of plain abdominal radiographs in the diagnosis of abdominal pain. Ann Intern Med 1982;97:257–261.
17. Lelcuk S, Klausner JM, Merhav A, et al. Endoscopic decompression of acute colonic obstruction. Ann Surg 1986;203:292–294.
18. Avots-Atotins K. Multifocal carcinoma of the colon. Surg Clin North Am 1986;66:793–800.
19. Isler JT, Brown PC, Lewis FG, Billingham RP. The role of preoperative colonoscopy in colorectal cancer. Dis Colon Rectum 1987;30:435–439.
20. Bode WE, Beart RW Jr, Spencer RJ, et al. Colonoscopic decompression for acute pseudo-obstruction of the colon (Ogilvie's syndrome). Am J Surg 1984;147:243–245.
21. Fausel CS, Goff JS. Nonoperative management of acute idiopathic colonic pseudo-obstruction (Ogilvie's syndrome). West J Med 1985;143:50–54.
22. Nanni G, Garbini A, Luchetti P, et al. Ogilvie's syndrome (acute colonic pseudo-obstruction). Dis Colon Rectum 1985;25:157–166.
23. Mivatvongs S, Vermeulen FD, Fang DT. Colonoscopic decompression of acute pseudo-obstruction of the colon. Ann Surg 1982;196:598–600.
24. Nano D, Prindiville T, Pauly M, et al. Colonoscopic therapy of acute pseudo-obstruction of the colon. Am J Gastroenterol 1987;82:145–148.
25. Spira IA, Rodrigues R, Wolff WI. Pseudo-obstruction of the colon. Am J Gastroenterol 1976;65:397–408.
26. Wanebo H, Mathewson C, Conolly B. Pseudo-obstruction of the colon. Surg Gynecol Obstet 1971;164:44–48.
27. Ponsky JL, Aszondi A, Perse D. Percutaneous endoscopic cecostomy: A new approach to nonobstructive colonic dilation. Gastrointest Endosc 1986;32:108–111.
28. Geelhoed GW. Colonic pseudo-obstruction in surgical patients. Am J Surg 1985;149:258–265.
29. Norton L, Young D, Scribner R. Management of pseudo-obstruction of the colon. Surg Gynecol Obstet 1974;138:595–598.
30. Gierson ED, Storm FK, Shaw W, Coyne SK. Caecal rupture due to colonic ileus. Br J Surg 1975;62:383–386.
31. Mungos J, Moossa AR, Block GE. Treatment of toxic megacolon. Surg Clin North Am 1976;56:95–102.
32. Fazio VLV. Toxic megacolon in ulcerative colitis and Crohn's disease. Clin Gastroenterol 1980;2:389–406.
33. Torsoli A. Toxic megacolon. Part 2: Prevention. Clin Gastroenterol 1981;1:117–121.
34. Moossa AR, Lavelle-Jones M, Scott MH. Management of acute presentations in inflammatory bowel disease. In: Gastrointestinal Emergencies. New York: Churchill Livingstone, 1987, pp 108–131.
35. Ballantyne GH, Brandner MD, Beart RW Jr, Ilstrup DM. Volvulus of the colon. Incidence and mortality. Ann Surg 1985;202:83–91.
36. Welch GH, Anderson JR. Acute volvulus of the sigmoid colon. World J Surg 1987;11:258–262.
37. Singh G, Gupta SK, Gupta S. Simultaneous occurrence of sigmoid and cecal volvulus. Dis Colon Rectum 1985;28:115–116.
38. Avots-Avotins K, Waugh D. Colon volvulus and the geriatric patient. Surg Clin North Am 1982;62:249–260.
39. Anderson JR, Welch GH. Acute volvulus of the right colon: An analysis of 69 patients. World J Surg 1986;10:336–342.
40. O'Mara CS, Wilson TH, Stonesifer GL, Cameron JL. Cecal volvulus. Ann Surg 1979;189:724–731.
41. Corman ML. Miscellaneous colon and rectal collections. In: Colon and Rectum Surgery. Philadelphia: JB Lippincott, 1984, pp 699–765.
42. Ballantyne GH. Review of sigmoid volvulus; history and results of treatment. Dis Colon Rectum 1982;25:494–501.
43. Wertkin MG, Aufses AH Jr. Management of volvulus of the colon. Dis Colon Rectum 1978;21:40–45.
44. Ballantyne GH. Review of sigmoid volvulus; clinical patterns and pathogenesis. Dis Colon Rectum 1982;25:823–830.
45. Anderson JR, Lee D. The management of acute sigmoid volvulus. Br J Surg 1981;68:117–120.
46. Agrez M, Cameron D. Radiology of sigmoid volvulus. Dis Colon Rectum 1981;24:510–514.
47. Willett C, Tepper JE, Cohen A, et al. Obstructive and perforative colonic carcinoma: Patterns of failure. J Clin Oncol 1985;3:379–384.
48. Steinberg SM, Barkin JS, Kaplan RS, Stablein DM. Prognostic indicators of colon tumors. Cancer 1986;57:1866–1870.
49. Kelley WE Jr, Brown PW, Lawrence W Jr, Terz JJ. Penetrating, obstructing, and perforating carcinomas of the colon and rectum. Arch Surg 1981;116:381–384.
50. Ohman U. Prognosis in patients with obstructing colorectal carcinoma. Am J Surg 1982;143:742–747.
51. Dutton JW, Hreno A, Hampson LG. Mortality and prognosis of obstructing carcinoma of the large bowel. Am J Surg 1976;131:36–41.
52. Phillips RKS, Hittinger R, Fry JS, Fielding LP. Malignant large bowel obstruction. Br J Surg 1985;72:296–302.
53. Aldridge MC, Phillips RKS, Hittinger R, et al. Influence of tumour site on presentation, management and subsequent outcome in large bowel cancer. Br J Surg 1986;73:663–670.
54. Umpleby HC, Williamson RCN, Chir M. Survival in acute obstructing colorectal carcinoma. Dis Colon Rectum 1984;27:299–304.
55. Schein CJ, Gemming RH. The prognostic implications of obstructing left colonic cancer. Dis Colon Rectum 1981;24:454–455.
56. Waldron RP, Donovan IA, Drumm J, et al. Emergency presentation and mortality from colorectal cancer in the elderly. Br J Surg 1986;73:214–216.
57. Wolmark N, Wienad HS, Rockette HE, and other NSABP investigators. The prognostic significance of tumor location and bowel obstruction in Duke's B and C colorectal cancer. Ann Surg 1983;198:743–750.

58. DeLeon ML, Schoetz DJ, Jr, Coller JA, Veidenheimer MC. Colorectal cancer: Lahey clinic experience, 1972–76. Dis Colon Rectum 1987;30:237–242.
59. Chapuis PH, Dent OF, Fisher R, et al. A multivariate analysis of clinical and pathological variables in prognosis after resection of large bowel cancer. Br J Surg 1985;72:698–702.
60. Vanek VM, Whitt CL, Abdu RA, Kennedy WR. Comparison of right colon, left colon and rectal carcinoma. Am Surg 1986;52:504–509.
61. Stewart J, Finan PJ, Courtney DF, Brennan TG. Does a water soluble contrast enema assist in the management of acute large bowel obstruction: A prospective study of 117 cases. Br J Surg 1984;71:799–801.
62. Koruth NM, Hunter DC, Krudowski ZH, Matheson NA. Immediate resection in emergency large bowel surgery: A 7 year audit. Br J Surg 1985;72:703–707.
63. Miller FB, Nikolov NR, Garrison N. Emergency right colon resection. Arch Surg 1987;122:339–343.
64. Corman ML. Carcinoma of the colon. Colon and Rectum Surgery. Philadelphia: JB Lippincott, 1984, pp 267–328.
65. Clark J, Hall HW, Moossa AR. Treatment of obstructing cancer of the colon and rectum. Surg Obstet Gynecol 1975;141:541–544.
66. Carson SN, Poticha SM, Shield TW. Carcinoma obstructing the left side of the colon. Arch Surg 1977;112:523–526.
67. Fielding LP, Stewart-Brown S, Blesorsky L. Large bowel obstruction caused by cancer: A prospective study. Br Med J 1979;2:515–517.
68. White CM, Macfie J. Immediate colectomy and primary anastomosis for acute obstruction due to carcinoma of the left colon and rectum. Dis Colon Rectum 1985;28:155–157.
69. Armsterdam E, Mayer K. Primary resection with colocolostomy for obstructive carcinoma of the left side of the colon. Am J Surg 1985;150:558–560.
70. Klatt GR, Martin MH, Gillespie JI. Subtotal colectomy with primary anastomosis without diversion in the treatment of obstructing carcinoma of the left colon. Am J Surg 1981;141:577–578.
71. Deutsch A, Zelikovski A, Sternberg A, Reiss R. One stage subtotal colectomy with anastomosis for obstructing carcinoma of the left colon. Dis Colon Rectum 1983;26:227–230.
72. Hughes ESR, McDermott FT, Polglase AL, Nottle P. Total and subtotal colectomy with anastomosis for obstructing carcinoma of the left colon. Dis Colon Rectum 1985;28:162–163.
73. Feng YS, Hsu H, Chen SS. One-stage operation for obstructing carcinoma of the left colon and rectum. Dis Colon Rectum 1987;30:29–32.
74. Nichter LS, Busuttil RW. Update on the management of de novo adult intussusception. Curr Surg 1983; May–June:186–193.
75. Nyhan W, Wilson N, Powers NG, et al. Specialty conference: Intussusception. West J Med 1986;144:722–727.
76. Agha FP. Review: Intussusception in adults. Am J Radiol 1986;146:527–531.
77. Nagendran T, Imm F, Butler K. Intussusception in adults. Ala Med 1986; November:28–30.
78. Felix E. Adult intussusception: A case report of recurrent intussusception and a review of the literature. Am J Surg 1976;131:758–761.
79. Hurwitz LM, Gertler SL. Colonoscopic diagnosis of ileocolic intussusception. Gastrointest Endosc 1986;31:217–218.
80. Schuind F, Gansbeke DV, Ansay J. Intussusception in adults—report of 3 cases. Acta Chir Belg 1985;85:55–60.
81. Fawaz F, Hill GJ. Adult intussusception due to metastatic tumors. South Med J 1983;76:522–523.
82. Zamboni WA, Fleisher H, Zander JD, Folse JR. Spontaneous expulsion of lipoma per rectum occurring with colonic intussusception. Surgery 1987;101:104–107.
83. Watson R, Quayle AR. Intussusception in pregnancy. Case report and review of the literature. Br J Obstet Gynecol 1986;93:1093–1096.
84. Nielsen PT, Bentsen N. Simultaneous occurrence of colo-colic intussusception and distal colon perforation. Acta Chir Scand 1983;148:107–108.
85. Gomes GA, Hernandez A, Plasencia G, Dove DB. Adult intussusception with autoamputation and preservation of bowel continuity. Dis Colon Rectum 1984;27:654–657.
86. Lambert ME, Knox RA, Schofield PF, Hancock BD. Management of the septic complications of diverticular disease. Br J Surg 1986;73:576–579.
87. Letwin ER. Diverticulitis of the colon. Am J Surg 1982;143:579–581.
88. Killingback M. Management of perforative diverticulitis. Surg Clin North Am 1983;63:97–115.
89. Krukowski ZH, Matheson NA. Emergency surgery for diverticular disease complicated by generalized and faecal peritonitis: A review. Br J Surg 1984;71:921–927.
90. Krukowski ZH, Koruth NM, Matheson NA. Evolving practice in acute diverticulitis. Br J Surg 1985;72:684–686.
91. Kyle J, Davidson AI. The changing pattern of hospital admissions for diverticular disease of the colon. Br J Surg 1975;62:537–541.
92. Rodkey GV, Welch CE. Colonic diverticular disease with surgical treatment. Surg Clin North Am 1974;54:655–675.
93. Classen JN, Bonardi R, O'Mara CS, et al. Surgical treatment of acute diverticulitis by staged procedures. Ann Surg 1976;184:582–586.
94. Liebert CW, DeWeese BM. Primary resection without anastomosis for perforation of acute diverticulitis. Surg Gynecol Obstet 1981;152:30–32.
95. Auguste LJ, Wise L. Surgical management of perforated diverticulitis. Am J Surg 1981;141:122–127.
96. Underwood JW, Marks CG. The septic complications of sigmoid diverticular disease. Br J Surg 1984;71:209–211.
97. Eisenstat TE, Rubin RJ, Salvatti EP. Surgical management of diverticulitis; the role of the Hartmann procedure. Dis Colon Rectum 1983;26:429–432.
98. Nagorney DM, Adson MA, Pembeston JH. Sigmoid diverticulitis with perforation and generalized peritonitis. Dis Colon Rectum 1985;28:71–75.

Trauma to the Colon and Rectum

C H A P T E R 1 2

Alexander J. Walt
Scott A. Dulchavsky

HISTORICAL PERSPECTIVE

No area within the field of surgery is static. However, the evolution of our current management of colonic and rectal injuries illustrates how slowly changes may occur and how the weight of tradition may impede the growth of new ideas. Yesterday's blasphemy has become today's tentative truth partly because of our improved ability to limit shock and infection. Furthermore, a willingness has emerged to challenge and disprove accepted beliefs with well-designed surgical protocols.

Almost 40 years elapsed before Woodhall and Ochsner's paper[1] on the feasibility and desirability of primary repair of colonic injuries was well accepted. The clinical research of the late 1970s, underpinned by improved technical training of residents in trauma centers, led to the acceptance of primary repair as the appropriate treatment in most cases of colonic injury. A significant change is that surgeons of today need first to justify their decision *not* to do a primary repair rather than a staged procedure. The slow transition to this view is partly attributable to the fact that mortality associated with colonic injuries has often been unfairly and incorrectly attributed to the colon, rather than to the extensive associated injuries that are so often present. Failure to examine available data critically has perpetuated excessively conservative practices.

In trauma, certain organs acquired, during earlier decades, reputations that engendered excessive caution—if not fear—in the minds of surgeons. One century ago the heart was considered inviolate, as is reflected by Billroth's famous statement that "Any surgeon operating on the heart is a fool." Yet by the early 1960s (preceding well-established aortocoronary bypass), stabs and gunshot wounds of the heart were being operated on with salvage rates in excess of 80%. The liver, often regarded as surgical *terra incognito*, has surrendered much of its menace, except when injury to the large juxtahepatic veins is present. Similarly, injuries of the colon and rectum, with current mortality rates of approximately 6% or less, are being approached with greater confidence, less conservatism, and more logic than in the past. When the causes of death are analyzed, two thirds are found to be the result of nonintestinal factors. Although injury to the large bowel continues to be distinguished by high morbidity rates, some of this problem is iatrogenic and attributable to the selection of colostomy or ileostomy in patients when these procedures are in fact avoidable.

World War II Experience

A brief exploration of the changing therapeutic saga of large bowel injury in the modern era begins with World War II, which produced influential reports backed by the full military authority of Ogilvie from the Western Desert and of Mason for the U.S. Forces. Ogilvie wrote

The treatment of colon injury is based on the known insecurity of suture and dangers of leakage. Simple closure of a wound to the colon, however small, is unwarranted; men have survived such an operation, but others

have died who would still be alive had they fallen into the hands of a surgeon with less optimism and more sense. Injured segments must either be exteriorized or functionally excluded by approximal colostomy.[2]

The implementation of this policy reduced the mortality rate from the injured colon by about one half.

Unfortunately, the environment in which this dogma developed is often not appreciated. In the desert and subsequently on the Italian front, a substantial delay between wounding and definitive operation at a field surgical unit was the standard circumstance. By the time the patient was operated on, gross contamination and established infection of the peritoneal cavity was the norm. Antibiotics were as yet unavailable (the first, penicillin, was provided in only small amounts as an experimental drug in 1944). Facilities in the field surgical units were relatively primitive, and casualties were not yet helicoptered back to sophisticated operating rooms. The patient was treated by a generation of surgeons unschooled in the lessons of today's urban violence and technically much less well trained. Above all, Ogilvie observed the disasters that occurred when these patients were cared for in understaffed and improvised units or, often worse, the deterioration that followed the transport of patients with freshly anastomosed colonic wounds over long distances and bumpy tracks. The rapid establishment of a colostomy and early evacuation of the patient were shown to be safer and more efficient from both clinical and military viewpoints.

This fear of the leaking anastomosis and peritonitis became deeply ingrained in combat surgeons. Nevertheless, on their return to civilian life, the generation of young World War II surgeons soon began to reexamine the military edict in the light of civilian needs; transport, hospital facilities, antibiotics, nursing care, and acquired surgical experience were all different and incomparably more favorable. By 1951, Woodhall and Ochsner were suggesting the desirability of primary anastomosis in selected cases of colonic injury to reduce hospital stay, morbidity, and need for multiple operations.[1] They stated that "the wartime practice of exteriorization of colon wounds has been carried over into civilian practice too wholeheartedly for the patients' greatest good. It is possible that with the use of antibiotics and modern supportive therapy the more radical methods of treating major colon wounds will find greater applicability."[1]

Experience After World War II

Unfortunately, the 1950s were soon interrupted by the Korean War, and the management protocols of the campaigns that had ended just 6 years earlier were

reinstituted. A new generation of surgeons were also temporarily "immunized" against the concept of primary repair. Nevertheless, in 1957, Pontius et al repeated the plea for primary colonic repair.[3]

During the 1960s there was a clinical analysis of the differences between military and civilian injuries.[4, 5] The safety of primary repair of most stab wounds and low-velocity missile injuries rapidly gained adherents, but soon the accelerated civilian use of guns, often of high velocity and causing extensive damage to multiple organs, reinforced the traditional caution associated with the care of military wounds. The prospect of having to account at morbidity and mortality conferences for any purported failure following a primary repair was chilling, even when the morbidity might not originate from the colon and would *not* have been avoided by a staged operation. Conservative thinking continued to promote the advantages of a defunctioning colostomy while discouraging or ignoring its disadvantages—temporal, psychological, economic, and surgical.

The 1970s was the decade during which serious challenges to conservative treatment became more evident. Large series of cases from major urban trauma centers began selectively to advance the cause of a more liberal use of primary repair. Contraindications became more clearly defined and were crystallized in the conclusions of Stone and Fabian in 1979, who advocated obligatory colostomy under defined conditions.[6] These conditions were (1) shock with preoperative blood pressure less than 80/60 mm Hg, (2) hemorrhage with intraperitoneal blood loss of more than 1,000 cc, (3) more than two intra-abdominal organs injured, (4) contamination with significant peritoneal soilage by feces, (5) operation begun more than 8 hours after injury, (6) colonic wound so destructive as to require resection, and (7) abdominal wall injury with major loss of substance requiring mesh replacement.

Nonetheless, firm beliefs—perhaps prejudices—continued to be expressed. Prominent among these was the belief that healing in the left colon was substantially different from that in the right colon, a view based mainly on the purported effects of increased collagenase in the descending colon of rabbits.[7] The concept of primary repair of the left colon, with or without resection, was thought by many to be outside the bounds of good judgment.

The 1980s were characterized by a few well-planned prospective randomized series of cases from single institutions, which brought a reasoned perspective to the problem (Table 12–1). The pioneering study of Stone and Fabian[6] was followed by others that confirmed and extended their original observations. The net result of this clinical research has been a gradual but steady loosening of old inflexibilities and a sub-

Table 12–1. COLON TRAUMA: MANAGEMENT TRENDS

Institution	Year	No. Patients	Knife:GSW:Blunt	Percentage Primary Repair	Percentage Exteriorization	Mortality
Charity	1957	128	38:59:3	38%	7.0%	19.0%
Baylor	1957	122	29:65:1	68%	16.0%	15.0%
Los Angeles County	1963	138	25:49:5	55%	7.0%	6.6%
Grady	1968	266	19:80:1	37%	34.0%	14.6%
Denver	1985	228	NA	49%	15.0%	3.0%
Wayne State	1987	239	16:76:5	44%	4.0%	9.3%
Baylor	1990	1006	25:72:2	61%	8.3%	10.4%

Combined trauma center data depict the patient mix, incidence of primary repair, and use of exteriorization in the previous decades. Note the generous early use of primary repair in the Baylor series.

GSW = gunshot wound; NA = not applicable.

stantially increased incidence of primary repair. In a world in which fear of medicolegal punishment for not performing staged procedures has long influenced practice, the data that establish primary repair as an acceptable standard of care that encourages more rapid recovery time have substantially changed surgical attitudes.

Now, in the 1990s, although some questions are unanswered, an extensive data base is available from which to develop surgical decisions. Obviously, the temptation to push the boundaries of primary repair beyond reasonable limits has to be resisted. Nevertheless, the great majority of colonic injuries seem not to need concomitant colostomy when technical competence and good clinical judgment are present.

As new technology and data broaden our understanding, few, if any, surgical problems are ever finally resolved. These factors are the subject of the following assessment of current approaches to colonic and rectal injuries, which constitute separate problems by virtue of their anatomic constraints.

COLONIC INJURIES

Wounding Agents

Colonic injury may be blunt or penetrating (most often from stabs, missiles, or intraluminal pressure). The anatomic and clinical pictures of each vary widely. Penetrating injuries are the most common types, but their relative incidence in any specific demographic area reflects the cultural characteristics of the population. Representative series are illustrated in Table 12–1.

Blunt Injuries

Morgagni, in his *Epistola* of 1761, described the clinical course of patients sustaining intestinal injury from blunt abdominal trauma. In his discourse, he warned against initial optimism and highlighted the progressive nature of these injuries in the initially stable patients. Blunt intestinal injuries occur in 3% to 10% of patients admitted with abdominal trauma.[8, 9] Although the small bowel and its mesentery are more frequently injured than the colon, the incidence of blunt colonic injury is increasing in part because of "seat-belt injuries" and a rise in the number of motor vehicle accidents. Blunt injury constitutes about 5% of all colonic injury

Automobile accidents account for over 90% of blunt colonic injuries, with the steering wheel and the seat belt immediately responsible. Other etiologic factors include the handle bars of cycles, and kicks and blows on the relaxed abdominal wall. A fractured lumbar vertebra, especially in conjunction with a hematoma of the anterior abdominal wall, should serve as a warning that the bowel may have been compressed between the two.

A significant blunt force is required to produce a colonic injury; therefore, associated organ injury is noted in more than 90% of patients with blunt colonic injury. The liver and spleen are the organs most frequently involved, and the mortality following their injury parallels the extent of associated organ injury. Injuries to the head, thorax, and skeleton are often present. Three mechanisms lead to nonpenetrating colonic injury: direct crush injuries, shearing forces, and burst injuries. Crush injuries to the colon occur most frequently and result from a direct compression of the colon between the anterior abdominal wall and the lumbar spine. This compression may produce serosal tears, hematoma formations, or complete lacerations. Injuries of this nature occur most frequently in the transverse colon and must be suspected in patients sustaining significant blunt abdominal trauma, particularly if there is an anterior abdominal hematoma, rectus muscle injury, or spinal fracture. Deceleration injuries of the colon involve shear stress at points of relative colonic fixation. Consequently, these injuries are noted in the splenic or hepatic flexures or at the distal sigmoid colon and may have associated mesenteric injury due to the tearing forces. Bursting injuries of the colon are similar to blunt duodenal and stomach injuries and involve a rapid increase in intraluminal pressure from the bursting force, frequently against a competent ileocecal valve. Bursting injuries of the colon most commonly involve the cecum.

Overall, blunt colonic injuries most frequently involve the transverse; the right colon is next most frequently involved, followed by the left colon. Transverse colonic injuries are most commonly serosal or mural hematomas; right and left colonic injuries are frequently full-thickness injuries.

The spectrum of injury varies widely. Serious injuries are almost equally divided between transections and perforations. Partial seromuscular tears, intramural hematomas, and contusions almost invariably heal spontaneously. A lurking threat is posed by an initially silent mesenteric tear, and gradual ischemia of the subtended colon wall may occur. Subtle abdominal symptoms may develop along with an insidious peritonitis occurring between the fourth and eighth postinjury days, when the gangrenous bowel perforates.[10] In such cases there may be little association between the severity of the injury and the subsequent degree of damage observed in the colon.

The diagnosis of blunt colonic injury is often made during laparotomy for associated organ injury. Occasionally, a bursting injury of the colon provides free air on preoperative abdominal radiography; however its absence does not preclude injury. Diagnostic peritoneal lavage (DPL) has proved invaluable in the rapid evaluation of patients with blunt abdominal trauma.[11] Bacterial or fecal material on DPL makes possible the diagnosis of colonic injury. Partial-thickness colonic injuries or mesenteric injuries may be entertained when the lavage red blood cell (RBC) count exceeds 100,000 cells/mm^3, although some surgeons prefer to use a smaller number as a guide.

Potential complications may arise from undiagnosed transmural colonic hematomas. Although the majority of these hematomas resolve without complication, liquefaction occasionally occurs and a colocutaneous fistula or an intra-abdominal abscess may result. Alternatively, colonic stricture may be noted at a variable postinjury interval, attributable to localized ischemia or exuberant fibrosis. Although the exact number of these complications is unknown, awareness of their occurrence encourages rational postinjury follow-up.

In a series of 35 patients at Wayne State University, multiple concomitant injuries occurred in about 90% of patients with blunt abdominal trauma. These injuries often dominate the clinical picture and initiate the laparotomy. In this series, other injured viscera included the spleen (nine), liver (eight), jejunum (six), ileum (five), blood vessels (four), kidney (three), pancreas (three), gallbladder (one), stomach (one), and duodenum (one). Extensive retroperitoneal hematomas and colonic mesentery tears both occurred in 12 patients. In addition, 15 of the 35 patients had head injuries, 16 had major fractures, and 9 had chest injuries.

Treatment of Blunt Injuries

The management of blunt colonic injuries depends on the condition of the colonic wall. Superficial simple tears respond well to primary repair. More difficult decisions must be made when associated extensive contusion is present or when ischemia follows mesenteric occlusion. All five patients in the Wayne State University who had ileocolostomies did well, although others reported leakage. Special care must be taken with primary anastomoses in the presence of widespread contusion, especially with concomitant intra-abdominal infection. Whenever there is doubt about the blood supply of the bowel, resection and temporary colostomy or ileostomy are advisable.

Associated Injuries in Penetrating Trauma

Associated injuries vary with the wounding agent, and these lesions may be intra- or extra-abdominal. The possibility of intra-abdominal injury being present must never be ignored when the entry wound is in the chest or buttocks, or even as distant as the cervical region in the case of gunshot wounds.

Associated injuries in representative series are delineated in Table 12–2. Many patients have more than one injured organ, and this possibility must also be excluded.

Table 12–2. ASSOCIATED INJURIES IN PATIENTS WITH COLONIC INJURY (n = 1600)

Small bowel	36.7%
Vascular	12.5%
Stomach	13.8%
Liver	18.1%
Pancreas	6.0%
Spleen	5.9%
Lung	11.7%
Kidney	12.5%
Extremity	10.1%

Data from combined series of Burch 1991,[26] George 1988,[29] George 1989,[23] Levison 1990,[21] Pontius 1957.[3]

Diagnosis in Penetrating Trauma

The diagnosis of colonic injury following penetrating abdominal trauma is usually made during laparotomy for peritoneal signs or hypotension. Routine laparotomy is advocated for any gunshot wound that has transgressed the peritoneal cavity and for a high-velocity wound in proximity to the peritoneal cavity, to avoid overlooking blast effects. Occasionally, in lateral or upper abdominal gunshot wounds, DPL is helpful to determine peritoneal penetration; a positive test finding mandates further evaluation or exploratory laparotomy. During laparotomy for trauma, a generous midline incision is essential for rapid and proper examination of the colon and intra-abdominal organs. The incision is made along the putative trajectory of the missile but also beyond, as bizarre unpredictable injuries may occur. The colon should be fully mobilized in areas of questionable injury. Any mesenteric hematomas must be assumed to conceal a colon injury until visual examination of the entire serosal surface proves otherwise.

Wounds of the Abdomen

The treatment of knife wounds of the abdomen has undergone a transition from mandated laparotomy to selective observation in hemodynamically stable, alert patients. Any unstable patient who has no extra-abdominal cause or one who has signs of peritoneal irritation should undergo emergent laparotomy.[12] Clinically stable cooperative patients may be safely observed by the surgical team for development of peritoneal signs. The precise value of DPL or computed tomography (CT) scan of the abdomen in questionable cases is disputed.[13] The criteria for positive DPL results in penetrating abdominal trauma ranges from 20,000 to 100,000 RBCs/mm^3 in various reports; the lower figure results in a higher negative laparotomy rate, whereas use of the higher figure may miss significant injuries. CT has been heralded as an organ-specific diagnostic modality to allow selective observation of stable patients following trauma. Unfortunately, the diagnostic sensitivity of the CT scan for hollow visceral injury is relatively poor, with a false-negative examination rate of up to 13%. Triple-contrast CT including intravenous, oral, and enema instillation of water-soluble contrast agent may improve these results in distal colonic injury, but more proximal lesions may still elude diagnosis. The accuracy of the CT scan in trauma is greatly influenced by the experience of the interpreter, which must be considered in making a decision.

The technique of laparoscopy is cautiously being assessed in trauma patients, as it may allow organ-specific diagnosis following penetrating or blunt abdominal trauma.[14] Furthermore, more advanced laparoscopic techniques may permit the repair of simple gastrointestinal and colonic injuries without laparotomy, although this approach is still investigational.[15] Exquisite judgment must be exercised in these patients, because complete laparoscopic visualization of the retroperitoneal portions of the colon is not possible. Any question of injury in these areas mandates laparotomy. The ultimate role of laparoscopy in the management of patients sustaining wounds of the abdomen still must be defined.

Wounds of the Flank and Posterior Abdomen

Penetrating wounds of the flank and posterior abdominal region may inflict occult injury on the extraperitoneal right or left colon.[16] Injuries at this location may initially appear innocuous owing to the paucity of abdominal findings afforded by their retroperitoneal location. Patients with stab wounds in the flank region have a 20% to 40% incidence of associated intra-abdominal organ injury, whereas wounds in the back have an 8% to 10% incidence of such injury. The lateral abdominal musculature affords little protection to the viscera; the kidneys and colon are in close approximation (2 to 3 cm) to the skin surface in nonobese individuals. Wounds in a more posterior location cause fewer problems, because the spine and paraspinous musculature provide a thicker defense requiring a wounding agent of 8 cm or longer to cause significant damage. A selective approach to stab wounds of the back and flank may be safely adopted in cooperative patients. As with anterior stab wounds, a deterioration of the abdominal findings mandates laparotomy. During exploration for wounds of the back and flank, the retroperitoneal colon must be fully mobilized to allow careful examination in the region of the knife's path to exclude posterior or intramesenteric colonic injury.

Wounds of the Extraperitoneal Colon

In an effort to avoid missing injuries of the extraperitoneal colon, a more aggressive approach in diagnosis has been suggested.[16] Although the occurrence of missed injuries with subsequent intramesenteric or intra-abdominal abscess formation is infrequent, these complications may be devastating when they occur. DPL is predictably disappointing following wounds to the flank and back with retroperitoneal organ injury, because the injury site is sequestered from the lavage fluid causing a false-negative interpretation of the effluent. A patient with suspected colon injury in this location may benefit from an abdominal CT scan with triple-contrast technique. The patient is given an oral and an intravenous contrast agent along with intracolonic radiopaque medium (Gastrografin). Although free perforation is rarely seen on this examination, more subtle abnormalities, such as colonic mesenteric hematoma or localized contrast extravasation, allow a presumptive diagnosis of colonic injury.

Wounds of the Rectum

Rectal injuries must be diligently sought in all patients who have penetrating pelvic injuries, severe pelvic fractures, or splaying injuries. Meticulous perineal examination is essential in these patients. Any trauma patient with hematochezia or guaiac-positive stool should be assumed to have a rectal injury. Sigmoidoscopy may be helpful when the rectum is clear of feces, but the examination is frequently hampered by a lack of adequate preparation. A high index of suspicion of rectal injury should mandate definitive treatment of the presumed injury.[17, 18]

Iatrogenic Wounds

The diagnosis of iatrogenic colonic injury following colonic endoscopy is obvious when other intra-abdominal organs are directly visualized.[19] Gradual air insufflation during the examination usually provides a generous pneumoperitoneum that makes the diagnosis obvious roentgenographically. Colonic injury should also be suspected if there is sudden pain during the procedure or delayed abdominal pain and discomfort. If there is any suspicion of bowel perforation following endoscopy, a water-soluble contrast enema allows the diagnosis to be made with certainty. When the lesion consists of a small tear caused by excessive pressure from the instrument in a prepared bowel, observation and antibiotics may be all that is necessary. If the perforation is caused by biopsy or fulguration, the lesion should be regarded as a stab wound, although some of these lesions are now followed conservatively.

Perforations associated with barium enemas are far more serious than purely instrumental perforations.[20] The combination of barium and feces is a potentially virulent mixture causing severe infection. Subsequent granulomas and widespread dense adhesions with resulting intestinal obstruction may follow. Most of these lesions are the result of problems with the large intrarectal balloon or enema tip and may take the form of extensive lacerations, which are often extraperitoneal. It is highly questionable whether a gently performed barium enema would perforate a diverticulum, as is sometimes claimed. Immediate operation is essential in order to cleanse the peritoneal cavity and prevent further leakage. Perforation of the colon through a colostomy by a catheter or an enema tip is extremely dangerous. Few patients survive, presumably because of delay.

Other Wounds

Extensive lesions may result from the passage of a jet of compressed air up the anal canal. This injury usually follows a prank when the nozzle is held a few inches from the victim's buttocks and the pressure suddenly turned on. It is estimated that about 4 lb/in^2 of pressure is needed to rupture the bowel; compressed air jets may generate up to 125 lb/in^2. The laceration of the bowel usually occurs in the rectosigmoid area and may extend for 10 cm or more. Early operative treatment is essential.

Rectal impalement by a wide variety of objects such as pickets, broomsticks, and hydraulic jacks has been described. These wounds may extend into any abdominal organ and even into the chest. The principles of treatment are the same as for all penetrating injuries. An additional caveat is that the object of the impalement should be left *in situ* while the patient is transported to the hospital and should be removed only at operation, under direct vision and with the abdomen open. This approach assists in identifying the injured organs, reduces fecal spillage, and facilitates immediate control of hemorrhage, which may otherwise be catastrophic on withdrawal of the impaling object.

Treatment of Penetrating and Blunt Injuries

The initial treatment of colonic and rectal injury is concentrated on stabilization of the patient with fluid resuscitation and on focused examination to preclude life-threatening injury. In patients with multiple injuries, concomitant extracolonic injuries may need immediate attention, especially when hemorrhage is continuing.

Antibiotics for covering enteric pathogens should be started preoperatively in patients suspected of having an intra-abdominal injury. The pathogenic organisms most often cultured in patients with colonic injury are *Escherichia coli*, enterococci, and *Bacteroides*. Although there is no unanimity about the initial selection of antibiotics, there appears to be a movement away from regimens including an aminoglycoside. The second-generation cephalosporins and newer synthetic penicillin combinations provide adequate coverage for the majority of pathogens associated with large bowel injury.

During laparotomy for trauma, a generous midline incision is essential for rapid, thorough examination of the colon and other intra-abdominal organs, especially along the trajectory of the missile. Any obviously contaminating material is removed, and the peritoneal cavity is irrigated with warm saline. The colon should be fully mobilized in questionable areas, and any mesenteric hematomas should be assumed to conceal a colonic injury until disproved by direct examination of the entire serosal surface. Maneuvers to obtain hemostasis take precedence over further exploration. Following identification of a colonic injury, an attempt should be made to limit temporarily further abdominal contamination with a running, absorbable suture for a simple penetrating injury, or forceps or staple exclusion for more extensive injury. The treatment of colonic injuries is then individualized by the severity of the injury.

FACTORS INFLUENCING PRIMARY REPAIR

Primary repair is the ideal goal of surgical treatment. Analysis of the many factors that militate against its success is vital.[21–26] Ultimately, success depends on an adequate blood supply to the suture line, sufficient oxygenation, appropriate nutrition, minimization of infection, and absence of excessive tension on any suture line. Other factors often discussed as having significant influence on the colon's ability to heal include concomitant shock, the age of the patient, the anatomic site of injury in the bowel, the time elapsed between injury and repair, the extent of injury, the extent and nature of concomitant lesions, the pre-existing condition of the patient, the amount of blood transfused, and the injury severity score. Most of these factors are inter-related and consequently difficult to disentangle with precision. In the last analysis, the surgeon's decision is guided by integrated clinical judgment that considers all these factors and gives relative weights to each as they apply to the specific patient on the operating table. These factors merit separate consideration.

Shock

Preoperative shock of less than 80 mm Hg has been said to be an absolute contraindication to primary repair.[6] The reduction of blood flow associated with hypotension, if sustained, may preclude healing of the anastomosis. However, any consideration of hypotension must take into account its duration as well as its depth preoperatively and how adequately pressure and flow are restored at the time of operation. In patients rendered normotensive following repletion of their blood volume, the initial blood pressure level is by no means an absolute contraindication to primary repair.

Age

It has been traditional to regard age as a potent factor in the determination of outcome. Although this is intuitively and logically understandable, age needs to be defined by physiologic rather than temporal criteria. Nelken and Lewis found no correlation between age and mortality.[27] Although aging diminishes the reserves of cardiopulmonary, renal, and other systems, these reductions, in the absence of significant established clinical deficits, do not affect the outcome of a primary anastomosis. In practice, a case may be made that the outcomes for older patients, all things considered, are more favorable with a single operation than with staged operations, which require multiple general anesthetics and hospital admissions. It can be argued with reason that older patients fare as well as younger patients at comparable initial operations but are much less able to cope with complications, should these occur.

Fecal Contamination

The degree of fecal contamination tends to parallel the size of the colonic injury, which in turn is usually related to the destructive qualities of the causative agent, the multiplicity of visceral injury, and the amount of blood lost.

There is uniform agreement that minor contamination has little effect on outcome but that substantial and continuing contamination may be associated with adverse clinical events, including death. Patients with much fecal spillage, especially when cleansing of the peritoneal cavity is delayed beyond 6 to 8 hours, are at an increased risk of morbidity and mortality. These factors have been examined by Burch and colleagues,[24] Flint and colleagues,[25] Nelken and Lewis,[27] Adkins and colleagues,[28] and George and associates,[29] but no universal agreement has emerged. The major question concerns to what extent, if any, the initial surgical procedure that is selected can be correlated with the morbidity and mortality that are inevitable in some of these severely ill patients. It is now recognized that there are no objective data to indict primary closure as producing greater morbidity, under these circumstances, than a defunctioning procedure. As a result, a number of experienced surgeons contend that performing a primary anastomosis when gross contamination is present may not be associated with any higher mortality or morbidity than performing a defunctioning procedure. To an extent, the past condemnation of primary repair seems to have been "guilt by association," but this procedure needs further testing. Until its validity is definitively established, caution is advisable.

Adkins found no correlation between the amount of spillage and outcome, and he concluded that the presence of feces is not a contraindication to primary repair.[28] However, Nelken and Lewis disagree.[27] It is sometimes difficult to distinguish the extent of contamination or infection that constitutes a standard, but most surgeons concur that in the presence of overt peritonitis, primary anastomosis should be avoided.

Anatomic Site of Injury

The site and extent of injury help to shape the decision of which operation is optimal. The influence of associated injuries and contamination is discussed elsewhere, but these entities exercise much less influence than in the past. The degree of bowel injury is an important factor and is well illustrated by Burch et al.[26] This group defined "extensive" colonic injury as the tearing of more than 50% of the bowel circumference or the presence of overt ischemia; all other injury was defined as "routine." In their series, 252 of 1,004 patients fell into the extensive group and 752 into the routine group. In the years 1985 to 1989, routine injuries of the right colon underwent primary repair in 98% of patients, of the transverse colon in 94%, and of the left colon in 89%. In contrast, extensive lesions of the right colon underwent primary repair in 71% of patients, of the transverse colon in 12%, and of the left colon in only 2%. The dramatic differences in these figures reflect the ease and perceived safety of right hemicolectomy, as opposed to left hemicolectomy. The figures also reflect the significant difference in the incidence of primary repair between so-called routine and extensive injuries. Although the concept that the left colon heals less readily than the right colon is now seriously questioned by many, caution still prevails. Between 1980 and 1988, our unit performed primary repair on 43 of 73 (58.5%) of lesions of the right colon, in contrast to 23 of 88 (26.1%) of the left colon.[30]

The treatment for retroperitoneal colonic injuries is similar to that for wounds of other locations. The colon must be generously mobilized to allow repair or colostomy without tension. If the diagnosis of an injury in this region is late, the chance of subsequent retroperitoneal or mesenteric sepsis mandates colostomy for maximal safety.

Degree of Injury

Traditional wisdom has decreed that primary repair is unjustifiable in the presence of severe injury. Modern

Table 12–3. PENETRATING ABDOMINAL TRAUMA INDEX (PATI)*

Grade	Description
I	Serosal
II	Single-wall
III	Less than 25% wall
IV	Greater than 25%
V	Wall and blood supply injury

*PATI is the risk factor times the injury estimate for all organs injured; in the case of the colon, the risk factor is arbitrarily fixed at 4.

From Moore EE, Dunn EL, Moore JB. Penetrating abdominal trauma index. J Trauma 1981; 21:439.

attempts to quantify the degree of injury and to correlate it with the results of different surgical approaches have altered this view. The indices that have been popularized are summarized in Table 12–3.

Moore and associates[31] and Nelken and Lewis,[27] applying the penetrating abdominal trauma index (PATI), have concluded that this index is accurate and useful in predicting that patients with a score of less than 25 have *fewer* complications with primary closure than when a colostomy is established. PATI was also found to be helpful in predicting costs and the possibility of complications.

Levison and colleagues, defining the pattern of practice in the Wayne State University series by injury severity score, abdominal trauma index, colon injury score, and Flint's colon score (Table 12–4), showed that in the 1980s a statistically significant trend toward primary repair at increasing levels of increasing injury is discernible, without any deterioration in results.[21] As conflicting results can still be found, we, like many others, remain cautious about performing primary anastomosis on the left colon when a large resection is necessary. However, others no longer regard this as a highly significant contraindication. Primary repair of mild to moderate colonic injuries on the right colon and increasingly on the left now constitute an acceptable, and indeed the appropriate, standard of care.

Table 12–4. FLINT COLON INJURY SCORE

Grade I	Isolated colon injury
	Minimal contamination
	No shock
	Minimal delay
Grade II	Through-and-through perforation
	Lacerations
	Moderate contamination
Grade III	Severe tissue loss
	Devascularization
	Heavy contamination

From Flint LM, Vital GC, Richardson JD, Polk H. The injured colon. Ann Surg 1981; 193:619.

The fundamental unresolved issue in colonic injury currently revolves around the role of a primary unprotected anastomosis following *resection* of a portion of the left colon. Even the trauma centers with the largest experience remain hesitant to advocate such an approach. Data on this decision are difficult to find; when extractable, however, the data suggest that anastomotic complications following resection of the left colon have a significantly higher rate. Although Burch and associates had only 13 fecal fistulas in 592 primary repairs (2.2%), it seems that 3 of these followed 14 resections with colocolostomy in contrast to the remaining 10, which occurred in 578 other primary repairs.[26] The interesting report from Trinidad of 57 primary repairs (of 61 consecutive colonic injuries) with only one leak, which closed spontaneously, does not specify the anatomic sites of injury or the number of patients who required resection.[32] If rational attempts are to be made to assess and then to test the boundaries of primary repairs, precise data concerning the site, extent, and circumstances of resection need to be detailed.

Nevertheless, primary repair and anastomosis on the left side in patients with serious injuries are slowly gaining in popularity among experienced surgical units. Deep and sustained shock, large amounts of fecal spillage, overt peritonitis, and serious concomitant intra-abdominal visceral injuries remain contraindications, but even some of these are now seriously challenged. In summary, the status of primary anastomosis following colonic resection of the left colon remains unclear, but it is the last major frontier in colonic trauma and is slowly giving way.

STATUS OF DEFUNCTIONING COLOSTOMY

With the increased confidence in the safety of primary repair of the colon, colostomies are now established in less than 30% of colonic injuries.[33] In contrast, colostomies continue to play a major role for rectal injuries, in which primary repair is seldom feasible.

Colostomy is indicated (1) when associated with rectal injuries; (2) when resection of the left colon for extensive lesions is performed, as few cases are currently thought to lend themselves to resection and primary anastomosis in this region; (3) when uncertainty exists about the quality of the colonic repair; (4) when an exteriorized repair breaks down or cannot be returned to the abdomen; (5) when in the presence of established peritonitis primary repair is deemed to be risky.

The concept of mandatory colostomy in any circumstance has undergone severe scrutiny, as colostomy has many drawbacks.[34] Among the obvious disadvantages are the esthetic unpleasantness, the difficulty that many patients have in caring for the colostomy, the associated complications, the prolonged hospitalization, the need for readmission for colostomy closure, the multiple anesthetics, the morbidity associated with both the establishment of the colostomy and the subsequent closure, the economic loss to the patient because of time away from work, the prolonged convalescence, the cost to society for the hospitalizations, and the loss of productivity.

It is increasingly recognized that patients who have colostomies also have an appreciably higher intraperitoneal and abdominal wound infection rate than do patients who have primary closures. In a revisionist concept, Nelken and Lewis compared 37 patients who had primary closures with 39 patients on whom colostomies were performed.[27] The injury severity score, penetrating abdominal trauma index, colon score, age, sex, degree of injury, shock, and delay between injury and operation were comparable. Although major morbidity rate was much lower in the primary closure group (11% versus 49%), the study was not randomized, and it is difficult not to suspect that the colostomy groups were selected because of disadvantageous clinical features at the time of laparotomy. Nevertheless, observations such as these and others are provocative in suggesting the critical need for a meticulous review of indications for colostomy in the individual case.

Until the early 1980s, colostomy was associated with a morbidity of up to 30% and occasional mortality. Results are much improved today, as the procedure is recognized to merit an experienced surgeon and as techniques have been refined.[33] In today's terms, the disadvantages and dangers of colostomy appear to have been exaggerated, and it is now regarded as a low-morbidity procedure, provided that it is technically well performed. At the same time, indications for colostomy have become more stringent.

ESTABLISHMENT OF COLOSTOMY

Colostomy comes in many forms. The so-called *Hartmann procedure* has an end-colostomy, and the distal bowel is closed after a segment of bowel has been resected. It is useful to project the potential difficulties of later reanastomosis, to leave as much distal bowel as possible, and to mark the area of closure so that it is easily identifiable at the time of definitive reanastomosis. When feasible, the *double-barrel colostomy*, in which the two ends of the colon are separated, is favored by some. When the colostomy is established, care should be taken to ensure that subsequent closure will be as easy as possible. Placement of the two limbs close to each other helps to facilitate the closure. A *loop colostomy*, although popular, has the disadvantage of being bulky and difficult for the patient to manage postoperatively. Its advantage is related to the fact that at the time of repair, only the anterior wall needs to be resutured, and the loop can be gently replaced in the peritoneal cavity. *Loop colostomy with the distal limb closed by staples or sutures* in order to remove the disadvantage of potential distal spillage is advocated by some. In this case, resection of the area of bowel with formal anastomosis of the two lumens is necessary, as in a formal colectomy.

Controversy has existed about the optimal time period between establishment and closure of a colostomy. This period is highly variable and depends on the patient's general progress. Unlike elective colostomies, which are frequently closed within 2 or 3 weeks, the patient who requires a colostomy for reasons of trauma often needs a longer convalescence while concomitant injuries heal and nutrition is restored. In a series at our institution in 1978, the median interval from construction to closure was 101 days.[34] In a study by Crass et al in 1981, the median interval was 103 days with a range of 36 to 902 days.[35] In the Louisville series, the mean time was 122 days.[33] The majority of colostomies can be closed in 4 to 6 weeks in patients who show no signs of sepsis and who are in a satisfactory state of nutrition with virtual recovery from the major effects of their injuries. Conversely, when widespread sepsis is present, the time before closure may need to be extended by many months. Colostomy closures should not be associated with any mortality, and the major morbidity rate of about 5% is caused by infection, fecal fistula, and obstruction.

There is no universal agreement about whether a barium enema is essential prior to colostomy closure. A review by Atweh et al suggested that barium enema was beneficial in evaluating colorectal injuries below the peritoneal reflection, as the initial injury is often not visualized at the first operation by virtue of the anatomy.[36] For injuries above the peritoneal reflection, some think that a barium enema is not routinely needed, as the results do not change the planned surgical procedure. Most surgeons continue to favor barium enema before colostomy closure in patients who have had repair of substantial wounds of the colon to exclude excessive narrowing or the presence of a fistula. This investigation can be done as an outpatient procedure, thereby obviating the expense of extra hospitalization.

In summary, attitudes about colostomies for traums have changed considerably. Colostomies are established much less often today, and when they are established, morbidity has been greatly reduced.

TREATMENT OF RECTAL INJURIES

The treatment of rectal injuries generates little controversy. Diverting colostomy and presacral drainage are the cornerstones of management. The pelvic anatomy and juxtarectal injuries may make exposure difficult, but the wound of the rectum should be repaired whenever possible. If extensive dissection is necessary to expose the area, the wound should be permitted to heal by secondary intention. Irrigation through the defunctioned rectal stump and a digitally dilated anus has many advocates and is customarily done, although the advantages are not unequivocally established. To ensure complete defunctioning, the proximal end of the rectum may be closed with a row of staples. A 3- to 5-cm incision just anterior to the coccyx allows blunt dissection into the retrorectal space and placement of Penrose drains or closed suction drainage, which can usually be removed in 1 week. In massive pelvic injury in which the rectum is devitalized, an abdominoperineal resection is unavoidable.

EXTERIORIZATION

Exteriorization of the repaired colon has had a checkered history with periods of acceptance and rejection. Exteriorization was practiced briefly in World War II. Enthusiasm was rekindled in the 1970s when Lou et al,[37] Robbs,[38] and Kirkpatrick[39] were keen protagonists. The success rate varies between 50% and 70%, but a definite learning curve exists. Support for exteriorization dwindled in the 1980s, even among previous enthusiasts. This is well illustrated in Burch's series of 751 patients with "routine" injuries, in whom exteriorization was performed in 72 of 465 between 1980 and 1984, but in only 2 of 286 patients between 1985 and 1989. Exteriorization has rarely been advocated for severe colonic injuries.

Experimentally, it has been shown that the exteriorized repair heals well, provided that the serosa is kept moist and obstruction is avoided. The immediate appeal of exteriorization is easy to understand; if the repair heals, it can be dropped back into the peritoneal cavity in 7 to 10 days; in the approximately 35% of patients in which it does not heal, a colostomy can be established painlessly at the bedside. Exteriorization is done when uncertainty exists about the future healing of an intra-abdominal anastomosis. Apart from the perceived advantage of guarding against an intraperitoneal leak, exteriorization in the 50% to 70% of patients in whom the technique is successful obviates the need for a colostomy, shortens the hospital stay, saves money, reduces discomfort, and permits an earlier return to work.

Unfortunately, exteriorization has some specific problems. As only mobile segments of the bowel lend themselves to this technique, the transverse colon is a prime candidate. Attempts to exteriorize the right or left colon are often fraught with difficulty and are associated with very bulky and unsightly exteriorized bowel. Correct technique is vital if obstruction is to be avoided and this entails a gradual curve of the exteriorized segment of bowel over a 4 to 5 cm fascial bridge to avoid acute kinking and consequent high, proximal intraluminal pressure. Local care of the exposed bowel includes regular moistening with saline and the application of petrolatum on gauze. A covering self-adhesive colostomy bag helps preserve humidity. Replacement of the successfully healed bowel in the peritoneal cavity may be difficult if it is exposed for more than 7 to 10 days. With the demonstration that primary repair or anastomosis is feasible and will heal well in the same group of patients for whom exteriorization was previously advocated, there would seem to be little need for exteriorization.

PRINCIPLES OF TECHNIQUE

Details of the various operations are to be found in various surgical texts. The broad principles associated with the surgery of colorectal injuries may be summarized as follows:

1. A vertical abdominal incision, usually midline, must be generous and ensure easy access.
2. In the presence of peritoneal contamination, morbidity is reduced if the skin and subcutaneous tissues are left open, to be closed by secondary suture between the postoperative days 4 and 7 in most cases.
3. Anastomoses should have good vascularity and should be tension-free. An inner running layer of 3–0 polyglycolic acid suture and an outer layer of 3–0 interrupted silk is used by most surgeons, but a single layer of polyglycolic acid has given equally good results for many. Other surgeons favor staples. Application of omentum to the suture line may be a helpful adjunct.
4. The abdomen should be well irrigated with warm saline to remove all particulate matter, but the addition of antibiotics to the fluid has not been proved helpful.
5. Drains are seldom necessary, and if used, must be justified by a specific identifiable reason.
6. The abdominal incision should be closed with precision. Interrupted or running no. 1 polyglycolic acid sutures or no. 2 nylon sutures are favored by many, but the care and technique are, within reason, more important than the suture selected.
7. Antibiotics are begun preoperatively in suspected colorectal injuries. They are continued intraoperatively and for a variable number of days beyond, depending on the specific circumstances. In many cases, antibiotics can be stopped within 48 hours.

PURPORTED INNOVATIONS

Fibrin Sealant

Methods to improve the safety of anastomoses have been explored over the past century. The easiest, cheapest, and most effective technique is the placement of omentum over the anastomosis, simulating nature's spontaneous method of sealing small gastrointestinal leaks. The search for an effective glue to reinforce the suture line or compensate for technical error has not yet been successful. The most recent hope has been the application of fibrin sealant, which is readily available and biologically compatible. Animal experiments have not been promising.[40, 41]

Intracolonic Bypass Tube

Use of an intracolonic bypass tube (ICBT; Coloshield) has been extended from the elective situation to the definitive management of nine colonic perforations that ordinarily would have been treated with a defunctioning colostomy (of the nine, three resulted from gunshot wounds, three from blunt injuries, two from stab wounds, and one from an air hose).[42] At least four of the nine patients had extensive, severe concomitant intra-abdominal injury, and all had gross contamination. No repair leaked and the bypass tube passed spontaneously in about 2 weeks. Many resist the concept of this intraluminal stent, and no prospective randomized study has been done yet. Until more experience has been gained, the ICBT—for use in trauma—must be regarded as investigative.

Intraoperative Evacuation of Colonic Feces

Substantial feces in the bowel has been postulated to be a potent cause of mechanical anastomotic disruption. It is also suggested that intraluminal feces may result in the transluminal migration of organisms, which then serve as a visible or invisible source of sepsis. Intraoperative irrigation of the bowel to permit primary anastomosis in elective surgery has been advocated in the United Kingdom.[43] This technique consists of the insertion of a large tube into the mobilized proximal colon, which is led into a sterile bag alongside the operating table. A large 14-French Foley catheter is inserted into the ileum about 5 cm proximal to the ileocecal valve. The balloon is inflated in the cecum and drawn against the ileocecal valve. Warm saline is then used to irrigate the colon in a prograde fashion, with feces moved along by sequential manual manipulation. This method was subsequently applied selectively to injured patients close to the Green Line (i.e., area between Christian and Muslim sections) in Beirut and was thought to increase significantly the feasibility and the success of primary anastomosis. The colon may be irrigated with liters of saline prior to anastomosis and the fluid siphoned off at the side of the operating table. Alternatively, Baker and associates have the bowel flushed in a prograde manner, after the anastomosis has been completed, with the fluid collected through a large tube previously inserted into the rectum.[44] This practice of on-table irrigation is regarded by most as time-consuming and esthetically displeasing. Furthermore, a prospective randomized study of a selected group of 172 patients has been reported, of whom 91 patients had prograde colonic lavage on the operating table in association with an unprotected colonic primary anastomosis. This study leads to the conclusion that prograde irrigation did not influence morbidity or mortality and so it is not worth doing.

Temporary Ligation and Replacement of the Colon

The Ben Taub Hospital group has reported treating 25 desperately ill patients with exsanguinating hemorrhage, coagulopathy, acidosis, and hypothermia by umbilical tape ligation of the colon, which is then dropped back into the peritoneal cavity.[26] The abdomens were then closed with towel clips following packing for hemostatic control. Three of the 25 patients were sufficiently resuscitated to return later to the operating room for conversion to a colostomy. Details of the background and outcome do not permit judgment of this approach, but the accepted establishment of an end-colostomy at the initial operation would seem to add virtually no complexity to the original operation and to have self-evident advantages.

SUMMARY

Colonic injury occurs in up to 10% of patients with penetrating abdominal trauma and severe blunt ab-

---

EDITORIAL COMMENT

Dr. Walt and his colleagues have long challenged conventional wisdom and traditional methods of care of the injured patient. Their advocacy of primary repair for colonic injuries is well taken; today colonic injuries are no longer automatically treated by exteriorization. Dr. Walt wisely cautions that primary repair should not be undertaken in the presence of shock, massive blood loss, multiple organ injury, significant contamination, delayed operation, or extensive destruction of the colon and/or abdominal wall. The editors endorse both the concept of primary repair of colonic injuries and the admonitions concerning its use.

For rectal injuries, conventional radiographs or CT scans utilizing a water-soluble contrast medium instilled into the rectum are valuable diagnostic aids and may disclose unsuspected perforations of the rectum or lower abdominal colon. The water-soluble contrast material is free from the hazards associated with barium. In treating patients with suspected rectal injuries (e.g., displaced pelvic fractures, missile injuries to the pelvis), rectal perforations may be diagnosed by using flexible endoscopy aided by irrigation. This is best accomplished while the patient is anesthetized for the treatment of other injuries.

---

dominal trauma. The diagnosis should be suspected in patients with penetrating abdominal injury or with peritoneal signs on examination. A high index of suspicion is required to diagnose less obvious retroperitoneal or nontransmural injuries in a timely fashion. DPL, CT, endoscopy, or laparoscopy may be helpful in selected patients, but the diagnosis of colonic injury is still made most often during exploratory laparotomy for associated injuries. Colonic injuries are amenable to careful primary repair in 60% to 70% of patients, and the trend toward primary repair continues. The purported difference between the left and right colon is increasingly challenged. Colostomy is reserved for severe destructive colonic injuries and for rectal injuries. The mortality rate associated with colonic and rectal injuries has decreased dramatically over the past decade and is attributable to the bowel injury *per se* in less than 5% of cases.

REFERENCES

1. Woodhall JP, Ochsner A. The management of perforating injury of the colon and rectum in civilian practice. Surgery 1951;29:305.
2. Ogilvie WH. Abdominal wounds in the western desert. Surg Gynecol Obstet 1944;78:225–238.
3. Pontius RG, Cresch O, DeBakey ME. Management of large bowel injury in civilian practice. Ann Surg 1957;146:291–295.
4. Vannix RS, Carter R, Hinshaw DB, Joergenson EJ. Surgical management of colon trauma in civilian practice. Am J Surg 1963;106:364–371.
5. Haynes CD, Gunn CH, Martin JD. Colon injuries. Arch Surg 1968;96:944–948.

6. Stone HH, Fabian TC. Management of perforating colon trauma: randomization between primary closure and exteriorization. Ann Surg 1979;190:430–436.

7. Hawley PR, Faulk WP, Hunt TK. Collagenase activity in the gastrointestinal tract. Br J Surg 1970;57:869–900.

8. Dauterive AH, Flancbaum L, Cox EF. Blunt intestinal trauma. Ann Surg 1984;201:198–203.

9. Strate RG, Grieco JG. Blunt injury to the colon and rectum. J Trauma 1983;23:384–388.

10. Stahl KD, Geiss AC, Bordan DL, et al. Blunt trauma and delayed colon injury. Curr Surg 1985;4–9.

11. Kreis DJ. Diagnostic peritoneal lavage. In: Spruce C, ed. Invasive Procedures in Critical Care. New York: Churchill Livingstone, 1985, pp 225–236.

12. Meyer AA, Crass RA. Abdominal trauma. Surg Clin North Am 1982;62:105–111.

13. Meyer DM, Thal ER, Weigelt JA, Redram HC. Evaluation of computed tomography and diagnostic peritoneal lavage in blunt abdominal trauma. J Trauma 1989;29:1168–1179.

14. Ivatury RP, Simon RJ, Seksler B, Bayard V, Stahle WM. Laparoscopy in the evaluation of the intrathoracic abdomen after penetrating injury. J Trauma 1992;33:101–109.

15. Birns MT. Inadvertent instrumental perforation of the colon during laparoscopy: Nonsurgical repair. Gastrointest Endosc 1989;35:54–55.

16. Peck JJ, Berne JV. Posterior abdominal stab wounds. J Trauma 1981;21:298–306.

17. Burch JM, Feliciano DV, Mattox KM. Colostomy and drainage for rectal injuries: Is that all? Ann Surg 1989;209:600–611.

18. Lavenson GS, Cohen A. Management of rectal injuries. Am J Surg 1971;122:226–230.

19. Christie JP, Marrazzo J. Miniperforation of the colon—not all postpolypectomy perforations require laparotomy. Dis Colon Rectum 1990;34:132–135.

20. Walt AJ. Injuries to the colon and rectum. In: Berk JE, ed. Bockus Gastroenterology. 4th ed. Vol. 4. Philadelphia: WB Saunders, pp 2575–2582.

21. Levison MA, Thomas DD, Wiencek RC, Wilson RF. Management of the injured colon: Evolving practice at an urban trauma center. J Trauma 1990;30:247–253.

22. Shannon FL, Moore EE. Primary repair of the colon: When is it a safe alternative? Surgery 1985;98:851–859.

23. George SM, Fabian TC, Voeller GR, et al. Primary repair of colon wounds. Ann Surg 1989;209:728–734.

24. Burch JM, Brock JC, Gevirtzman L, et al. The injured colon. Ann Surg 1986;203:701–711.

25. Flint LM, Vital GC, Richardson JD, Polk H. The injured colon. Ann Surg 1981;193:619–623.

26. Burch JM, Martin RR, Richardson RJ, et al. Evolution of the management of the injured colon in the 80's. Arch Surg 1991;126:979–984.

27. Nelken N, Lewis F. The influence of injury severity on complication rates after primary closure or colostomy for penetrating colon trauma. Ann Surg 1989;209:439–447.

28. Adkins RB, Zirkle PK, Waterhouse G. Penetrating colon trauma. J Trauma 1984;24:491–499.

29. George SM, Fabian TC, Mangiante EC. Colon trauma: Further support for primary repair. Am J Surg 1988;156:16–20.

30. Levison MA, Walt AJ. Colonic trauma. In: Fazio V, ed. Current Therapy in Colon and Rectal Surgery. Philadelphia: BC Decker, 1989, pp 329–333.

31. Moore EE, Dunn EL, Moore JB. Penetrating abdominal trauma index. J Trauma 1981;21:438–445.

32. Naraynsingh V, Ariyanayagam D, Pooran S. Primary repair of colon injuries in a developing country. Br J Surg 1991;78:319–320.

33. Livingston DH, Miller FB, Richardson JD. Are the risks after colostomy closure exaggerated? Am J Surg 1989;158:17–20.

34. Smit R, Walt AJ. The morbidity and cost of the temporary colostomy. Dis Colon Rectum 1978;8:558–561.

35. Crass RA, Trambaugh RF, Kudsk KA. Colorectal foreign bodies and perforation. Am J Surg 1981;142:85–88.

36. Atweh NA, Vieux EE, Ivatury R, et al. Indications for barium enema preceding colostomy closure in trauma patients. J Trauma 1989;29:641–642.

37. Lou MA, Johnson AP, Atik M. Exteriorized repair in the management of colon injuries. Arch Surg 1981;116:926–929.

38. Robbs JV. The alternative to colostomy for the injured colon. S Afr Med J 1978;53:95–99.

39. Kirkpatrick JR. The exteriorized anastomosis: Its role in surgery of the colon. Surgery 1977;82:362–365.

40. Van der Hamm AC, Kort WJ, Weijma IM, et al. Effect of fibrin sealant on the healing colonic anastomosis in the rat. Br J Surg 1991;78:49–53.

41. Oka H, Harrison RC, Burhenne HJ. Effect of a biologic glue on the leakage rate of experimental rectal anastomosis. Am J Surg 1982;143:561–564.

42. Ravo B. Colorectal anastomotic healing and the intracolonic bypass procedure. Surg Clin North Am 1988;68:1267–1294.

43. Dudley HAF, Radcliffe AG, McGeehan D. Intraoperative irrigation of the colon to permit primary anastomosis. Br J Surg 1980;67:80–81.

44. Baker LW, Thomson SR, Chadwick SDJ. Colon wound management and prograde colonic lavage in large bowel trauma. Br J Surg 1990;77:872–876.

Prolapse of the Rectum

CHAPTER 13

Roger R. Dozois
Santhat Nivatvongs

Prolapse of the rectum, or procidentia, is a rather uncommon disorder of still-obscure etiology characterized by full-thickness eversion of the rectal wall either into the lower rectum or the anal canal (incomplete or so-called hidden or occult prolapse) or through the anus and protruding externally (complete prolapse). The segment of protruding rectum typically appears as a series of concentric mucosal rings.

In this chapter, the pathophysiologic mechanisms that may favor this condition and its anatomic and physiologic consequences as well as the modalities of preoperative evaluation and diagnosis are discussed briefly. A greater emphasis is placed on the choice of operation, the selection of patients for a given surgical procedure, the preoperative and postoperative management, and the technique of the various operations we prefer in most instances. The difficult problem of when and how to manage the commonly associated incontinence is also discussed.

PATHOPHYSIOLOGY

The exact cause of rectal procidentia remains unclear. The condition tends to predominate in the following groups: in women, varying from three to ten women for one man[1]; in patients with the habit of straining excessively when defecating; and in those with chronic mental disorders. Pregnancy cannot be etiologically implicated, because the condition is also seen in men, and indeed one half of the women afflicted by procidentia are nulliparous.[2] Cineradiographic studies strongly support the concept that rectal prolapse is the result of intussusception or infolding of the rectum initiated either 6 to 8 cm from the anal verge[3] or, more likely, at the higher level of the rectosigmoid; the latter concept was ingeniously demonstrated by Theuerkauf, Beahrs, and Hill in 1970.[4] By attaching radiopaque metal clips to the everted, prolapsed bowel, these researchers have shown that the intussusception process begins near the rectosigmoid junction. As it progresses caudally, the intussusceptum gradually pulls the upper rectal wall away from its sacral and lateral moorings. With continued straining, the bowel continues to roll from inside out until the mucocutaneous junction initially and the rectal wall itself eventually evert completely outside the body.

This progressive and sequential phenomenon explains why some patients have occult prolapse and why the sigmoid mesentery may elongate, the cul-de-sac may deepen, and the pelvic floor musculature may increasingly weaken. Most cases seem to be explicable on the basis of intussusception, but further evidence is needed, especially from early cases, to explain the initial formation of the intussusceptum. Thus far, the initial cause of the process of intussusception remains unknown.

ANATOMIC AND PHYSIOLOGIC CONSEQUENCES

In the past, many anatomic anomalies often seen in patients with rectal prolapse, such as an abnormally deep rectovaginal or rectovesical pouch, a lack of rectal fixation, a lax pelvic floor muscle, a redundant rectosigmoid and sigmoid colon, and a poor anal sphincter tone, were blamed as the causative factors. As can easily be surmised from the description of the intussusception process, it is more than likely that many of these anatomic findings may, in fact, be the result of the prolonged prolapsing of the rectum rather than its cause. Many clinical observations support this contention. For instance, a deep pelvic pouch or enterocele is not always present in a patient with prolapse.

Evidence against the concept of pelvic floor musculature weakness also comes from cinegradiographic studies of voluntary contraction of these muscles, which indicate a normally moving pelvic floor in many such cases.[5] Studies of anorectal function and the dynamics of defecation indicate that patients with rectal prolapse have impaired voluntary and involuntary sphincter activity, decreased functional rectal capacity, and abnormal continence.[6, 7] Spencer has noted that the rectal inhibitory reflex may be absent or obtunded in many such patients, possibly because of the inability of the sphincter to relax or to sense the increased rectal pressure necessary to initiate the reflex.[8] Recurring and long-standing protrusion of the bulky intussusceptum through the anal orifice could certainly explain, at least in part, the weakened sphincter tone. Indeed, the fecal incontinence frequently observed preoperatively in a patient with prolapse is often reversed by correction of the prolapse without any direct attempt to surgically strengthen the pelvic floor muscles.

Excessive abdominal straining appears to be a key factor in the pathogenesis of a series of events and anatomic changes that eventually lead to complete rectal prolapse. On straining, the anterior rectal wall is normally pressed firmly against, but not into, the upper anal canal. If straining is excessive, the pelvic floor musculature weakens and then descends, stretching the puborectal and the sphincter apparatus.[9] This leads to a funnel-shaped outpouching of the pelvic floor, a condition now recognized as the descending perineum syndrome.

Because the force of expulsion is applied mostly against the anterior rectal wall, the wall tends to follow through in the anal canal and may become irritated, inflamed, and even ulcerated, a condition known as solitary ulcer syndrome. Eventually this sequence will lead to incomplete and then complete prolapse. Thus, descending perineum syndrome, solitary rectal ulcer, and occult prolapse may all be clinical conditions heralding complete rectal prolapse. Chronic stretch injuries to the puborectal muscle and external sphincter may lead to their denervation[10] and contribute to the incontinence caused by other mechanical factors.

DIAGNOSIS AND PREOPERATIVE EVALUATION

Symptoms and Signs

The early manifestations of rectal prolapse may be innocuous and often consist of vague anorectal discomfort during defecation. Difficulty in initiating defecation and the sensation of incomplete evacuation are common. When asked, some patients admit to using digital manipulations to help evacuate the rectal contents. In many instances, a history of constipation and excessive straining can be obtained. In complete prolapse, the protrusion of the rectum may be noted only as a mass during and after severe straining and defecation. As time passes, prolapse can be precipitated by exertion, coughing, sneezing, or even walking. With a more pronounced and more prolonged problem, there is a greater likelihood that the patient will also complain of fecal and occasionally urinary incontinence. Indeed, by the time the diagnosis of rectal prolapse is secured, as many as 50% of the patients have fecal incontinence. In patients with occult prolapse, pressure and a sensation of incomplete evacuation after defecation may be the only complaints.

The diagnosis can most often be confirmed by simply asking the patient to mimic defecation and to strain on the toilet seat. Typically, the everted segment has circular mucosal folds (Fig. 13–1). In the case of occult prolapse, the diagnosis is more difficult to establish. On endoscopy, patients may have redness of the rectal mucosa or even a solitary ulcer anteriorly 6 to 8 cm from the anal verge. In fact, the diagnosis of occult prolapse should be entertained in the patient with benign rectal ulcers, colitis cystica profunda, or localized proctitis.[11] When the patient is sitting and straining on the toilet, the perineum may descend or bulge outward in a funnel-shaped fashion. The diagnosis may be confirmed by defecography (Fig. 13–2).

The condition of complete rectal prolapse must be distinguished from that of mucosal prolapse in which the anal canal mucosa alone protrudes through the anal orifice, appearing as linear furrows. In mucosal prolapse, the characteristic bulging of the anus, or of the perineum and sulcus between the anus and the protruding bowel is absent.

Barium Enema and Defecography

Opacification of the colon and rectum may not be necessary in patients with obvious complete prolapse, other than to rule out associated pathologic processes of the colon. In patients with incomplete or hidden prolapse, it may be most useful as a process of exclusion and as reassurance of the patient (see Fig. 13–2). Careful physical examination is sufficient to establish the diagnosis in most instances of complete prolapse.

Conventional anal manometry may be the most appropriate means of documenting the degree of damage in patients with incontinence or to help predict postoperative functional results. In some patients, anal manometric results may help in planning the surgical

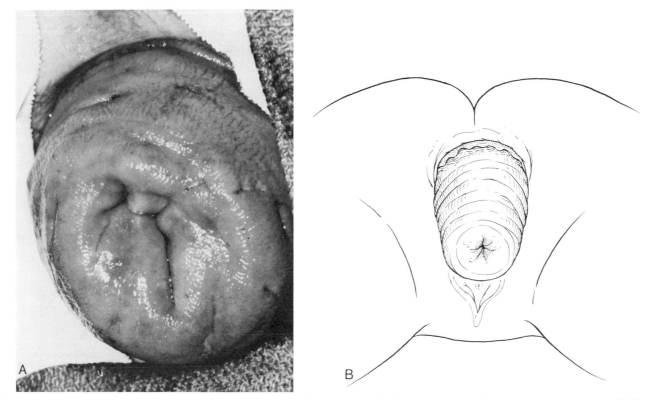

Figure 13–1. Complete rectal prolapse. *A,* The everted rectal wall appears as a tubular mass made up of several concentric mucosal folds. *B,* A schematic representation of rectal prolapse.

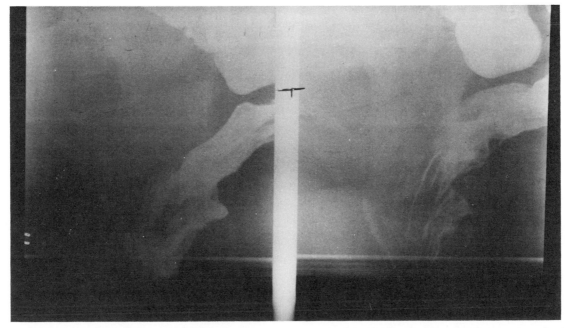

Figure 13–2. Occult rectal prolapse. Defecography showing intussusception of distal sigmoid and proximal rectum into distal rectum.

procedure, that is, to add anterior plication of the puborectal muscle at the time of perineal proctectomy or to perform a postanal repair after anterior resection and rectal fixation have failed to reverse the problem of incontinence.

SURGICAL TREATMENT

In adults the disease is progressive, and once the diagnosis is established, surgical correction is indicated. More than 100 operative procedures have been described to correct rectal prolapse, which suggests that none is entirely effective and satisfactory. Many procedures represent variations of a given basic procedure, and all are designed to correct the anatomic defect perceived to be responsible for the prolapse.[1]

In our current practice, we employ three procedures to surgically treat adult patients with complete rectal prolapse. These include (1) transperineal rectosigmoidectomy, (2) anorectal mucosectomy with rectal wall musculature plication, and (3) transabdominal sigmoid resection with rectopexy.

Selection of Procedure

The choice of procedure is tailored according to the patient's age, the general health status, and the degree of prolapse. As a general rule, procedures involving the perineal approach offer greater safety and correct the prolapse, at least over the short term, and are therefore more suitable for older and/or less healthy patients. If the prolapsing rectal segment is shorter than 3 to 4 cm, we prefer to employ a modification of the so-called Delorme procedure consisting of anorectal mucosectomy with plication of the muscular coat of the rectum.[12] If the prolapse is longer than 3 to 4 cm and a perineal approach is preferred, a transperineal rectal amputation of the Altemeier type is used.[13] By contrast, procedures that involve a transabdominal approach may offer greater opportunity for prolonged correction of the defective process, but they are associated with greater risks of morbidity and mortality and should therefore be reserved for the otherwise healthy patient.

Surgical Technique

Bowel Preparation

Regardless of the technique chosen, a complete overnight bowel cleansing together with antibiotic therapy is used. Unless the procedure is contraindicated, the large intestine is washed with 4 liters of bowel-cleansing solution ((GoLYTELY) taken orally starting the day before surgery (1:00 to 6:00 P.M.).[14] Neomycin (2 g) and metronidazole (2 g) are given orally at 7:00 P.M. and 11:00 P.M. the night before surgery. Alternatively, in debilitated patients a combination of repeated tap water enemas and cathartics can be used.[14] Patients with severe incontinence should be prepared with GoLYTELY, as they may not be able to retain enemas.

Transperineal Rectosigmoidectomy

Because many of the patients referred to us for corrective surgery of rectal prolapse are elderly, frail women with a rather long prolapsed segment, this procedure, initially championed in this country by Altemeier and associates, is often used.[13] A Foley catheter is placed in the bladder. In most patients, general anesthesia is preferred, although in high-risk patients spinal anesthesia or, much more rarely, local anesthesia of the anal sphincteric area[15] can be satisfactory. The patient is placed in the lithotomy position in gynecologic stirrups (Fig. 13–3), and the table is slightly tilted in a Trendelenburg position. The anorectal area and the perineum are thoroughly prepared with a 5% solution of povidone-iodine (Betadine) and the prolapsing segment pulled out maximally with Babcock clamps (Fig. 13–4).

The prolapsing segment is then sequentially amputated by means of electrocautery. The mucosa, submucosa, and muscularis propria of the protruding outer rectal wall are incised circumferentially, starting 2.0 cm proximal to the dentate line (distally on the everted segment) (Fig. 13–5). The inner portion of the prolapsed bowel then comes into view, including the peritoneal sac anteriorly (see Fig. 13–5). In most instances, the sac is opened, its contents pushed cephalad into the peritoneal cavity, and the redundant peritoneum excised with scissors (Fig. 13–6). The vessels and fatty tissue of the mesorectum or mesosigmoid are then carefully clamped, transected, and ligated circumferentially with 3-0 chromic catgut (see Fig. 13–6). The mesorectum or mesosigmoid should not be transected too far proximally from the anal verge to prevent interfering with the blood supply of the future anastomosis. The remaining peritoneum of the resected sac is now sutured to the anterior wall of the sigmoid or rectum with continuous 3-0 chromic catgut (Fig. 13–7).

The residual inner rectal or sigmoid tube is then transected full thickness, with either the scissors or the electrocautery. The two cut segments are then approximated together with four quadrant sutures of 3-0 Vicryl (Fig. 13–8). Two to three additional sutures of interrupted 3-0 Vicryl are then placed between the two

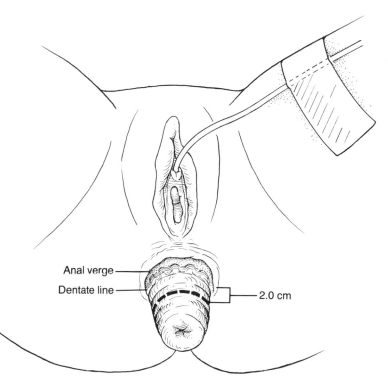

Figure 13–3. Perineal rectosigmoidectomy. The patient is placed in the lithotomy position in stirrups, and a catheter is inserted in the bladder. Note the dotted line indicating level where the mucosal dissection will be initiated.

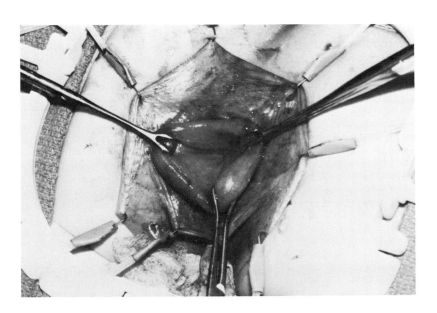

Figure 13–4. Perineal rectosigmoidectomy. The surgeon has placed Babcock clamps on the prolapsing segment, which is shown being pulled out to assess extent of prolapse. Note "lone star" retractor placed to expose the dentate line area.

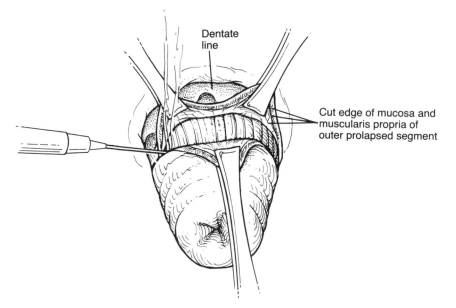

Figure 13–5. Perineal rectosigmoidectomy. An initial circular incision is made anteriorly through the mucosa and muscularis propria of the outer prolapsed segment 1.5 to 2.0 cm proximal to the dentate line using electrocautery. Note the partial exposure of the muscularis propria of the inner prolapsed segment.

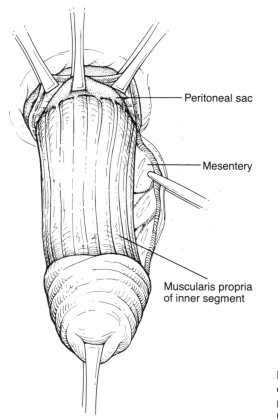

Figure 13–6. Perineal rectosigmoidectomy. The incision is extended circumferentially and the outer prolapsed segment pulled, exposing the muscularis propria of the inner prolapsed segment, the peritoneal sac anteriorly, and the mesentery posteriorly.

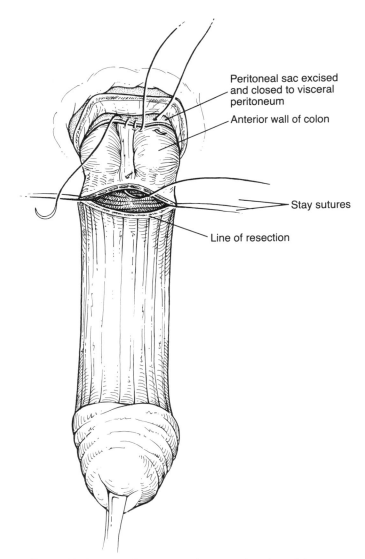

Peritoneal sac excised
and closed to visceral
peritoneum

Anterior wall of colon

Stay sutures

Line of resection

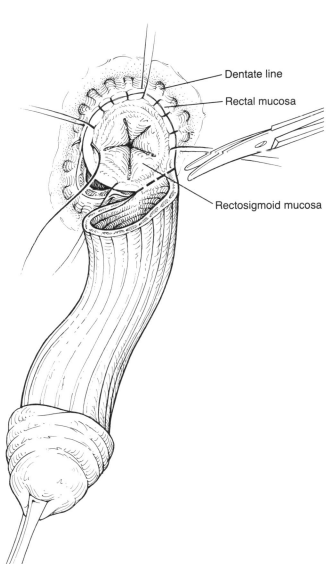

Dentate line

Rectal mucosa

Rectosigmoid mucosa

Figure 13–7. Perineal rectosigmoidectomy. The edges of the remaining peritoneal sac are sutured together to the anterior muscular wall of the prolapsing inner segment of bowel with continuous 3-0 chromic catgut. After the mesentery has been serially divided between clamps and tied with 3-0 silk and meticulous hemostasis completed, the remaining prolapsed sigmoid and/or rectum is transected with scissors or with the electrocautery. The transection is completed anteriorly and laterally sufficiently to place three anchoring sutures of 3-0 Vicryl between the proximal and distal portions of the divided bowel.

Figure 13–8. Perineal rectosigmoidectomy. The remainder of the prolapsing segment is transected, and a fourth (posterior midline) anchoring suture is placed. The anastomosis may then be completed with a continuous 3-0 Vicryl suture.

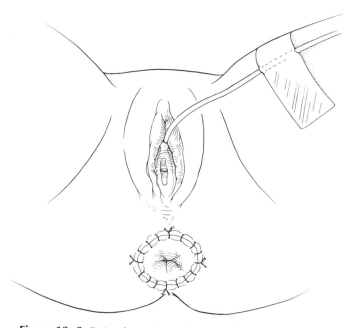

Figure 13–9. Perineal rectosigmoidectomy. Alternatively, the anastomosis may be completed with additional interrupted sutures of 3-0 Vicryl placed between each of the four quadrant sutures; the anastomosed segment is then gently eased back into the anal canal.

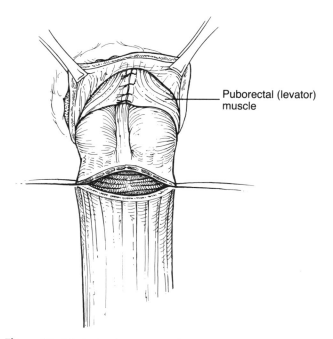

Puborectal (levator) muscle

Figure 13–10. Perineal rectosigmoidectomy. In patients with severe, incapacitating incontinence, the puborectal muscle may be approximated anteriorly using interrupted sutures of stout, nonabsorbable material.

segments of bowel in each quadrant to complete the anastomosis. The anastomosed segment can now be gently eased endoanally (Fig. 13–9).

If the patient has incapacitating incontinence as assessed clinically and manometrically prior to operation, the puborectal muscle is approximated anteriorly with interrupted 2-0 Vicryl sutures prior to completion of the anastomosis (Fig. 13–10). An alternative approach is to add a posterior rectopexy and to proceed with a postanal repair, all done by way of the perineal approach.[16]

Anorectal Mucosectomy with Rectal Wall Musculature Plication

This procedure with its modifications is most often referred to as the Delorme procedure, named after the French surgeon who initially described it in 1900.[12] It is used infrequently in our practice and is limited to high-risk, elderly patients with short-segment prolapse (3 cm or shorter). The procedure consists of shortening the protruding rectal muscular wall by plicating it after the denuding of its mucosal lining.

A Foley catheter is inserted into the bladder prior to placing the anesthetized patient in the prone jackknife position. The rectal ampulla is irrigated with a 5% solution of povidone-iodine first and then with water until the rectum is clear of stool. A mucosectomy of the protruding segment is then carried out in a manner similar to that for ileal pouch–anal anastomosis.[17] To minimize bleeding and facilitate the dissection, the mucosa of the distal anal canal is infiltrated submucosally with a solution of 0.25% bupivacaine (Marcaine) containing 1:200,000 epinephrine.

Exposure of the anal canal area can be maximized by using two Gelpi retractors placed at right angles to each other and a small Richardson retractor (Fig. 13–11), or the newly described "lone star" retractor (Fig. 13–12).[18] Starting about 1 cm proximal to the dentate line, the mucosa is circumferentially dissected free from the underlying internal sphincter and muscularis propria (Fig. 13–13). As the dissection proceeds cephalad, a tube of mucosa is gradually developed while gentle traction is applied caudally on the mucosal tube with the help of a Richardson retractor appropriately placed between the muscle wall and the mucosal tube. The dissection is extended until the rectum can no longer be easily pulled outward (Fig. 13–14). The proximal portion of the mucosal tube can then be transected (Fig. 13–15). Sutures of 3-0 Vicryl sequentially incorporate the uppermost transected mucosa and muscularis propria, multiple areas of the denuded muscularis propria placed in a zigzag, left-to-right manner, and

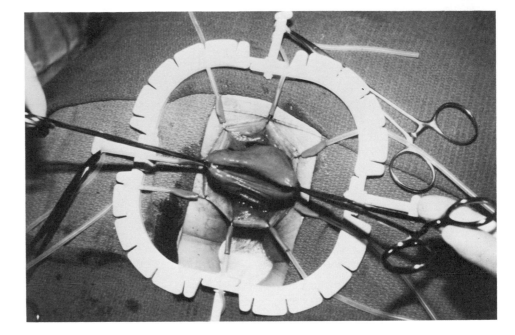

Figure 13–11. Anorectal mucosectomy. The patient is placed in the prone jackknife position, and the buttocks are taped to increase anal exposure. The amount of prolapse is assessed by the surgeon with clamps placed on the redundant segment, which is pulled aborally. A lone star retractor has been used to expose the anal area.

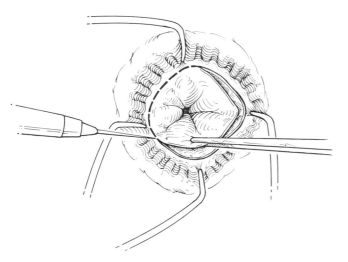

Figure 13–12. Anorectal mucosectomy. Retractors used to efface the anus and expose the dentate line area may include the lone star retractor (as shown in Fig. 13–4 and 13–11) or two Gelpi retractors placed at right angles to each other. (From Dozois RR. Ileal pouch-anal anastomosis. Surg Rounds 1987;10:38–48.)

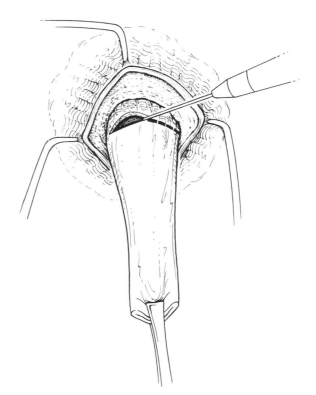

Figure 13–13. Anorectal mucosectomy. The mucosectomy is initiated with the electrocautery starting 1.5 cm proximal to the dentate line and extended circumferentially and proximally.

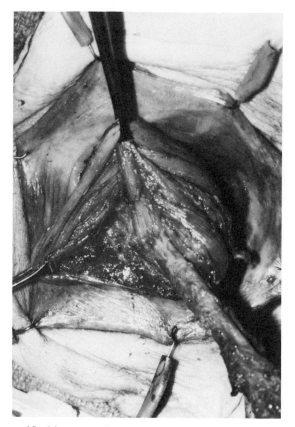

Figure 13–14. Anorectal mucosectomy. The "mucosectomy," or stripping of the mucosa from the underlying muscularis propria, is extended cephalad for a distance of 10 to 15 cm or until the rectum can no longer be pulled outward. The mucosal "tube" is then amputated at the level of the future proximal side of the anastomosis.

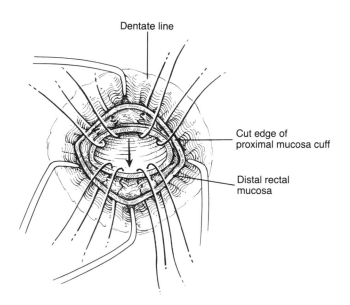

Dentate line

Cut edge of proximal mucosa cuff

Distal rectal mucosa

Figure 13–15. Anorectal mucosectomy. Interrupted sutures of 2-0 Vicryl are then placed between the mucosa and underlying muscle of proximal (amputated) and distal (above dentate) segments, taking several bites of rectal wall muscle in between in a "zigzag" fashion.

the distal cut end of the anal canal mucosa (Fig. 13–16). After eight such sutures have been placed and tied, the proximal and distal ends of the mucosa are approximated together, resulting in a concertina-like plication of the rectal muscular wall. Additional sutures can then be placed between the proximal and distal segments to complete the anastomosis. The pleated muscular wall shortens the rectum, thereby eliminating the prolapse (Fig. 13–17). A petroleum jelly (Vaseline) gauze pack can be placed across the anastomosis for 24 to 48 hours.

Postoperative Care

Both transperineal proctosigmoidectomy and anorectal mucosectomy with plication of the rectal wall are extremely well tolerated by the elderly and even very frail patient. Pain is minimal or absent. An oral liquid diet can usually be resumed the day after the operation, and the patient rapidly advanced to a normal diet. The Foley catheter can be removed the next day. Stools are kept soft but formed with a combination of bulk-forming agents and fecal softener and laxative (Peri-Colace). Most patients are discharged from the hospital within 5 days after the operation.

Sigmoid-Colonic Resection with Rectopexy

With the patient under endotracheal general anesthesia and in the supine position, the abdominal wall is cleansed with a solution of 5% povidone-iodine. A Foley catheter is inserted into the bladder. Ankle straps are used to help maximize the Trendelenburg positioning. Thromboguards (Meda Sonics, Mountain View, CA) are applied on the lower extremities to reduce the postoperative risk of thromboembolism. The abdominal cavity is entered through a lower midline incision extending to the pubis. After careful abdominal exploration, the patient is placed in the exaggerated Trendelenburg position, and the small bowel loops are packed away from the pelvis by means of a long pack. A Balfour retractor together with a bladder blade helps maximize exposure. Beahrs and coworkers have underscored four principles that should be adhered to when one performs an anterior resection for rectal prolapse:[19]

1. Dissect the rectum from the hollow of the sacrum down to the level of the levators, incising the lateral ligaments.

2. Remove sufficient sigmoid to maintain tautness of the rectum.

3. Perform the anastomosis at a point that allows for easy restoration of colorectal continuity.

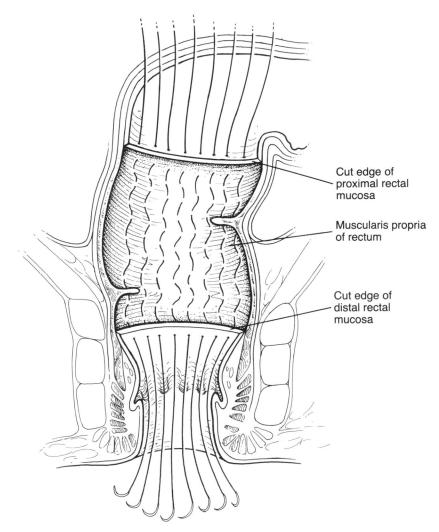

Cut edge of
proximal rectal
mucosa

Muscularis propria
of rectum

Cut edge of
distal rectal
mucosa

Figure 13–16. Anorectal mucosectomy. The sutures are then tied starting with the four quadrant-anchoring ones and continuing with the ones placed in between.

4. Suspend the rectum in a manner that avoids excessive tension on the anastomosis.

The lateral peritoneal attachments of the usually very redundant sigmoid colon are first incised. Rectal dissection and mobilization are then carried out in a manner similar to that for low anterior resection, except that the lateral stalks are severed closer to the rectal wall.

We believe that postoperative adhesions of the mobilized rectum favor fixation of the rectum to the sacrum more than any other maneuvers or material advocated by various authors for "fixing" the rectum to the sacrum. The pelvic peritoneum is incised close to the rectal wall on either side to unite the rectovesical or rectouterine sulcus.[20] The rectum is then mobilized posteriorly to the anococcygeal ligament and anteriorly to below the prostate in men or the lower one third of the vagina in women. The "air dissection" technique described by Beahrs and colleagues facilitates the pos-

terior portion of the dissection and helps develop a natural plane between the posterior rectum and the anterior sacrum with its venous plexus.[21] The laxity of the rectal moorings usually noted in these patients facilitates this dissection. The lateral stalks are then severed on both sides close to the rectal wall, preferably by means of electrocautery.

The completely mobilized rectum is pulled cephalad into the abdomen. The endopelvic fascia and peritoneum on each side of the rectum are sutured to the periosteum and presacral fascia of the middle to upper sacrum, by using two or three interrupted sutures of 2-0 Prolene on each side to hold it firmly in position. The sutures are not tied until all have been put in place (Fig. 13–18). A substantial portion of the redundant sigmoid colon is then prepared for resection. After lifting the superior hemorrhoidal vessels anteriorly and away from the clearly visualized left ureter, they are clamped, transected, and ligated.

After both the distal and the proximal bowels to be

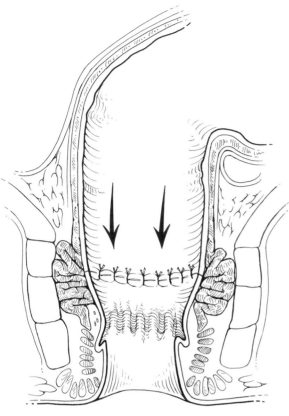

Figure 13–17. Axial schematic appearance of anastomosis above dentate line with plicated rectal wall.

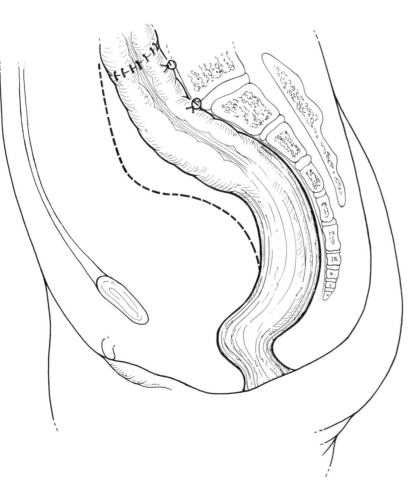

Figure 13–18. Completed anterior resection with rectopexy. The redundant sigmoid colon has been excised. The rectum has been mobilized to the pelvic diaphragm, and elevated and fixed to the presacral fascia. The colorectal anastomosis is above the sacral promontory.

anastomosed have been bared, the surgeon places a curved, noncrushing Foss clamp across the rectum 2 to 3 cm distal to the proposed site of resection. The surgeon then places a Pemberton right-angle clamp just proximal to the curved shod, places a sponge under the area of the bowel to be transected to minimize contamination, and severs the bowel against and just below the angle clamp using an angle-shaped scalpel. Again, the bowel should be transected at a level immediately superior to the level of the promontory to permit an easy end-to-end hand-sewn anastomosis. The clamped, transected bowel is rotated upward and placed into an open pack, which is folded over and clamped snugly around the bowel to avoid contamination of the surgical field.

The proximal bowel is then sequentially clamped with a noncrushing shod clamp (proximally) and an angle crushing clamp (distally). The bowel is transected sharply near the latter clamp over a sponge with the scalpel. Both cut ends of the lumen are cleansed with povidone-iodine–soaked sponges.

The surgeon (standing to the left of the patient) then places seven sutures of 3-0 silk through the seromuscular layers of the transected sigmoid colon and rectum (two corner sutures, one middle suture, and two sutures on each side between the middle and the corner sutures). After the posterior row of silk sutures has been placed, the two curved shods are approximated, the knots tied, and the silk cut close to the knots. A mucosal layer of 3-0 chromic catgut is then placed in an over-and-over inverting fashion starting on the medial side of the bowel, approximating anatomically the mucosa and submucosa of the posterior wall first. As the surgeon approaches the lateral sigmoid and rectal walls, the stitch is locked to minimize purse-stringing the lumen.

The surgeon proceeds medially and anteriorly with a running over-and-over mucosal inverting suture. At this point, when the anastomosis has been circumferentially inverted, the chromic sutures are tied together outside the lumen. The anterior seromuscular layers of the proximal and distal bowel are then approximated with interrupted sutures of 3-0 silk, burying the mucosal layer. The sutures are cut as tied.

The pelvic floor is then reconstructed by approximating the incised peritoneal surfaces with continuous 3-0 Vicryl sutures. The abdomen is closed in layers using interrupted 0 Vicryl in the fascia and subcuticular 3-0 Vicryl on the skin.

Postoperative Care

The patient is maintained on intravenous fluids for 3 to 5 days postoperatively. Then oral alimentation is resumed and gradually increased over 2 to 3 additional days. The urinary catheter placed preoperatively is removed 4 days postoperatively at about the time when bowel functions return. The patient is usually dismissed 7 to 9 days postoperatively.

EDITORIAL COMMENT

We wholeheartedly agree with the author's decision not to include, in the recommended procedures for correction of prolapse of the rectum, the various operations using synthetic material to fix the rectum to the sacrum. Although they are appealing because of technical simplicity, these procedures are fraught with complications including stenosis, obstruction, and erosion with perforation and sepsis. Correction of any of these complications is difficult and may require multiple operations and diversion of the fecal stream.

The etiology of prolapse of the rectum is unclear, but we have been impressed by the common association of episiotomy as a possible causative factor in prolapse in young women. This association implicates an injury to the pelvic diaphragm and therefore suggests that repair of the muscle is in order. Furthermore, there is debate as to whether the prolapse of the rectum is an intussusception or a hernia. On the basis of our observations of the perineal repair of Altemeier, it appears that the condition is *both* a rectosigmoid intussusception into the rectum *and* a sliding hernia of the cul-de-sac through the pelvic diaphragm (levator ani). The perineal repair is the only operation that corrects the anatomic abnormalities: resection of the rectosigmoid and anterior repair of the levators correct the hernia. In addition, a rectocele is commonly present with prolapse, and a levator repair may be elected to correct this defect and to re-establish a perineal body.

Although technically more intricate than an anterior resection, the perineal repair avoids laparotomy and intraperitoneal colon resection while remedying the observable anatomic defects.

We agree that the mucosectomy-plication operation is appropriate for small prolapses. We differ slightly with the authors' technique of perineal repair. Our circumferential incision is placed at least 2 cm (distal on the everted segment) from the dentate line. This preservation of 2 cm of full thickness of rectum appears to preserve proprioception, and thus eventual fecal control, more effectively.

Management of Persistent Anal Incontinence

By the time rectal prolapse is recognized and treated, as many as 50% of the patients already have become incontinent of stool and gas. Contrary to previous beliefs, the incontinence results less from the recurring transanal protrusion of the rectum with repeated mechanical stretching of the sphincter apparatus[1] than from the prolonged stretching and ensuing damage of the pudendal innervation of the sphincter.[10] This may explain why not all incontinence problems are reversible. Because the continence of as many as 50% to 75% of incontinent prolapse patients improves over a period of 6 to 12 months after surgical correction of the prolapse,[1, 22] direct surgical repair of the continence mechanisms is not attempted at the time of abdominal repair. If necessary, the postanal repair can be used with some degree of success at a later date in patients with persistent, incapacitating incontinence.[22, 23]

In patients who had a transabdominal repair, we prefer to defer such an attempt to correct the incontinence for at least 12 months. If a transperineal rectosigmoid amputation has been done, we can approximate the levators anteriorly with relative ease prior to anastomosis. However the clinical results of the postanal repair leave much to be desired,[23–25] and ultimately a permanent colostomy may be required for some patients with incapacitating incontinence. It seems on the basis of results in patients with idiopathic incontinence, that the type of approach (anterior or posterior) is irrelevant.[26]

CONCLUDING REMARKS

Surgical correction of complete rectal prolapse is imperfect, as can be deduced from the myriad operations that have been proposed over the years to alleviate this cumbersome and humiliating ailment. In most instances, we favor anterior resection for several reasons. Most surgeons are familiar with the technique of anterior resection, which can be done safely in most patients. Construction of the anastomosis at a comfortable level just above the promontory helps reduce further complications. Simple suturing of the stalks to the presacral fascia is technically easy to perform and avoids complications resulting from foreign materials, such as obstruction or perforation with Marlex mesh[27] or disk space infection from nylon strips.[28] For the older and more debilitated patient, we have more recently opted for a transperineal approach, which is safer but technically more complex. These techniques should therefore be employed only by surgeons familiar with their technical intricacies.

None of the operations provides perfect results, but the transabdominal anterior resection appears to be most satisfactory in a great proportion of the patients, even over the long term.[29] Nevertheless, it has been clearly demonstrated that the success rate of any type of surgical repair and the risk of recurrence have a linear relationship to the length of follow-up.[29] The long-term results of transperineal repairs may be less satisfactory over the long term than those obtainable with a transabdominal approach, and they will need to be assessed carefully over time. However because they are reserved for the elderly patients, their greater safety may more than compensate for the possibly greater risk of eventual recurrence.

ACKNOWLEDGMENT. The authors are indebted to B.J. Huebner for the preparation of this manuscript.

REFERENCES

1. Wassef R, Rothenberger DA, Goldberg SM. Rectal prolapse. Curr Probl Surg 1986;23:402–451.
2. Jurgeleit HC, Corman ML, Coller JA, Veidenheimer MC. Procidentia of the rectum: Teflon sling repair of the rectal prolapse, Lahey Clinic experience. Dis Colon Rectum 1975;18:464–467.
3. Brodén B, Snellman B. Procidentia of the rectum studied with cineradiography: A contribution to the discussion of causative mechanism. Dis Colon Rectum 1968;11:330–347.
4. Theuerkauf FJ Jr, Beahrs OH, Hill JR. Rectal prolapse: Causation and surgical treatment. Ann Surg 1970;171:819–835.
5. Fry IK, Griffiths JD, Smart PJG. Some observations on the movement of the pelvic floor and rectum with special reference to rectal prolapse. Br J Surg 1968;53:784–787.
6. Neill ME, Parks AG, Swash M. Physiological studies of the anal sphincter musculature in fecal incontinence and rectal prolapse. Br J Surg 1981;68:531–536.
7. Metcalf AM, Loening-Baucke V. Anorectal function and defecation dynamics in patients with rectal prolapse. Am J Surg 1988;155:206–210.
8. Spencer RJ. Manometric studies in rectal prolapse. Dis Colon Rectum 1984;27:523–525.
9. Parks AG, Porter NH, Hardcastle J. The syndrome of the descending perineum. Proc R Soc Med 1966;59:477–482.
10. Parks AG, Swash M, Urich H. Sphincter denervation in anorectal incontinence and rectal prolapse. Gut 1977;18:656–665.
11. Failes D, Killingback M, Stuart M, De Luca C. Rectal prolapse. Aust NZ J Surg 1979;49:72–75.
12. Delorme R. Sur le traitement des prolapsus du rectum totaux par l'excision de la muqueuse rectale ou rectal-colique. Bull Mem Soc Chir (Paris) 1900;26:498–518.
13. Altemeier WA, Culbertson WR, Schowengerdt C, Hunt J. Nineteen years' experience with the one-stage perineal repair of rectal prolapse. Ann Surg 1971;173:993–1001.
14. Wolff BG, Beart RW Jr, Dozois RR, et al. A new bowel preparation for elective colon and rectal surgery: A prospective, randomized clinical trial. Arch Surg 1988;123:895–900.
15. Goldberg SM, Gordon PH, Nivatvongs S. Principles of anesthetic management in anorectal surgery. In: Essentials of Anorectal Surgery. Philadelphia: JB Lippincott, 1980, pp 58–68.
16. Prasad ML, Pearl RK, Abcarian H, et al. Perineal proctectomy, posterior rectopexy, and postanal levator repair for the treatment of rectal prolapse. Dis Colon Rectum 1986;29:547–552.
17. Dozois RR. Technique of ileal pouch–anal anastomosis. Perspect Colon Rectal Surg 1989;2:85–94.
18. Roberts PL, Schoetz DJ Jr, Murray JJ, et al. Use of new retractor to facilitate mucosal proctectomy. Dis Colon Rectum 1990;33:1063–1064.
19. Beahrs OH, Theuerkauf FJ Jr, Hill JR. Procidentia: Surgical treatment. Dis Colon Rectum 1972;15:337–346.
20. Frykman HM. Abdominal proctopexy and primary sigmoid resection for rectal procidentia. Am J Surg 1955;90:780–788.
21. Beahrs OH, Kiernan PD, Hubert JP. An Atlas of Surgical

Techniques of Oliver H. Beahrs. Philadelphia: WB Saunders, 1985, pp 256–272.

22. Parks AG. Anorectal incontinence. Proc R Soc Med 1975; 68:681–690.

23. Keighley MRB, Matheson DM. Results of treatment for rectal prolapse and fecal incontinence. Dis Colon Rectum 1981; 24:449–453.

24. Miller R, Bartolo DCC, Locke-Edmunds JC, Mortensen NJMcC. Prospective study of conservative and operative treatment for faecal incontinence. Br J Surg 1988;75:101–105.

25. Yoshioka K, Keighley MRB. Critical assessment of the quality of continence after postanal repair for faecal incontinence. Br J Surg 1989;76:1054–1057.

26. Miller R, Orrom WJ, Cornes H, et al. Anterior sphincter plication and levatorplasty in the treatment of faecal incontinence. Br J Surg 1989;76:1058–1060.

27. Keighley MRB, Fielding JWL, Alexander-Williams J. Results of Marlex mesh abdominal rectoplexy for rectal prolapse in 100 consecutive patients. Br J Surg 1983;70:229–232.

28. Loygue J, Nordlinger B, Cunci O, et al. Rectopexy to the promontory for the treatment of rectal prolapse: Report of 257 cases. Dis Colon Rectum 1984;27:356–359.

29. Schlinkert RJ, Beart RW Jr, Wolff BG, Pemberton JH. Anterior resection for complete rectal prolapse. Dis Colon Rectum 1985;28:409–412.

Special Operations on the Colon and Rectum

CHAPTER 14

Fabrizio Michelassi
Tommaso Balestracci

APPENDECTOMY AND MANAGEMENT OF APPENDICEAL ABSCESS

Appendectomy

Indications

Indications to perform an appendectomy include acute appendicitis, interval appendectomy following conservative treatment of an appendiceal abscess, mucocele of the appendix, and small carcinoids of the appendix without metastases to ileocecal lymph nodes. A right hemicolectomy is the procedure of choice in the presence of either a carcinoid of the appendix larger than 2 cm or a carcinoid with lymph node metastases, and for an adenocarcinoma of the appendix.

Preoperative Preparation

Patients undergoing appendectomy require fluid resuscitation and appropriate perioperative antibiotics. A nasogastric tube should be inserted if there is gastric distention or ileus.

Operative Technique

Once the patient is anesthetized, the abdomen is inspected and palpated for evidence of a mass that might have not been appreciated while the patient was awake. Although many different incisions for an appendectomy have been described, we prefer a transverse incision over the palpable mass or over the point of maximum tenderness (Fig. 14–1). The incision is lateral to the rectal sheath, although this can be incised if exposure is not adequate. A muscle-splitting technique is used to gain access to the abdominal cavity, separating the fibers of the external and internal oblique muscles and the transverse abdominal muscle (Fig. 14–2). The peritoneum is opened in a transverse direction, and cultures for aerobic and anaerobic organisms are obtained if free fluid is present. Two or three retractors are then inserted in the wound and the anterior wall of the cecum is grasped. By following the anterior tenia and by rocking the cecum in a craniocaudal direction, the appendix is delivered to the incision (Fig. 14–3). If the appendix cannot be delivered this way, digital exploration of the right lower quadrant may reveal an inflammatory mass. In this situation, the appendix is mobilized by gentle finger dissection; one should note the retroperitoneal structures that may be intimately adherent to the inflamed appendix, such as the right ureter, the right gonadal vein, and the right common iliac vessels. Alternatively, it may be necessary to divide inflammatory adhesions by sharp dissection to avoid rupturing a friable, gangrenous appendix with blunt dissection. The mesoappendix is then divided by serially applying hemostats and ligating each with interrupted fine silk sutures.

Once the base of the appendix is free it is clamped with two straight hemostats. The specimen is removed after transecting the appendix between the clamps (Fig. 14–4). The appendiceal stump is ligated with an absorbable suture, and the mucosa of the appendiceal stump is lightly electrocoagulated. If the wall of the

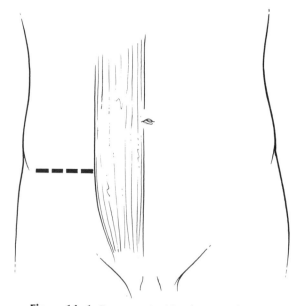

Figure 14–1. Transverse incision for appendectomy.

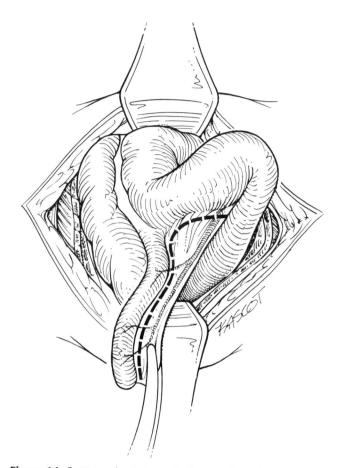

Figure 14–3. View of anterior wall of cecum through the transverse incision after placement of retractors, with mobilization of the appendix and delivery into the wound.

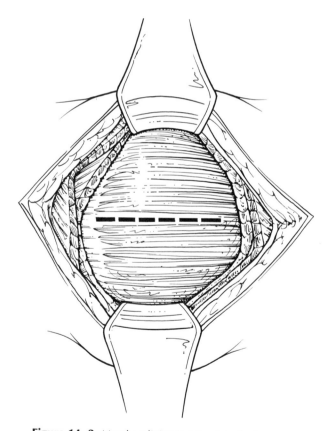

Figure 14–2. Muscle-splitting incision into the transverse abdominal muscle.

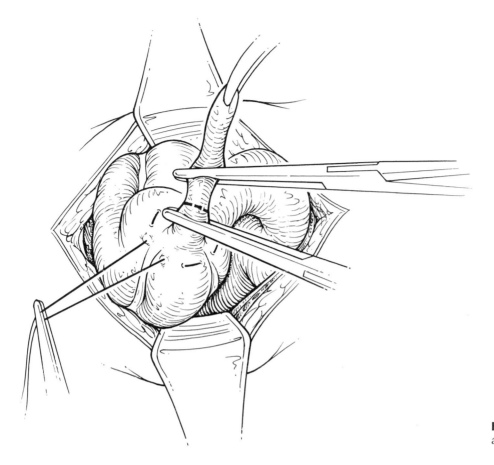

Figure 14–4. Division of the appendix.

cecum is not edematous and thickened, the appendiceal stump may be buried under a fine silk pursestring suture inserted around the appendiceal stump, 1 cm away from it (Fig. 14–5). The stump can be buried by means of other methods, such as Z-stitches or interrupted Lembert stitches. The cecum is then returned to the abdominal cavity, and the right lower quadrant and pelvis are irrigated copiously. In the absence of a perforated appendicitis or an appendiceal abscess, one should inspect the distal ileum in search of a Meckel's diverticulum in need of removal. The abdominal incision is closed in layers, and the skin edges are approximated with a subcuticular running stitch. If an appendiceal abscess or a gangrenous perforated appendix is present, the skin edges are left open for local wound management and approximated 4 to 5 days after operation, by means of plastic adhesive strips.

If the cecum cannot be mobilized because of inflammatory adhesions and the appendix cannot be brought to full exposure, the base of the appendix may be divided between clamps and the appendix removed in a retrograde fashion to sequentially obtain adequate control of the mesoappendix.

If the diagnosis of appendicitis was incorrect and the appendix is normal, the appendix is removed to prevent confusion later, and an orderly abdominal exploration is performed. The cecum, terminal ileum, pelvic organs, and upper abdominal cavity are inspected in search of neoplasia of the right colon, perforated diverticulitis of the cecum or sigmoid colon, regional enteritis, foreign-body perforation of the terminal ileum, Meckel's diverticulitis, mesenteric adenitis, tubo-ovarian abscess, ectopic pregnancy, ovarian tumor, or twisted ovary. The upper abdominal cavity is also explored for acute cholecystitis or perforated peptic ulcer. Less likely entities, such as a rupturing abdominal aneurysm, retroperitoneal or rectus sheath hematoma, amebic perforation of the cecum, or tubercular ileitis, should be entertained when the more common entities are ruled out. The goal of the exploration is either to identify the cause of the patient's complaints or to be certain that no other lesions are present before closing the abdominal incision. To facilitate inspection of the pelvis, the lateral portion of the rectus abdominis muscle can be divided; if disease is remote from the right lower quadrant, the incision can be extended medially into a transverse infra-umbilical one. Alternatively, the incision can be closed and a different approach to the abdominal cavity employed.

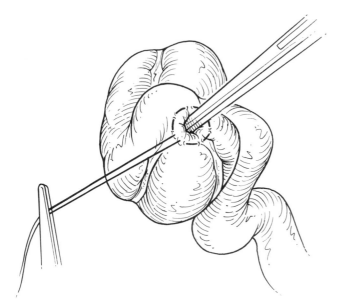

Figure 14–5. Inversion of the appendiceal stump with a pursestring suture.

Postoperative Care

In the absence of perforation or peritonitis, antibiotics may be discontinued postoperatively. Patients in this situation usually do not require nasogastric suctioning; their diets can be advanced rapidly, and usually they are discharged within 2 to 4 days after the operation. In the presence of a perforation or peritonitis, the proper broad-spectrum antibiotic coverage for aerobic and anaerobic organisms is instituted at the time of operation and continued for 5 to 7 days. These patients usually require nasogastric suctioning initially and until bowel activity is resumed. If the wound has been packed open, the dressing should be changed every 4 to 6 hours to achieve mechanical débridement and to determine when secondary closure can be accomplished.

Complications

Wound infection is the most common complication after appendicitis. As soon as infection is detected, the superficial wound must be opened and the abscess drained. The wound usually heals with an excellent cosmetic appearance, even by secondary intention. Because of the muscle-splitting incision, evisceration or incisional hernias are extremely rare.

A postoperative intra-abdominal abscess may occur as a sequela of perforation and peritonitis. This requires open or percutaneous drainage. Occasionally, a pelvic abscess may be managed by transrectal or transvaginal drainage (Figs. 14–6 and 14–7).

Postoperative paralytic ileus occasionally develops into a mechanical obstruction in the presence of a slowly resolving peritonitis. The intestinal obstruction is initially treated with continuous nasogastric or nasoenteric suctioning and antimicrobial therapy for the continuing peritonitis. Laparotomy is entertained only for a complete or unresolving partial obstruction.

Dehiscence of the stump or rupture of the cecal wall may result from slippage of the appendiceal stump ligature, necrosis of the cecal wall from a periappendiceal abscess, erosion by a drain, or unrecognized regional enteritis. An immediate laparotomy with a cecostomy and, more commonly, a resection with ileostomy are the procedures of choice.

Management of Periappendiceal Abscess

A small percentage of patients may present with findings consistent with a localized periappendiceal inflammation. If these patients are not obstructed, are tolerating liquids, and are in otherwise good general health, they may be treated nonoperatively with intra-

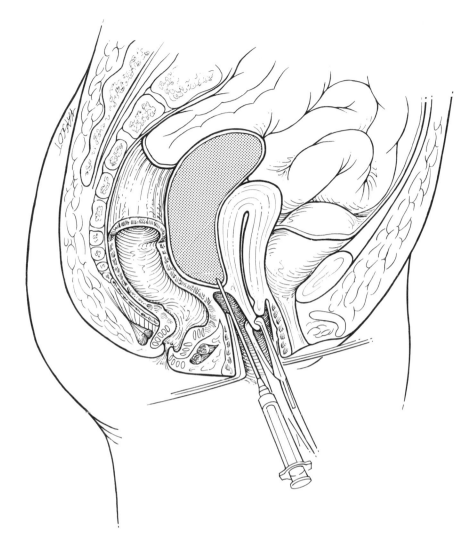

Figure 14–6. Transvaginal drainage of a pelvic appendiceal abscess.

venous antibiotics and observed for abatement of their symptoms and eventual resolution within 7 to 10 days. If at any time during this period symptoms or findings progress, patients should undergo urgent appendectomy. Otherwise, they are discharged to return in 6 to 8 weeks time for an elective interval appendectomy.

If patients who have findings consistent with localized periappendiceal abscess present with abdominal distention, intestinal obstruction, or worsening sepsis or belong to a high-risk group, such as elderly or medically compromised patients, a trial of intravenous antibiotics should not be performed. These patients should undergo an urgent appendectomy and drainage of a periappendiceal abscess as soon as they are resuscitated.

Urgent operation, if required, is accomplished through the same transverse incision described for acute appendicitis. If it becomes apparent that the abscess abuts against the anterior or lateral abdominal wall, the peritoneum is opened in that specific location to accomplish drainage of the abscess without entering the abdominal cavity. However, if the abscess is not readily available, the remainder of the peritoneal cavity is protected by laparotomy pads before the abscess is drained. Also, care is exercised to avoid disturbing any inflammatory adhesion between loops of intestine and omentum in order to protect against widespread contamination. Once the abscess is drained, if the base of the appendix is visible and an appendectomy appears feasible, the appendix should be removed and the stump ligated. In children, a consistent effort to perform an appendectomy should be made in order to avoid continued soilage by feces through the lumen of the relatively wide appendiceal base. If the appendectomy is postponed, an interval appendectomy should be performed 6 to 12 weeks later, depending on the duration of purulent or fecal drainage from the abscess cavity. The abscess cavity is drained with a large drain or a sump drain, which exits through a separate incision. The drain is left in place until no further discharge is collected and the original abscess cavity has totally obliterated.

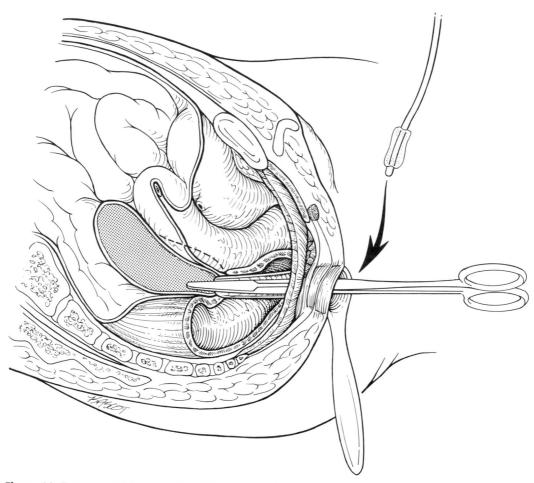

Figure 14–7. Transrectal drainage of a pelvic appendiceal abscess.

When the abscess is in the pelvis and can be palpated on rectal or vaginal examination as a bulge, it can be drained transrectally through the anterior rectal wall (see Fig. 14–7) or transvaginally through an incision in the posterior fornix (see Fig. 14–6). To facilitate these approaches, the bladder is emptied with a catheter and the patient is placed in the lithotomy position. Transrectal and transvaginal drainage are not recommended for children. These procedures are restricted to fully developed adults.

CECOSTOMY

Indications

Cecostomy, a procedure widely used in the past, is rarely performed today because it does not provide complete fecal diversion, only decompression. A transverse colostomy, when appropriate, accomplishes effi-

cient decompression and diversion, and it allows for proper mechanical cleansing of the obstructed bowel.

Tube cecostomy should be considered in the following patients: those with a reduced cecal volvulus at high risk of recurrence, in whom resection of the cecum is not desirable; patients with "pseudo-obstruction" of the colon (Ogilvie's syndrome), in whom an exploratory laparotomy was performed for presumptive mechanical obstruction and none was found or in whom repeated colonoscopies have failed to decompress the distended colon and signs of impending cecal perforation develop; occasionally, patients with a left-sided colonic anastomosis, to prevent gaseous distention of the proximal colon; patients with a large intestinal obstruction; patients with a perforation of the cecum, either secondary to a mechanical obstruction or due to iatrogenic injury during the performance of an appendectomy when the wall of the cecum is indurated and friable; patients with an impending perforation of the cecum secondary to a mechanical obstruction of the colon; and rarely patients with stump leakage or cecal wall rupture in the first few days after an appendectomy. In many of these situations most surgeons prefer a colostomy or favor immediate resection with an end-ileostomy. The most appropriate indication for a cecostomy, therefore, is a distended cecum with serosal tears or patches of ischemic necrosis; such areas of necrosis are used for the cecostomy site itself.

Preoperative Preparation

Because these operations are sometimes done urgently in the presence of a large bowel obstruction, the patient must be fully resuscitated before the operation begins. When the cecostomy is performed as an independent procedure, one must preoperatively locate the cecum so that the incision is precisely placed and the size of the incision is minimized. This can be easily achieved preoperatively by obtaining a supine abdominal x-ray film with a marker at the umbilicus.

Operative Strategy

A tube cecostomy or a skin-sutured cecostomy can be fashioned. A tube cecostomy is more easily and expeditiously performed, and after it is no longer needed, the resulting fistula usually closes spontaneously soon after the tube is withdrawn. Conversely, it requires significant nursing care and frequent irrigation and often becomes obstructed by semisolid fecal material. A skin-sutured cecostomy is a better decompressing and cleansing stoma that requires much less nursing care, although it requires formal surgical closure when no longer needed.

A cecostomy in a massively dilated, unprepared, fragile cecum carries the possibility of fecal contamination of the abdominal cavity and wound. Precautions should be taken (1) by using laparotomy pads and gauzes to isolate the cecostomy from the remainder of the abdominal cavity and the wound, (2) by preparing two independent suction devices before the cecotomy is performed so as to have one suction device ready when the other suction is overwhelmed or plugged, and (3) by using copious irrigation if contamination occurs. In the case of the skin-sutured cecostomy, the cecum should be sutured to the abdominal wall before being opened.

Good communication between the surgeon and the anesthesiologist is essential to avoid a sudden increase in the intra-abdominal pressure while the dilated cecum is handled and sutured to the fascia of the abdominal wall. Often, the cecal wall is thin and fragile because of the distention of the viscus and will tear easily if not handled gently.

Operative Technique

Tube Cecostomy

If the cecostomy is performed without laparotomy, a 6-cm transverse incision is selected over the dilated cecum as localized preoperatively by an abdominal radiograph (Fig. 14–8). After adequate mobilization, the cecum is inspected. If a necrotic patch is detected on the anterior or lateral wall, this area is selected for the cecostomy. Two concentric 2-0 silk seromuscular pursestrings are then applied on the wall of the cecum. If necessary, an attempt is made to decompress part of the intraluminal gaseous contents by using a 16-gauge needle attached to suction (Fig. 14–9). The needle puncture should be placed through the center of the area that will be used for the stoma. A large (30- to 32-gauge) Foley, mushroom, or Malecot catheter is then selected. The large size of the tube helps ensure prolonged patency. Although a Foley catheter is easier to insert and secure, the internal diameter of a mushroom or a Malecot catheter is larger than the internal diameter of a similar-size Foley catheter. The selected tube is passed through a separate stab incision. It is then inserted in the cecum and secured in position by tying the two pursestrings (Fig. 14–10). The cecum is then secured to the abdominal wall with a series of nonabsorbable sutures placed around the cecostomy (Fig. 14–11). It is easier to insert and tie the lateral sutures first, as they are the most difficult ones to reach. An omental flap, if available, can also be placed around the cecostomy as a further ensurance against contamination. The transverse incision is then closed in layers, and the decision to close the skin or to leave it open to heal by secondary intention is based on the amount of contamination that has occurred during the procedure. The tube is secured to the skin of the interior abdominal wall with several stout sutures to avoid accidental displacement in the immediate postoperative period.

With the abdomen open during an exploratory laparotomy, the tube cecostomy is facilitated by the greater access to the cecum, the easier mobilization of the viscus, and the avoidance of an incision in the right lower quadrant, which may sometimes interfere with the tube cecostomy. It is also much easier to isolate the cecum from the remainder of the abdominal cavity by using laparotomy pads to minimize eventual contamination. The technique of cecostomy is otherwise the same.

Skin-Sutured Cecostomy

The right lower quadrant transverse incision, subsequent exploration of the cecum, and detection of sites

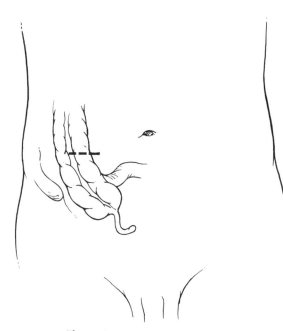

Figure 14–8. Incision for a cecostomy.

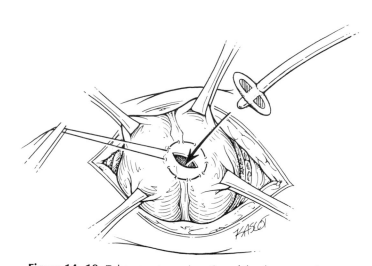

Figure 14–10. Tube cecostomy: insertion of the decompressing cecostomy tube, pursestring suture.

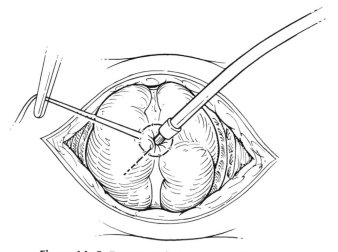

Figure 14–9. Temporary decompression of the cecum.

of ischemic necrosis are steps common to the skin-sutured cecostomy as well as the tube variety. After adequate mobilization, the wall of the cecum is then sutured to the abdominal wall with interrupted 3-0 seromuscular silk sutures placed all around the incision at an interval that will produce a waterproof seal and prevent any fecal contamination of the peritoneal cavity on opening of the cecal wall. This layer of sutures is placed so as to allow an adequate portion of cecal wall to herniate through the abdominal wound to allow for eventual fixation to the skin without tension. The incision in the anterior wall of the cecum is made only after the subcutaneous edges of the wound have been protected with gauze. Availability of two suction devices will further minimize contamination. A transverse incision is then carried out in the middle of the exposed cecal wall (Fig. 14–12), and the edges are then sutured to the skin with interrupted 4-0 chromic catgut on an atraumatic needle (Fig. 14–13). A proper stoma appliance is immediately fitted around the cecostomy to protect the surrounding skin.

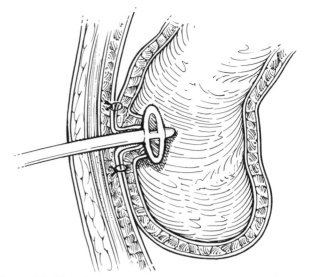

Figure 14–11. Tube cecostomy. The cecum is sutured to the interior abdominal wall.

Postoperative Care

The skin-sutured cecostomy is treated as any other stoma by applying a proper appliance around it to protect the surrounding skin. A tube cecostomy needs frequent irrigation with saline to maintain its patency.

Complications

Peristomal sepsis or detachment of the cecum from the anterior abdominal wall with resultant fecal peritonitis is a complication of both the tube and the skin-sutured cecostomy. A pericecostomy cellulitis is frequently seen in tube cecostomies when fecal material leaks around the tube. A rare complication of tube cecostomy is failure to close spontaneously after withdrawal of the tube, whereas a more common complication of the skin-sutured cecostomy is significant prolapse.

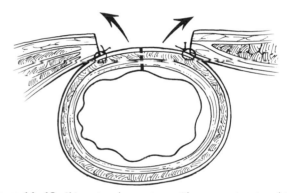

Figure 14–12. Skin-sutured cecostomy. The cecum is sutured to the abdominal wall. A transverse incision is made in the middle of the exposed cecal wall.

POLYPECTOMY

Indications

Because of the well-established techniques of colonoscopic polypectomy for pedunculated polyps and the availability of colonoscopic electrocoagulation or neodymium-yttrium aluminum garnet (Nd-YAG) laser photoablation for sessile polyps, the operation of colotomy and polypectomy is infrequently indicated today. It is necessary, however, when colonic polyps are

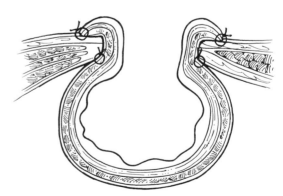

Figure 14–13. Skin-sutured cecostomy. The cecum is opened and sutured to the abdominal skin.

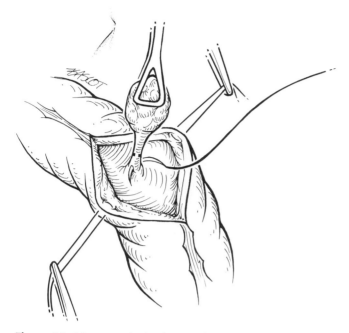

Figure 14–14. Longitudinal colotomy after the application of stay sutures and removal of a polyp after controlling its blood supply.

inaccessible to the colonoscope, when they are sessile and too large for endoscopic removal, or when during an extracolonic or colonic operation a polyp is located that has not been suspected or endoscopically removed preoperatively and does not lend itself to en bloc removal with the major specimen. In some of these instances, when the palpatory findings suggest malignant transformation or a large sessile polyp is on the mesenteric side of the colonic lumen, a segmental colectomy is the procedure of choice.

Preoperative Preparation

Operative polypectomy is rarely accomplished today as a primary procedure. Therefore, the preoperative preparation is consistent with the lesion to be approached. If polypectomy is to be performed for a colonic resection, the patient is prepared with a mechanical cleansing of the colon. If the operation is to be performed for extracolonic pathology, the incidental operative polypectomy should be done only in the presence of a mechanically prepared large intestine.

A colonoscopy or preferably a double-contrast barium enema is required to precisely identify the location of the polyp and to diagnose the presence of synchronous lesions that may influence or alter the operative approach.

Operative Technique

The colon is inspected and palpated to locate the polyp and to determine whether other polyps are present. Inspection of the serosal surface at the base of the polyp and the nearby mesenteric lymph nodes must be carried out for evidence of neoplastic invasion. In addition, transmural palpation of the polyp should be used to judge its mobility and consistency. If the assessment is consistent with a benign pedunculated polyp, the colonic segment harboring the polyp is isolated from the remainder of the colon by applying noncrushing intestinal clamps proximally and distally. A longitudinal colotomy is performed along the anti-mesenteric tenia (Fig. 14–14) after the abdominal cavity has been protected with laparotomy pads and a 3-0 silk stay suture has been applied on either side of the tenia. The polyp is then grasped, and the stalk is clamped and suture-ligated after the removal of the polyp (Fig. 14–14). If the stalk of the polyp is wide, several interrupted 3-0 absorbable sutures may be necessary to obtain closure of the mucosal defect and adequate hemostasis. A frozen section is obtained to rule out malignant degeneration invading the stalk, which would require a formal segmental resection. The colotomy can be closed in a transverse direction

(Fig. 14–15) by using 3-0 Dexon sutures in a running Connell stitch for the inner layer and interrupted 3-0 silk Lembert sutures for the outer layer.

Complications

The most common postoperative complication is hemorrhage from the stalk of the polyp or from the colotomy. Meticulous hemostasis at the time of the polypectomy reduces the incidence of this complication.

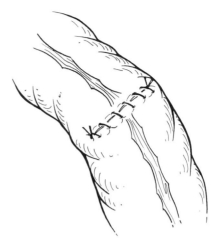

Figure 14–15. Closure of colotomy in a transverse fashion.

FULGURATION OF RECTAL TUMORS

Indications

Fulguration should be restricted to tumors of the lower and middle rectum. To be amenable to fulguration, a tumor must be completely visible and exposed through a transanal approach. Fulguration should be reserved for very poor risk and elderly patients and for patients with demonstrated distant metastasis. The inability to stage the lesion restricts this procedure to the aforementioned groups or to selected patients who have benign polyps with small foci of malignancy and to a few patients with tiny, mobile cancers. For patients who refuse a colostomy and are not suited for any other form of sphincter-saving resection, fulguration is an option, as are local excision, laser therapy, and endoluminal radiotherapy.

Preoperative Preparation

The preoperative preparation is similar to the one obtained for local resections of rectal lesions. The colon is mechanically cleansed with oral osmotic solutions and occasionally with laxatives and enemas. Perioperative antibiotics are administered.

Operative Technique

The patient is placed in the dorsal lithotomy position for tumors of the posterior wall, and in the prone or jackknife position for tumors of the anterior rectal wall. Exposure is facilitated by the Parks retractor or by using two or three long, narrow Deaver retractors (Fig. 14–16). By using the electrocautery, the tumor and a margin of normal mucosa is electrocoagulated or excised by a loop in a repeated sweeping fashion (Fig. 14–16). Constant suctioning of the rectal ampulla is necessary to evacuate debris, liquid, and smoke. By

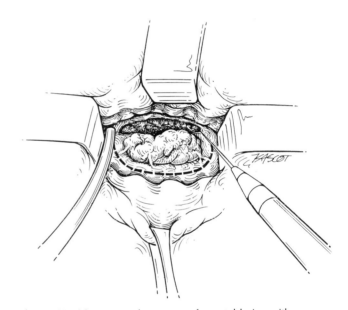

Figure 14–16. Transanal exposure of a rectal lesion with an electrocautery excision.

way of irrigation, curettage, or suctioning, the charred tumor surface is cleansed, and further electrocoagulation made possible. Exposure of the underlying muscle layer or the extrarectal fat is an indication that the tumor has been removed. Although electrocoagulation of a rectal mass can be done on the posterior wall as deeply as necessary, care must be exercised on the anterior wall or with higher lesions that may extend above the peritoneal reflection in order to avoid perforation into the vagina, urethra, or peritoneal cavity.

Postoperative Care

In the absence of complications, the patient is discharged 1 or 2 days after the operation and is followed with monthly proctoscopies in order to assess the need for further fulguration.

Complications

The most common complication is bleeding, which may require operative intervention through a transanal approach with either suture ligation or further electrocoagulation of the bleeding point. Other complications include rectovaginal fistula, rectourethral fistula, and penetration into the abdominal cavity as a result of aggressive local electrocoagulation. Repeated fulgurations of large (occupying more than one third of the rectal circumference) lesions may lead to stenosis of the rectum, necessitating the colostomy that was originally refused.

LASER TREATMENT OF RECTAL LESIONS

The three main types of lasers available are the carbon dioxide, argon, and Nd-YAG laser. The different wavelengths generated by these lasers determine the characteristics of the beam, the depth of penetration into tissues, and the kind of resulting tissue damage.

The laser of choice for colorectal carcinomas is the Nd-YAG laser. This laser is used in either a noncontact or a contact mode, and it vaporizes tissues. In the past, the laser was used in a noncontact mode, which made the therapeutic application imprecise with deep penetration of energy and tissue necrosis that were difficult to control. Technical improvements have made it possible to use the same laser in the contact mode, which requires lower energy and causes less tissue damage.

Success with the endoscopic use of the Nd-YAG laser has been reported in palliating obstructing rectal lesions and restoring patency of intestinal lumen. From one to six outpatient sessions over 7 days are usually required for successful palliation. With its ability to reestablish a lumen and control hemorrhage, the Nd-YAG laser therapy may become a substitute for surgical colostomy in the unresectable obstructing colorectal adenocarcinoma or for the debilitated or medically compromised patient.

POSTERIOR PROCTOTOMY FOR RECTAL LESIONS

Indications

Excellent exposure of lesions of the anorectum may be obtained by means of a transanal approach. By pulling the rectosigmoid down into the rectal ampulla, even high lesions can sometimes be approached transanally. If the lesion is large, sessile, and 7 to 10 cm from the anal verge, the choices are a low anterior resection and anastomosis, a trans-sphincteric approach according to York-Mason, or a trans-sacral approach. The low anterior resection and anastomosis are described in Chapter 9. The transanal and trans-sphincteric approaches are described in Chapter 18. This discussion covers the trans-sacral approach or posterior proctotomy.

The posterior approach can be used in treating benign lesions of the rectum that are too high above the anal verge and too large or sessile to be excised transanally. The posterior approach can also be employed for selected cases of small, mobile, low-grade, early malignant lesions of the middle and lower rectum when a low anterior resection or an abdominal perineal resection is to be avoided because of age, concomitant systemic diseases, or refusal of a permanent colostomy by the patient.

The sacral approach is also appropriate in the elderly patient with borderline continence. By avoiding mechanical and forceful anal dilatation, one assures patients that their continence will not deteriorate.

Preoperative Preparation

The colon and rectum are mechanically cleansed with oral osmotic solutions, laxatives, and occasional enemas as well as by dietary restrictions. The mechanical preparation of the colorectum in these cases is no different from that used for other operations on the left side of the colon and rectum. A preoperative colonoscopy or double-contrast radiograph is necessary to disclose other synchronous lesions that may influence the operative approach.

Operative Technique

The patient is placed in the prone position with the chest supported by pillows and the pelvis placed over a Wilson frame. Pillows are placed under the thighs and legs, and points of pressure are systematically avoided by shifting or increasing protection with plastic padding, blankets, and pillows. The intergluteal crease may be opened in the obese patient by attaching adhesive tape to the buttocks and the lateral rail of the operating table.

A vertical incision is made from a point overlying the third sacral vertebra to a point immediately behind the anus (Fig. 14–17). After deepening the incision down to the sacrum (Fig. 14–17), the anococcygeal raphe is isolated and incised longitudinally. Detaching the raphe from the coccyx allows exposure of Waldeyer's fascia. The sacrotuberous and sacrospinous ligaments can then be divided from their insertion to the last two sacral and first coccygeal vertebrae, thereby allowing for the coccyx and the fifth sacral vertebra to be removed (Fig. 14–17) by means of Rongeur forceps. Bone wax can be used to control bleeding from the surfaces resulting from the severed vertebrae. Waldeyer's fascia is then divided in the midline (Fig. 14–18) to expose the rectum underneath. Starting as distally as possible, one prepares the rectal wall by teasing away the retrorectal fat and by electrocoagulating small perirectal vessels. The degree of mobilization of the distal rectum depends on the size and location of the lesion to be removed and on whether the lesion should be removed along a submucosal plane or with a full-thickness wedge or sleeve resection. Small, benign polyps without clinical evidence of malignant degeneration can be removed along a submucosal plane. Large villous adenomas with a clinically suspicious site of malignant transformation or early adenocarcinomas should be handled by way of a full-thickness removal. For extensive and circumferential villous adenomas, a sleeve or segmental resection may be preferable.

The rectal wall should be opened longitudinally (Fig. 14–19) at a site separate from the lesion after stay sutures have been applied. If the lesion is to be removed along the submucosal plane, it may be advantageous to inject the submucosa with saline with or without epinephrine (1:400,000). The lesion can then be removed with a 1-cm margin of normal surrounding mucosa by means of sharp scissor dissection. Hemostasis is obtained with the electrocautery or with interrupted sutures. If the mucosal defect is small, it can usually be repaired primarily; if the remaining mucosal defect is large, it can be left denuded, although in this situation a wedge or sleeve resection is preferred. Following excision of the lesion, the rectum is closed longitudinally in two layers.

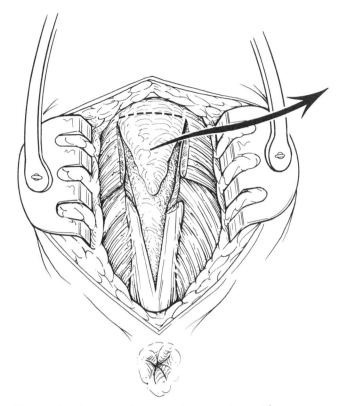

Figure 14–17. Incision for a posterior proctotomy with exposure of the sacrum and anococcygeal raphe, and excision of the coccyx.

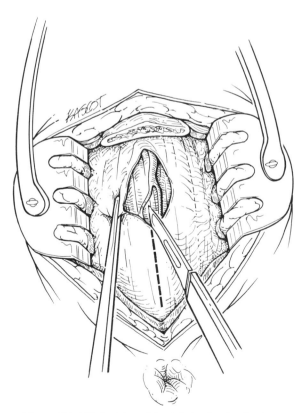

Figure 14–18. Incision of the inferior levator fascia.

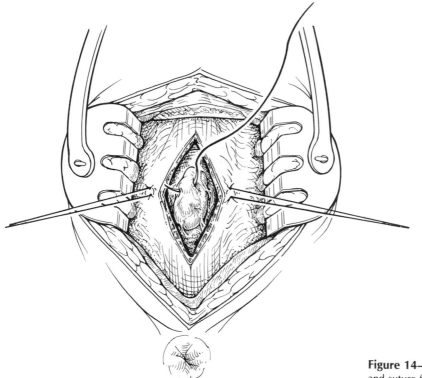

Figure 14–19. Longitudinal incision in the posterior rectal wall and suture fixation of the tumor.

The presacral space is then drained, and the drain is exited through a separate incision. Waldeyer's fascia is closed and the anococcygeal raphe is reconstructed. The superficial subcutaneous tissue is approximated while both dead space and the creation of fat necrosis are avoided. The skin is then closed with interrupted vertical mattress sutures.

Postoperative Care

The suction drain is left in place until there is no further discharge. The skin sutures are left for 7 to 10 days. Bowel movements are delayed for 5 to 7 days by using a low-residue diet and oral codeine as the pain medication of choice. The patient is usually discharged after the presacral drain is removed.

Complications

Hemorrhage from the polypectomy site may occur in the immediate postoperative period or after several days. If it is seen in the immediate postoperative period, it is usually the result of incomplete hemostasis at the time of operation; if it occurs up to 1 week later, it is usually attributable to detachment of the eschar or to a partial dehiscence. In all cases the hemorrhage may be self-limited or may require emergency intervention via a transanal approach. Delay in wound healing may result from the persistence of subcutaneous dead space after closure or from the formation of fat necrosis. Should a dehiscence occur and a fecal fistula manifest itself, a totally diverting transverse colostomy should be performed until the fistula has healed.

EDITORIAL COMMENT

The operations described in this chapter are basic staples on the menu of the surgeon. Because of their fundamental nature and ill-perceived simplicity, they are often delegated to the least experienced surgeon, particularly in teaching hospitals. Hence, these procedures are frequently poorly done and associated with major complications. For each operation there are subtle variations or presentations that deserve comment.

The "decision tree," or algorithm, for periappendiceal inflammation or abscess can be difficult. An obvious intra-abdominal abscess with associated fever or leukocytosis is best treated by extraperitoneal drainage. A walled-off perforation without spread of peritonitis or discernible abscess formation may be initially treated by nonoperative means, as the authors suggest. This is a difficult clinical decision: Is this a true abscess or a sealed perforation with phlegmon? This decision has been made considerably easier by computed tomographic scan, and small abscesses that were previously not diagnosed clinically are now readily demonstrated and localized for drainage. The utilization of axial tomography precisely defines the nature of the inflammatory process, and as a result, nonoperative management is now uncommon.

A tube cecostomy to supplement or to "protect" a low pelvic anastomosis is an ill-conceived concept, usually without merit. The authors have specifically detailed the few and shrinking indications for cecostomy.

One of the frustrations in performing a polypectomy or a segmental colectomy for a small polyp that has been biopsied or subtotally excised by colonoscopy is the surgeon's inability to find the exact site of the polyp or its remaining stalk. Empiric resections based on colonoscopic measurements are notoriously inaccurate. A practical solution is to have the endoscopist tattoo the polyp site by injection of India ink or another suitable dye into the bowel wall at the site of the polyp. This is an aid for localization that avoids the necessity of opening the bowel for inspection or endoscopy with resultant contamination.

Fulguration appears to be an all-inclusive term for local ablation of a rectal tumor by various techniques of electrocauterization ranging from "branding" to electrical scalpel excision. Fulguration may be used curatively for small tumors whose boundaries have been precisely demonstrated by transrectal ultrasonography. We prefer to perform this as a serial, layered excision of the tumor by a loop cautery with a combing technique. By this method the layers of the rectum can be accurately identified and serial specimens obtained for histologic examination to confirm adequate removal. For larger tumors multiple fulgurations may be necessary.

Posterior proctotomy is an excellent diagnostic, as well as therapeutic, maneuver. Villous adenomas, particularly those at 6 to 8 cm from the anal verge and situated anteriorly, are particularly appropriate for removal by this technique. A whole-mount histologic examination of the entire specimen is obtained. If the tumor is benign or harbors only intraepithelial malignancy, nothing other than surveillance need be done. If an invasive malignancy is diagnosed, an appropriate "cancer operation" may then be performed.

BIBLIOGRAPHY

Appendectomy and Management of Appendiceal Abscess

Buck JR. Acute appendicitis. In: Cameron J, ed. Current Surgical Therapy. 1st ed. Philadelphia: BC Decker, 1984.

Chassin JL: Appendectomy. In Chassin JL, ed. Operative Strategy in General Surgery: An Expositive Atlas. New York: Springer-Verlag, 1984.

Colombani PM. Acute appendicitis. In: Current Surgical Therapy. 3rd ed. Philadelphia: BC Decker.

Condon RE. Appendicitis. In Sabiston DC Jr, ed. Textbook of Surgery. 13th ed. Philadelphia: WB Saunders, 1986.

Dudgeon DL. Acute appendicitis. In: Cameron J, ed. Current Surgical Therapy. 2nd ed. Philadelphia: BC Decker, 1986.

Ellis H. Appendix. In: Schwartz S, Ellis H, eds. Maingot's Abdominal Operations. 9th ed. Norwalk, CT: Appleton & Lange, 1989.

Walt AJ. The appendix. In Nora PF, ed. Operative Surgery. Principles and Techniques. 3rd ed. Philadelphia: WB Saunders, 1990.

Cecostomy

Aldrete JS. Diverting and venting colostomy techniques and colostomy closure. In: Nyhus L, Baker R, eds. Mastery of Surgery. 1st ed. Boston: Little, Brown & Company, 1989.

Chassin JL. Operations for colon obstruction. In: Chassin JL, ed. Operative Strategy in General Surgery: An Expositive Atlas. Vol 1. New York: Springer-Verlag, 1984.

Laser Treatment of Rectal Lesions

Sankar MY, Joffe SN. Laser surgery in colonic and anorectal lesions. Surg Clin North Am 1988;68:1447–1469.

Posterior Proctotomy for Rectal Lesions

Parks AG, Nicholls RJ. Perianal endorectal operative techniques. In: Dudley, Pories, Carter, eds. Operative Surgery, Alimentary Tract and Abdominal Wall. 4th ed. St. Louis: C. V. Mosby, 1983.

OPERATIONS ON THE ANUS AND PERIANAL REGION

Common Ailments of the Anorectal Region

C H A P T E R   1 5

Elliot Prager

This chapter addresses the surgical approaches to a number of pathologic conditions affecting the anorectum. It represents how and why I perform a given procedure. My exclusion of alternative techniques should not be interpreted as a denigration of any other method. However, I am comfortable with and confident of only operations with which I have extensive experience. Presented here is the distillate of my preferences.

HEMORRHOIDS

To the average layperson (and, unfortunately, to many physicians) any anorectal symptom is indicative of hemorrhoids. The sophisticated treating surgeon must ensure that the patient's symptoms can be properly attributed to this condition. Bleeding associated with pain on defecation, for example, usually suggests a fissure. Other symptoms, such as itching and irritation, are nonspecific and may be a consequence of other anorectal problems or dietary factors (commonly caffeine and vitamin C) or may be due to overaggressive attempts at anal cleansing. Hemorrhoid treatment is not successful in these situations. One must also differentiate between the symptoms of internal hemorrhoids—prolapse, painless bleeding, and mucous leakage—and those of external hemorrhoids—swelling, pain, and difficulty with hygiene.

After examination confirms the presence of hemorrhoids and their probable association with the symptoms, one then explains the alternatives for management. With the exception of their bleeding to the point of causing anemia, hemorrhoids rarely pose a signifi-

cant health hazard. The patient may reasonably accept or reject treatment. The goal of therapy is to ameliorate the patient's symptoms but not necessarily to achieve a cure. Because hemorrhoids are varicosities of the anal canal, other veins may eventually become varicose and possibly symptomatic. With the exception of proctectomy, I know of no guaranteed "cure."

Internal Hemorrhoids

My preferred treatment of symptomatic internal hemorrhoids is rubber band ligation. Infrared coagulation is especially suitable for small or nonpliant hemorrhoids or for those in the area of previously treated hemorrhoids. Even if there is an external component, most symptoms are usually attributable to the internal hemorrhoids. Treatment in the office is a simple and effective approach to alleviating the primary complaint.

Thrombosed Hemorrhoids

Whether to excise a thrombosed hemorrhoid is usually determined by the duration of symptoms. Within the first few days after the episode, pain is relieved more effectively and more quickly by excision. If the pain has already subsided or has significantly improved, one can assure the patient that without any active treatment the lumps will resolve in 3 to 6 weeks. If this is a recurrent thrombosis, subsequent thromboses are more likely, and excision is again a preferred treatment. If the thrombosed hemorrhoid has already eroded the skin, one can usually evacuate the clot through the

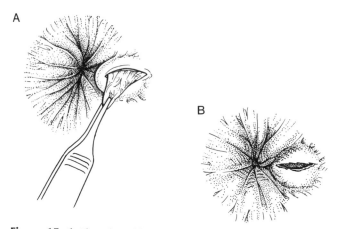

Figure 15—1. Thrombosed hemorrhoid with superficial erosion *(B)*. The clot is easily removed *(A)* through the erosion *(B)* with forceps or a small clamp.

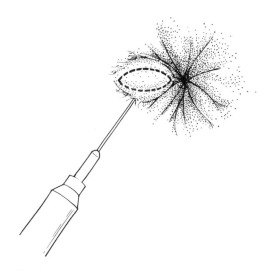

Figure 15—2. Infiltrate the thrombosed hemorrhoid with local anesthetic and outline an elliptical incision.

opening with minimal discomfort to the patient, enlarging the wound as necessary (Fig. 15–1).

Technique of Thrombosed Hemorrhoid Excision

The area is infiltrated with 0.5% bupivacaine (Marcaine) in epinephrine, 1:200,000. An elliptical incision is outlined, which ideally results in a 1- to 2-mm gap in the skin so that the edges of the wound do not coapt and allow a seroma or hematoma to form (which would reproduce the pain and swelling) (Figs. 15–2 to 15–4). For this reason incision alone with evacuation is contraindicated. One should not extend the dissection into the internal hemorrhoidal complex, so as to avoid significant bleeding. Electrocoagulation is helpful for bleeding vessels, and the wound is left open. A single gauze pad placed between the buttocks without tape is an adequate dressing. The patient is advised to start sitz baths the following morning, for 10 to 15 minutes, two to three times per day. Complications of the procedure include re-formation of clot, bleeding, and failure to heal (fissure). This last complication can usually be prevented by avoiding midline incisions, especially in the anterior position, if possible.

In the case of thrombosed prolapsed hemorrhoids with or without gangrene, I strongly recommend admission to the hospital and urgent hemorrhoidectomy. Resolution of symptoms and return to work are quicker than when the conservative approach (bed rest, stool softeners, pain medications, and sitz baths) is employed. Usually, the latter treatment is eventually followed by a hemorrhoidectomy anyway. Urgent or emergent surgery will, in fact, make the patient more comfortable almost immediately.

Hemorrhoidectomy

I recommend this procedure in the case of symptomatic internal and external hemorrhoids or when office therapy fails to alleviate symptoms. If prolapse is a significant symptom, one must ensure that the patient has a true hemorrhoid prolapse and not a full-thickness procidentia. If the history is suggestive, one should examine the patient sitting on the toilet after evacuating an enema in order to determine the extent and nature of the protrusion.

Preparation

A single sodium biphosphate (Fleet) enema on the morning of surgery to clear the rectal ampulla is adequate for cleansing. A more vigorous clean-out may delay postoperative bowel evacuation and prolong the hospitalization. The perianal area should not be shaved unless the patient is exceptionally hirsute, because when the hairs grow back they will be uncomfortable in the stubble stage.

Anesthesia

Local, regional, or general anesthesia can be successfully employed.

Position

I prefer that the patient be placed in the prone jack-knife position with the kidney rest maximally elevated and with a Trendelenburg position sufficient to allow me to stand straight and look down on the operative field. In order to visualize the perianal area optimally, 3-inch tapes should be placed slightly behind the lateral midline of the anal area and directed approximately at a 30-degree angle forward. Ater cleansing with povidone-iodine (Betadine) and applying drapes one should examine the external hemorrhoidal groups and, with a Hill-Ferguson retractor in place, visualize the internal hemorrhoidal groups. Then one plans which hemorrhoids will require excision and which ones may involve a submucosal dissection.

At this point one can inject the perianal tissues encompassing the external hemorrhoids with 10 ml of a 1:100,000 or 1:200,000 solution of epinephrine. I prefer the premixed 0.5% Marcaine with 1:100,000 epinephrine so as to obtain some long-lasting regional anesthesia. The individual hemorrhoidal groups up to the proximal hemorrhoidal vascular pedicle are injected with an additional 10 to 15 ml of solution (Fig. 15–5). When the internal hemorrhoids are being injected, a retractor or a finger is placed into the anal canal in order to check that the needle does not penetrate the mucosa and enter the lumen. After the infiltration is completed, a gauze pad is placed in the anal canal, and while a second gauze pad is held externally, the solution is gently rubbed into the tissues for 2 minutes. This allows the epinephrine a chance to infiltrate the tissues and thereby to work effectively.

At this point the operation can begin. I prefer a closed hemorrhoidal technique with excision of redundant mucosa and skin. I believe that the closed technique (as opposed to open hemorrhoidectomy) is more likely to avoid two major postoperative complications: pain and stricture. A closed hemorrhoidectomy ensures that raw surfaces are obviated and that after all the wounds are sutured, one can assess the capacity of the anal passage rather than guess at its future appearance after open wounds have contracted and healed.

A Hill-Ferguson retractor is placed into the anal canal and the most prominent hemorrhoidal group

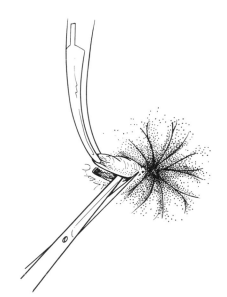

Figure 15–3. Sharply excise the thrombosis.

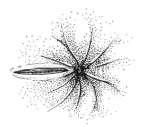

Figure 15–4. The edges of the wound should gap by 1 to 2 mm.

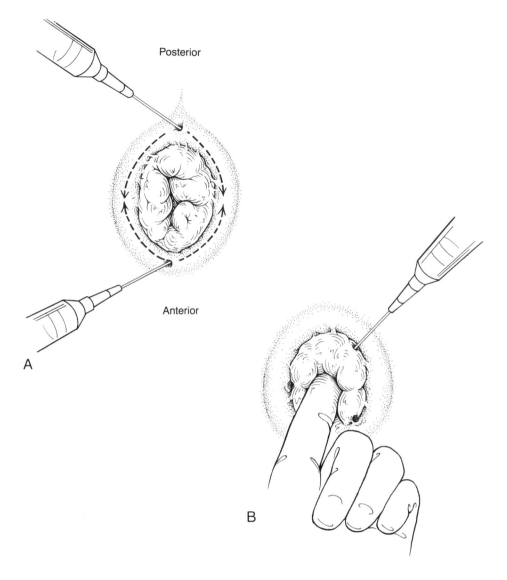

Figure 15–5. *A* and *B*, Infiltrate external and internal hemorrhoids with a local anesthetic containing epinephrine.

managed first. Parallel incisions are made on either side, extending from the base of the pedicle to a point on the perianal skin beyond the subcutaneous external sphincter edge and encompassing all the external hemorrhoid (Fig. 15–6). If the external component is wide, a distal ellipse may be used. The skin is grasped with a hemostat and retracted upward by the first assistant while the surgeon distracts the edges of the wound with the fingers of the nondominant hand. Dissection proceeds proximally with care taken to expose and preserve the internal and external sphincter muscles (Fig. 15–7). All tissue superficial to the sphincter is essentially hemorrhoid and may therefore be excised. As one pulls the hemostat upward, the muscles are tented up in a coniform configuration. Dissection is easiest at the apex of this cone, because the muscle then falls back. Lateral dissection should be at the lateral margin of the incision, rather than at the medial, in order to maximize hemorrhoid removal without

sacrificing additional skin and mucosa (Fig. 15–8). One should continue to be aware of the previously made incision, because the anatomy is distorted by pulling up on the pedicle and distracting the edges.

At the termination of the dissection, the pedicle is transfixed at its most proximal point. I prefer to use 3-0 catgut on a ⅝ circle needle. The needle is passed through the pedicle toward the lumen, rather than into the muscle wall, and the suture tied on either side. The hemorrhoid is transected and a hemostat placed on the short end under no tension so that the tied pedicle assumes its natural position in the anorectum (Fig. 15–9). With the same 3-0 suture, two throws are placed deeply, but not widely, to secure the pedicle and tied again to the short end, which then can be cut (Fig. 15–10).

If the operative plan does not involve nearby incision, at this point submucosal and subcutaneous dissection of adjacent hemorrhoidal tissue is appropriate.

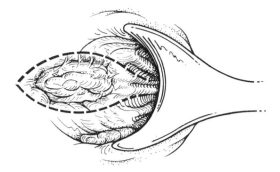

Figure 15–6. Outline the incision prior to dissection, because retraction distorts the anatomy.

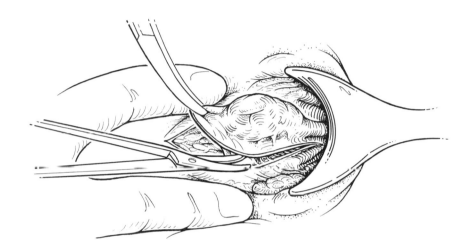

Figure 15–7. The operation consists of dissecting all tissue superficial to the sphincter muscle.

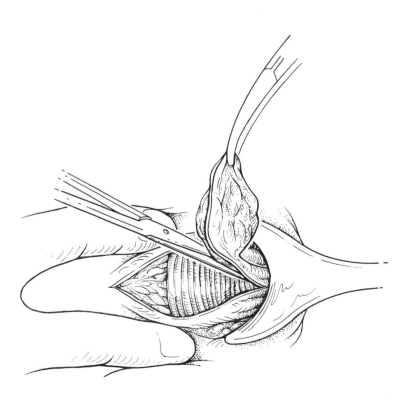

Figure 15–8. Internal and external muscle exposed as dissection proceeds proximally.

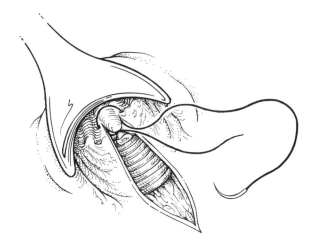

Figure 15–9. Transfixed pedicle.

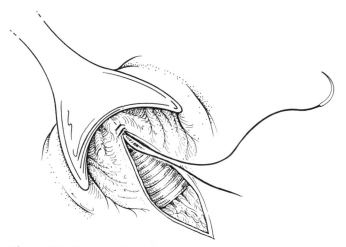

Figure 15–10. Two additional passes of the suture ensure control of the hemorrhoidal artery and vein pedicle.

In order to do this, a hemostat is placed on the mucocutaneous edge and tented up. The hemorrhoidal tissue is grasped with forceps and dissected off the overlying skin and mucosa and the underlying muscle (Fig. 15–11). If a large opening is made in the skin or mucosa, closing with a 4-0 plain suture will suffice; small rents can be ignored. After completing adjacent hemorrhoidal dissection, the same 3-0 suture is run, carefully avoiding wide bites (Fig. 15–12). One must properly align the mucocutaneous junction in order to avoid an ectropion, which can lead to leakage and irritation. The remaining hemorrhoids are excised in a similar fashion and in order of decreasing size. After major hemorrhoidal groups are removed, external skin tags can be trimmed and closed. Isolated small internal hemorrhoids can be either banded in the operating room or managed in the office at a later time.

My preference is to recommend partial internal lateral sphincterotomy concomitant with hemorrhoidectomy. I believe that this procedure markedly decreases postoperative pain. If the patient agrees to this procedure, I perform it before the closure of the left lateral group. If there is no true lateral group, I do the procedure in the most lateral aspect of the incision closest to the right or left lateral position (Fig. 15–13). It is essential that one refer to hemorrhoidal position by relating it to anterior, posterior, midline, lateral, right, or left, rather than two o'clock, three o'clock, and so on. The latter nomenclature is incomprehensible unless the patient's position is also explicitly stated, and even then it is somewhat confusing.

At the end of the procedure, a Hill-Ferguson retractor is used to check all the pedicles and suture lines for hemostasis. If it is possible to introduce a medium retractor, it is clear that stenosis is not a concern. Finally, a ¼-inch Penrose drain is placed about 3 to 4 inches into the anorectal canal and cut, with about 1 inch left protruding from the anal orifice. This drain acts as a wick, and in the case of significant bleeding in the immediate postoperative period, blood will steadily drip out to announce the hemorrhage. Otherwise, multiple units can accumulate in the colon until they stimulate an evacuation with the chaos accompanying 1,500 cc of blood and clot in the bed. Dressing consists of a single folded gauze sponge over the cleft and one or two unfolded 4 × 4-inch gauze pads over that, all held in place by two pieces of 1-inch tape without any tension on the buttocks. A large dressing secured with overlapping strips of 3-inch tape compressing the buttocks medially will limit mobility and often raise large painful skin blisters. Intrarectal packing is also to be decried. Not only is its removal painful, but its presence is uncomfortable and will never compensate for inadequate operative hemostasis.

Fluids should be restricted postoperatively. One should prevent continual questions by the nursing staff about voiding or any mention or appearance of a catheter. If the patient wants to void but cannot do so, a trial of bethanecol chloride (Urecholine) is appropriate prior to catheterization.

The patient can be offered a regular diet immediately after surgery and ambulation encouraged when anesthesia wears off. Injectable pain medication as well as oral analgesia is ordered on an as-needed basis. I do not employ stool softeners or cathartics. The former create a pasty stool that sticks to suture lines as well as the surrounding tissues and is irritating and difficult to clean. Cathartics are poorly controlled once taken, and a prolonged bout of frequent loose stools is painful and may disrupt the incisions. On the morning after surgery the dressing and the Penrose drain are removed and 10- to 15-minute sitz baths taken three times a day. The patient may be discharged after the first bowel movement, regardless of whether it is spontaneous or induced. If the patient has no bowel movement by the third postoperative day, the rectum is gently digitalized to ensure that there is no obstruction and then a sodium biphosphate enema is administered.

I have performed this operation in the ambulatory surgery setting for motivated patients and have been surprised by the smooth postoperative recovery period. More experience may show that many, if not most, hemorrhoidectomies may be done in this way.

The preceding discussion has already alluded to several postoperative complications. In the following discussion, the common ones are more completely listed with a description of what can be done to avoid or treat them.

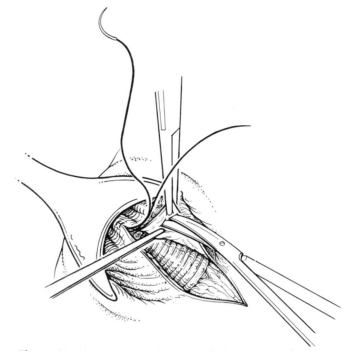

Figure 15–11. Submucosal dissection of adjacent hemorrhoids helps avoid stricture.

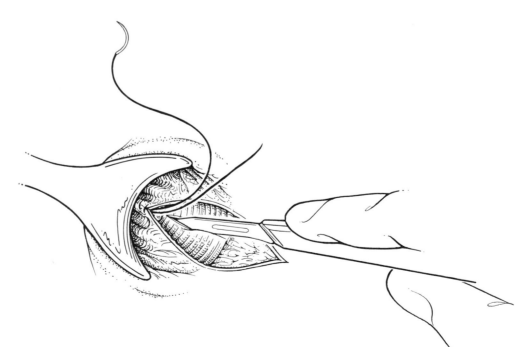

Figure 15–12. Partial internal sphincterotomy done in the left lateral position.

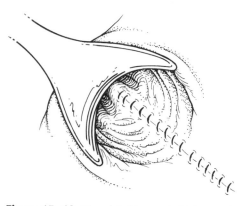

Figure 15–13. Completed hemorrhoidal wound closure.

Postoperative Complications

Bleeding

If the patient does not have a coagulopathy, significant bleeding most often occurs from a hemorrhoidal pedicle or less commonly from an artery in the base of the wound. It is best not to manage this complication at the patient's bedside. Lighting, assistance, position, and anesthesia are unequal to the challenge. The patient should be returned to the operating room and a determination made as to which incision or incisions are bleeding. These should be opened as indicated, and hemostasis secured. Bleeding can also occur 8 to 12 days postoperatively. This is usually caused by the disappearance of a ligature from an unthrombosed hemorrhoidal pedicle artery. The patient should be examined in the office or the emergency room and, if still bleeding, taken to the operating room.

Urinary Retention

Fluids should be restricted intraoperatively and postoperatively, medication to somnolence avoided, and the patient not harassed about voiding. Bethanecol chloride may be tried if the patient cannot void and is uncomfortable. On the morning after the operation, the patient is allowed to enter the sitz bath and encouraged to void while relaxed in the bath. If all fails, straight catheterization can be used; once is usually enough.

Pain

Usually, pain is easily controlled with oral agents. I have found a combination of proproxyphene napsylate–acetaminophen (Darvocet-N) 100 mg and ibuprofen (Motrin) 400 mg every 4 hours to be surprisingly effective. If the patient experiences prolonged, extreme pain, it is important to check for pressure from a distended bladder, an ampulla distended with stool, or a frank hematoma. Occasionally ecchymosis alone causes pain.

Infection

This complication is more theoretical than real. During 20 years in practice, I have had one patient form an abscess under one closed hemorrhoidal group. Treatment consists of drainage in the office under local anesthesia.

Long-Term Complications

Stricture. Stricture is best treated by careful avoidance. When the closed technique is employed, one is aware—incision by incision—of the size of the anal canal, and the patient should not suffer this complication. If it does occur, it is treated as outlined in the discussion of anal stricture further on.

Recurrent Hemorrhoids. Recurrent hemorrhoids is a misnomer. Removed hemorrhoids never grow back, but other veins in the anal canal may become varicose. Recurrent symptoms are usually referable to internal hemorrhoids, and these can almost always be treated in the office. One should educate the patients postoperatively about prevention, most importantly instructing them not to use the toilet as a library. Prolonged sitting on the toilet with relaxed sphincters will increase pressure in the hemorrhoidal veins.

Ectropion. Ectropion can be avoided by sewing the pedicle in its proper location, rather than distally in the anal canal, and by properly aligning the two wound edges when closing the incision. If ectropion is present and troublesome, treat by excision as illustrated in Figure 15–14.

Skin Tags. The complication of skin tags may result from not removing enough redundant skin or may be

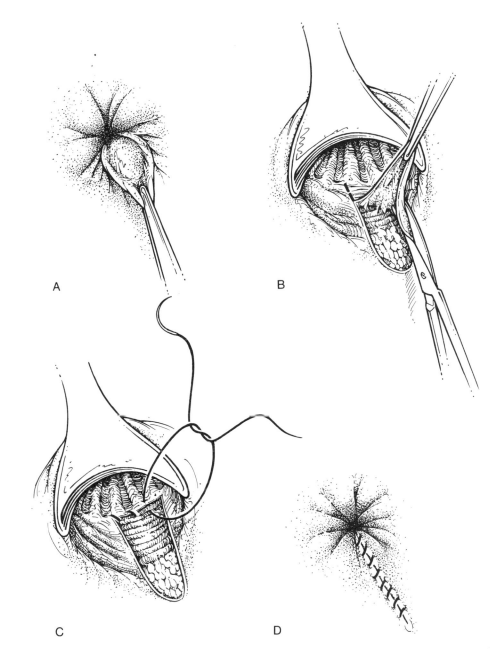

Figure 15–14. *A*, Mucosal ectropion. *B*, Excise to dentate line. *C*, Suture mucosa down at level of dentate line. *D*, Suture mucocutaneous defect if the base is not too broad, or leave open and allow to heal in.

a consequence of healing of the incision. Some patients complain of irritation and difficulty in cleansing. I first suggest that they avoid dry toilet paper and instead wash gently with cotton balls moistened with tap water. If this is not effective, the tags can be removed in the office after the patient has been given local anesthesia.

FISSURE-IN-ANO

In my practice the most common pathologic condition of the anorectum requiring surgery is anal fissure. It is also the most commonly overlooked anal abnormality. Frequently a patient with a classic history of pain and bleeding on defecation tearfully describes an examination done with finger and instrument. Pain was inflicted, but the correct diagnosis was not made. In fact the method of examination described is unnecessary and contraindicated. The diagnosis can be readily made without causing undue discomfort by gently spreading the buttocks and examining the distal anal canal. Surgery is indicated for the patient with a chronic fissure or the patient with an acute fissure for whom conservative measures (bulk agents, baths, steroid suppositories) over a 2- to 3-week period have failed.

Operative Treatment

Internal anal sphincterotomy is a simple and effective approach for the surgical management of anal fissure. Reported cure rates generally exceed 90%. It is not necessary to excise the fissure, and I deplore the concept of anal dilatation. The latter technique, when effective, probably owes any success to excessive trauma to both the internal and external sphincter, risking subsequent problems with bowel control.

Partial sphincterotomy can be accomplished in the lithotomy, lateral decubitus, or prone jackknife position. It can be performed with short general anesthesia or with regional or local anesthesia. Local anesthesia is suggested for doing this operation in the office. I have found this to be relatively nontraumatic with cooperative women (who are more comfortable in stirrups) but less applicable in men.

Surgical options for performing partial sphincterotomy include the following:

1. *Open versus closed technique.* The advantage of an open sphincterotomy is direct visualization of the internal and subcutaneous external sphincters as well as the intersphincteric groove. One is therefore more likely to divide the proper muscle (the internal sphincter). The disadvantages of the open technique are the longer time needed to perform it and its association with a suture line that causes discomfort. The closed technique is rapidly performed and avoids an incision and suture repair. However it is more difficult to learn because of the need to manually, rather than visually, appreciate the intersphincteric groove and internal sphincter.

2. *Single versus multiple sphincterotomies.* To avoid persistence of the fissure I have found that it is necessary to perform full-thickness sphincterotomy extending at least as proximal as does the fissure. Multiple shorter incisions or incisions of less than full thickness do not address the problem as well.

3. *Lateral sphincterotomy versus sphincterotomy at the fissure site.* Dividing the internal sphincter at the base of the fissure is certainly a simple procedure, one that self-evidently demarcates the extent of incision needed. Midline incision, however, especially in anterior midline sphincterotomy in women, is associated with an increased risk of incontinence as well as the occurrence of keyhole deformities and associated leakage.

4. *Right lateral versus left lateral sphincterotomy.* A left lateral sphincterotomy is usually easier for right-handed surgeons to perform when the patient is in the lithotomy position. Theoretically, however, this is directly under the usual major hemorrhoidal group. On the right side, the hemorrhoidal artery and vein split into anterior and posterior groups, and the right lateral position should therefore be relatively avascular.

In summary, my preference is a right, lateral, partial, internal submucosal sphincterotomy performed in the lithotomy position.

If the procedure is performed in the office with a local anesthetic, 10 ml of 0.5% bupivacaine with epinephrine 1:200,000 is injected around the circumference of the anus. Then 2 ml of the same solution is injected into the base of the fissure and into the right lateral intersphincteric groove. The operation then proceeds as if the patient had undergone a general anesthetic.

A Hill-Ferguson retractor is introduced into the anal canal and the fissure examined. Additional abnormalities are identified if evident. The right lateral area is exposed, and the intersphincteric groove carefully palpated (Fig. 15–15). This is the most important part of the operation. The groove must be properly located in order to ensure appropriate muscle division. The location may be variable, and care should be taken not to mistake the lateral border of the external sphincter for the intersphincteric groove. The relative position of the fissure itself is helpful, because it overlies the internal sphincter. By noting its location, one can extrapolate to the position of the internal sphincter at the right lateral site. If it is impossible to ascertain the location of the intersphincteric groove with confidence, one ought to employ the open technique in order to visualize both muscles clearly. The surgeon who has little experience with the technique should consider the open approach, at least initially.

After locating the intersphincteric groove, one inserts a cataract knife (52N Beaver blade) or a no. 15 blade flat into the groove, turning it toward the internal muscle and toward the lumen (Fig. 15–16). A finger is placed in the lumen to give a sense of the position of the mucosa, and the distal full thickness of the internal sphincter is cut for a distance at least as long as the length of the fissure (Fig. 15–16). The knife is withdrawn and the efficacy of the operation checked; simultaneously any undivided fibers are broken by applying pressure to the right lateral aspect with the index finger (Fig. 15–17). Finally, the integrity of the mucosa is checked. If there is a rent in the mucosa, it can be closed with a continuous 4-0 chromic catgut suture. A balled-up 4 × 4-inch gauze pad is placed against the puncture wound and kept in place manually as the patient's legs are lowered. One can then remove manual pressure, since the buttocks provide compression once the legs are abducted. Recovery room nurses are instructed to remove the gauze in 20 to 30 minutes.

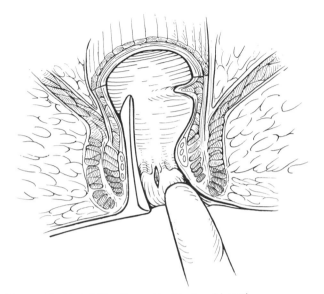

Figure 15–15. Midline fissure identified and lateral intersphincteric groove palpated.

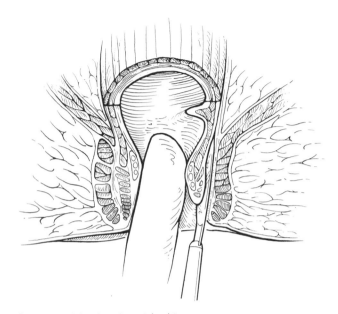

Figure 15–16. Closed partial sphincterotomy.

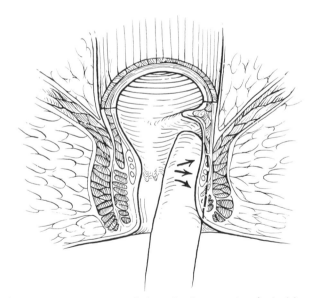

Figure 15–17. Pressure with the index finger against the incision will divide uncut internal sphincter fibers.

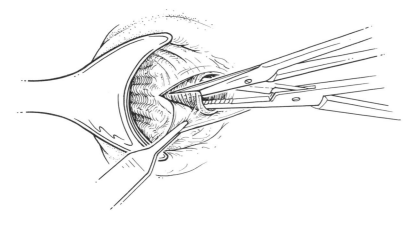

Figure 15–18. Open partial sphincterotomy.

Acetaminophen and sitz baths may be taken for pain and the patient seen in 3 weeks. I do not recommend stool softeners or cathartics.

The open technique involves an incision in the right lateral position just long enough to expose the intersphincteric groove and the length of the muscle that one intends to cut (Fig. 15–18). A clamp is spread in the groove to separate the two muscles and then the internal sphincter cut with a straight scissors (Fig. 15–18). I obtain hemostasis with cautery and close the incision with a continuous 4-0 chromic catgut suture. Instructions and follow-up are the same as those for closed sphincterotomy.

Perioperative Complications

Bleeding

Minor bleeding from the puncture wound is frequently noted. This almost always stops with direct pressure. Among my more than 1,000 closed sphincterotomy patients, only one required admission and overnight observation for bleeding. He was placed on bed rest with a gauze compression dressing and was discharged the following day.

Infection

An abscess at the sphincterotomy site complicates 1% of procedures. It is probably the result of an opening made in the mucosa and not appreciated at the time of surgery. Treatment by incision and drainage can easily be done in the office under local anesthesia. Some of these patients develop an anal fistula. It is always an extrasphincteric type and can readily be managed by office fistulotomy.

Pain

Within a few hours of the surgery, the patient should feel good. Commonly a bowel movement on the fol-

lowing day is pain-free. The fissure is usually healed within 3 weeks.

Long-Term Complications

Incontinence

Incontinence is a complication reported in 5% to 8% of most studies. It usually occurs in women over 50 years of age and is primarily incontinence of flatus or a liquid stool. It is difficult to evaluate the true incidence of this complication, because a number of women over 50 years of age have impairment without anal surgery. If incontinence is caused by transection of the external sphincter, repair is indicated. If no muscle disruption is evident, perineal muscle strengthening exercises may be initiated and a bulk agent added. If only the internal sphincter has been cut and the edges are still distracted, I have repaired the muscle with some improvement noted.

Persistence

I prefer this term to recurrence. The usual reasons for persistence are failure to cut a sufficiently long segment of the internal sphincter, failure to cut the full thickness of the internal sphincter, or transection of a portion of the external sphincter with the mistaken belief that the internal sphincter was being cut. Persistence may result from underlying inflammatory bowel disease, other granulomatous disease, venereal disease, or neoplasm. If any suspicious lesion is present at the time of the surgery, one should biopsy the edges of the fissure. If inflammatory bowel disease is suspected, endoscopy and a contrast study should be performed. I have had three patients whose persistent fissures predated the appearance of intestinal Crohn's disease by 1 to 5 years.

Anal fissure can cause severe disability, but if proper attention is given to the principles outlined, the patient

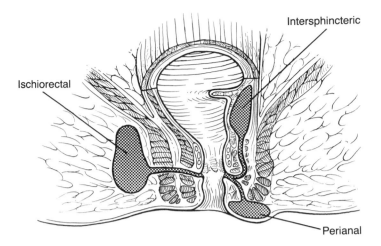

Figure 15–19. Location of perianal, ischiorectal, and intersphincteric or submucosal abscesses.

should obtain almost immediate relief from a simple and easily tolerated procedure.

ABSCESS AND FISTULA

Anorectal abscess and fistula are inter-related conditions and therefore are discussed together. An anorectal fistula is usually the consequence of an abscess originating from an infection in the anal glands; this is the cryptoglandular theory. Possible exceptions are fistulas in patients with inflammatory bowel disease, cancer, and other inflammatory processes such as diverticulitis and trauma. Not all septic processes of the perianal area are associated with diseases of the intestine. Hidradenitis suppurativa, infected sebaceous cysts, pilonidal sinus disease, a Bartholin duct abscess, and even urinary tract infection may be present in this region. For the purpose of this chapter, the discussion is confined to abscess and fistula derived from anal gland infection.

Abscess

Regardless of whether abscesses are perianal, ischiorectal, or intra-anal (submucosal or intersphincteric) in location (Fig. 15–19), all must be drained. This statement may seem self-evident, but it is not uncommon for me to see a patient treated by a physician or surgeon with antibiotics in the hope that a "suspected" abscess will become "evident," or an appreciated abscess "more mature." The skin of the buttocks is thick, and an ischiorectal fossa abscess may never truly "point." Swelling, induration, and tenderness to palpation are highly suggestive of an underlying abscess. Once the diagnosis is suspected, it is imperative to establish drainage or to prove that no abscess is pres-

ent. This can be accomplished with the aid of a local anesthetic instilled in the area in question and by aspiration with a 16- or 18-gauge needle. It is often necessary to insert the needle deeply in order to locate the abscess. This is especially true if it is located in the postanal space or ischiorectal fossa.

Once the diagnosis has been established, either by means of inspection or by needle aspiration, the abscess must be drained. Most patients prefer not to be inconvenienced by immediate hospitalization; therefore I usually prefer to drain the abscess, after administering a local anesthetic, in the office. This approach generally eliminates the possibility of one-stage drainage and fistulotomy, a technique performed in the operating room. Approximately 70% of patients require subsequent fistulotomy after abscess drainage. Therefore, in anticipation of a possible fistulotomy, the drainage incision should be made as close to the anal opening as is possible (Fig. 15–20). This consideration ensures the shortest possible tract, should fistulotomy ultimately be required.

Technique

The area is infiltrated with bupivacaine 0.5%, a long-acting anesthetic, with epinephrine 1:100,000, and a no. 11 knife blade is used to puncture the skin down to the abscess cavity. As stated, if I am uncertain about the location, I aspirate first. Once the cavity is reached, a cruciate incision is made in the skin, and then forceps and scissors are used to trim the edges of the wound to leave a circular or oval defect (Fig. 15–21). Finally, the cavity is explored with forceps, a clamp, or an index finger, and an attempt is made to break up any loculations that may be present. Packing is contraindicated because the primary purpose is to promote adequate drainage. A drain is also unnecessary, since the patient should have an ample opening over the cavity. A dressing to protect the patient's underclothes

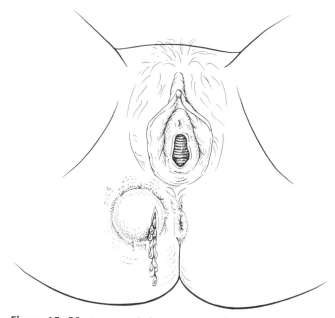

Figure 15–20. A perirectal abscess is drained as close to the anal canal as is practical.

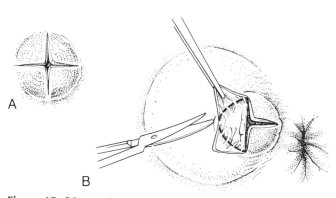

Figure 15–21. *A* and *B*, To ensure adequate drainage of the abscess, a skin defect is created that will take some time to heal.

is sufficient. The patient is instructed to take sitz baths three times daily, starting that evening or the following morning. Antibiotics are unnecessary except in severely diabetic or immunocompromised patients. These patients, in any case, should be treated in the hospital. Patients are asked to return to the office in about 2 weeks so that they can be checked for healing and examined for the presence of a fistula.

An intra-anal abscess, either submucosal or intra-sphincteric, may be particularly difficult to diagnose because inspection will be entirely normal. However digital examination usually reveals swelling and tenderness or may be impossible to accomplish because of pain. If one suspects an intra-anal abscess and adequate evaluation cannot be accomplished in the office, it is imperative to administer an anesthetic to facilitate further evaluation. Severe anal pain in the absence of a fissure is considered to be caused by an abscess until this is disproved.

With the patient under anesthesia, a submucosal abscess is usually obvious, but an intersphincteric abscess may be more subtle. Probing for the latter abscess with a large-bore needle in a firm, slightly indurated area should demonstrate the abscess (Fig. 15–22). Once located, the abscess should be entirely unroofed. Bleeding can be controlled by electrocautery, but I often run a continuous catgut suture around the edges of the wound for security (Fig. 15–23). Postoperatively the patient is instructed to take sitz baths three times a day and to return to the office on a weekly schedule so that the wound can be checked and the cavity examined to ensure healing from the base.

Complications

Complications of abscess incision and drainage are few. They include bleeding, persistent sepsis, fistula, and Fournier's gangrene.

Bleeding. This is rarely of significance and usually comes from the skin. It can be controlled with electrocoagulation or by suture.

Persistent Sepsis. If the abscess is inadequately drained, the patient continues to have pain, possible fever, and discharge. A second drainage procedure may be required, possibly performed in the operating room with a general or regional anesthetic.

Fistula. This is more a consequence than a complication. If a fistula does develop following the treatment of an abscess, it should be operatively corrected in order to avoid the recurrence of an abscess.

Fournier's Gangrene. This life-threatening complication may be a consequence of delay or inadequate drainage. The condition is most likely to be seen in diabetic individuals or in otherwise debilitated patients. Wide débridement, broad-spectrum antibiotic coverage, and meticulous wound care are necessary; fecal diversion may also be required. Mortality rates are reported to be as high as 33%.

Fistula-in-Ano

The operative treatment of fistula-in-ano is a potential "minefield" challenging surgeons to employ their skills at the height of their abilities. One who only occasionally enters this area should consider not venturing at all because of two important concerns. First, the best opportunity to treat the patient and to cure the fistula is at the initial surgery. At this time the possibility of creating a false passage or an artificial internal opening is minimized. The surgeon must determine the amount of muscle traversed by the tract, the level of the internal opening relative to the sphincter, and the necessity for esoteric measures (e.g., seton insertion). Second, inappropriate sphincter division or the creation of false tracts that subsequently require extensive muscle division may result in incontinence of flatus or feces. This is not to imply that a properly done fistulotomy avoids incontinence. Every fistulotomy carries the risk of some degree of impairment (although the risk can be minimized by the experienced surgeon), and all patients undergoing this operation should be so counseled.

Despite the above cautions, neglect is not an alternative. Without surgical correction, a patient with fistula may suffer recurrent abscesses and may develop new tracts and additional secondary openings. Subsequent attempts at surgical cure may be more difficult, and continence problematic. Once the diagnosis of a fistula is established, nothing is gained by inordinate delays in treatment. However a fistula is not considered an emergency, and even a few months may be permitted to pass if the patient considers this interim to be necessary.

Technique

This discussion addresses the treatment of only inter-sphincteric, trans-sphincteric, and horseshoe fistulas (Fig. 15–24). These represent more than 90% of the presentations of anal fistula. The operation can be performed under any anesthetic. I find the lithotomy position to be the best one for an anterior fistula and the prone (jackknife) position optimal for posterior and horseshoe fistulas. The initial step is to define the tract. The secondary opening should be visible externally; digital examination or anoscopy may reveal the primary (internal) opening (Fig. 15–25).

One should keep Goodsall's rule in mind: A secondary opening anterior to the midtransverse plane is associated with a radially located primary opening. However a secondary opening in the posterior location

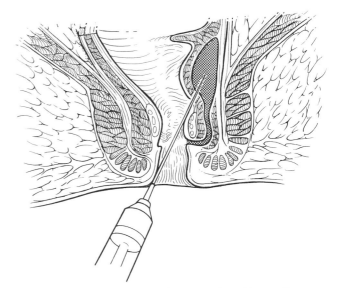

Figure 15–22. Intersphincteric abscess confirmed by needle aspiration.

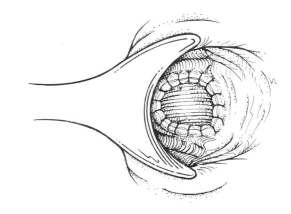

Figure 15–23. Unroofing an intersphincteric abscess and suturing the wound edges for hemostasis.

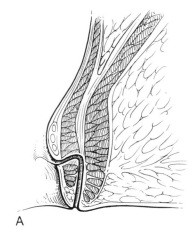

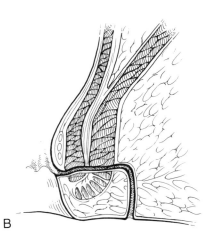

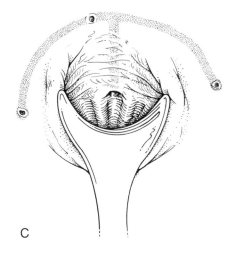

Figure 15–24. *A,* Intersphincteric fistula. Surgery will divide internal sphincter only. *B,* Trans-sphincteric fistula. Both internal and external sphincters are divided by properly performed fistulotomy. *C,* Horseshoe fistula primary opening is seen in the midline. Secondary openings are present in midline position as well as right and left lateral positions.

usually tracks around to the posterior midline (Fig. 15–26). A common exception to this is a horseshoe fistula, which classically has a posterior anal midline internal opening and secondary openings in the anterior perianal areas. If a primary opening cannot be palpated or visualized, I gently probe through the secondary opening and usually find the primary opening by this technique. If the probe fails to come through the primary opening but is palpated or visualized directly beneath the mucosa at the level of the crypts, I am confident in completing the fistulotomy by easing it through the mucosa. If it fails to approach the mucosa, several maneuvers are available to define the fistula.

Many surgeons rely on injecting dye, milk, or hydrogen peroxide and then look for colored fluid or air bubbles at the primary opening (Fig. 15–27). I occasionally use hydrogen peroxide but avoid inserting dye, because the tissues stain and the anatomy can be obscured. If the primary opening is identified by the injection technique, a second probe is placed through it to connect with or to pass by the first probe (Fig. 15–28).

Another approach is to open the fistula over the probe to the point of apparent blockage. Frequently the direction of the proximal tract is then evident, and it can be probed (Fig. 15–29). Alternatively one can pull on the distal tract and draw the remainder of the fistula taut. This may cause the primary opening to retract, thereby allowing the surgeon to unroof the remainder (Fig. 15–30).

An important caution is that not all fistulas are straight single tracts. Some have a branch off the main tract, often extending cephalad and parallel to the rectum. The reason for this branching is evident on considering the etiology of fistulas. A large abscess cavity spontaneously or surgically drained may collapse yet leave a cephalad extension (Fig. 15–31). This extension, if unrecognized, presents a significant danger, and subsequent improper treatment may result in a false passage and a fistula encompassing all of the sphincter mechanism (Fig. 15–32).

Once the primary and secondary openings are defined, I place a probe through the entire tract and determine the extent of sphincter involved (Fig. 15–33). In general, the initial surgical attempt does *not* involve dividing the puborectalis muscle. Therefore, I am comfortable dividing the entire tract. An exception to this is an anterior fistula in a woman. In this situation I prefer seton division, because muscular support is so limited in this area. If the anesthetic cannot permit assessment of the extent of muscle involvement, a seton can be placed and the patient re-examined after the anesthetic has worn off. If I believe that the fistula transverses too much muscle for safe division, I divide the internal sphincter and place a seton loosely about

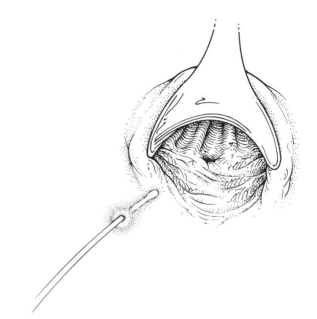

Figure 15–25. Probe passing through the secondary opening toward primary opening.

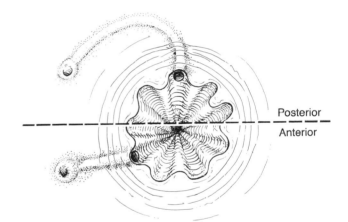

Figure 15–26. Secondary openings anterior to the midtransverse plane connect radially to primary openings. Secondary openings posterior to the midtransverse plane will connect to a primary opening in the posterior midline. Notable exceptions may be horseshoe fistulas.

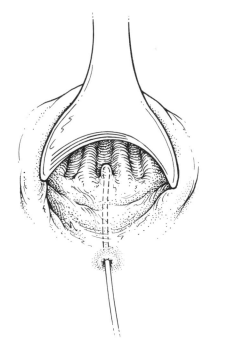

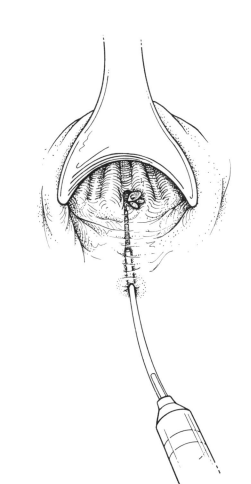

Figure 15–27. Injecting hydrogen peroxide through the secondary opening produced bubbles, which identify the primary opening site.

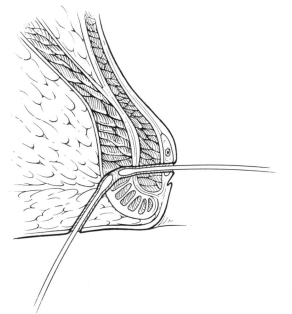

Figure 15–28. Entire fistula tract defined by separate probes placed through primary and secondary openings.

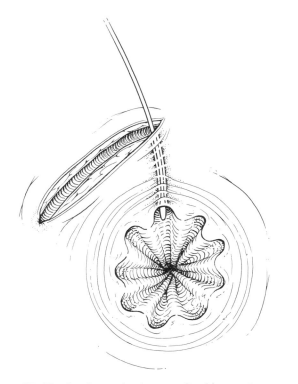

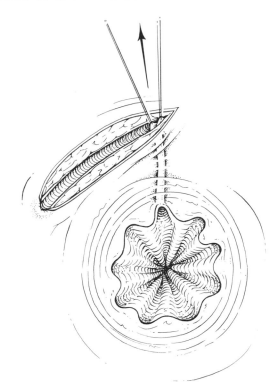

Figure 15–29. Sharply angulated tract outlined by opening up to the acute turn and then probing remaining tract.

Figure 15–30. The primary opening is identified by retracting the fistula tract and observing the point of mucosal pucker.

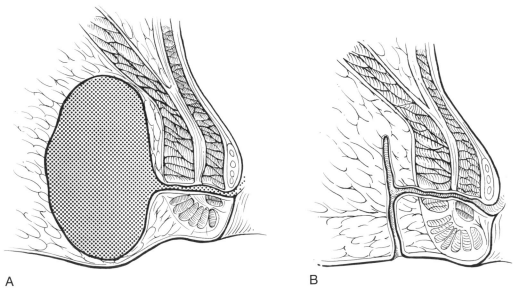

A

B

Figure 15–31. *A*, Large ischiorectal fossa absceses. *B*, Resultant fistula tract following drainage of the abscess.

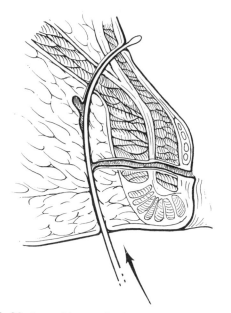

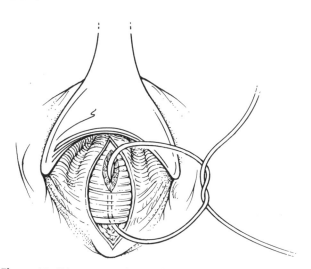

Figure 15–34. Mucosa, skin, and internal sphincter have been divided, and a seton placed about the external sphincter encompassed by the fistula tract.

Figure 15–32. Extrasphincteric fistula caused by improperly probing tract.

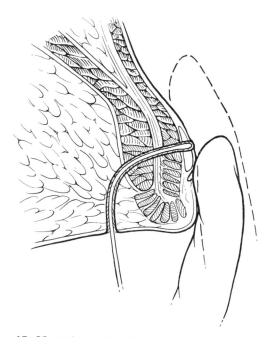

Figure 15–33. With a probe defining the fistula tract, a digital examination can determine the extent of sphincter involvement.

the external sphincter (Fig. 15–34), progressively tightening this after the remainder of the wound has healed.

After the entire tract of an uncomplicated fistula is defined, a cautery is used to open it over a probe, and then the external wound is fashioned with gentle sloping side walls (Fig. 15–35). The base is not excised but is allowed to remain as the tough fibrous residual portion of the fistula (Fig. 15–36). I prefer fistulotomy to fistulectomy (excising the fibrous tract), since a much smaller wound results and healing time is considerably shortened. I use electrocautery for hemostasis and place a povidone-iodine–moistened sponge into the fistulotomy wound.

The patient is seen in the office the following morning, and the loose pack is removed—if it has not already fallen out. The wound is examined by running an index finger along the length of the base, and the patient is shown how to do this for self-examination. The patient is asked to take two or three warm baths each day and to digitalize (i.e., palpate) the wound once at each bath. The patient is seen at weekly intervals until healing is complete. The concept is that the wound heals from the base and the skin edges are not allowed to appose. If the latter occurs, the fistula has, in essence, recurred (Fig. 15–37). Because proper healing should be the surgeon's main objective, careful postoperative care is as necessary as the operation itself. All of the preceding approaches are appropriate to uncomplicated fistulas.

The operation for a horseshoe fistula differs in that the entire tract is not opened. With the patient in the prone jackknife position, a probe is placed into the primary opening and the proximal tract as far as the postanal space is opened, and the side walls are trimmed (Fig. 15–38). An attempt is then made to pass a clamp from the secondary opening to the postanal space and to pull a gauze sponge through the tract (Fig. 15–39), running the sponge back and forth to curette the tract. Next, the sponge is removed and a ¼- or ½-inch Penrose drain placed through the horseshoe limb and secured to itself (Fig. 15–40). The postanal space and proximal fistulotomy are packed loosely with a povidone-iodine–moistened sponge. Postoperative care is the same as that described for uncomplicated fistula. Each drain is left in for 2 to 3 weeks. After removal, the tracts are probed with a cotton-tipped applicator at the patient's weekly visits. The horseshoe limb generally closes 1 to 3 weeks after the drains are removed, and the midline opening is healed shortly after that.

Complications

Incontinence. All patients should be warned prior to surgery that there is a possibility of impaired control of flatus or of loose stool if a part of the sphincter

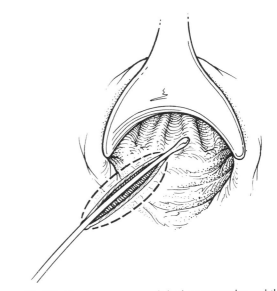

Figure 15–35. Fistulotomy accomplished over a probe and the wound edges beveled.

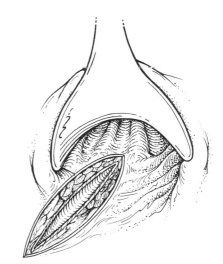

Figure 15–36. Fistulotomy wound demonstrating the posterior wall of the fistula tract at the base of the wound.

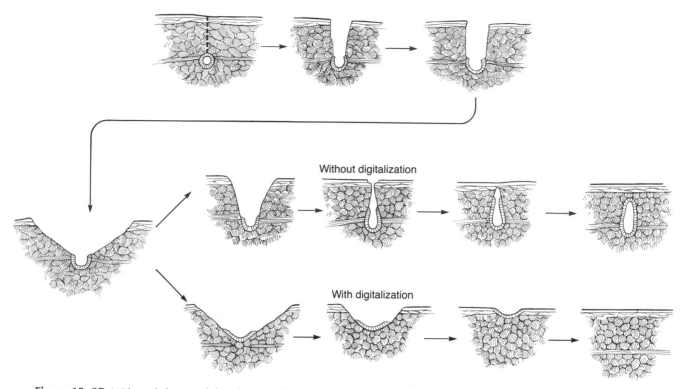

Figure 15–37. Without daily wound digitalization, there is the danger of apposition of the skin edges and recurrence of the fistula.

Without digitalization

With digitalization

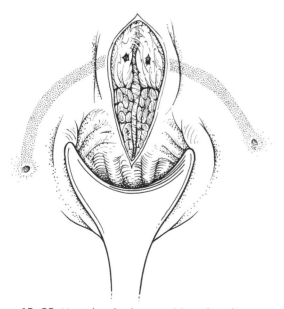

Figure 15–38. Horseshoe fistula opened from the primary opening to the postanal space.

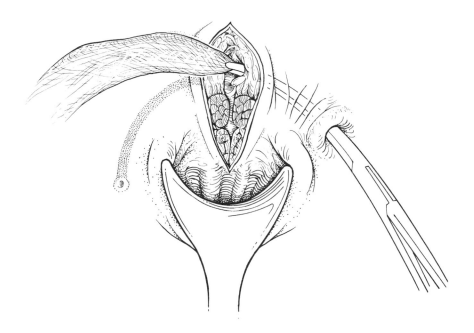

Figure 15–39. Limbs of horseshoe fistula curetted with gauze.

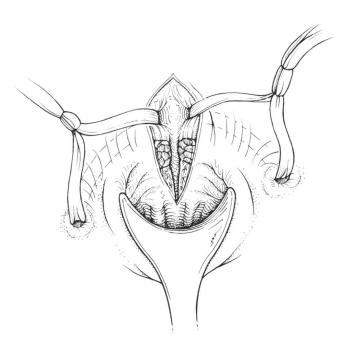

Figure 15–40. Penrose drains placed about the limbs of the horseshoe fistula.

mechanism is divided. This possibility should particularly be emphasized in women. However, incontinence of formed stool should not occur unless the entire sphincter mechanism has been divided. *The best treatment is prevention.* Most extrasphincteric fistulas are iatrogenic; that is, they result from the inappropriate passage of the probe into the rectum above the levators. The surgeon performing the initial operation for a fistula *must not* create a false passage. Once the patient has become incontinent following disruption of the sphincter, it is necessary to reconstruct the muscles for correction.

Recurrence or Persistence. This complication is best treated by prevention. The importance of the postoperative care in the management of fistulas cannot be sufficiently emphasized. In the case of recurrence, reoperation is obviously necessary.

PILONIDAL ABSCESS AND SINUS

Numerous surgical procedures are described for the treatment of pilonidal abscess and sinus. As with other conditions necessitating surgical treatment, this implies that none is entirely satisfactory. The technique that I favor virtually to the exclusion of all others is recommended for its simplicity, cost savings, and low rate of recurrence.

Abscess

An acute pilonidal abscess is drained in the office with a local anesthetic. The incision is made as close to the midline as possible in order to limit the length of the subsequent sinusotomy wound. A cruciate incision is made and then the edges trimmed to produce a round or oval defect (Fig. 15–41). Packing is avoided. The patient is instructed to take two to three warm baths each day. After all the inflammation has subsided, definitive surgery can be scheduled at the patient's convenience.

Pilonidal Sinus

Sinusotomy is my preferred operation for quiescent pilonidal disease. Depending on the extent of disease and the patient's fortitude, this can be accomplished in the office with a local anesthetic or in the outpatient surgery department by using a regional or general anesthetic.

The patient is placed in the prone (jackknife) position, and the buttocks are taped apart. The sacral area is shaved carefully. All visible sinus openings are probed thoroughly in an attempt to outline the full extent of the disease. With a probe in place, each sinus is opened and all cavities unroofed (Fig. 15–42). The edges of the wound are beveled to create a gentle slope, thus avoiding any overhanging edges. One should see a continuous fibrous base. Any interruptions, crevices, or folds should be investigated to uncover an unopened pocket. Granulation tissue is removed from the base by means of either a curette or a gauze sponge. The electrocautery is used for hemostasis, and the wound is loosely packed with a povidone-iodine–moistened sponge. Dry sterile dressings cover the packing, and the patient is asked to return to the office the following day with someone who can assist in wound care. This individual is shown how to dress the wound twice daily according to the following protocol:

1. During or following a 10- to 15-minute warm bath, the gauze dressing is removed.

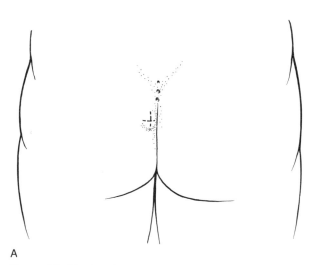

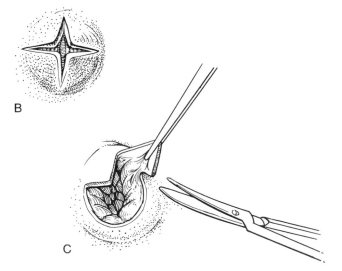

Figure 15–41. *A* to *C*, Unroofing a pilonidal abscess.

2. The open wound is irrigated with a Water Pik utilizing one container of water at a force that does not produce pain.

3. The wound is repacked with a povidone-iodine–moistened sponge.

4. A dry, sterile dressing is applied.

5. The patient is cautioned to avoid riding a horse, bicycle, motorcycle, or truck and is instructed not to perform any floor exercises on the back.

The patient is seen at weekly intervals. Granulation tissue is removed by rubbing with gauze or applying silver nitrate. The skin around the wound edges is shaved as necessary. Even if the wound seems to be healed, pressure is applied to the scar to ensure that the entire depth of the wound is firmly healed. When one is confident that the wound is healed, the patient is asked to return in 1 month in order to test the operative site once again.

Complications

Delayed healing. Occasionally I have a patient whose wound appears clean and healthy but is not healing. Although culture does not disclose any unusual organism, by placing the patient on oral erythromycin, 333 mg three times daily for 1 to 4 weeks, healing often results.

Recurrence. Most instances of recurrence are, in fact, persistence of the original pilonidal problem. Treatment consists of thorough unroofing and reinstitution of wound care as already described. Occasionally, however, a fistula-in-ano is mistaken for pilonidal sinus disease. Every patient should undergo careful examination to be certain that there is no connection with the anal canal.

CONDYLOMA ACUMINATUM

Condyloma acuminatum is one of the frustrating problems commonly seen in surgical practice. A cure with one treatment is seldom possible, and often a half dozen or more sessions are required. This fact must be made clear to the patient at the outset in order to enlist cooperation and understanding. At the first office visit, I suggest always asking male patients whether they are homosexual. The mode of transmission of this disease is explained and it is recommended that their partners be evaluated and treated if necessary. The requirement of human immunodeficiency virus and serologic testing is also discussed.

Treatment

If the patient has only a few external warts, a 25% solution of podophyllin is applied with the wooden end of a cotton-tipped applicator; the cotton-tipped end wipes the surrounding normal tissue (Fig. 15–43). The patient is instructed to wash the treated area thoroughly 90 minutes later. The patient is asked to return in 7 to 10 days, at which time new or persistent warts are similarly treated. If there are none following two successive visits, the patient is asked to return in 6 weeks; if free of warts at that time, the patient is dismissed from care.

If there are many external warts or a combination of external and internal anal warts, (one need not be concerned about warts extending into the rectal area), I prefer that the treatment be undertaken in the outpatient surgery department with a general anesthetic. The patient is placed in the lithotomy position and the needlepoint coagulator employed. One or two warts should be excised for pathologic examination, and the remainder coagulated. I try to limit the coagulant to the epidermis, because the virus does not extend into the dermis. After all condylomata have been fulgurated, the necrotic tissue can be gently picked off with a hemostat and the base lightly coagulated.

Postoperative care consists of a nonnarcotic analgesic and warm baths twice daily. The patient is seen in the office at 10 days. At this time recurrent external warts are treated with podophyllin, and anal canal warts are fulgurated after the patient has been given a local anesthetic, if necessary. Subsequent visits are timed as outlined above. If at any time the number of warts increases greatly, it is advisable to return the individual to outpatient surgery for fulguration of all visible disease.

ANAL STENOSIS

Anal stenosis is a recognized complication of hemorrhoidectomy and other operations of the anal canal. Anal stenosis may also occur in the elderly patient who has had decades of loose stools as a result of taking laxatives or mineral oil. Many patients adapt to and easily tolerate a significant degree of stenosis. I believe

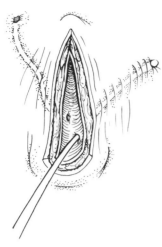

Figure 15–42. Pilonidal sinusotomy is preferable to sinusectomy. All tracts must be identified and opened.

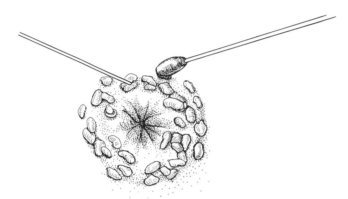

Figure 15–43. Podophyllin application to external warts.

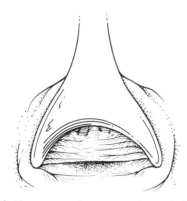

Figure 15–44. The retractor demonstrates bowstringing of the stricture.

that surgical correction is indicated when the patient seeks remedy for pain or the inability to defecate easily.

Technique

For patients with severe stenosis or those who have persistent or recurrent stenoses following operative correction, I use an advancement or rotation flap technique. For most patients, however, I employ a much simpler operative procedure performed in the outpatient surgery department. The patient is prepared with a single sodium biphosphate enema and placed in the dorsal lithotomy position. A digital examination assesses the degree of stenosis in the relaxed, anesthetized patient. Care is taken to exclude a fissure. If there is a fissure and no stenosis is evident, an internal anal sphincterotomy is indicated. If there is a stenosis with or without fissure, stricturoplasty and partial internal sphincterotomy are performed.

With a Hill-Ferguson retractor in the anal canal, the narrow stricture band is readily identified (Fig. 15–44). A vertical incision is made in the right lateral position 7 to 10 mm in length on either side of the stenotic area (Fig. 15–45). The full thickness of the internal sphincter is divided for the length of the incision, and the surrounding subcutaneous and submucosal tissues are undermined for 3 to 5 mm (Fig. 15–46). The vertical incision is closed in a transverse fashion with interrupted 3-0 atraumatic catgut sutures (Fig. 15–47). This theoretically increases the circumference of the anal canal by 14 to 20 mm. When the degree of stenosis warrants, this procedure is repeated in the patient's left lateral position, with the sphincterotomy omitted. Postoperative care includes gentle washing after bowel movements with cotton balls moistened with tap water (rather than wiping with dry paper), a mild analgesic, and a visit to the office at 3 weeks.

Complications

Persistence or Recurrence. In approximately 10% of patients, this procedure for anal stenosis fails. If this happens, rotation or advancement flap is indicated.

Ectropion. I have had two patients with minor ectropions and a resultant mucous discharge. Both controlled the symptoms by placing a tuft of dry cotton against the anal opening. If operation is necessary, perform it as illustrated in Figure 15–14.

I have had no patients who experienced bleeding or abscess formation following this procedure, although both complications are possible.

SOLITARY RECTAL ULCER

Solitary rectal ulcer is usually associated with the symptoms of bleeding, tenesmus, discharge of mucus, and a feeling of incomplete evacuation. On physical examination, a solitary ulcer or occasionally multiple ulcers are found, or a mass may be demonstrated that on biopsy usually demonstrates the changes associated with colitis cystica profunda. The underlying common finding seems to be trauma to the mucosa leading to submucosal fibrosis and ulceration or cyst formation. Thus, solitary ulcer and colitis cystica profunda may be related manifestations of a common pathologic process. Trauma may consist of digital insertion or repeated use of enemas or may be associated with straining repeatedly and for prolonged periods of time during defecation. In addition, prolapse—either complete prolapse or an internal intussusception—is also associated with this pathologic change.

Therapy depends on the presence or absence of an intussusception. If intussusception is present, treatment of this underlying cause is usually curative. My operative preference is a low anterior resection (described elsewhere in this text). For individuals in whom no intussusception can be demonstrated, conservative measures that consist of increased fluids, dietary fiber, and counseling not to strain is successful in approximately 70% of patients. Those patients who fail to respond present a difficult treatment problem. Often these patients have paradoxical contraction of the sphincter mechanism during defecation, and occasionally a course of biofeedback treatment helps. In individuals with a significant and symptomatic mass of colitis cystica profunda, transanal rectal resection may be indicated.

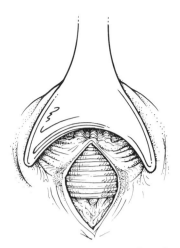

Figure 15—45. Longitudinal incision in the lateral position, 7 to 10 mm proximal and distal to the stricture.

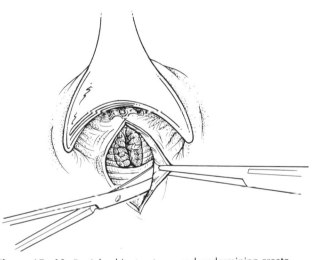

Figure 15—46. Partial sphincterotomy and undermining create enough relaxation for closure without tension.

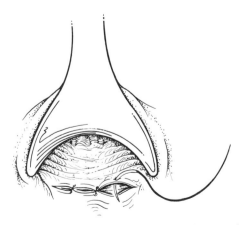

Figure 15—47. Horizontal closure of the wound.

EDITORIAL COMMENT

Fistulotomy or fistulectomy for fistulas that traverse the entire sphincteric complex may result in impaired continence. As Dr. Prager points out, the course of the tract and its exact relationship to the sphincter must be accurately determined prior to the operative procedure. In those cases in which the tract traverses the entire sphincter, or the majority of it, after division of the mucosa, skin, and internal sphincter, a seton is utilized for the external sphincter. For complex or neglected fistulas (e.g., those often in association with Crohn's disease), treatment may require temporary diversion of the fecal stream, multiple fistulotomies, and perineal and sphincter repair as staged procedures.

An attractive alternative to the described method of pilonidal sinusotomy is to "marsupialize" the wound by suturing the edges of the defect either to the fibrous tissue at the base of the sinus or to the presacral fascia. This technique results in a smaller defect and reduced healing time.

Anal Incontinence

C H A P T E R   1 6

Robert W. Beart, Jr.
George E. Block

Anal incontinence of feces can have multiple presentations and implications. Problems noted by the patient may be limited to liquid stool or gas. Incontinence may not include gross loss of stool, and patients may be bothered only by a slight mucous discharge.[1] Unfortunately most physicians are not comfortable with or knowledgeable about the management of continence disorders. Proper treatment for these problems requires an understanding of the normal anatomy and physiology of the anorectal area and colon as well as the techniques of assessment that are currently available. In an effort to discern the problem, and therefore the solution, a careful history, physical examination, and selective testing are necessary.

ANORECTAL ANATOMY

The "tail muscles" are adapted in the human to form the pelvic support structures and the anal sphincter mechanisms.[2] Phylogenetically, the anococcygeal raphe of the human is the tail of lower animals. In humans, these muscles form the levator support floor (ileococcygeal and pubococcygeal muscles).

Anatomic studies of the external sphincter date from 1715; yet it has defied consistent and consensual description.[3] Anatomically, the anal canal is the part of the proctodeum lying between the anal valves and the anal verge. The surgical anal canal is 2 to 6 cm long and extends from the puborectal muscle to the anal verge. Because of the significance of the puborectal muscle for the mechanisms of continence, it is unclear why this area has traditionally been excluded from the anatomic definition of the anal canal. In normal anatomy, the anal orifice is positioned in the middle of a line drawn between the ischial tuberosities. The anus is easy to dilate, and even a neonate's anus easily admits a 2-cm proctoscope for examination.

The anal canal consists of voluntary and involuntary muscles. The smooth (involuntary) muscle of the internal sphincter begins at the dentate line and variably extends to the anal verge. The internal sphincter is a thickening of the inner circular muscle of the colon. The groove between the internal and external muscles is palpable, particularly when the anus is dilated and the muscle on tension, just inside the anal verge. Some fibers from the longitudinal layer of colon muscle may interdigitate with the internal sphincter. These longitudinal fibers also terminate in the ischiorectal and perirectal fat on the deep aspects of the perianal skin. The longitudinal fibers help tie together the various muscles and perimuscular tissue.

Components of the external anal muscle (voluntary) include the external sphincter and the components of the pelvic floor or levator ani muscle. The external anal muscle is similarly tethered to the skin by fibers from the longitudinal muscle of the colon. The internal sphincter is tethered anteriorly to the perineal body and posteriorly to the anococcygeal raphe. A few fibers of the external sphincter are found subcutaneously, but their function is not entirely clear.

The levator ani muscles arise from the walls of the true pelvis. They fill the outlet of the bony pelvis and support the intra-abdominal contents. The components of the levator ani muscles include the iliococcygeal, pubococcygeal, and puborectal muscles. The middle of these muscles, the pubococcygeal muscle, attaches to the anus and rectum to seal the pelvic floor around the outlet of the rectum. The puborectal muscle is deficient anteriorly but is intimately adjacent to the rectum laterally and posteriorly (Fig. 16–1). It angulates the

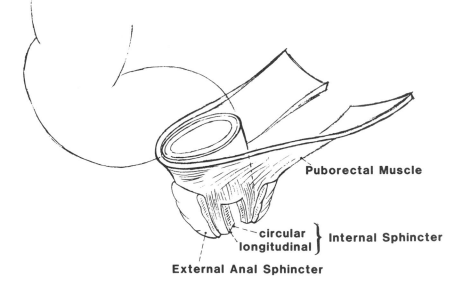

circular
longitudinal } **Internal Sphincter**

Puborectal Muscle

External Anal Sphincter

Figure 16–1. Angulation of the rectum as effected by the puborectal muscle. The puborectal sling around the rectum is illustrated, and its relationship to the internal and external sphincters is depicted.

rectum anteriorly against the anal canal and thus holds the lower rectum anteriorly and cephalad.

The second, third, and fourth sacral segments are the nerve centers that serve the rectum, anus, bladder, and urethra. Together with higher brain centers, these parasympathetic segments are responsible for urinary and fecal continence. These segments also serve cutaneous sensation in the anal canal and perianal skin. The sympathetic supply arises from the second, third, and fourth lumbar segments. The sympathetic and parasympathetic fibers join at the level of the ischial spine to form two nervi erigentes, which supply short branches directly to the rectum and anus.

The pudendal nerve, arising from the anterior divisions of the second, third, and fourth sacral nerves, runs through the Alcock canal. It supplies branches to the iliococcygeal and pubococcygeal muscles and to the puborectal muscle. The perineal branch of the fourth sacral nerve courses through the ischiorectal fossa to innervate the puborectal sling and external sphincter. Bilateral loss of all sacral nerves S2 to S4 leads to complete incontinence along with loss of the anorectal reflex mechanisms and sensitivity.

Duthie has mapped the nerve endings in the anal canal. He found conventional receptors that sense pain, touch, cold, and pressure as well as unconventional receptors from the anal verge to 1.0 to 1.5 cm above the dentate line.[4] No receptors were found in the rectal mucosa. The role of sensation in the rectum seems unclear, but it may be limited to sensing distention and initiating relaxation of the anal sphincters.[5, 6]

PHYSIOLOGY OF CONTINENCE

The internal anal sphincter is tonically contracted and initiates the act of defecation by reflexive relaxation in response to rectal distention. The frequency of rectal pressure waves is greater in the rectum than in the sigmoid colon, and therefore stool is likely to be propelled upward to an area of lesser pressure, leaving the rectum empty. After spinal anesthesia is administered or in paraplegia, the internal sphincter profile is not diminished, which demonstrates the importance of this muscle to maintaining continence.[7]

The puborectal muscle and anal sphincters function as a unit.[8] No motor activity is present in the pelvic floor muscles at rest. There is an increase in activity of these striated muscles of the pelvic floor during speaking, coughing, taking a deep breath, or touching the rectum. The most prominent feature in lateral radiographic films is the sharp 80-degree angle between the anal canal and the rectum. This angle is maintained by the puborectal muscle. The puborectal muscle is highly sensitive to alterations of pressure in the abdominal cavity and in the rectum.[9] This sensitivity may be lost after a pull-through procedure is performed, if the rectal cuff is short.

If the rectum is filled with intestinal contents, tension receptors in the rectal wall are stimulated and interpreted by cortical centers as fullness and the need to defecate. Simultaneously, there are reflexive relaxation of the external sphincters and contractions of the external anal sphincter and the puborectal muscle. These muscles are voluntarily relaxed when defecation is socially convenient.

The main function of the colon is water absorption; the main purpose of the rectum is to delay the passage of intestinal contents. This is achieved by means of the voluntary sphincters and the pressure gradient that runs against the direction of normal peristalsis.

The mechanism of defecation is fairly clear. Various reflexes, including the gastrocolic and ileocolic reflexes, as well as the voluntary abdominal wall contractions, initiate the "call" to defecation by promoting the filling of the rectum with colon contents. Intrarectal pressure stimulates the receptors in the rectum and puborectal muscle, and one experiences the need to defecate. Simultaneous relaxation of the internal sphincter allows a sample of rectal contents to enter the anal canal, where the hypersensitive mucosa discriminates among flatus, liquid, and solid. The reflexive contraction of the external sphincter and puborectal muscle prevents expulsion of stool. If expulsion is not permitted, pressure gradients of the rectum propel the contents to a more proximal segment. An intrarectal pressure between 25 and 30 mm Hg stimulates a reflexive inhibition of the sphincters. The external sphincter is brought into action to supplement the puborectal muscle in arresting defecation. If flatus under high pressure is expelled through a mildly occluded anus, a flutter-valve action results with an accompanying characteristic noise.

This discussion has covered the anatomy, physiology, and mechanisms of a noncontroversial system. However one must also note the conflict in the innervation, degree of activity, sensitivity, physiologic measurements, and ultimately the mechanisms of continence. The information presented here is logical and makes it possible to conceptualize abnormalities in a way that helps define therapeutic alternatives.[9, 10]

Ultimately, continence is maintained by the following: the ability to sense and distinguish impending evacuation as well as the ability to distinguish the nature of the rectal contents; the ability of the rectum to store feces through adaptive compliance and accommodation; the maintenance of outlet resistance by voluntary contraction of the puborectal muscle and external anal sphincter; and the motivation to respond appropriately. The timing of voluntary defecation is primarily related to environmental and social factors; however prolonged rectal distention ultimately overcomes voluntary sphincter tone and produces inhibition of voluntary and reflexive external sphincter tone.

MECHANISMS OF ANAL INCONTINENCE

Once trained during infancy in the social graces of continence, most of us think little about the mechanisms involved. At any time, however, various problems can disrupt continence. This disruption is a distressing social and personal handicap. It is estimated that 4 or 5 of every 1,000 individuals may suffer from varying degrees of incontinence. This frequency may double among the elderly. Incontinence is a problem that compromises rehabilitation of the injured elderly population and sometimes limits home care. Alternatively, it may result in the individual being housebound

Table 16–1. CLASSIFICATION AND CAUSES OF ANAL INCONTINENCE

Neurologic Cerebral
  Dementia
  Cerebrovascular disease
  Hydrocephalus
  Cerebral tumors
  Multiple sclerosis
Spinal Cord
  Trauma
  Spinal cord compression (tumors, myelopathy)
  Multiple sclerosis
  Spinal cord ischemia
Lower Motor Neuron Pathway Lesions; Conus Medullar Lesions
  Structural abnormalities
  Multiple sclerosis
  Ischemia
  Degenerative multisystem atrophy
Cauda Equina
  Lumbosacral spinal trauma
  Lumbar intervertebral disk prolapse
  Lumbar canal stenosis
  Ankylosing spondylitis
Peripheral Nerves
  Diabetic neuropathy
  Intrapelvic tumor
  Endometriosis
  Pudendal neuropathy (straining or childbirth)
Local Sphincter Pathology
  Congenital anorectal anomalies
  Obstetric anal sphincter tears
  Sphincter trauma
  Perianal suppuration
  Rectal or anal neoplasms
Multifactorial
  Acute or chronic confusional states
  Drug intoxication
  Fecal impaction
  Physical immobility
  Neural aging
Enteric
  Acute or chronic diarrheal illness

From Mathers S, Swash M. Faecal incontinence. Int Disabil Studies 1988; 10:164–168.

because of the social embarrassment of incontinence experienced in public. There are many causes of incontinence (Table 16–1). Most lists of incontinence mechanisms do not address the quality of the stool. It is reasonable to assume that if we are continent for liquid urine, we should also be continent for liquid stool; however it is also clear that solid stool is much easier to retain than liquid stool. Therefore liquid stool should be considered at least a partial contributor to incontinence problems, but other contributing components should be sought.

EVALUATION OF ANAL INCONTINENCE

Evaluation of a patient with anal incontinence begins with a thorough history. The physician should keep in mind the embarrassment that many patients feel when discussing bodily functions. Specific questions may be necessary to elicit the appropriate response. For instance, one must differentiate between urgency with an associated loss of stool and true incontinence. Patients with incontinence usually do not sense impending stool, whereas those with urgency sense the stool but cannot reach a facility quickly enough.

Incontinence can be classified as minor (mucous leakage without gross fecal loss), moderate (occasional gross fecal loss), or severe (gross fecal loss with little control, usually requiring a pad). The history must cover the usual bowel habits, including time, frequency, and severity of incontinence events as well as any associated symptoms, such as abdominal pain, prolapse, or perianal discomfort. Diseases such as diabetes, neuropathies, and medications taken by the patient should be recorded. The time at which incontinence occurs should be noted (at night or with stress, or in relationship with dietary intake, stool quality, or position, and so forth). In females a history of multiple childbirth or injury at childbirth should be noted. A history of anal trauma or surgery may be relevant.

Associated urinary incontinence may suggest a pelvic floor weakness or a spinal lesion. Anal pain may suggest anal pathology such as a fissure or a tumor. The date of onset may help establish whether this is a congenital problem or one related to a specific event in the patient's background. A history of mucosal or rectal prolapse suggests a mechanical problem that may be primary or secondary. A long history of constipation and straining should alert the physician to the problem of traction pudendal neuropathy.

Psychiatric screening has been recommended with fecal incontinence.[11] It is unclear to what degree psychiatric disturbances are a result of—or a cause of—continence disorders. Generally, incontinent patients do not differ from controls when evaluated for anxiety or depression. However patients who have poor results from surgery have significantly higher hospital anxiety and depression anxiety scores than those who obtained clinical benefit.

At the time of physical examination, the physician should note if the patient wears a pad or the clothing is stained. The anus is inspected for conformation and patulousness, scarring, growths, or changes of inflammation. Sensation is assessed with a pin and cotton swab, and an anal wink reflex is elicited by perianal stroking. Perineal descent or prolapse may be noted when the patient is asked to strain. Digital examination of the anus is carried out while the resting tone and squeeze pressures are noted. Scarring, deformity, and growths may also be noted on digital examination. The physician should look for fecal impaction, which is one

Table 16–2. PHYSICAL EXAMINATION

Anal conformation
Anal sensation
Anal reflex
Anal canal tone
Perineal descent (extent)
Anal canal conformation (scarring, defects)
Anal squeeze
Puborectal tone and tenderness
Presence of prolapse
Evidence of impaction

of the relatively common causes of incontinence in the geriatric patient.[12–14] Endoscopic evaluation of the anus and rectum, to look for evidence of neoplastic or inflammatory changes, concludes the physical examination (Table 16–2).

Manometric evaluation can help to identify the nature and severity of the incontinence.[8, 15–18] Among 208 patients the most frequent cause of incontinence was idiopathic[107]; there were 57 iatrogenic injuries and 33 obstetric injuries. About 70% of patients with idiopathic incontinence experienced no urge, compared with 38% with iatrogenic incontinence and only 3% with obstetric incontinence. Prolapse was noted in 58% of patients with idiopathic incontinence. Anal resting and squeeze pressures varied widely.[15]

Increased understanding of the mechanisms of fecal continence has produced a number of valuable diagnostic tests (Table 16–3). We believe most of these tests are appropriate only for preoperative assessment. Defecography can assess the anorectal angle and occult problems such as prolapse. Anal manometry is used to quantitate the extent of muscular and reservoir function. This information is valuable only for comparison with postcorrection data. Electromyography and pudendal latency studies help to define the absence of neurologic function, but the absence may be temporary and reversible following surgical correction. As we gain more experience with these tests, we hope they will become useful for predicting the appropriateness and success of various therapeutic alternatives.[13, 19, 20]

Table 16–3. ANAL INCONTINENCE TESTING

Anal manometry with compliance and capacity
Anal electromyography
Transit time
Pudendal latency
Defecography
Saline infusion
Balloon pull-through

MANAGEMENT OF ANAL INCONTINENCE

Management of anal incontinence centers on the recognition that if the stool is kept formed and the rectum empty, significant incontinence can rarely occur, in spite of the quality of sphincter function. Dietary modification and antidiarrheal medication should help to achieve fecal continence. Psyllium-containing products can be taken to thicken the stool. Virtually all patients presenting with any degree of fecal incontinence are first offered a conservative program of muscle-strengthening exercises, psyllium stool-thickening products, and transit-slowing medications (Table 16–4). Only patients who fail the regimen are candidates for more aggressive intervention. Patients should be instructed to take enough psyllium to thicken their stools and told not to follow the package directions, which encourage them to drink large amounts of water.

If psyllium and constipating agents are not adequate to control the patient's symptoms, a more complete evaluation is necessary. At this point, one orders anal manometry with compliance, defecating proctography, and an anal electromyographic study with pudendal nerve latency. The purpose of the studies is to identify a surgically correctable abnormality. An anatomic defect might be readily identifiable on physical examination, and these studies will confirm that there is no additional abnormality prior to correction. On the basis of the results, varying problems will be addressed with a variety of surgical procedures, or surgery will be rejected as a therapeutic alternative.

In an effort to compare surgical with conservative management of anal incontinence, Miller and associates compared 20 patients given conservative management with 26 patients selected for surgical correction.[21] Of the conservative group, 40% had successful results, compared with 65% of the operative group. They noted improvement of resting and squeezing anal canal pressures following surgical repair. Scheuer and coworkers similarly concluded that postanal repair restores anatomy rather than function.[22, 23]

Injured Sphincter

If a disrupted sphincter is identified, surgical correction is reasonable. Whether the injury is secondary to perineal sepsis, anal surgery, or birthing injury, repairs are generally successful.[24] Ctercteko and coworkers reported 60 cases of anal sphincter repair. Satisfactory continence was attained in 86%. A diverting colostomy was utilized in 33%, but this does not seem necessary for a successful repair. Results were less satisfactory if there was evidence of neurogenic incontinence. These investigators favored a direct overlapping sphincter repair.[25]

Among 19 patients who required surgical repair of an obstetric sphincter tear some months or years after injury, 9 (47%) had evidence of pudendal nerve damage at preoperative anorectal physiologic investigation.[26] The result of surgical repair was excellent in eight of ten patients, in whom there was no evidence of nerve damage, whereas only one of nine patients with nerve damage had a satisfactory response. Thus the functional result of delayed anal sphincter repair is partly dependent on whether the nerve supply is intact.

Operative Techniques

Anal Sphincter Repair

Repair of the external voluntary sphincter is a discrete anatomic repair of the injured muscle. The sphincteric injury is usually a result of obstetric trauma that was unrecognized or imperfectly repaired, extensive fistulotomy, or (occasionally) direct trauma. The repair may be undertaken as an isolated procedure, or more commonly it may be done together with the repair of residual abnormalities of trauma, such as a keyhole deformity of the anal orifice.

The patient is prepared for this operation as for any major colorectal procedure, with a thorough mechanical bowel preparation supplemented by prophylactic antibiotics. The incision site depends on the site of injury and/or associated injuries. Anterior repairs are more common, and for these a semicircular incision is made anterior to the anal verge. In the female patient the incision is made between the anus and the posterior vaginal fourchette, posterior to the perineal body. If a coexistent abnormality, such as a keyhole deformity, is to be simultaneously corrected, the anterior curved

Table 16–4. ANAL INCONTINENCE THERAPEUTIC ALTERNATIVES

Stool thickening (psyllium)
Transit slowing (loperamide, codeine)
Biofeedback: Muscle exercises and strengthening
Sphincter repair
Rectal reconstruction
Sphincter replacement
    Thiersch
        Wire
        Gracilis muscle
        Silastic
    Artificial sphincter

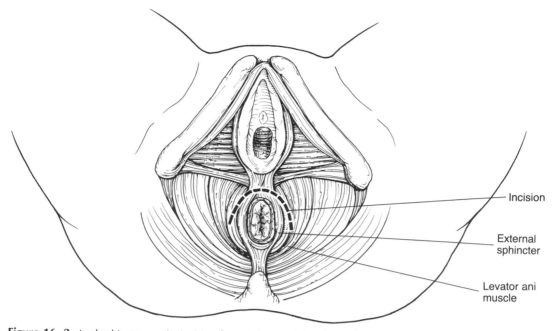

Figure 16–2. Anal sphincter repair. Incision for anterior repair in relationship to the underlying muscles of the perineum.

incision is made at the mucocutaneous junction, and any existing scar is excised. For posterior repairs the incision is placed between the coccyx and the anal verge.

Dissection with electrocautery is the most convenient method for this repair. Dissection, either anterior or posterior, is continued down through the subcutaneous tissue and scar to the wall of the anal canal. Care must be taken not to perforate the anorectum to avoid postoperative sepsis with dehiscence of the repair and formation of a fistula.

If a keyhole deformity exists, the mucocutaneous junction is dissected in order to free the bowel wall (internal sphincter) approximately 30 degrees on each side of the defect until an intact tube of bowel is demonstrated. At this point the V-shaped cleft in the bowel wall is repaired in one or two layers until a perfect cylinder of bowel exists (Fig. 16–2).

The external (voluntary) sphincter is identified. Its recognition may be facilitated by means of an electric neuromuscular stimulator. The scarred muscle may exist as a complete circular investment of the anal canal or as an incomplete sphincter with retraction from the site of injury. The sphincter muscle is then freed from underlying scar tissue for 1.0 to 1.5 cm on either side of the injury. The scar tissue is divided and trimmed so that a fibrotic scar exists on either edge of the sphincter muscle to be repaired. These ends are brought to the midline to assess tension. If undue tension or compromise of the lumen of the canal exists, additional circumferential dissection to free the voluntary sphincter from the underlying internal sphincter

is performed to provide adequate muscle length for a tension-free repair. In performing this maneuver one must take care not to dissect the area external to the sphincter at the horizontal median, to avoid damaging the pudendal nerves. Injury to these nerves may be avoided by identification with an electric nerve stimulator (Figs. 16–3 and 16–4).

After proper identification and freeing of the two ends of the injured sphincter, repair is accomplished. Repair may be effected by either an end-to-end method or an overlapping technique. The overlapping technique is preferred if enough muscle remains for a tension-free repair. In this method the scar end of the muscle is approximated one on top of the other with an overlap of from 5 to 8 mm. One should use stout (3-0 or larger) vertical mattress sutures of material that will not be absorbed during the healing process. If suturing frays the scarred end of the muscle, the suture may be tied through absorbable small pads. Pull-out wires similar to those utilized in the repair of flexor tendons have been advocated by some but are rarely necessary (Figs. 16–5 and 16–6).

Following repair, the anal canal is inspected visually and digitally to ensure an adequate lumen and to rule out inadvertent perforation. Hemostasis is scrupulously obtained, aided by the application of a topical solution of 1:100,000 epinephrine. The wound is closed in layers with absorbable suture, and great care is exercised not to leave a dead space, in order to prevent a catastrophic wound infection. Particular attention is paid to skin closure. Subcuticular closures are to be avoided, because these fragile closures are often disrupted merely

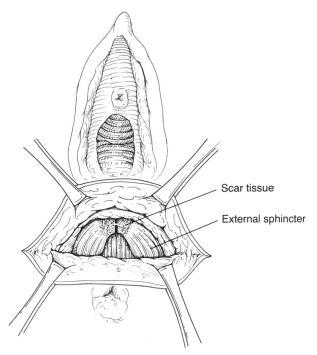

Scar tissue

External sphincter

Figure 16–3. Anal sphincter repair. Elevation of full-thickness skin flaps with identification of external sphincter and scar tissue at the site of injury.

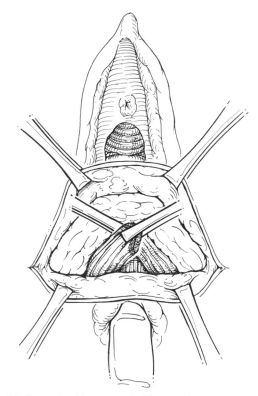

Figure 16–5. Anal sphincter repair. The circular sphincter is reapproximated around the rectum to assess for tension and/or compromise of the lumen.

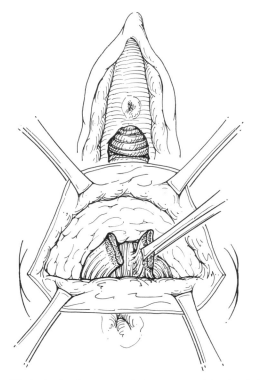

Figure 16–4. Anal sphincter repair. Dissection of the divided external sphincter with freeing of the muscle in order to afford a tension-free repair.

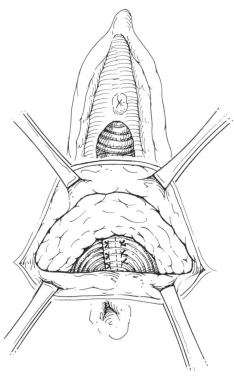

Figure 16–6. Anal sphincter repair. The repair is completed by vertical mattress sutures in an overlapping technique and utilizing stout nonabsorbable sutures.

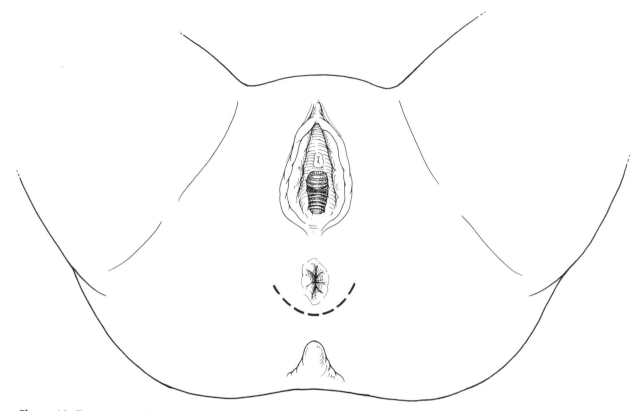

Figure 16–7. Posterior anal reconstruction (proctopexy). The line of incision is shown between the anal orifice and the coccyx.

by sitting, particularly in obese patients. Interrupted sutures using Lembert or mattress techniques are recommended. Postoperatively, the patient is not maintained on a liquid diet or constipated by codeine-containing compounds. Rather, a near-normal diet is gradually resumed, although roughage is avoided for 3 to 4 weeks. Stool softeners such as docusate sodium (Colace) are also utilized. After 3 weeks have passed, the patient is instructed to initiate daily sphincter-strengthening exercises until normal function is obtained.

Posterior Sphincteroplasty with Suture of Puborectal Muscle (Proctopexy)

The posterior repair, as practiced today, was devised by Parks. The operation is initiated by a posterior curved incision anterior to the coccyx (Fig. 16–7). The plane between the internal and external sphincters is identified, and this plane is opened so as to lift the anal canal forward with its intact internal sphincter up to the level of the puborectal muscle. This dissection is accomplished from the midline posterior well anterior to the three o'clock and nine o'clock positions of the anal canal (Fig. 16–8). The underlying puborectal sling is then plicated by stout interrupted nonabsorbable sutures (Fig. 16–9). This plication repairs the

laxity of the puborectal sling and the patulousness of the anal canal.

Following plication of the puborectal sling, the external sphincter can be similarly tightened around the anal canal to overcome the preoperative patulous condition. The skin and subcutaneous layers are closed in the usual manner.

Posterior and anterior repairs have been recommended for anal incontinence. Evaluation of these procedures continues. Yoshioka and Keighly evaluated 104 patients with postanal repair[27]; 60% noted urgency after surgery, 76% still leaked feces, and 52% continued to wear pads. Maximal resting and squeezing anal pressures did not change significantly after the operation. They concluded that the quality of continence after anal repair is poor. They subsequently concluded that patients who did not improve after operation could have been detected preoperatively by their low resting, squeezing, and straining anal pressures as well as by videoproctographic evidence of increased pelvic floor descent.[28]

Miller and associates have compared the effectiveness of anterior sphincteroplasty and levatorplasty in the treatment of fecal incontinence, regardless of etiology.[29] Some 14 patients with traumatic sphincter injuries and 16 with idiopathic fecal incontinence underwent surgery. A satisfactory result was obtained in 71% of the traumatic group and in 62% of the idiopathic group. In both groups, a good result was associated with a significant increase in the maximum voluntary contraction pressure. In Miller's experience, the approach (anterior or posterior) and the anorectal angle are irrelevant to the outcome of surgery for idiopathic fecal incontinence. Success appears to be more closely related to improved sphincter pressure and anal sensation. Womack and colleagues similarly noted that postanal repair need not be restricted to patients with widening of the anorectal angle, because its beneficial effects did not appear to be related to reducing the angle.[30]

Stricker and colleagues reported on 76 patients having sphincter repairs for incontinence.[31] They concluded that women with anterior sphincter defects were most effectively treated with anoplasty skin closure combined with deep external sphincter plication. The posterior proctopexy was most valuable in patients who had intact external sphincters and incontinence that had no recognizable cause or that followed repair of rectal prolapse.

Neurogenic Incontinence

If the sphincter is inadequate for repair, either secondary to destruction or denervation, several alternatives are available. A polyester-impregnated silicone elastomer sling can be used to encircle the anus and works much like a Thiersch wire.[32] Obviously, this is not a dynamic sphincter, but it does increase outlet resistance. Several procedures have been described using autologous tissues to achieve the same result. Gracilis muscle can be wrapped around the anus to achieve outlet obstruction.[33–35] This is not a dynamic sphincter and functions much like the Silastic wrap. Yoshioka and Keighley noted postoperative sepsis in five of six patients who had a gracilis sling, in spite of a diverting colostomy in two patients. Functional results were poor in all patients, and ultimately all required colostomy.[18] Williams and colleagues have utilized an implanted electrical stimulator in an attempt to convert the gracilis muscle to a slow-twitch fatigue-resistant muscle.[36] They demonstrated conversion, which enabled the neosphincter to mount a sustained contraction.

Onishi and associates described a gluteus maximus muscle wrap with the advantage of being a voluntary muscle that may achieve a degree of dynamic function.[37] Shono and others described an experimental free muscle transplant that involved microneurovascular techniques.[38] Up to 80% of normal function was obtained after transplantation. Electromyographic and histologic studies documented normal patterns of muscle fibers and function without fibrotic degeneration.

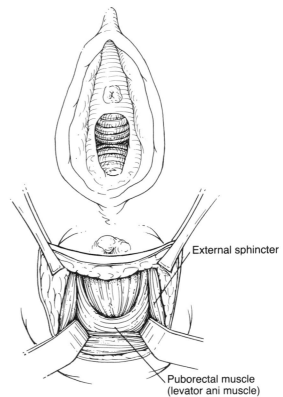

External sphincter

Puborectal muscle
(levator ani muscle)

Figure 16–8. Posterior anal reconstruction (proctopexy). Dissection is carried down between the internal and external sphincters so that the puborectal sling is visualized to the extent shown.

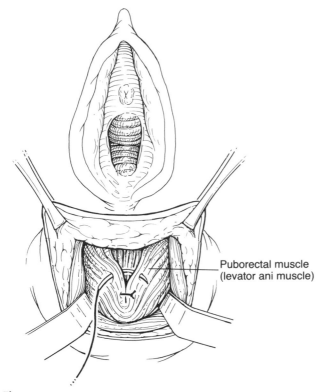

Figure 16–9. Posterior anal reconstruction (proctopexy). Plication of the puborectal sling with stout nonabsorbable sutures. After plication is complete, the external sphincter may be similarly plicated if the anus is patulous.

Puborectal muscle (levator ani muscle)

Rectal Prolapse

Most patients with incontinence associated with rectal prolapse notice improvement following correction of the rectal prolapse.[39] The small proportion who remain incontinent may benefit from sphincter repair at a later date.[40] The exact method of sphincter repair remains controversial. Postanal repair may be preferable in the absence of a specific demonstrable sphincter defect. Henry and Hunter and colleagues think it is the procedure of choice if the patients have levator neuropathy and loss of the anorectal angle.[41, 42] This approach is attractive because it is minimally invasive and relatively free of major complications. Experience is necessary in performing this repair to avoid a stricture by making the repair too tight or failure by making the repair too lax. In the incontinent patient with severe perineal atrophy, an abdominal wall stoma may be easier to manage than a perineal "stoma."

Crohn's Disease

Many have been discouraged from operating on patients with rectal Crohn's disease. Increased understanding of the mechanisms of continence and surgical techniques has led to improved results. Scott and others reported on a group of six patients with anorectal Crohn's disease, who had undergone anal surgery that resulted in incontinence.[43] Five of six patients had excellent results. Anal sphincter repair in a highly selected group of patients can be associated with good results without wound breakdown or fistula formation.

SUMMARY

Historically, anal incontinence has been poorly understood and treated. Increasing knowledge of the anatomy and physiology of continence has advanced the testing procedures that help to predict the appropriate therapeutic alternatives for a given problem. Incontinence can be a multifactorial problem; the physician must possess sophisticated clinical skills and diagnostic alternatives to guide selection of the appropriate treatment.

REFERENCES

1. Lieberman DA. Common anorectal disorders. Ann Intern Med 1984;101:837–846.
2. Holschneider AM, Freeman NV. Anatomy and function of the normal rectum and anus. Birth Defects 1988;24:125–154.

3. Dalley AF II. The riddle of the sphincters. The morphophysiology of the anorectal mechanism reviewed [erratum appears in Am Surg 1987; 53:398]. Am Surg 1987;53:298–306.
4. Duthie HL. Progress report. Anal continence. Gut 1971; 12:844–852.
5. Kuijpers JH. Anatomy and physiology of the mechanism of continence. Neth J Med 1990;37:S2–S5.
6. Cherry DA, Rothenberger DA. Pelvic floor physiology. Surg Clin North Am 1988;68:1217–1230.
7. Dubrovsky B, Filipini D. Neurobiological aspects of the pelvic floor muscles involved in defecation. Neurosci Biobehav Rev 1990;14:157–168.
8. Schuster MM. The riddle of the sphincters. Gastroenterology 1975;69:249–262.
9. Dickinson VA. Maintenance of anal continence: A review of pelvic floor physiology. Gut 1978;19:1163–1174.
10. Wald A. Disorders of defecation and fecal continence. Cleve Clin J Med 1989;56:491–501.
11. Fisher SE, Breckon K, Andrews HA, Keighley MR. Psychiatric screening for patients with faecal incontinence or chronic constipation referred for surgical treatment. Br J Surg 1989;76:352–355.
12. Smith ED, Stephens FD, Holschneider AM, et al. Operations to improve continence after previous surgery. Birth Defects 1988;24:447–479.
13. Read NW, Sun WM. Anorectal manometry, anal myography and rectal sensory testing in anorectal conditions. Indian J Gastroenterol 1990;9:75–80.
14. Read NW. Functional assessment of the anorectum in faecal incontinence. [Discussion]. Ciba Found Symp 1990;151:119–135.
15. Kuijpers HC, Scheuer M. Disorders of impaired fecal control. A clinical and manometric study. Dis Colon Rectum 1990;33:207–211.
16. Parks AG. Anorectal incontinence. Proc R Soc Med 1975;59:477–482.
17. Staples C, Henschke P. Faecal incontinence. Aust Fam Physician 1989;18:972–976.
18. Yoshioka K, Keighley MR. Clinical and manometric assessment of gracilis muscle transplant for fecal incontinence. Dis Colon Rectum 1988;31:767–769.
19. Mathers S, Swash M. Faecal incontinence. Int Disabil Studies 1988;10:164–168.
20. Holschneider AM. Function of the sphincters in anorectal malformations and postoperative evaluation. Birth Defects 1988;24:425–445.
21. Miller R, Bartolo DC, Locke-Edmunds JC, Mortensen NJ. Prospective study of conservative and operative treatment for faecal incontinence. Br J Surg 1988;75:101–105.
22. Read NW. Mechanisms of flatulence and diarrhoea. Br J Surg 1985;72:S5–S6.
23. Scheuer M, Kuijpers HC, Jacobs PP. Postanal repair restores anatomy rather than function. Dis Colon Rectum 1989;32:960–963.
24. Bielefeldt K, Enck P, Wienbeck M. Diagnosis and treatment of fecal incontinence. Dig Dis 1990;8:179–188.
25. Ctercteko GC, Fazio VW, Jagelman DG, et al. Anal sphincter repair: a report of 60 cases and review of the literature. Aust N Z J Surg 1988;58:703–710.
26. Laurberg S, Swash M, Henry MM. Delayed external sphincter repair for obstetric tear. Br J Surg 1988;75:786–788.
27. Yoshioka K, Keighley MR. Sphincter repair for fecal incontinence. Dis Colon Rectum 1989;32:39–42.
28. Yoshioka K, Keighley MR. Critical assessment of the quality of continence after postanal repair for faecal incontinence [erratum appears in Br J Surg 1990;77:356]. Br J Surg 1989;76:1054–1057.
29. Miller R, Orrom WJ, Cornes H, et al. Anterior sphincter plication and levatorplasty in the treatment of faecal incontinence. Br J Surg 1989;76:1058–1060.
30. Womack NR, Morrison JF, Williams NS. Prospective study of the effects of postanal repair in neurogenic faecal incontinence. Br J Surg 1988;75:48–52.
31. Stricker JW, Schoetz DJ Jr, Coller JA, Veidenheimer MC. Surgical correction of anal incontinence. Dis Colon Rectum 1988;31:533–540.
32. Labos S, Rubin RJ, Hoexter B, Salvati EP. Perineal repair of rectal procidentia with an elastic fabric sling. Dis Colon Rectum 1980;23:467–469.
33. Bruining HA, Bos KE, Colthoff EG, Tolhurst DE. Creation of an anal sphincter mechanism by bilateral proximally based gluteal muscle transposition. Plast Reconstr Surg 1981;67:70–73.
34. Corma ML. Follow-up evaluation of gracilis muscle transposition for fecal incontinence. Dis Colon Rectum 1980;23:552–555.
35. Pickrel KL, Broadbent TR, Masters FW, et al. Construction of a rectal sphincter and restoration of anal continence by transplanting gracilis muscle. Report of four cases in children. Ann Surg 1952;135:853–862.
36. Willams NS, Hallan RI, Koeze TH, et al. Construction of a neoanal sphincter by transposition of the gracilis muscle and prolonged neuromuscular stimulation for the treatment of faecal incontinence. Ann R Coll Surg Engl 1990;72:108–113.
37. Onishi K, Maruyama Y, Shiba T. A wrap-around procedure using the gluteus maximus muscle for the functional reconstruction of the sphincter in a case of anal incontinence. Acta Chir Plast 1989;31:56–63.
38. Shono T, Nagasaki A, Goto S, Ikeda K. Experimental free muscle transplantation to the anus using microsurgical technique—a new treatment for anal incontinence. Z Kinderchir 1989;44:352–356.
39. Henry MM. Fecal incontinence and rectal prolapse. Surg Clin North Am 1988;68:1249–1254.
40. Wong WD, Rothenberger DA. Surgical approaches to anal incontinence [Discussion]. Ciba Found Symp 1990;151:246–59.
41. Henry MM. Pathogenesis and management of fecal incontinence in the adult. Gastroenterol Clin North Am 1987;16:35–45.
42. Hunter RA, Saccone GT, Sarre R, et al. Faecal incontinence: Manometric and radiological changes following postanal repair. Aust N Z J Surg 1989;59:697–705.
43. Scott A, Hawley PR, Phillips RK. Results of external sphincter repair in Crohn's disease. Br J Surg 1989;76:959–960.

Rectovaginal Fistula

C H A P T E R   1 7

Theodore R. Schrock

Rectovaginal fistulas are tracts between the epithelial surfaces of the rectum and vagina. They account for less than 5% of rectal fistulas.[1] Symptoms are distressing, and operative repair is advisable if conditions permit.

CLASSIFICATION

Rectovaginal fistulas may be classified in various ways. Perhaps the most familiar grouping is by location along the 7- to 9-cm length of rectovaginal septum. *Low fistulas* are the most common type. They arise at or just above the dentate line and enter the vagina near the posterior vaginal fourchette. *High fistulas* connect the middle one third of the rectum and the posterior vaginal fornix. *Middle rectovaginal fistulas* are found at some point between the low and high varieties. Fistulas emerging from the anal canal distal to the dentate line are termed *anovaginal*. Fistulas that originate at the dentate line, although anovaginal by strict criteria, are generally placed in the *low rectovaginal* category.

Rectovaginal fistulas can be distinguished by size. Small fistulas are less than 0.5 cm in diameter, medium fistulas are 0.5 to 2.5 cm, and large fistulas are more than 2.5 cm.

Still another classification integrates position, size, cause, and surgical approach.[2] *Simple rectovaginal fistulas* are located in the lower one half of the vaginal septum; they are small to medium in size, have a traumatic or an infectious cause, can be repaired by way of a perineal approach, and do not require a colostomy. *Complex fistulas* involve the upper half of the vaginal septum. They are large; they result from irradiation, inflammatory bowel disease, or neoplasm;

they must be repaired through the abdomen; and often a colostomy is needed.

ETIOLOGY

Reported causes of rectovaginal fistulas vary greatly among institutions. Trauma and cryptoglandular infections share the lead in most series, but inflammatory bowel disease is a more frequent cause in some specialist referral centers.

Congenital Etiology

Congenital rectovaginal fistula is invariably associated with an imperforate anus. The rectum ends as a blind pouch above the levators and communicates with the perineum through a fistula to the vagina. Congenital anomalies are not discussed further here.

Traumatic Etiology

Traumatic disruption of the rectovaginal septum during childbirth is a common cause of rectovaginal fistula.[3] Complete disruption of the perineum and the anal sphincters can occur as an extension of a midline episiotomy or as a laceration in the absence of an episiotomy. Rarely, pressure necrosis during prolonged labor causes a rectovaginal fistula with an intact perineal body. A majority of obstetric injuries are recognized and repaired at childbirth, but if infection develops, wounds break down and fistulas are established. The sphincter components of the repair may remain substantially or partially intact, and continence is preserved. In other instances, extensive dehiscence results in incontinence in addition to a rectovaginal fistula.

Surgical trauma can cause rectovaginal fistulas. Abdominal or vaginal hysterectomy, proctectomy, local excision of rectal neoplasms, snare polypectomy, and fulguration of condylomata are among the procedures that can give rise to this complication. Trapping of the posterior vaginal wall in an end-to-end stapler during anterior resection of the rectum is a relatively recent development.

Impalement injuries may heal with a residual rectovaginal fistula. Violent assault is another cause. Chemical burns to the vagina are seen occasionally. Foreign bodies (including surgical sponges) introduced into the vagina or rectum may erode through the septum into the adjacent structure. Fecal impaction, if untreated, can necrose the rectovaginal septum.

Infections

Cryptoglandular infections, the origin of most anorectal abscesses and fistulas, are responsible for some rectovaginal fistulas. Vaginal delivery may precipitate a cryptoglandular infection, and if it erupts into the vagina, a fistula results. Chlamydial infections of the lymphogranuloma venereum types can cause rectovaginal fistulas. Tuberculosis is rarely etiologic. A pelvic abscess in the pouch of Douglas may drain into both rectum and vagina and establish a fistula; this situation too is exceptionally rare.

Inflammatory Bowel Disease

Both Crohn's disease and ulcerative colitis may be associated with rectovaginal fistulas, but anorectal Crohn's disease is more likely to be directly responsible. Crohn's disease tends to involve the full thickness of the bowel, and it often erodes into adjacent structures.

Neoplasm

Extension of carcinoma of the rectum, cervix, vagina, or bladder may produce a rectovaginal fistula. Leukemia and other hematologic disorders, such as aplastic anemia and agranulocytosis, are other causes.

Irradiation

Radiotherapy to the pelvis for the treatment of gynecologic, rectal, or bladder cancer may cause tissue necrosis that results in a rectovaginal fistula. Most of these fistulas are of the high variety, because they ensue after treatment of cervical or endometrial cancer. Fistulas appear after an interval of a few months to 2 years after treatment. Usually there are symptoms of radiation proctitis before the fistula develops. The presence of persistent or recurrent cancer is a concern and must be ruled out.

DIAGNOSIS

Symptoms depend on the cause, location, and size of the rectovaginal fistula. Escape of flatus through the vagina may be the only symptom of a small fistula, but with a larger one stool also passes into the vagina. Vaginitis can be severe. Associated incontinence is particularly distressing in women with extensive disruption of the sphincter.

Examination should establish the presence of the fistula and its position, size, and relation to the sphincters. Abscess cavities should be sought. Integrity of the sphincters and underlying conditions, such as irradiation injury or Crohn's disease, should be evaluated. Vaginitis may be apparent. Large fistulas are visible and palpable from the rectal or vaginal sides or from both sides, and a probe shows the course of the tract. Small fistulas may be difficult to find, and this is particularly true of the less common middle or high fistulas. If necessary, a vaginal tampon is inserted, and half-strength hydrogen peroxide containing a few drops of methylene blue is instilled into the rectum. The anus is plugged for about 10 minutes, and at that time the vaginal tampon is removed and inspected. If there is no stain on the tampon, either there is no fistula at all or one should consider a fistula from some structure other than the rectum (e.g., bladder, colon, small intestine.)[4] Occasionally the presence of a fistula cannot be established until an examination is performed while the patient is under anesthesia. The condition of the tissues—soft or indurated—must be evaluated. Associated rectal stenosis should be noted.

Endoscopy of the rectum is directed toward identification of diseases such as Crohn's disease. Colonoscopy is indicated in some instances. Barium enema x-ray studies, vaginograms, and fistulograms may be needed in some instances. Anal manometry is helpful in evaluating integrity of the sphincter.

SURGICAL TREATMENT

Foreign bodies, including nonabsorbable sutures, should be removed if they contribute to the persistence of the fistula. Abscesses need drainage, antibiotics may be necessary, and local skin care measures are helpful.

Small fistulas that result from obstetric injuries may heal spontaneously. Fistulas from cryptoglandular or other infections may heal with appropriate drainage and antibiotics. Large traumatic fistulas and those resulting from irradiation, Crohn's disease, or neoplasms rarely, if ever, close without operative intervention.

Timing of Operation

Operative repair of traumatic fistulas should be delayed until inflammation has resolved and the tissues are soft and pliable. Operation in the presence of inflammation is certain to fail. Some surgeons arbitrarily wait for up to 6 months after injury before attempting repair, but that interval is unnecessary if the tissues have recovered earlier. One should individualize the timing on the basis of the findings.

The patient should be in good general condition. Many patients with fistulas are young and otherwise healthy. However some individuals are malnourished, and the elderly often have associated conditions that need attention.

Inflammatory bowel disease should be as well controlled as possible. Decisions to repair rectovaginal fistulas in Crohn's disease are difficult to make. These issues are discussed further in this chapter.

Irradiation-induced fistulas do not heal spontaneously. A colostomy may allow inflammation and induration in the rectovaginal area to resolve; these tissues may need several months—even up to 1 year—to soften as much as possible before repair is attempted.[5]

Preparation

A full mechanical and antibiotic bowel preparation should be given. Douches may help clear vaginitis. Systemic antibiotics are administered perioperatively. A bladder catheter is inserted after anesthesia is induced. Surgeons vary in their preferences for general, regional, or local anesthesia.

Approaches

Four approaches are commonly employed for repair of a rectovaginal fistula: perineal, anal, vaginal, and abdominal.[6] Abdominal procedures are used for high or middle fistulas. Low fistulas are treated by one of the other methods. Gynecologists usually place the patient in lithotomy position and perform a vaginal repair. Anal or perineal procedures are preferred by general and colorectal surgeons. Although a fistula

may result from obstetric trauma, the rectum is the more significant contributor to persistence of a fistula. The rectum is the high-pressure side of the system (25 to 85 cm H_2O), and the vagina is the low-pressure side (atmospheric).[7] An anal approach provides the greatest exposure of the rectal side of the fistula, which must be repaired precisely.

The general principles of surgical repair include excision of unhealthy tissue, hemostasis, avoidance of tension on suture lines, and, if possible, avoidance of contiguous suture lines.

PERINEAL REPAIRS

Fistulotomy with Layer Closure

Low rectovaginal and anovaginal fistulas have been treated by fistulotomy alone, but this procedure is inadvisable if the tract encompasses more than a trivial amount of perineal body or muscle because of the risk of incontinence. However a fistulotomy can be done to convert the defect to a complete perineal tear, and a layer closure of the wound is carried out. This method is chosen for women with a low rectovaginal fistula associated with significant sphincter disruption. Fistulotomy with layer closure obliterates the fistula tract and repairs the sphincters.

The patient is placed in the lithotomy position. Tissues overlying the fistula are divided, and the fistula is thus converted to a complete perineal laceration (Fig. 17–1). The edges of the tract are excised, and the vaginal wall is sharply dissected from the remnants of the perineal body and the wall of the anal canal (Fig. 17–2). I prefer scissors dissection rather than scalpel, and hemostasis is achieved by means of electrocautery. The stumps of the external sphincter and the internal sphincter retract laterally during healing after injury, and these structures are dissected out with care to avoid injury to the vascular supply entering posterolaterally. The scarred ends are preserved because they hold sutures well. The rectal mucosa and anoderm are closed with fine interrupted sutures of absorbable material, and the knots are buried into the lumen of the anal canal (Fig. 17–3).

The internal sphincter is reapproximated with interrupted 3-0 absorbable sutures, and the external sphincter is sutured in the midline with interrupted 2-0 material (Fig. 17–4). An overlapping technique may be used (see further on). Sometimes the internal sphincter cannot be separately identified because it is fused to the external sphincter, and both structures are repaired together.

The remnants of the perineal body are joined anterior to the anal canal with interrupted 2-0 sutures (Fig. 17–5). One must be careful to make this approximation

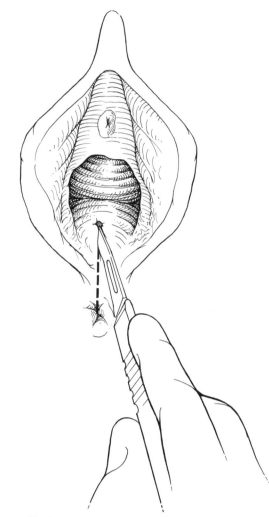

Figure 17–1. Fistulotomy with layer closure. A midline incision converts the rectovaginal fistula to a complete perineal laceration.

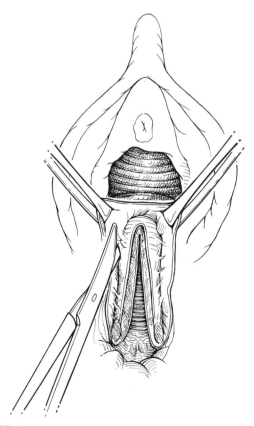

Figure 17–2. The vaginal wall is sharply dissected from the remnants of the perineal body and the wall of the anal canal.

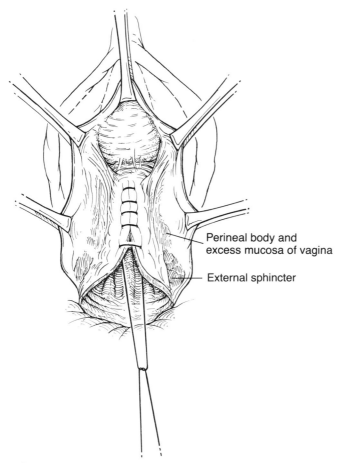

Perineal body and
excess mucosa of vagina

External sphincter

Figure 17–3. The rectal mucosa and anoderm are closed with fine interrupted absorbable sutures.

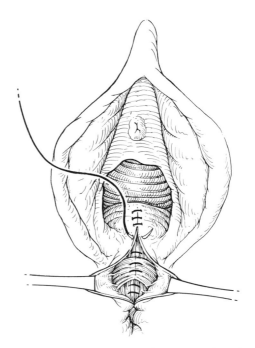

Figure 17–5. The vaginal mucosa is closed with a fine absorbable suture.

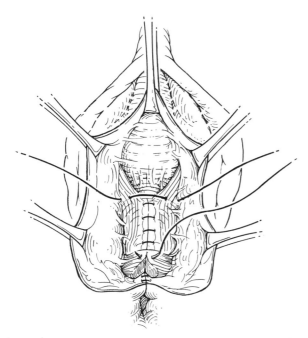

Figure 17–4. The internal and external sphincters are sutured in the midline.

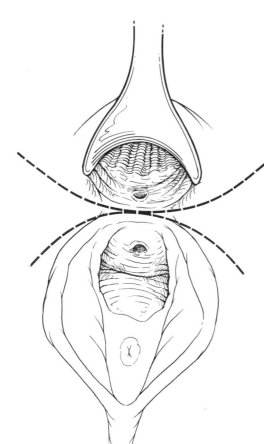

Figure 17–6. Excision of fistula with layer closure. Intersecting curved incisions are made in the perineum.

symmetric. The vaginal mucosa is closed with a continuous fine absorbable suture. A small drain is placed if a cavity remains.

Excision of Fistula with Layer Closure

This perineal operation works well for a woman who has an ectopic anus (placed too close to the vagina) that is either congenital or a consequence of obstetric injury.[4] Fecal incontinence is often present, and both problems are resolved in a single procedure.

The operation is performed with the patient in the prone position. Either a curved incision parallel to the anus or a cruciate incision is made in the perineum (Fig. 17–6). Cruciate incisions are useful because the procedure is completed as a Z-plasty, which further separates the anus and vagina.[4] One must be careful not to devascularize the skin by placing the two curved incisions too close together.

A Hill-Ferguson retractor is kept in the anal canal throughout the procedure in order to avoid creating a stenosis. Some surgeons infiltrate the rectovaginal septum with a local anesthetic containing dilute epinephrine, but I have not found that step necessary or helpful.

The rectum is separated from the vagina, and the stumps of the sphincters are identified. The fistula tract is transected as the dissection proceeds upward. The levator ani muscles (mainly the puborectal muscle) are brought together in the midline with one or two layers of interrupted sutures of 2-0 absorbable material (Fig. 17–7). The external sphincter muscles are reapproximated either directly (Fig. 17–8) or as an overlapping pants-over-vest repair (Fig. 17–8A).[2] The overlapping masses of sphincters are joined with mattress sutures at two points, with all sutures placed to be tied on the same side. The redundant vaginal mucosa and the fistula tract are excised as indicated in Figure 17–8. The skin flaps are mobilized and closed as shown in Figure 17–9 to complete the Z-plasty. A small drain may be left for 2 to 3 days if there is a subcutaneous space.

Postoperative care after either of these procedures is performed traditionally has the aim of preventing defecation for about 5 days. One recommended program is as follows: loperamide two tablets, codeine 60 mg, and deodorized tincture of opium (15 drops), each given four times daily.[4] After 5 days, medications are discontinued and bowel movements are resumed. Many of us no longer follow this practice, choosing instead to initiate stools early rather than risk impaction that could prove difficult.[6] A regular diet and oral bulk are prescribed immediately, and a laxative is given if there is no stool by the second day.[6] Sitz baths are comforting. Ambulation is permitted immediately, and

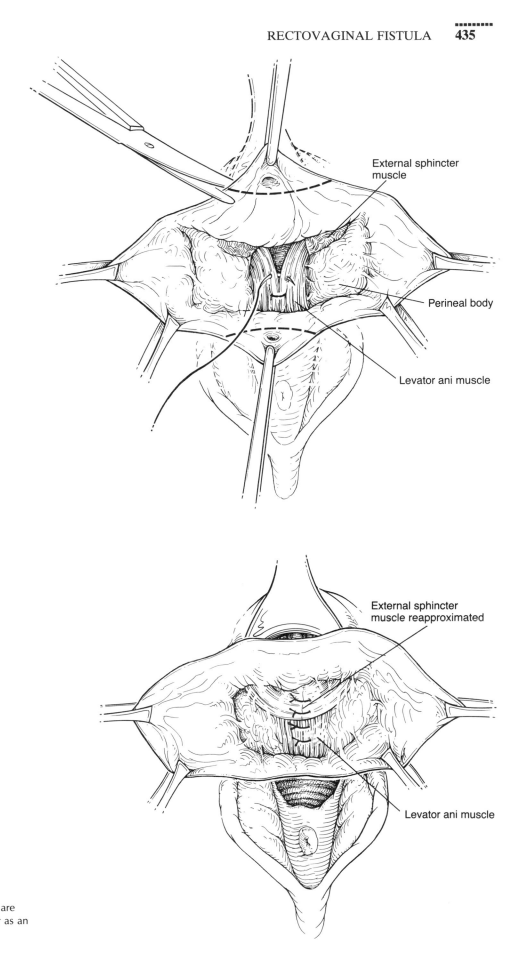

Figure 17–7. The levator ani muscles are sutured together in the midline.

Figure 17–8. External sphincters are approximated directly as shown or as an overlapping repair.

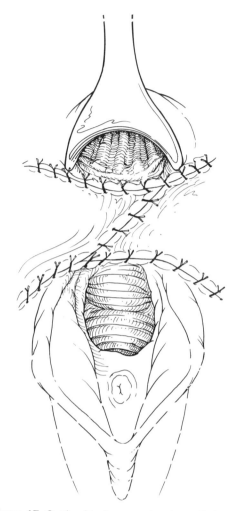

Figure 17–9. The skin flaps are closed as a Z-plasty.

the patient is discharged after the first bowel movement. The patient is instructed not to use tampons or to have intercourse and to avoid strenuous activities for 6 weeks.[6]

ANAL REPAIRS

Excision of Fistula with Layer Closure

This procedure involves a sliding rectal flap, but it is thinner than the flaps in the advancement procedures described further on.[7]

Transanal excision with layer closure is depicted in Figure 17–10.[6, 7] The patient is prone, and the operation is done using general, regional, or local anesthesia. The anus and vagina are prepared with povidone-iodine. A large Hill-Ferguson retractor is inserted.[7] Transverse elliptical excision of the fistula is carried through the full thickness of the rectum and vagina to and including the vaginal orifice of the fistula (Fig. 17–10B and C). The mucosa and submucosa of the rectum are dissected cephalad for at least 4 cm. Lateral dissection is carried out as far as possible to expose the levator muscles for the repair.

The defect in vaginal mucosa is left open for drainage, but the connective tissue of the vaginal wall is approximated transversely (or longitudinally if it comes together more easily) with 3-0 sutures (Fig. 17–10D). Next, two or three layers of 2-0 sutures bring muscle from the lateral region into the midline. This muscle, the external sphincter and levators, builds a strong bar of tissue to separate the vaginal fistula orifice from the rectal mucosa. The rectal mucosal flap is then advanced over the repair of the septal defect and sutured to the distal edge of the elliptical incision with 3-0 sutures (Fig. 17–10E). The intent is to offset the suture lines as shown in Figure 17–10G. The rectal mucosal and vaginal septal suture lines may be contiguous if care is not taken to avoid this occurrence. Also, there will be tension on the suture line of the flap if mobilization is inadequate. Despite these potential pitfalls, reported results are good (see further on).

Sliding Flap Advancement

Sliding rectal advancement flaps to close rectovaginal fistulas have been described by various authors.[8–11a] Although there were substantial differences in techniques in the past, modifications have been made so that surgeons disagree only in details. The essential steps common to all of these repairs include the following: excision of the scarred fistula tract, at least on the rectal side; repair of the septal defect, with the vagina

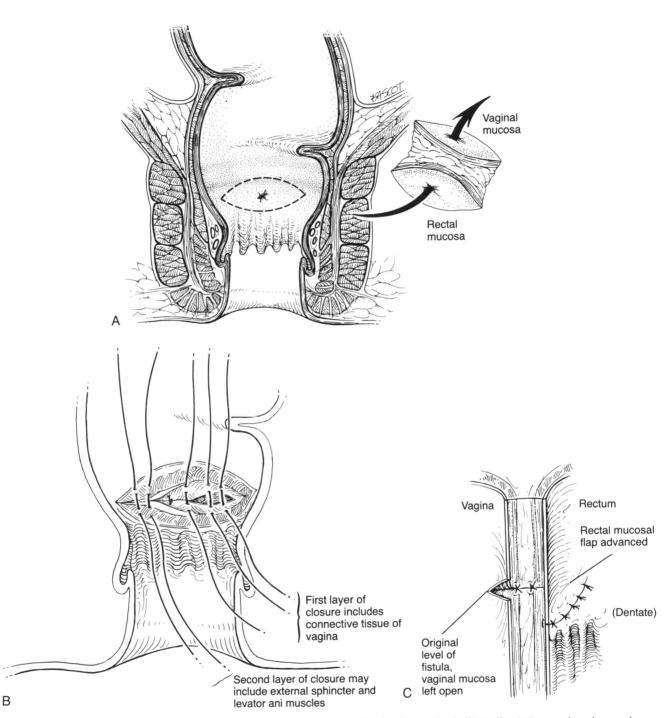

Figure 17–10. *A,* Excision of fistula with layer closure. The full thickness of the fistula is excised elliptically. *B,* Two or three layers of sutures approximate connective tissue of the vaginal wall and the musculature. *C,* The rectal mucosal flap is advanced to offset the suture lines.

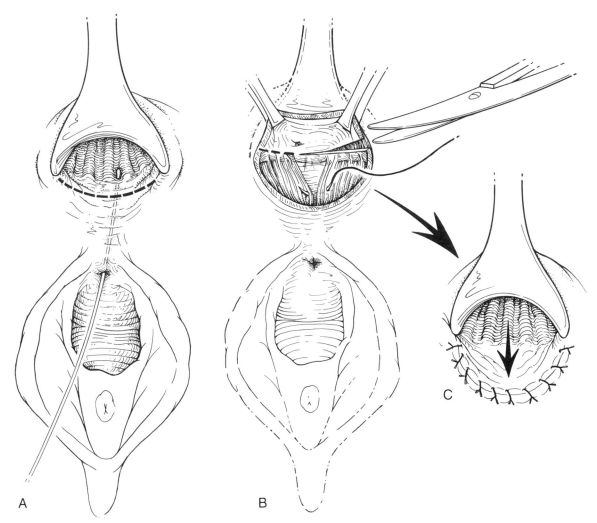

Figure 17–11. *A,* Sliding flap advancement. A semicircular incision is made in the anoderm of the anterior anal canal. *B,* After mobilization of the rectal wall, the fistulous portion is excised. The levators are sutured in the midline. *C,* The rectal flap is then advanced and approximated to the anoderm.

left open for drainage; suture approximation of the sphincters in the midline; and mobilization of a full-thickness flap of anterior rectal wall to cover the repair.[6]

The method depicted in Figure 17–11 is modified from that described by Russell and Gallagher.[11] The patient is prone. A Hill-Ferguson retractor is placed in the anal canal (Fig. 17–11*A*). With a no. 15 scalpel blade, a 3.0- to 4.5-cm semicircular incision is made in the anoderm of the anterior anal canal several millimeters below the dentate line (Fig. 17–11*B*). A sharp scissors dissection continues through the underlying internal sphincter muscle all the way to the posterior wall of the vagina.

The full-thickness flap of rectal wall is then mobilized cephalad (Fig. 17–11*C*). The flap must be at least 4 cm long, and dissection should be carried laterally around one half of the circumference. The rectovaginal

fistula is divided as the flap is mobilized. Allis clamps or skin hooks on the end of the flap help keep tension on the tissue to facilitate the dissection. Numerous tiny vessels are controlled by cautery. The dissection plane is difficult to identify at first because of scarring, particularly in the midline, but as dissection proceeds above the fistula, undisturbed tissue is encountered and the planes develop easily.

As the procedure was originally described, no repair of sphincters was included.[11] The vaginal side of the fistula was left open, and the full-thickness flap was simply advanced and sutured after excision of the rectal fistula orifice as indicated in Figure 17–11*C*. However, in accordance with the general principles previously listed, I prefer to repair the septal defect, leaving the vagina open and then bringing muscle (levators mainly) from a lateral position into the midline with 2-0 sutures. If the muscles are not approximated, a cavity is left

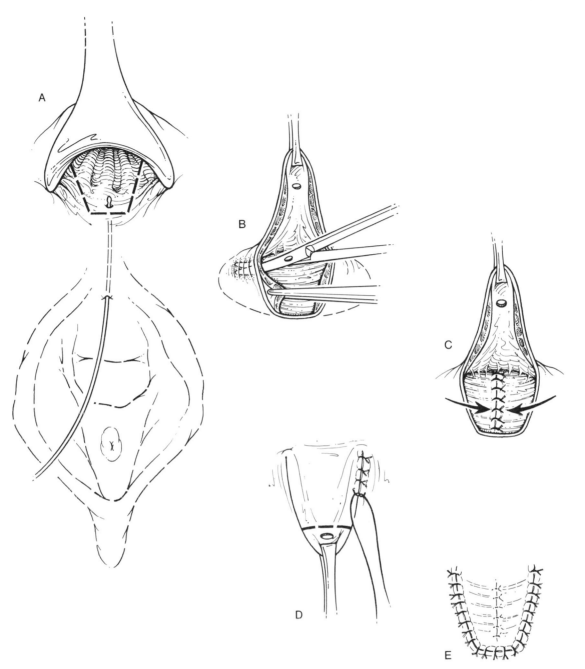

Figure 17–12. *A* to *E,* Another method of endorectal flap advancement. A rectal flap of this shape must have a base twice the width of the apex. Rectal mucosa is elevated laterally, musculature is approximated in the midline, the fistula is excised, and the flap is advanced and closed.

between the endorectal flap and the vaginal septum. This cavity can accumulate fluid and lead to infection, despite leaving the vagina open for drainage. The rectal wall is pulled downward, the fistula is excised, and the flap of healthy tissue is sutured (Fig. 17–11C).

Another variation on the endorectal flap advancement technique is shown in Figure 17–12.[2] Its principal difference from the method just described is the creation of a flap with the shape shown in Figure 17–12B.

The base of this flap must be at least 4 cm cephalad to the fistula, and it should be twice the width of the apex to ensure adequate blood supply; this point is crucial. The flap of mucosa, submucosa, and full thickness of the circular muscle of the rectum (internal sphincter in the lower portion) is then raised from apex to base. In the process, the fistula is transected (Fig. 17–12C). The authors do not describe midline approximation of the levator muscles. Instead the rectal mucosa is ele-

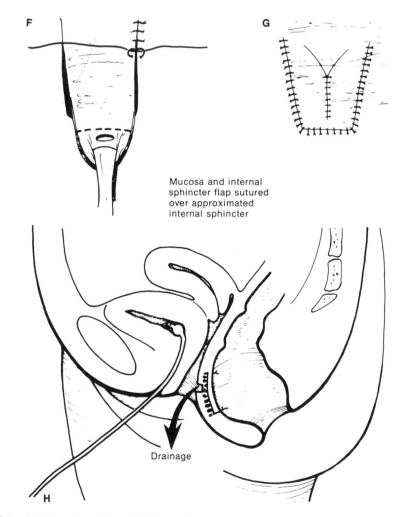

Mucosa and internal
sphincter flap sutured
over approximated
internal sphincter

Drainage

Figure 17–12 *Continued F* to *H*, Mucosal and internal sphincter flap are sutured over approximated internal sphincter (*F to H*, From Corman ML. Colon and Rectal Surgery. 2nd Ed. Philadelphia: JB Lippincott, 1989, p 153–165.)

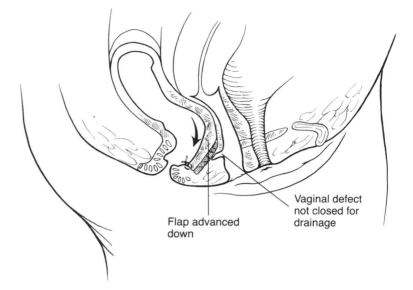

Vaginal defect
not closed for
drainage

Flap advanced
down

Figure 17–12 *Continued I,* Sagittal view of the advancement flap with the vaginal defect opened for drainage.

vated from the lateral incisions (Fig. 17–12*D*), and the internal sphincter is brought together in the midline (Fig. 17–12*E*). This step is possible only because of the two lateral extensions of the incision in the anterior rectal wall; it cannot be done with only a semicircular incision of the sort shown in Figure 17–11.

The flap is then advanced without tension, the rectal orifice of the fistula is excised (Fig. 17–12*F*), and the interrupted 3-0 absorbable sutures are used to attach the flap (Fig. 17–12*G*). The final arrangement of the advancement flap with respect to the original fistula site is shown in Figure 17–12*H*. The vaginal orifice of the fistula is left open for drainage.

Both techniques of rectal flap advancement use full-thickness rectal wall flaps with less risk of tension and necrosis than the mainly mucosal flap already described for excision of fistula with layer closure.

VAGINAL REPAIRS

Gynecologists routinely repair rectovaginal fistulas through the vagina.[12] Excision and layer closure, much as already described for an anal procedure, is a common vaginal technique. The disadvantage of the vaginal approach is that the most critical part of the repair, closure of the rectal wall, is performed through the vaginal defect in the depths of the wound. Furthermore, the sutures that approximate rectal wall, muscle, septum, and vaginal mucosa all overlie one another, and contiguous suture lines predispose the patient to recurrence of the fistula.

Vaginal repair by inversion with a pursestring suture has little place in the operative armamentarium. Mar-

tius described a method in which bulbocavernosus tissue was mobilized to be interposed between the layers of a rectovaginal fistula repair.[13] This technique is not described here, but it is appropriate for a few patients with complex irradiation injuries. Vaginal repair of high fistulas is sometimes performed by gynecologists, but most surgeons believe that high fistulas are more successfully approached through the abdomen. Colpocleisis is denudation of the vaginal epithelium with obliteration of the remaining space. It is not used much today, but in the past it played a larger role in the management of fistulas caused by irradiation.

ABDOMINAL REPAIRS

A temporary colostomy is not required for anal or perineal repairs of low or middle rectal fistulas caused by trauma or infection. If the fistula is high or complicated, or if it is caused by irradiation, neoplasm, or Crohn's disease, a diverting colostomy may be helpful. If a colostomy is established in a patient with irradiation injury, the perineum is allowed to heal for several weeks or months before rectovaginal fistula repair is undertaken.

Abdominal operation is preferred for repair of high rectovaginal fistulas, the sphincters being preserved whenever possible. In simple cases the rectum and vagina are sharply separated, and the defects in the walls of both structures are sutured. It is helpful to place omentum between the rectum and vagina to separate the suture lines.

In many instances, including most of the irradiation-induced fistulas, the rectal wall is not healthy enough

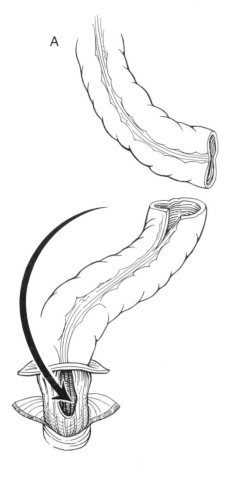

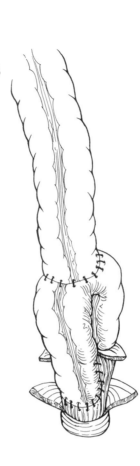

Figure 17–13. *A* and *B*, The onlay graft procedure to close defects in an irradiated patient. The proximal end of the rectosigmoid is split and folded downward for anastomosis to the distal rectum at the fistula site. Continuity is restored by end-to-side anastomosis.

simply to close the defect. Anterior resection with rectal anastomosis distal to the vaginal suture line is performed, and if standard anastomotic techniques are not feasible, endoanal anastomosis may be necessary.[14] Rectal mucosa is stripped transanally and the proximal colon is brought down inside the cuff. The end-to-end stapler facilitates the anastomosis.

The onlay graft procedure shown in Figure 17–13 uses the colon to close defects in the distal rectum in patients with irradiation-induced rectovaginal fistulas.[5] The sigmoid is divided, and a colostomy is established. The rectosigmoid is split and folded on itself so that the open end is sutured to the rectum around the large distal defect. This may require both abdominal and perineal approaches. At a subsequent operation, the colostomy is taken down and anastomosed to the top of the rectosigmoid loop. This procedure is conceptually simple, but patients with irradiation-induced rectovaginal fistulas may not heal well. The rectal fistula site and the rectosigmoid colon that covered it probably were heavily irradiated in this situation.

Some patients with a rectovaginal fistula in association with a badly diseased or damaged rectum are best treated by proctectomy. Fistulas associated with malignancy, irradiation, and Crohn's disease are often in this category.

RESULTS

Repair should be successful in 85% to 90% of low rectovaginal fistulas in uncomplicated cases.[4, 10, 11] Rates of success are still good after repair of a recurrent fistula if only one previous operation has been performed.[12] Results are less predictable if there were two or more prior repairs. Recurrence is the result of postoperative infection or dehiscence of suture lines related to intrinsically poor healing properties of the tissue, ischemia, excessive tension, or underlying anorectal disease. Patients with fecal incontinence associated with rectovaginal fistulas are improved after repair, but perfect continence may not return.[4]

RECTOVAGINAL FISTULAS IN CROHN'S DISEASE

Although anorectal complications of Crohn's disease may improve with medical therapy, rectovaginal fistulas rarely heal permanently. 5-Aminosalicylic acid (5-ASA) enemas and systemic therapy, including metronidazole, may help. An operation should not be carried out in the presence of active Crohn's proctitis, and it may be advisable for the patient to accept the situation, at least for a while. Some patients with Crohn's disease live comfortably with small, minimally symptomatic, rectovaginal fistulas.

When Crohn's disease is in remission and the anorectum is grossly normal or nearly so, rectovaginal fistula repair can be carried out in symptomatic patients. The decision can be difficult, and the best course is not always clear.

The preferred procedure is a rectal advancement flap. Successful healing is achieved in up to 60% of patients.[8, 9, 15–17] Factors predictive of failure include other anal pathologic problems and active small bowel Crohn's disease and not closing the fistula tract in layers.[11] Incontinence is not a problem after these operations. If the repair breaks down and the fistula recurs, however, it may be larger than before.

Flaps of gracilis or inferior gluteus have been employed to correct rectovaginal fistulas in patients with Crohn's disease, but experience is limited.[18] A rectovaginal fistula is rarely the only reason—and seldom the principal reason—for proctectomy or proctocolectomy in Crohn's disease.[8, 17] Patients with active Crohn's proctocolitis may have a rectovaginal fistula, but it is the unresponsiveness of the disease in general that motivates consideration of extirpative operations.

EDITORIAL COMMENT

The perineal complications of Crohn's disease are often neglected by surgeons who elect a nihilistic approach to this aspect of the disease. Hence, we commonly encounter patients with well-established rectovaginal or rectoperineal fistulas or complex fistulas and abscesses whose drainage will result in a cloaca. Many of these patients could have avoided the extensive soft tissue destruction if the basic principles of drainage and fistulotomy had been applied in a timely fashion.

The repair of a rectovaginal or rectoperineal fistula in the Crohn's disease patient is based on several principles: (1) the mucosa of the rectum should be free of the *gross* changes of Crohn's disease other than the presence of the internal os at the dentate line; (2) the fistula must be symptomatic to a degree that is unacceptable to the patient; (3) the patient must be aware that *new* fistulas may occur in the future; (4) irrespective of the operative technique employed, all repairs depend on separation of the rectal and vaginal repairs by interposed soft tissue—usually the levator muscles and the perineal body.

In complex repairs, particularly for fistulas in which considerable perineal sepsis is present, fecal diversion prior to repair is essential. The diverting colostomy is closed when the repair is well healed.

For patients with extensive fistulas, severe perineal sepsis and/or sphincteric destruction, *and* evidence of gross Crohn's disease in the rectum, proctectomy is the only reasonable choice. For these patients we divide the operation into two stages. At the first stage the intra-abdominal Crohn's disease is resected with a permanent end-stoma. The rectum is removed so as to establish a short Hartmann pouch of no more than 4 to 5 cm in length. The perineal abscesses are drained and the fistulas are laid open as the final step of the first procedure. The perineum is allowed to heal, and after approximately 6 to 8 weeks, perineal proctectomy is accomplished with primary closure of the perineum. This technique allows the surgeon to avoid contamination of the abdomen and pelvis from the perineum and also allows a primary closure of the perineum at the second operation.

REFERENCES

1. Laird DR. Procedures used in treatment of complicated fistulas. Am J Surg 1948;76:701–708.
2. Buls JG, Rothenberger DA. Anal and rectovaginal fistulas: Repair of the low fistula. In: Kodner IJ, Fry RD, Roe JP, eds. Colon, Rectal, and Anal Surgery. St Louis: CV Mosby, 1985, pp 63–75.
3. Tancer ML, Lasser D, Rosenblum N. Rectovaginal fistula or perineal and anal sphincter disruption, or both, after vaginal delivery. Surg Gynecol Obstet 1990;171:43–46.
4. Corman ML. Colon and Rectal Surgery. 2nd ed. Philadelphia: JB Lippincott, 1989, pp 153–165.
5. Bricker EM, Johnston WD. Repair of postirradiation rectovaginal fistula and stricture. Surg Gynecol Obstet 1979;148:499–506.
6. Hoexter B. Rectovaginal fistula. In: Fazio VW, ed. Current Therapy in Colon and Rectal Surgery. Philadelphia: BC Decker, 1990, pp 28–32.
7. Greenwald JC, Hoexter B. Repair of rectovaginal fistulas. Surg Gynecol Obstet 1978;146:443–445.
8. Cohen JL, Stricker JW, Schoetz DJ, et al. Rectovaginal fistula in Crohn's disease. Dis Colon Rectum 1989;32:825–828.
9. Crim RW, Fazio VW, Lavry IC. Rectal advancement flap repair in Crohn's patients—factors predictive of failure. Presented to American Society of Colon and Rectal Surgeons, St Louis, 1990.
10. Lowry AC, Thorson AG, Rothenberger DA, Goldberg SM. Repair of simple rectovaginal fistulas. Influence of previous repairs. Dis Colon Rectum 1988;31:676–678.
11. Russell TR, Gallagher DM. Low rectovaginal fistulas. Approach and treatment. Am J Surg 1977;134:13–18.
11a. Rothenberger DA, Christenson CE, Balcos EG, et al. Endorectal advancement flap for treatment of simple rectovaginal fistula. Dis Colon Rectum 1982;25:297–300.
12. Lescher TC, Pratt JH. Vaginal repair of the simple rectovaginal fistula. Surg Gynecol Obstet 1967;124:1317–1321.
13. Hibbard LT. Surgical management of rectovaginal fistulas and complete perineal tears. Am J Obstet Gynecol 1978;130:139–141.
14. Parks AG, Allen CLO, Frank JD, McPartlin JF. A method of treating post-irradiation rectovaginal fistulas. Br J Surg 1978;65:417–421.
15. Heyen F, Winslet MC, Andrews H, et al. Vaginal fistulas in Crohn's disease. Dis Colon Rectum 1989;32:379–383.
16. Morrison JG, Gathright JB Jr, Ray JE, et al. Results of operations for rectovaginal fistula in Crohn's disease. Dis Colon Rectum 1989;32:497–499.
17. Radcliffe AG, Ritchie JK, Hawley PR, et al. Anovaginal and rectovaginal fistulas in Crohn's disease. Dis Colon Rectum 1988;31:94–99.
18. Hecker WC, Holschneider AM, Kraeft H. Surgical closing of rectovaginal, rectourethral, urethrovaginal and vesicocutaneous fistulas by means of interposition of the gracilis muscle. Chirurgerie 1980;51:43–45.

SECTION IV

SPECIAL CONSIDERATIONS

Intestinal Stomas:
Construction and Care

C H A P T E R   1 8

Stephen R. Gorfine

Irwin M. Gelernt

Joel J. Bauer

The surgical creation of an "artificial anus" or intestinal stoma has been practiced since the eighteenth century.[1] Patients subjected to this form of therapy usually suffered from advanced intestinal obstruction, often caused by distal colonic malignancy. Survival beyond the postoperative period was rare. As technical capabilities and postoperative management improved through the eighteenth and nineteenth centuries, eventual recovery and return to health became more common. However, the dearth of effective pouching techniques and a general lack of patient information made life with a stoma arduous at best.[2]

It was not until the middle of this century that effective modalities for enterostomal creation and management began to develop in earnest. The past 50 years have seen dramatic improvements in surgical and anesthetic techniques, nutrition, and antibiotics. Similarly, advances in patient education, enterostomal therapy, and manufactured stomal appliances have brought well-devised intestinal stomas into the surgical "mainstream."

The feature common to all enteral stomas is the surgical establishment of a new mucocutaneous junction. Although exteriorization of almost any segment of the gastrointestinal tract is technically feasible, ileostomies and colostomies constitute the majority of intestinal stomas. The typical stoma serves one of three purposes: intestinal decompression, fecal diversion, or fecal elimination. The need for the stoma may be temporary or permanent.

PREOPERATIVE PERIOD

The preoperative preparation of all potential ostomates includes a number of features. Psychological and physical issues must be addressed. Preoperative counseling from the surgeon and enterostomal therapist is vitally important. A preoperative visit from a volunteer of the local chapter of the United Ostomy Association can help relieve anxiety and advance patient acceptance.

Thorough mechanical and antibiotic bowel preparation is indicated in all but emergent situations.[3] The enterostomal therapist (ETRN) or surgeon should mark the skin of the proposed site of the stoma in all patients.[4] The mark should be indelibly made by ink, tattoo, or scratch-mark so that it will not be obscured at the time of operation.

The area chosen should be easily accessible to the patient, distant from bony prominences, and free from scars, creases, and depressions that would interfere with effective pouching.[5] Selection of an appropriate site is important, especially for the permanent stoma. When possible, one should ask the patient to stand, sit, bend at the waist, and wear clothing in order to ascertain that the stoma and pouch will not conflict with these activities. The selection must be tailored to the individual's needs.

COLOSTOMY

Numerous types of colostomies have been devised to meet various surgical needs. The patient's disease and, to a lesser degree, the surgeon's preference usually dictate the choice of stoma. The most common technical variations are the end, loop, end-loop, and "blowhole" colostomies.

Colostomy Construction

End-Colostomy

An end-colostomy is usually constructed from the sigmoid colon or the descending colon. End-colostomy is indicated when disease or surgical resection of the distal rectum or anus precludes colorectal or coloanal anastomosis. Pelvic or distal rectal malignancy is the most common underlying process.[6] A temporary end-colostomy is also frequently employed in the staged operative management of perforating diverticular disease. Occasionally, penetrating rectal trauma, Crohn's disease of the anus or rectum, or severe perianal suppurative disease, such as Fournier's gangrene, requires treatment by temporary or permanent fecal diversion.

OPERATIVE TECHNIQUE

As stated, preoperative bowel preparation and stomal marking whenever possible are strongly recommended. Most end-colostomies are placed in the left lower quadrant, at the middle of the left rectus abdominis muscle. Alternate sites, including the lower pole of the abdominal incision, are possible but in our opinion are less desirable.[7] Whenever possible, the abdominal skin incision should be sufficiently distant from the colostomy site that eventual scarring will not interfere with pouching (Fig. 18–1).

The colonic segment chosen for the stoma often depends on the underlying pathologic process. The bowel must reach the anterior abdominal wall without tension, and it must have an adequate blood supply. If possible, it should not have been included in a field of radiation. Furthermore the segment should be pliable and free of diverticula and muscular hypertrophy. Fulfillment of all these requirements often precludes choosing the sigmoid colon, even when it is available.

When the sigmoid colon is unsuitable, the descending colon is used.

In all patients the colon must be adequately freed from its retroperitoneal attachments. This is accomplished by division of the white line of Toldt. The splenic flexure occasionally requires mobilization to achieve optimal free length when the descending colon is chosen. If further mobility of the descending colon is required, the inferior mesenteric vessels can be divided at their origin.[7] Once the stomal segment is optimally mobilized, it is transected with the linear stapler. Epiploic appendices are removed by means of electrocautery from the distal 3 to 4 cm of the stomal end.

The abdominal wall on the marked side is stabilized by grasping the cut edges of the peritoneum, fascia, and skin with towel clips placed at the level of the mark. The center of the mark is grasped with a Kocher clamp or an Allis clamp, and traction is applied away from the abdominal wall. A circle of skin of 2 to 3 cm in diameter is excised by means of electrocautery.

The surgeon applies upward pressure to a laparotomy pad placed against the peritoneal surface of the colostomy site while an assistant maintains medial traction at the cut edge of the abdominal wound. The subcutaneous fat is left in place, and Scarpa's fascia is divided sharply. Blunt dissection is continued to the level of the rectus abdominis muscle sheath. The anterior rectus sheath is opened by a 2-cm cruciate incision made with electrocautery. The rectus abdominis muscle is split in the direction of its fibers, and each portion is retracted away from the middle. Care is exercised to avoid damaging the inferior epigastric vessels that are between the rectus muscle and the posterior rectus sheath. The posterior rectus sheath or transversalis fascia and peritoneum are divided transversely with electrocautery, thereby exposing the intra-abdominal pad. The defect in the abdominal wall should be large enough to admit two fingers easily (Fig. 18–2).

The stomal limb may be brought to the abdominal wall defect either by passing it directly through the peritoneal cavity ("intraperitoneal colostomy") or by tunneling it beneath the peritoneal membrane ("extraperitoneal colostomy"). The advantage of the extraperitoneal approach lies in lower incidences of parastomal herniation, prolapse, and retraction.[8] However, eventual closure of an extraperitoneal stoma is considerably more difficult than that of an intraperitoneal stoma. Therefore, extraperitoneal tunneling is recommended for the permanent end-stoma only.[9]

When an extraperitoneal stoma is fashioned, the tunnel is begun at the point of colonic mobility. The cut edge of peritoneum is lifted at the left gutter, and a tunnel to the abdominal wall wound is created by

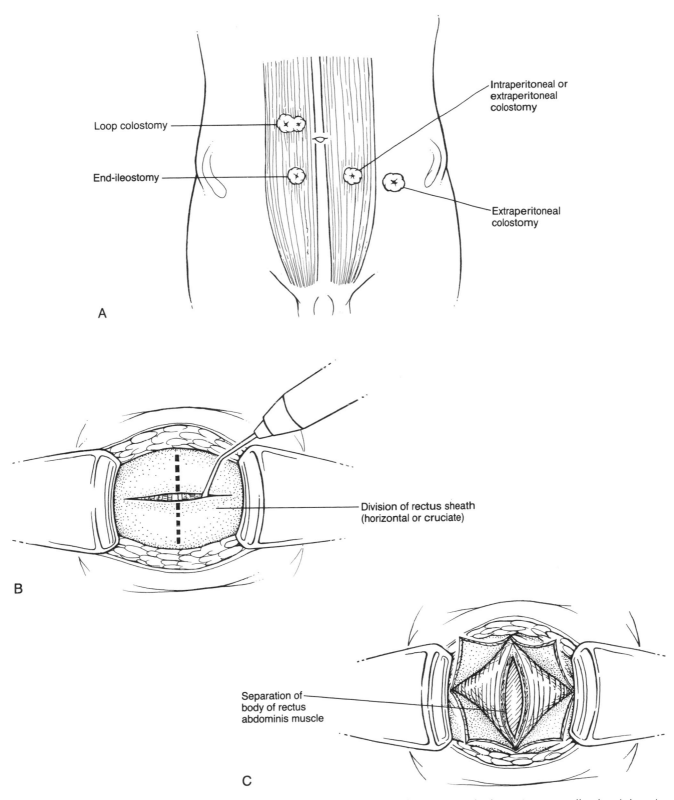

Figure 18–1. Stomal sites and construction. *A*, Preferred sites of stomal placement. Ileostomies and colostomies are usually placed through the rectus abdominis muscle to avoid parastomal hernias. Stomas should not be placed near scars, skin folds, or bony prominences. *B*, Construction of stomal sites. After a disk of skin is excised, the anterior rectus sheath is incised in either a horizontal or a cruciate fashion. *C*, Construction of stomal sites. The rectus abdominis muscle is split longitudinally.

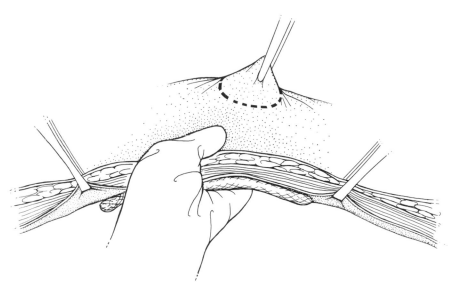

Figure 18–2. Construction of stomal site. The full thickness of the abdominal wall is grasped with Allis forceps or towel clips, so that a true vertical incision may be made, symmetrically traversing all layers. The surgeon's hand, aided by a sponge or pad, indicates the boundaries of the rectus abdominis muscle, and a skin disk is excised over this point.

blunt dissection. A Babcock clamp is passed through the abdominal wall and the tunnel, and the stapled edge of the colon is grasped. The colon is then eased through the retroperitoneum and out the abdominal wound. Care is taken during this manuever to avoid twisting the colonic mesentery (Fig. 18–3).

If the intraperitoneal route is chosen, the stapled end of the colon is simply brought through the abdominal wall. The colon is transected at the point where the stomal end reaches the abdominal wall with neither tension nor redundancy. Again, care is taken to avoid twisting the segment while pulling it through the stomal aperture, because rotation of the segment compromises its blood supply. In the intraperitoneal position, the mesentery of the exteriorized segment is fixed to the parietal peritoneum with a running, absorbable suture. This eliminates the possibility of internal herniation around the stomal limb (Fig. 18–4).

Once the colonic segment is exteriorized, the abdominal contents are returned to anatomic position, and the abdominal cavity is lavaged. The exit points of any drains should avoid the peristomal area. The abdominal incision is closed by means of standard technique.

Maturation of the stoma is performed immediately after the abdomen is closed. The incisional wound is covered with sterile towels. The colonic staple line is excised with electrocautery leaving approximately 1 cm of colon above skin level. Hemostasis at the cut edge should be perfect. The cut edge of the colon is fixed to the skin of the abdominal wall with absorbable 3–0 sutures. The full thickness of the colonic wall must be included in each suture. The skin sutures need not be confined to the dermal layer but may include the epidermis. Usually 8 to 12 sutures will suffice. When completed, the stoma should be flush with or should slightly pout from the abdominal wall. The colostomy

should be pouched with a simple clear plastic appliance to permit easy inspection. The incision is then dressed according to the surgeon's preference (Fig. 18–5).

In situations in which liquid colostomy effluent can be expected, the stoma should be everted so that it protrudes slightly from the abdominal wall. To accomplish this, transection of the exteriorized end should leave about 2 cm of bowel above skin level. Eversion is accomplished by placing four three-point sutures at the twelve, three, six, and nine o'clock positions. These sutures pass through all colonic layers at the cut edge, the seromuscular bowel wall at the level of the skin, and the skin edge. Suture placement must be aligned so as to prevent twisting of the stoma. One or two simple sutures placed from the cut edge of the colon to the skin margin in the intervals between the three-point sutures complete the maturation. Colostomy pouching and wound dressing are performed as before.

MUCOUS FISTULA

On occasion the surgeon may find that colonic resection leaves two intestinal ends unsuitable for anastomosis, because of local or systemic considerations. In this situation, the proximal bowel is matured in the standard fashion as an end-stoma. The distal end, if long enough to reach the anterior abdominal wall, can be matured as a separate, distal stoma or mucous fistula. The mucous fistula can be matured at a second abdominal stoma site, as described, or it can be brought out through the lower pole or upper pole of the main abdominal incision and matured there.[10] Pouching of this stoma is usually not necessary, as it produces only a small amount of mucoid discharge.

Many surgeons believe that end-colostomy with mucous fistula offers the advantages of relative ease of colocolostomy and absolute fecal diversion. In the case

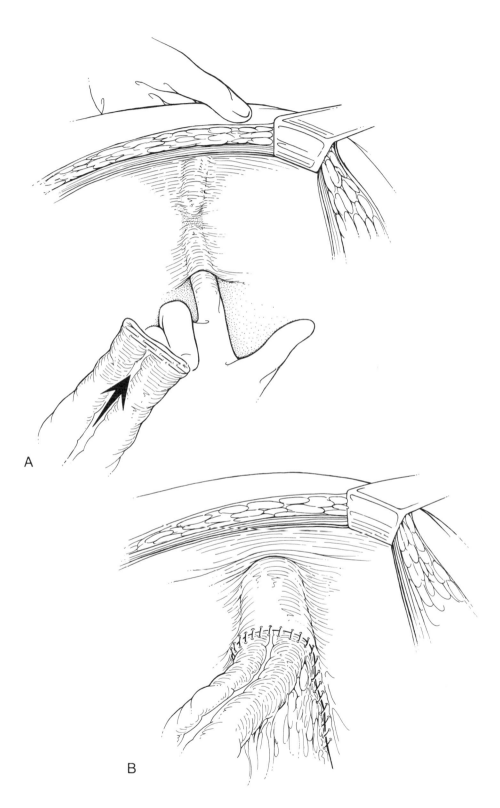

A

B

Figure 18–3. Construction of an extraperitoneal colostomy. *A,* An extraperitoneal tunnel is made by blunt dissection to the site of the stoma. The closed end of the colon is then brought through this tunnel, exiting at the stomal site. *B,* The peritoneal defect is sutured to the bowel wall, and the remaining mesenteric-peritoneal defect is closed.

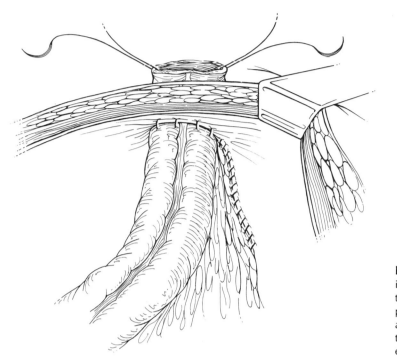

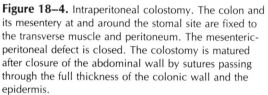

Figure 18–4. Intraperitoneal colostomy. The colon and its mesentery at and around the stomal site are fixed to the transverse muscle and peritoneum. The mesenteric-peritoneal defect is closed. The colostomy is matured after closure of the abdominal wall by sutures passing through the full thickness of the colonic wall and the epidermis.

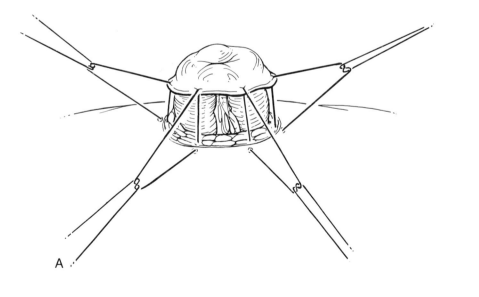

A

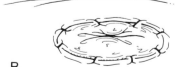

B

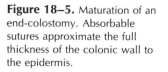

Figure 18–5. Maturation of an end-colostomy. Absorbable sutures approximate the full thickness of the colonic wall to the epidermis.

of end descending colostomy and rectosigmoid mucous fistula, the mucous fistula generally is more easily prepared for hand-sewn anastomosis than is a Hartmann pouch. However, transanal circular stapling techniques have virtually eliminated the problem of the "difficult" rectal segment.[11] Additionally, skin-level loop colostomies have conclusively been shown to divert completely.[12, 13] Finally, a successful mucous fistula requires a length of distal bowel adequate to reach the anterior abdominal wall easily. This requirement is most often lacking when a mucous fistula would be most valuable.[10] Therefore the role of the separate mucous fistula has been almost completely superseded by anastomosis and proximal loop diversion or by end-stoma and Hartmann closure.[11]

Loop Colostomy

Maturation of the apex of a loop of colon brought to the anterior abdominal wall creates a loop colostomy. In contrast to an end-stoma, the mesentery of the exteriorized segment is left undivided. The circumference of the bowel at the stoma may be partially or totally divided. Loop colostomy provides the advantages of rapid construction, certain blood supply, and easy closure.

Loop colostomy is commonly employed for temporary fecal diversion.[13] For example, distal colonic obstruction unsuited for immediate resection is most expediently managed by decompression by means of a double-barrel loop transverse colostomy. Protection of the tenuous distal anastomosis is another common, but less frequent, reason for diversion by loop transverse colostomy.[14]

Loop sigmoid colostomy is a possible therapeutic alternative in the management of rectal diseases not expected to require resection. Examples of these diseases include penetrating rectal trauma, Crohn's disease involving the anorectum, and radiation proctitis. Full preoperative bowel preparation and preoperative patient education whenever possible are recommended. The proposed stoma site should be marked indelibly on the skin in every case.

DOUBLE-BARREL COLOSTOMY

The double-barrel loop colostomy is most commonly fashioned from the transverse colon. The sigmoid colon is a possible but less often chosen alternative. The choice of operative incision depends on the full extent of the proposed procedure. The presence or absence of colonic obstruction also influences the choice of approach. Whenever possible, full exploration of the abdominal contents should be performed. When a limited procedure is planned, usually in the patient with colonic obstruction, preoperative confirmation of

this diagnosis should be obtained by endoscopic or radiographic means.

Operative Technique. In the limited procedure, the abdomen is entered through an 8- to 10-cm transverse incision overlying the upper portion of the right rectus abdominis muscle. The transverse colon is located and delivered into the operative wound. The loop should reach the anterior abdominal wall without tension.

The apex of the loop is freed of omentum and epiploic appendages for a distance of 5 to 10 cm proximally and distally. The length of the cleared segment should be twice the thickness of the abdominal wall pannus. The size of the aperture can be kept to a minimum by reducing the amount of tissue passing through the abdominal wall.

The apex of the loop is identified, and a clamp is passed through the mesentery at the colonic margin. A soft rubber drain is passed through the mesenteric defect and brought around the colon. The loop is exteriorized through the incision. The gastrocolic ligament is divided between clamps if mobility is insufficient (Fig. 18–6).

The colon is maintained at skin level by a glass, plastic, or rubber support or by a fascial or skin bridge traversing the mesenteric defect.[15] In the former circumstance, the drain is replaced by the support. The support is secured to the abdominal wall by a loop of rubber tubing or sutures. The fascia is closed snugly, but not tightly, around the loop by sutures placed at the corners of the wound. The skin edges are similarly reapproximated if the wound is large. Alternatively, the apical mesentery can be divided from the colon for a distance of 4 to 5 cm. The supporting fascial bridge is created by reapproximating the fascia through the mesenteric defect.

The colostomy is matured immediately. A small longitudinal incision is made through the anterior tenia, and the lumen is entered. Gas and stool are aspirated. The colotomy wound is lengthened longitudinally for a distance of about 5 cm. Care is taken to avoid damaging the posterior colonic wall. The edges of the colon, incorporating all colonic layers, are sutured to the abdominal wall skin with 3–0 long-term absorbable sutures. A simple appliance is fixed around the stoma.

As an alternative to immediate maturation, the loop of colon can be vented through an indwelling catheter. In this situation, the loop is brought out and fixed to the abdominal wall, as already described. Before the colon is opened, a pursestring suture of 2–0 silk is placed at loop's apex. The colonic wall is divided with electrocautery in the center of the pursestring. Gas is aspirated; then a 28-French rubber catheter is inserted into the colonic lumen and directed proximally. The pursestring is tied, thereby securing the catheter in

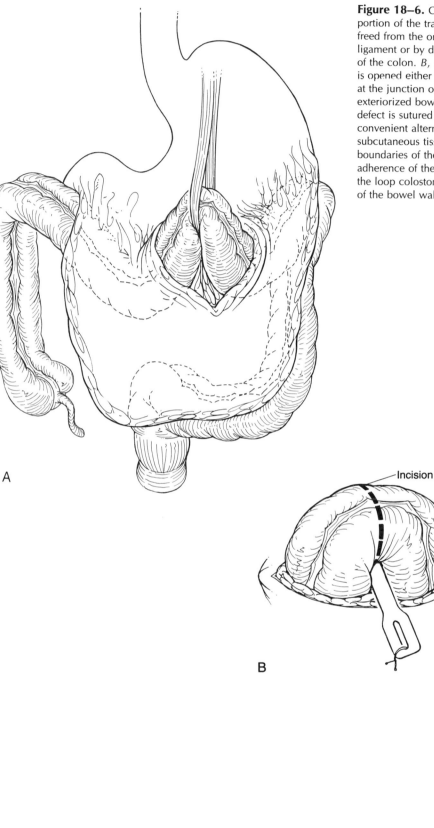

Figure 18–6. Construction of a loop colostomy. *A,* The portion of the transverse colon chosen for the colostomy is freed from the omentum, either through the gastrocolic ligament or by dissection of the omentum off of the free face of the colon. *B,* After exteriorization of the colon, the colon is opened either longitudinally along the tinea or transversely at the junction of the middle and distal one third of the exteriorized bowel. A supporting rod through the mesenteric defect is sutured to the skin adjacent to the stoma. A convenient alternative is to tunnel the supporting rod in the subcutaneous tissue so that it exits the skin outside the boundaries of the appliance, thus allowing 360 degrees of adherence of the appliance to the skin. *C,* The two orifices of the loop colostomy are matured by suturing the full thickness of the bowel wall to the cutaneous defect.

A

Incision

B

C

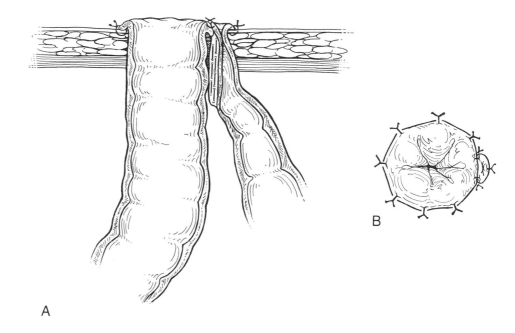

Figure 18–7. End-loop colostomy. *A,* The sigmoid loop, which had previously been divided by a stapler cutting device, is brought out through the abdominal wall. The staple line of the proximal stoma is excised. The distal stoma is allowed to retract into the stomal site, so that only a corner of the bowel is visible above the skin surface. The staples in this small area are then excised. *B,* The large and the small stoma are then matured in the usual fashion.

place. A second pursestring is placed outside the first and is also secured. The catheter is left for bedside drainage for 24 hours.

On the second postoperative day, the catheter is removed and the colostomy matured. This can be done at the bedside by enlarging the anterior colonic wall defect with electrocautery. Care is taken to avoid injury of the posterior colonic wall. This is most effectively accomplished by sliding a clamp into the colotomy and gently lifting the anterior wall off the posterior wall. The bowel wall is divided between the jaws of the clamp. The cut colonic edges generally do not require suture to the abdominal skin.

End-Loop Colostomy

The end-loop colostomy incorporates the best features of both loop stomas and end-stomas. It is readily created, easy to manage, and easy to close.[16] The overall complication rate is low at 12.6%.[17] It is most appropriate for the sigmoid position when colostomy closure is anticipated.

OPERATIVE TECHNIQUE

The sigmoid loop is mobilized in standard fashion. The apex of the loop should reach the anterior abdominal wall without tension. The preoperatively marked stoma site is prepared as described previously. The stomal defect in the abdominal wall should comfortably admit two or three fingers.

The apex of the loop is freed of epiploic appendages. The mesentery is pierced at the colonic margin. The linear cutter-stapler is passed through the mesenteric defect and fired. The entire proximal end and the antimesenteric corner of the distal end are grasped with Babcock clamps, and they are brought through the abdominal wall defect. Some authors recommend "crossing" the intestinal limbs so that the functioning proximal end is inferior to the more cranial, defunctionalized distal limb. We have found that this configuration adds no benefit and can contribute to significant postoperative morbidity. We therefore recommend bringing out the limbs with the functional proximal end superior to the distal limb. The main abdominal incision is closed in standard fashion. The wound is then covered for colostomy maturation (Fig. 18–7).

The proximal bowel end is opened 1 cm above skin level by excising the staple line with electrocautery or scissors. Hemostasis should be perfect. This end is then fixed to the abdominal wall skin with four 3–0 absorbable sutures placed through all colonic layers and the skin edge. Placement of these sutures should avoid the inferior stomal lip where it abuts the antimesenteric corner of the distal limb. This corner is then excised about 1 cm from its point. The resulting opening should be no more than 1 cm in diameter. The small distal stoma is fixed to the larger proximal stoma by two 3–0 absorbable sutures passed through the skin edge, then through all colonic layers of the distal and proximal limbs; finally it is passed back through the skin. Maturation of both stomas is completed by sutures between those already placed. When complete, the distal stoma is hardly visible beneath the larger proximal stoma. A single, clear plastic appliance is placed over both.

"Blow-Hole" Colostomy or Cecostomy

Blow-hole colostomy and cecostomy are reserved almost exclusively for the obstructed, critically ill patient. These stomas usually produce liquid output that is corrosive to the surrounding skin. Pouching is often difficult. The stomas do not completely divert the fecal stream. Often they are no more quickly or safely constructed than a well-formed loop transverse colostomy or loop ileostomy. For these reasons we have essentially abandoned them.

OPERATIVE TECHNIQUE

An 8- to 10-cm abdominal incision is made over the dilated colonic segment. No effort is made to deliver the distended bowel out of the abdominal cavity. The peritoneum is sutured to the bowel with 3–0 absorbable seromuscular sutures. A second layer of 3–0 sutures fixes the fascia to the seromuscular layer. The seal between the colonic and abdominal walls should be watertight. A large-bore needle affixed to suction tubing and connected to suction is passed through the bowel wall. Gas and stool are aspirated. The needle hole is then enlarged by transversely incising the anterior colonic wall. More adequate decompression is performed with suction. The cut edge of the anterior colonic wall is then sutured to the edge of the skin with 3–0 absorbable sutures. A clear plastic pouch is applied over the stoma.

Continent Colostomy

Despite intense efforts, the search for the continent colostomy has been disappointing. Various techniques have been proposed, including magnetic,[18] hydrophilic,[19] and inflatable occlusion devices[20]; muscle transposition[21]; and valved stomas.[22] All are designed to restrict the egress of stool from the stoma. Unfortunately, these techniques are too often surgically difficult or cumbersome to use, or do not result in acceptable continence for most patients. For this reason most surgeons recommend irrigation techniques rather than barrier methods.

Colostomy Closure

Any colostomate with an intact anal sphincter is technically a candidate for colostomy closure. However the patient's age, overall health, and nutritional condition as well as the status and prognosis of the underlying disease process must be considered before any surgery is undertaken. Thoughtful discussion with the patient and those involved in the patient's care should precede surgical planning. Debility or poor prognosis may render some patients poor candidates for stomal closure.

The size and compliance of the remaining rectum and the adequacy of the anal sphincters are also important in determining a patient's suitability for stomal closure. A small, noncompliant rectum contributes to fecal urgency and tenesmus. Incompetence of the sphincters leads to a degree of incontinence. A combination of both factors results in functional impairment that is greater than that caused by either factor alone. If doubt exists about the functional adequacy of the anorectum, manometric analysis is recommended. Conversion from a well-functioning abdominal stoma to an unmanageable perineal colostomy offers no benefit to the patient.

In virtually all patients, preclosure contrast radiography or colonoscopic evaluation of the remaining colon and rectum is strongly suggested. The need for evaluation depends on the disease entity that led to the original stomal surgery. The purpose of these studies is to ensure that the remaining colorectum is disease-free and/or adequately healed.

We defer closure for a minimum of 6 weeks from the initial surgery. This delay allows the stomal end of the colon to become free of inflammation, induration, and edema. A longer delay is indicated in patients in whom the first operation was performed for intraperitoneal sepsis resulting from colonic perforation.[23] The length of the delay is less important than meticulous attention to detail at the time of surgery.[24] Stomal closure is always an elective procedure. Each patient should receive optimal medical preparation before surgery. Thorough mechanical and antibiotic preparation of the colon and rectum is mandatory.[25] Defunctionalized distal segments can be lavaged via the mucous fistula or the anus, or both.[26] A 1% solution of neomycin or kanamycin is recommended for this purpose. An iodophor or a chlorhexidine scrub of the abdominal wall should be performed on the night before surgery.[27]

In the operating room the appliance is removed from the stoma, and any residual adhesive is cleaned from the peristomal skin with acetone or adhesive remover. The iodophor or chlorhexidine scrub of the abdominal wall and peristomal skin is repeated.

End-Colostomy

The surgical plan for closure of the end-colostomy varies, depending on the previous management of the distal segment. The stoma must always be mobilized from its attachments to the skin and returned to the abdominal cavity. A mucous fistula, if present, also needs to be taken down and prepared for anastomosis.

Operative Technique. Traditionally, after the abdomen is entered, the stoma or mucous fistula is mobilized by circumferentially incising the peristomal skin 1 or 2 mm from the mucocutaneous junction. Dissection is continued sharply in the subcutaneous space until the fascia is encountered. Fascial adhesions are divided, and the muscle is retracted. Finally, the peritoneum is freed from the colonic serosa. The open end of the bowel is covered with a sterile glove or rubber dam and is passed through the abdominal wall defect into the abdominal cavity.

Alternatively, passage of the open bowel through the abdominal wall can be avoided by the following technique. After the abdominal skin and peristomal area have been painted with iodophor, the abdominal skin is dried with pads. The abdomen and stoma are covered with an adherent plastic drape (Steri-Drape). The abdomen is entered, usually through the previous scar. The stomal limb is identified. The mesentery of this segment is divided between clamps at the level of the anterior parietal peritoneum. The stomal segment is transected with the linear stapler at the point of its entry into the abdominal wall. The closed bowel end is then free within the abdominal cavity. The small intramural segment of colon is removed from the abdominal wall by circumferential dissection just before the main abdominal incision is closed. Colocolostomy between the stomal and distal segments is performed by sutured or stapled anastomosis, according to standard principles. In patients in whom a small Hartmann pouch has been left distally, a transanal, circular, stapled anastomosis is performed faster and more easily.[28]

End-Colostomy and Hartmann Pouch

Operative Technique. Patients undergoing end-colostomy and Hartmann pouch procedures should be placed in the perineolithotomy position before the start of surgery. Extreme flexion of the hips or knees is unnecessary. The stoma is mobilized as previously described. The pelvic dissection need only expose enough of the top or anterior aspect of the rectal segment to accommodate the stapler cartridge. Locating the rectal wall and inserting the stapler in difficult cases can be facilitated by transanal sigmoidoscopic transillumination.[29]

Once the rectal wall has been identified, a site for the anastomosis is cleared of surrounding structures. The proximal bowel should reach the rectum without tension. The staple line at the proximal colonic end, if present, should be removed with electrocautery. A pursestring suture, applied with staples, or a hand-sewn whipstitch is placed at the bowel end. Every effort should be made to use the largest possible circular stapler.[30] The limiting factor is usually the diameter of the proximal bowel end. Many techniques for dilatation of this end have been described.[31-33] Injection of a few milliliters of 1% lidocaine solution into the colonic smooth muscle usually permits easy

passage of the largest anvil.[33] The anvil is secured by the pursestring or whipstitch suture.

The trocar is placed in the shaft of the stapler, then withdrawn into the instrument. The anus is gently dilated, and the stapler is passed into the rectal segment. The staple cartridge is pressed against the area previously cleared, and the trocar and shaft are advanced through the rectal wall. The trocar is removed from the shaft. The bowel end containing the anvil is brought into the pelvis. The anvil is fitted into the shaft, and the stapler closed. Care is taken to avoid catching any of the surrounding structures in the closing instrument. The stapler is fired. The instrument is opened, carefully passed through the anastomosis, and withdrawn from the anus. Two complete circles of colon and rectum should be recovered from the stapler.

The integrity of the anastomosis can be checked sigmoidoscopically. The proximal colon is occluded with a noncrushing clamp, and the pelvis is filled with saline. The sigmoidoscope is advanced to the level of the anastomosis. There should be no observable anastomotic bleeding and no escape of insufflated air, which would be visible as bubbles arising in the pelvic saline.

Once colocolostomy has been successfully completed, the colostomy defect in the abdominal wall is closed. The fascial edges are reapproximated with no. 1 or 0 long-term, absorbable sutures. These are most easily placed from outside the abdominal wall, once the skin and subcutaneous tissues have been retracted. Closure is performed vertically or transversely, depending on which direction offers the least wound tension. The abdominal contents are returned to anatomic position, and the incision is closed in the preferred fashion. The skin at the stoma site is either packed open or loosely approximated with nylon skin sutures.[34]

Loop Colostomy

In general, a loop colostomy is more easily closed than an end-stoma.[34] The reasons for this lie in the proximity of the bowel ends and the intact blood supply. Formal laparotomy is only rarely necessary.

Operative Technique. In all patients, both stomal limbs must be completely mobilized from their attachments to the abdominal wall. This can usually be accomplished through a circumstomal incision. Dissection is continued into the abdominal cavity, and any peristomal adhesions are divided. The bowel ends are delivered onto the abdominal wall, and the wound edges are protected with pads or towels. Any skin and devitalized tissue adherent to the bowel wall are excised with electrocautery. The ends should be soft and well vascularized and should lie in proximity to each other without tension. This sometimes requires complete excision of the portion that formed the stoma.

Local factors and the surgeon's preference determine the type of anastomosis to be performed. Choices include hand-sewn or stapled primary end-to-end anastomosis after resection of the stomal ends, hand-sewn or stapled closure of the colostomy defect, or functional end-to-end stapled anastomosis. All should yield similarly satisfactory results, provided that the colonic ends are free of inflammation, tension, and ischemia.[24]

Colostomy Complications

Major or minor problems complicate the course of up to 44% of all colostomies.[35] Many minor difficulties, such as peristomal irritation, can be solved by patient education and intensive enterostomal therapy. Others, such as high stomal output, often respond to dietary manipulation. Significant complications often require surgical correction.

Colostomy complications can arbitrarily be divided into two groups: early and late. Early complications tend to occur within the 30-day postoperative period. These include stomal ischemia, retraction or separation, infection, and bleeding. Late complications can occur at any time during the life of the colostomate. Common late complications include parastomal herniation, prolapse, and stenosis.[36]

Early Complications

ISCHEMIA

Insufficient blood supply to the distal colon causes stomal ischemia or even gangrene. This problem is more common in end-colostomies. Insufficient colonic mobilization leading to stomal tension, overly vigorous "stripping" of the mesentery, and a thick abdominal wall all contribute to its genesis.[37] The stoma appears dusky, cyanotic, or even black, rather than the normal pink, on the first or second postoperative day.

The extent of the ischemic process can be ascertained by gently inserting an empty glass test tube in the stoma and observing the mucosa with the aid of a bright light. If the mucosa is dusky or frankly gangrenous to below the level of the fascia, urgent colostomy revision is indicated. If the ischemic process is limited to the subcutaneous portion of the colon, immediate reoperation is usually not necessary. However, the ischemic stoma frequently becomes stenotic or retracted.[37] These complications often require elective revision.

HEMORRHAGE

Early postoperative bleeding from the lumen of the stoma is an uncommon event. When it occurs, it often signifies stomal or juxtastomal ischemia.[38] This is usually evident when the mucosa is inspected, as previously described. Stomal mucosal lacerations or ulcerations can also be visualized by means of this technique. Bleeding from these sources is usually self-limited in the patient with adequate coagulation parameters.

Bleeding from the colostomy can also be caused by a gastrointestinal lesion proximal to the stoma. In the early postoperative period, these can include surgical errors such as laceration or devascularization of a more proximal segment or inadequate hemostasis of a proximal suture or staple line. "Medical" bleeding from gastritis or ulcer diathesis is also possible and requires exclusion. The evaluation as well as the management of this complication should parallel that in any patient with gastrointestinal bleeding. However, rapid blood loss leading to hypovolemic shock or an ongoing transfusion requirement in the immediate postoperative period is usually most effectively handled by emergent re-exploration.

More commonly, early postoperative bleeding arises from the mucocutaneous junction. This bleeding is often caused by transected cutaneous or mesenteric vessels at or just under the skin of the stoma site. They can be adequately managed by the placement of a small 3–0 chromic catgut figure-eight suture at the bleeding point. If this maneuver fails in the setting of a transrectus colostomy, one should suspect disruption of the inferior epigastric vessels. Persistent bleeding from this source often requires operative management.

Bleeding from the stoma after the perioperative period has passed is a less common event. Irritation or frank laceration caused by an ill-fitting appliance is the most frequent cause. This problem is usually solved by reassessing pouching materials and techniques. In patients with Crohn's disease or carcinoma, recurrent disease as a cause of bleeding must be excluded.

An infrequent but particularly troublesome form of late stomal bleeding deserves mention. Patients with portal hypertension can develop an extensive network of microcirculatory portosystemic shunts in the peristomal skin. This problem can involve either a colostomy or an ileostomy.[39, 40]

Unlike esophageal varices, the colocutaneous varices are small, numerous, and prominent in the dermal and subcutaneous layers of the skin, rather than in the submucosal layer of the bowel. The peristomal skin is thin and shows a mottled, violaceous discoloration. The abdominal wall resembles a target with the stomal "bull's eye" surrounded by a bluish halo.

Bleeding is sporadic, unexpected, and vigorous.[41] The patient can lose blood at a very rapid rate. The patient typically feels nothing but notices that the appliance has filled with red blood. The site of bleeding is usually located on the peristomal skin, within 1 or 2 mm of the mucocutaneous junction. In our experience, bleeding from a mucosal site is uncommon.

Patients with this complication must be carefully instructed in its emergency management. The appliance and faceplate are carefully removed, and direct pressure is applied to the stomal area with a folded hand towel. This procedure allows the patient to reach the office or hospital without incurring even more severe blood loss.

Often bleeding has ceased by the time the patient comes to medical attention. If not, the source is obvious. Control in the emergency situation is best achieved, in our experience, by suture ligation. Absorbable, 2–0 figure-eight sutures placed parallel to the stomal circumference are most effective. Blood loss during this procedure can be significant, because the needle sites also tend to bleed. Injectional sclerotherapy has been attempted by others in this situation with some success.[42]

If the bleeding has already stopped at the time of examination, the site is often visible as a small, cherry-red papule. Cautery with silver nitrate or electrosurgical current, or an attempt at suture ligation will almost certainly renew bleeding. Observation without further intervention is warranted.

The best definitive management of this problem involves resolution of the portal hypertension by intra- or extrahepatic portosystemic shunting[41] or by liver transplantation.[43] If none of these options is viable, mucocutaneous disconnection or stomal revision by relocation offers a temporarily solution.[44]

RETRACTION AND SEPARATION

Disruption of the mucocutaneous junction is most apt to occur by the end of the first postoperative week. It almost always results from a technical error committed at the time of stomal creation. Contributing factors include peristomal infection, stomal ischemia, and inadequate colonic mobilization leading to tension in the stomal limb.[9]

Retraction below the level of the fascia requires immediate operative repair. Partial dehiscence often heals by secondary intention with appropriate local wound care. Systemic antibiotics are indicated when an element of cellulitis is present. Stenosis is a frequent sequela.

INFECTION

Infection at the stoma site involves the abdominal wall skin or subcutaneous tissues. Cellulitis that appears before the stoma begins to function is caused by bacterial seeding of the colostomy aperture at the time of surgery. This complication is most easily managed by débridement of devitalized tissue and by drainage of any parastomal collection that is present. Systemic antibiotics are indicated for all but the most localized processes.

Diabetic, steroid-dependent, and otherwise immu-nocompromised patients are more prone to a devastating mixed-organism infection of the deeper subcutaneous tissues and fascia. This rapidly spreading, necrotizing fasciitis presents with signs of systemic toxicity, peristomal erythema, and thin, serosanguineous drainage from the mucocutaneous junction. This complication, although infrequent, carries a disproportionately high mortality rate. The keystones of management are early recognition and aggressive surgical treatment. Broad-spectrum antibiotics, wide débridement of devitalized tissue, and relocation of the stoma are almost always required.[45]

Late Complications

PARASTOMAL HERNIA

Paracolostomy herniation is one of the most common late complications of colostomy.[46] Small hernias often contain the juxtastomal colonic wall. Larger hernias can contain intra-abdominal contents, such as omentum, small bowel, and colon. Hernias can cause pain, obstructive symptoms, problems with pouching, and difficulty in wearing clothes. Smaller hernias are more likely than larger ones to incarcerate and cause strangulation. A paracolostomy hernia increases the risk of colonic perforation during colostomy irrigation, especially if a catheter is used.

In general, parastomal hernias are best managed by surgical repair. Stomal binders or belts in conjunction with special faceplates may ameliorate, but not permanently correct, problems with pain and the ability to wear certain kinds of clothing. Nonsurgical therapy is usually reserved for patients whose overall health or prognosis is poor or for those who have undergone numerous procedures resulting in extensive abdominal wall scarring or deformity. It is also valuable as a temporizing measure prior to a planned colostomy closure.

Direct fascial suture of the defect after excision of the sac is possible in some patients. This method of treatment is reserved for small hernias. The incidence of recurrence increases with the size of the hernia. Effective surgical repair of a large or recurrent paracolostomy hernia usually involves relocation of the stoma and closure of the old defect.[47]

Preoperative preparation for this operation, as for any stomal surgery, includes antibiotic and mechanical bowel preparation, and careful selection and marking of the new stoma site. It is sometimes possible to relocate the new stoma via the hernia itself, thus obviating the need for formal laparotomy. This approach is feasible especially if the midline is chosen for the new site. Management of the hernia itself follows standard principles. Synthetic mesh is useful for closing extremely large defects or for reinforcing the parastomal region when relocation is not practical.[48] Mesh

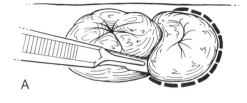

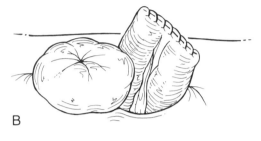

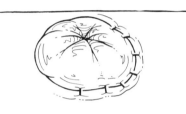

Figure 18–8. Conversion of a loop colostomy to an end-colostomy, usually for prolapse. *A,* The defunctionalized loop is dissected free from the skin, and the bridge of colon connecting the two loops is divided. *B,* The end of the distal limb is closed and replaced into the abdominal wall as a long Hartmann pouch. The fascial defect is closed. *C,* The medial wall of the proximal loop is then matured to the cutaneous defect in the usual fashion.

increases the chance of wound infection and later fistula formation, however.

PROLAPSE

Stomal prolapse occurs more frequently with loop colostomies than with end-stomas or end-loop stomas.[17, 49] Contributing factors include an overly large fascial defect, emergency surgery for distal obstruction, and mobility of the stomal mesentery.

Loop Colostomy. Some investigators report prolapse as the most common complication of loop colostomy.[50, 51] The prolapse usually involves intussusception of the efferent limb, although either limb or both limbs may be affected.

It is almost always possible to reduce the prolapsed stoma manually so that elective repair can be undertaken after standard bowel preparation. Bed rest, iced astringents, and patience are often necessary. The best definitive treatment of stomal prolapse is reversal of the colostomy. If this is not possible, the procedure must be tailored to the individual patient. Laparotomy is often unnecessary, and general anesthesia can frequently be avoided.

If colostomy closure is not feasible, conversion from a loop stoma to an end-, end-loop, or double-barrel colostomy is preferable. The stoma should be reduced before surgery if possible. Both limbs of the stoma are freed to the level of the peritoneum through a circumstomal skin incision. The loop and redundant proximal and distal colon are delivered through the stomal defect.

The type of reconstructed stoma selected depends on local circumstances and the surgeon's preference. In almost all cases the fascial defect requires narrowing prior to final maturation of the chosen stoma.

Operative Technique. If the original stoma was created because of unresolvable complete or partial distal obstruction, some type of mucous fistula is mandatory. In this situation, we prefer the end-loop stoma to the double-barrel variant, because the former is more easily pouched.[17] The redundant proximal and distal colon are divided with the linear stapler-cutter 1 or 2 cm above skin level. The mesentery of the excluded loop is divided, and the colonic segment is removed. The fascia is closed about the bowel with heavy, long-term absorbable sutures. A double-barrel or end-loop colostomy is fashioned as previously described.

If distal obstruction is not present, conversion to a true end-stoma is recommended. The redundant colon is transected proximally 1 or 2 cm above skin level.

The distal portion is closed with staples or sutures and returned to the abdominal cavity as a long Hartmann pouch. Resection of distal redundancy is not necessary. The fascial defect is narrowed with heavy, long-term absorbable sutures so that the fascia snugly approximates the protruding colon. The proximal lumen is matured as a standard end-stoma (Fig. 18–8).

In patients in whom preoperative reduction is not possible, the prolapsed stoma is "unrolled" after all layers of the everted colonic wall are circumferentially incised 1 or 2 cm from the mucocutaneous junction. This approach gives access to the intussuscepted colon that is immediately subjacent. One or both limbs may be found. The colon can be further unrolled or resected just above skin level.

An alternate technique for managing the prolapsed loop colostomy involves a modification of the Delorme procedure for treatment of rectal prolapse. We have found this technique more cumbersome and less successful than those already described.

End-Colostomy. The approach to the prolapsed end-stoma is essentially the same as that for prolapsed loop colostomies.

Operative Technique. For the mature stoma, a circumferential incision is begun in the mucosa of the everted colon, approximately 1 cm from the mucocutaneous junction. If the stoma is less than 6 months old, the incision is made at the mucocutaneous junction. The colon is unrolled, and the redundant mesentery is ligated and divided. The protruding portion of colon is shortened by excision to within 5 cm of the skin surface. The fascia is closed around the colon, if necessary, and the new stoma is matured as previously described (Fig. 18–9).

STRICTURE

Stomal stricture results from technical errors committed at the time of colostomy creation. The patient presents with obstructive symptoms when narrowing exceeds a critical level. Stenosis frequently involves the mucocutaneous junction or the subcutaneous segment of colon. Less commonly, the fascial defect is too tight. Simple digital examination establishes the point of stenosis. Surgical repair, rather than stomal dilatation, is the preferred management.

Treatment of stomal stricture by formal revision of the stoma is recommended, unless the point of narrowing is clearly limited to the peristomal skin. Stenotic scar formation occasionally recurs if treated by simple excision. In these cases, repair by Z-plasty offers a better solution (see further on). Z-plasty trades stomal length for increased stomal diameter. It is therefore an unsuitable technique for the stenotic and retracted colostomy, unless the colon can be mobilized at the time of repair.

Operative Technique. Stomal revision is begun through a circumstomal incision. Dissection is continued to the peritoneum, thereby liberating the entire stomal limb. The colon can usually be delivered at least 2 or 3 cm into the wound. If this is not possible or the length obtained is inadequate, formal laparotomy is indicated so that further colonic mobility can be obtained. In either case, the length of colon brought through the old stoma site should be sufficiently long so that the stenotic portion can be excised and a new stoma fashioned. The stoma is matured in the usual manner with 3–0 long-term absorbable sutures.

ILEOSTOMY

As with colostomy, ileostomy surgery has evolved dramatically since its first application in the nineteenth century.[52] The earliest ileostomies were used to treat patients with obstructing proximal colonic malignancies. In the beginning of the twentieth century, ileostomy creation for "bowel rest" in patients with chronic ulcerative colitis was described.[53] At that time, ileostomy was a procedure of last resort, carrying an associated mortality rate of nearly 30%.[54] Stomal management was nightmarish.[55] The first practical ileostomy appliance did not appear until 1944.[56]

The first ileostomies were often complicated by an early obstructive syndrome referred to as "ileostomy dysfunction."[57] This syndrome resulted from an obstructing serositis of the exteriorized limb. The elegant contributions of Brooke[58] and Crile and Turnbull[59] solved this problem, and their technique of ileostomy creation remains the standard. Currently, ileostomy is most commonly employed in the management of inflammatory bowel disease. Multiple stomal variants have been perfected to serve different needs.

Unlike a colostomy, an ileostomy almost constantly discharges liquid stool. Output averages 400 to 700 ml/day and rarely varies more than 20% with dietary manipulation.[60] The effluent causes irritation if left in contact with the skin. For these reasons, all ileostomies, with the exception of the continent ileostomy, require a "spout" protruding from the abdominal wall to effect adequate pouching. Technical variants include the end-, loop, loop-end, and continent ileostomies.

Ileostomy Construction

Preoperative preparation for ileostomy should be undertaken in conjunction with the enterostomal therapist whenever possible. Selection of the best-possible stoma site can avert many potential problems. The

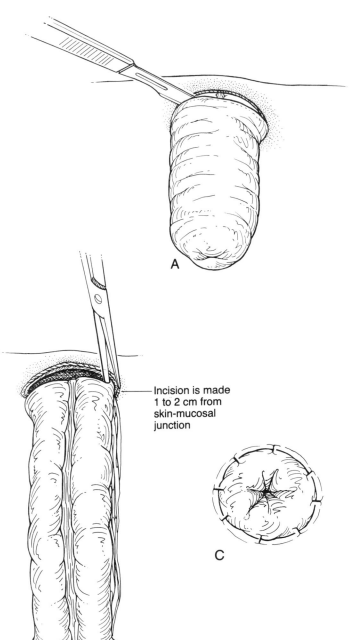

Incision is made
1 to 2 cm from
skin-mucosal
junction

A

B

C

Figure 18–9. Repair of a prolapsed end-colostomy. *A*, A circular incision is made in the mucosa of approximately 1 cm distal to the mucocutaneous junction. The prolapsed colon is then "unrolled," and the redundant mesentery is ligated. *B*, The redundant mesentery and bowel wall are then divided. The protruding portion of the colon is shortened to within 4 to 5 cm of the skin surface. The fascia is closed around the colon if necessary. *C*, The new stoma is matured in the usual fashion.

area chosen should be easily accessible to the patient, at a distance from bony prominences, and free from scars, creases, and depressions that might interfere with effective pouching.[5] When possible, the patient should be asked to stand, sit, bend at the waist, and wear clothing in order to ascertain that there is no conflict between these activities and the chosen site. The area selected should be indelibly marked on the abdominal skin. Mechanical and antibiotic bowel preparation is also part of the preoperative regimen in the case of an elective operation.

End-Ileostomy

End-ileostomy or Brooke ileostomy is the "gold standard" with which other types of ileostomy are compared. It is usually performed in conjunction with colectomy, ileocolectomy, or ileal resection.

OPERATIVE TECHNIQUE
In all patients with benign disease, the line of ileal transection should be as close to the colon or to the limit of diseased intestine as is possible. Preservation of the ileocolic vessels is encouraged whenever possible, especially if inflammatory disease exists or if restorative proctocolectomy is contemplated. The ileum is divided with the linear cutter-stapler. Any antimesenteric fat is trimmed away with electrocautery.

The technique for creation of the stomal aperature is essentially the same as that described for the colostomy. Towel clamps are used to stabilize the cut edges of the peritoneum, fascia, and skin on the marked side of the abdomen. The center of the mark is grasped with a Kocher or an Allis clamp, and traction is applied away from the abdominal wall. A circle of skin measuring 2 cm in diameter is excised with electrocautery.

The surgeon applies upward pressure to a laparotomy pad placed against the peritoneal surface of the ileostomy site while an assistant maintains medial traction on the abdominal wall. The subcutaneous fat is left in place, and sharp and blunt dissection is continued to the level of the rectus abdominis muscle sheath. The anterior rectus sheath is opened by a 2-cm cruciate incision made with electrocautery. The rectus muscle is split in the direction of its fibers, and medial and lateral portions are retracted away from the middle. Care is exercised to avoid lacerating the inferior epigastric vessels located posterior to the rectus muscle. The posterior rectus sheath or transversalis fascia and peritoneum are divided vertically with electrocautery, thereby exposing the intra-abdominal pad. The defect in the abdominal wall should be large enough to admit two fingers.

The stoma is fashioned from the terminal 5 to 6 cm of ileum. The finished stoma need protrude only 2 to 3 cm from skin level. The mesentery of the stomal segment often requires division or resection, so that the ileum can comfortably be brought through the abdominal wall without bowing or tension. This procedure can be accomplished without interruption of the blood supply if the vessels are first identified by transilluminating the mesentery. If restorative proctocolectomy is planned for a later time, division of vascular arcades should be avoided whenever possible (Figs. 18–10 and 18–11).

Extraperitoneal end-ileostomy has been advocated for the permanent end-stoma. The technique is similar to that of extraperitoneal colostomy. The ileum is brought to the abdominal wall aperture through a tunnel under the right parietal peritoneum. The advantage of this technical variation lies in the lowered risk of small bowel volvulus around the stomal limb. This type of stoma, however, is much more difficult to mobilize for closure or revision.[9] It is also more difficult to clear of obstructing undigested fiber when necessary.

Intraperitoneal ileostomy remains our procedure of choice. A Babcock clamp is passed from outside into the abdominal cavity through the abdominal wall defect. The stapled ileal end is grasped and gently pulled onto the abdominal wall. Care should be exercised to prevent tearing the mesentery or twisting the intestine. About 5 cm of ileum is exteriorized in this fashion (Fig. 18–12).

Before the abdominal wound is closed and the stoma matured, the free edge of the ileal mesentery is sutured to the right parietal peritoneum. This partitions the abdominal cavity, effectively preventing small bowel volvulus. The mesenteric edge is brought in proximity to the parietal peritoneum by removing any retractors opening the abdominal cavity. A running 3–0 long-term absorbable suture is placed from the point where the ileum enters the abdominal wall to the falciform ligament. Care is taken to ensure that none of the mesenteric vessels is pierced or ligated with this suture. The abdominal wound is closed according to the surgeon's preference.

Maturation of the stoma is performed after the skin of the main abdominal incision is closed. The wound is covered with sterile towels. The staple line is sharply excised from the terminal ileum. Bleeding from the cut edge should be brisk, and the mucosa pink. After adequate blood supply to the terminal end has been ascertained, meticulous hemostasis is induced with electrocautery.

The stoma is matured by eversion. This is achieved by placing four, three-point sutures of 3–0 long-term, absorbable material. The first two sutures are placed on either side of the mesentery. The third and fourth are placed at points of the ileal circumference opposite the first two (Fig. 18–13).

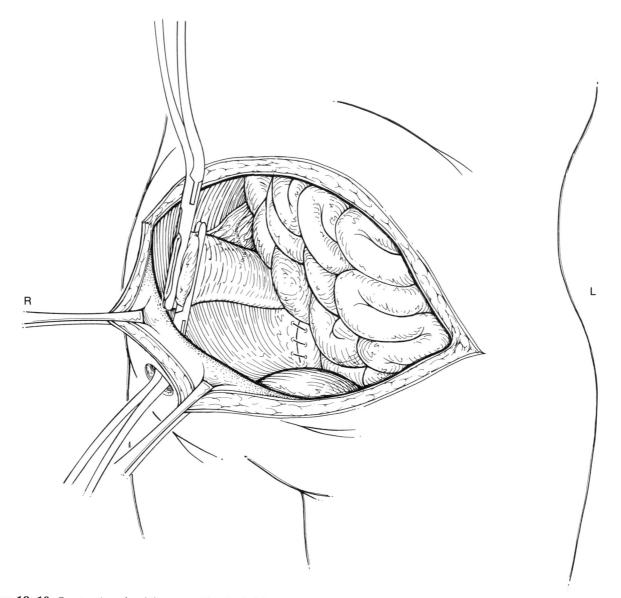

Figure 18–10. Construction of end-ileostomy. The divided ileum is delivered through the previously prepared stomal defect with noncrushing clamps so that the cut mesentery of the terminal ileum is at the right oblique of the patient. The protruding ileum extends approximately 4 cm from the skin edge so that when everted on itself it will be approximately 2 cm in height.

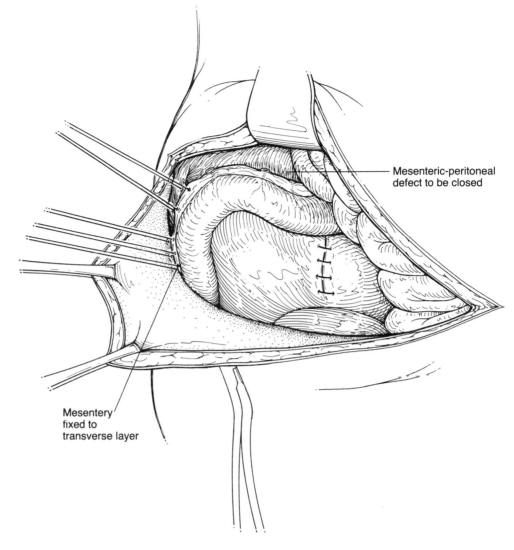

Figure 18–11. Construction of intraperitoneal ileostomy. The mesentery of the ileum is sutured to the transverse layer at the edge of the stomal defect in the abdominal wall with stout nonabsorbable sutures. Usually, two to three sutures suffice, and this guards against ileostomy prolapse. The remaining mesenteric-peritoneal defect is then serially closed to obliterate the defect in the right gutter and to obviate the occurrence of paraileostomy hernia.

Each suture is first passed through all layers of the cut edge of ileum, then through the seromuscular layer of the stoma at skin level, and finally through the dermal layer of skin. The seromuscular bites of all four sutures should be at the same level relative to the skin and should be approximately 4 cm from the cut edge. None of the sutures is tied until all are in place. The edge of the bowel should roll over and down as the sutures are tied. The complete stomal circumference is approximated to the skin edge by placing 3–0 sutures between the four anchoring sutures. Usually, six to eight more sutures will be required. These are passed through all layers of the ileal edge, then through the subcuticular layer of the skin. Penetration of the epidermis should be avoided to prevent ectopic implantation of ileal mucosa and hypertrophic scar formation along the suture tracts. The completed stoma should protrude 2 or 3 cm from the abdominal wall. A clear plastic, one-piece pouch is applied, and the main wound is dressed.

Loop Ileostomy

Loop ileostomy is most commonly constructed in conjunction with restorative proctocolectomy.[61] Less frequently, this type of stoma is indicated to effect emergency decompression of an obstructing proximal colon lesion or to protect a tenuous proximal colonic suture line.[62] It is also valuable for the unusual situation in which an end-stoma does not comfortably reach the skin surface through a fatty abdominal wall.

OPERATIVE TECHNIQUE

The loop of ileum chosen for the stoma should reach the anterior abdominal wall without tension. All layers of the abdominal wall are placed under tension, and a

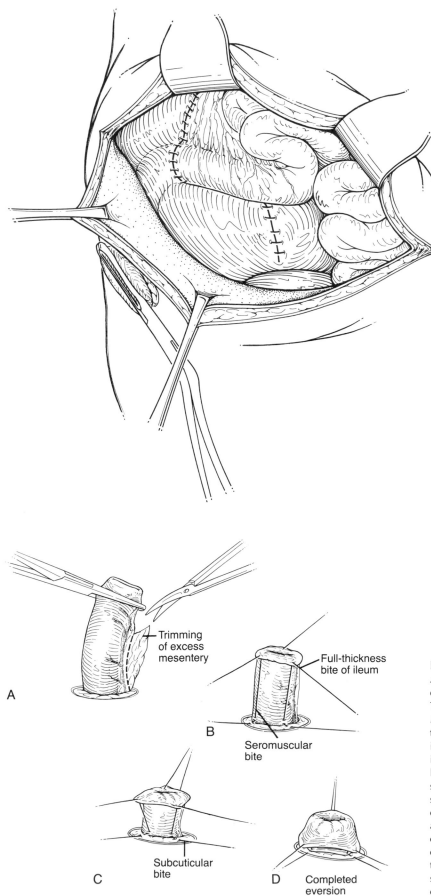

Figure 18–12. Construction of an extraperitoneal ileostomy. A tunnel is made from the incised pelvic peritoneum to the site immediately underlying the proposed stoma. The ileum is then tunneled through this defect to exit at the previously marked stoma. As in the intraperitoneal ileostomy, the mesentery of the small bowel is fixed to the transversalis fascia adjacent to the stomal defect. The peritoneum is then brought down over the ileostomy and its mesentery, thus obliterating the gutter defect on the right. Any mesenteric-peritoneal defect remaining is then closed as shown.

A

Trimming of excess mesentery

B

Full-thickness bite of ileum

Seromuscular bite

C

Subcuticular bite

D   Completed eversion

Figure 18–13. Construction of Brooke ileostomy. *A*, The ileal mesentery is trimmed so as to avoid excess mesenteric tissue at the site of the stoma. The terminal arcade is scrupulously preserved. *B*, The first sutures are placed at positions twelve, three, six, and nine o'clock. The sutures incorporate the full thickness of the end of the ileum and a bite of the seromuscular wall at the level of the abdominal wall, and exit in a subcuticular manner through the skin. *C*, The sutures are serially tied to effect eversion. The original protrusion of the ileostomy was approximately 4 cm. Tying these sutures with eversion results in a 2-cm stoma. *D*, Following eversion with the stay sutures, the construction of the ileostomy is completed by sutures through the subcuticular layer of the skin and the full thickness of the outer layer of the everted ileostomy.

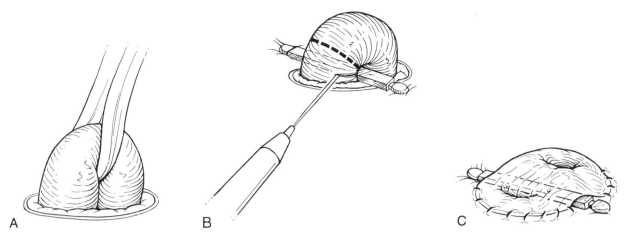

Figure 18–14. Construction of loop ileostomy. *A,* The loop stoma is brought through the fascial cutaneous defect with a Penrose drain so that there is no tension. *B,* The ileostomy is partially divided on the anterior surface at the junction of the middle and distal one third. *C,* The ileostomy is matured over the rod in a method similar to that for the construction of an end-ileostomy.

2-cm disk of skin is excised from the anterior abdominal wall at the previously marked site. The subcutaneous fat is resected as a cylinder to the level of the fascia. The fascia is incised, and the rectus abdominis muscle split. In contrast to the opening for the end-ileostomy, the defect for the loop stoma should generously accommodate two fingers.

The mesentery of the stomal loop is pierced at the bowel margin, and a rubber drain is passed through this hole to encircle the bowel. The tubing is passed through the abdominal wall defect, and the ileal loop eased through the abdominal wall. Although some researchers advocate twisting the loop so that the proximal end is dependent,[63] we have found that this maneuver seems to promote intestinal obstruction. We believe that the loop is more easily brought out as it lies anatomically, with the proximal limb superior to the distal limb. In either case, the surgeon must be certain which limb is proximal and which distal. Maturation of the wrong end while leaving the proximal end flush, leads to intractable pouching problems.

The apex of the loop should extend about 5 cm beyond the level of the skin. The rubber drain is removed and replaced by a glass or plastic rod. The rod is held in place by suturing it to the abdominal skin or by passing a piece of rubber tubing from end to end. If the rod is sutured, it should be eccentrically placed with a larger aperture left for the proximal stoma. The abdominal incision is closed in standard fashion and covered with a sterile towel.

The stoma is matured immediately. The loop is placed on gentle traction away from the abdominal wall. A partially circumferential incision is made through the wall of the distal ileal limb just above skin level. This incision should extend from mesenteric border to mesenteric border. The proximal end is everted by placing four three-point sutures of 3–0 long-term absorbable material. This is most easily accomplished by placing two paramesenteric sutures first. Each should pass through the cut ileal edge, then through the seromuscular layer at skin level, and finally through the dermis of the stomal opening. These sutures should penetrate the skin close to the rod on the side of the proximal limb. Two more three-point sutures are similarly placed on the antimesenteric side of the proximal limb. The proximal limb everts when all four sutures are tied. The stoma is completed by placement of 3–0 sutures between those already in place. The distal lumen is also fixed to the dermis with simple 3–0 long-term absorbable sutures. The mesenteric border of the loop should fit snugly, not tightly, against the rod when the stoma is complete. All skin sutures should be confined to the dermal layer. The completed stoma is pouched in the operating room. The rod is ready for removal when it slides back and forth easily under the stoma, usually in 7 to 10 days (Fig. 18–14).

End-Loop Ileostomy

The end-loop ileostomy is a rodless variant of the standard loop stoma. It is used in the same settings as the standard loop ileostomy. The end-loop variant is more easily pouched in the early postoperative period because of its smaller size and absent rod. This advantage fades once the rod is removed from the standard loop ileostomy. Proponents of the end-loop stoma also claim that this arrangement offers more complete diversion because of a smaller distal lumen.[17]

OPERATIVE TECHNIQUE

The stomal opening in the abdominal wall is created as previously described. The ileal loop chosen for the stoma is divided with the linear cutter-stapler. The mesentery abutting the point of transection is divided for a distance of about 10 cm. This permits the proximal limb to be drawn out of the abdominal cavity without "dragging" the distal limb along with it.

The proximal end and the antimesenteric corner of the distal end are brought out through the abdominal wall defect. The proximal limb should extend 5 cm

above skin level. The main abdominal wound is closed in standard fashion and covered with a sterile towel.

The staple line of the proximal limb is resected with electrocautery. The "point" of the antimesenteric distal corner is removed with heavy scissors. The proximal end is matured in the same fashion as a standard end-ileostomy. The small, distal lumen is sutured to the dermis as a mucous fistula. Two transition sutures are placed at the points where the proximal and distal lumina touch each other. These sutures pass through the dermis, through the proximal ileal wall, through the distal ileal wall, and back through the dermis. The finished stoma is pouched in the same fashion as that for an end-stoma.

Continent Ileostomy

The continent ileostomy, or Kock pouch, introduced by Professor Nils Kock in the 1960s was the culmination of a decades-long search for an alternative to the standard ileostomy.[64] Unlike an end-ileostomy or its variants, the continent ileostomy consists of an internal reservoir, valve mechanism, and flush stoma. Fecal waste is eliminated via a catheter passed into the reservoir through the stoma.

Continent ileostomy is a therapeutic option primarily for patients with chronic ulcerative colitis and familial adenomatous polyposis coli. It is the only alternative to standard ileostomy after colectomy when the anal sphincter mechanism has been destroyed by surgery or disease. Although the need for reservoir ileostomy has diminished with the advent of restorative proctocolectomy by ileal pouch–anal anastomosis, some patients still choose continent ileostomy as a primary or secondary procedure.[65] Careful patient education and selection continue to be of paramount importance. The contraindications to continent ileostomy have not changed: Crohn's disease, emergency surgery, suboptimal immunologic or nutritional status, short-bowel syndrome, extreme youth or age, obesity, and inability to intubate the pouch because of mental or physical impairment.[66]

Preoperative management includes mechanical and antibiotic bowel preparation, enterostomal counseling, and marking of the proposed stoma site. The continent stoma traverses the midportion of the rectus abdominis muscle, but it is placed lower in the iliac fossa.

OPERATIVE TECHNIQUE
The abdomen is entered via a midline incision. Proctocolectomy, if indicated, is performed in the standard fashion. Every effort is made to preserve the maximal ileal length. The terminal ileum is transected at the cecal margin. If a standard ileostomy is present, it should be freed from the skin and reduced into the abdominal cavity.

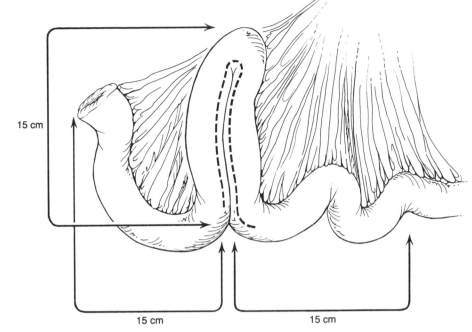

15 cm

15 cm   15 cm

Figure 18–15. Construction of a Kock pouch. Schematic representation. The terminal ileum is utilized so that four segments of ileum are involved in the construction. The most distal portion measures approximately 15 cm and will be the efferent limb of the pouch. The middle portion is two loops of ileum, each measuring 15 cm in length, which will be the body of the pouch. The most proximal portion is the afferent limb, which also measures 15 cm.

The continent ileostomy is constructed from the terminal 45 cm of ileum. The most distal 15 cm becomes the nipple valve and stoma (the "outflow tract"), and the adjacent 30 cm becomes the reservoir. The antimesenteric border of the ileum is grasped with a Babcock clamp 30 cm from the cut end. This distance should actually be measured with a scalpel handle or a sterile ruler. The bowel is folded on itself with the 30-cm point resting at the apex of the loop. We have found that sutures are preferable to staples in pouch construction, because the suture lines stretch as the pouch matures. Staple lines remain as constricting rings when the pouch dilates (Fig. 18–15).

The antimesenteric borders of the ileum proximal and distal to the 30-cm mark are joined by a running suture of 2–0 long-term absorbable material. Each limb is opened with electrocautery, thereby creating two longitudinal enterotomies running parallel to the suture line. The incision in the afferent limb is continued proximally 2.5 cm beyond the distal termination of the incision in the efferent limb. This procedure allows the afferent and efferent limbs to be separated once the pouch is closed. Both enterotomies are continued to the tip of the loop, where they meet. A second layer of 2–0 long-term absorbable sutures joins the two cut edges. This leaves a U-shaped pouch of small bowel open toward the inflow and outflow tracts (Fig. 18–16).

The nipple valve is constructed from the 10 cm of distal ileum immediately adjacent to the pouch. Once intussuscepted, the valve will be 5 cm long. This segment is prepared for intussusception by thinning its mesentery and denuding its serosal surface. Mesenteric bulk is reduced by excising the fat between the vessels. Extreme care is taken to avoid injury to the blood supply. The serosal surface is denuded of peritoneum by rubbing it with a fine rasp and scoring it with electrocautery. We have also found that scattered subserosal injections totaling 5 ml of a solution of 100 mg/ml of tetracycline are helpful. Three 2–0 silk sutures are placed on both sides of the mesenteric border in such a fashion that, when tied, they maintain the intussusception. These sutures are passed proximally and distally, equidistant from the point of intussusception, 3, 5, and 7 cm apart (Figs. 18–17 and 18–18).

A Babcock clamp is passed into the outflow tract from the pouch side to grasp the midpoint of the valve. As the ileum is intussuscepted by gentle traction into the pouch, the previously placed silk sutures are sequentially tied. The valve is further stabilized by three rows of staples placed on either side of the mesentery and the antimesenteric border. These are most easily placed with a *bladeless* linear stapler-cutter. Six to eight 3–0 silk sutures are passed through all layers of the valve to stabilize the intussusception further. A row of interrupted 3–0 silk sutures fixes the base of the valve to the surrounding pouch wall at its point of exit (Figs. 18–19 and 18–20).

The pouch is closed by bringing the apex of the U to the apex of the enterotomy in the afferent limb. A double layer of 3–0 long-term absorbable sutures closes the enterotomy and completes the pouch. Competence of the valve is tested by occlusion of the inflow tract with an intestinal clamp. A bullet-nosed catheter is

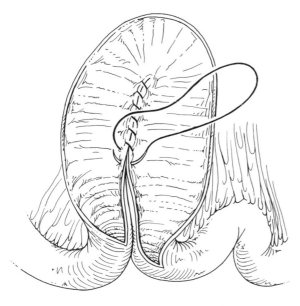

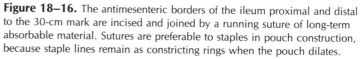

Figure 18–16. The antimesenteric borders of the ileum proximal and distal to the 30-cm mark are incised and joined by a running suture of long-term absorbable material. Sutures are preferable to staples in pouch construction, because staple lines remain as constricting rings when the pouch dilates.

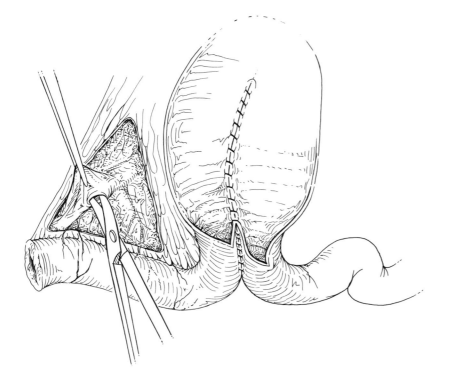

Figure 18–17. The nipple valve is constructed from 10 cm of the distal ileum immediately adjacent to the pouch. Once constructed, the valve will be 5 cm long. This segment is prepared for intussusception by thinning its mesentery and denuding its serosal surface. Extreme care is taken to avoid injury to the blood supply. The pouch's inner layer has been completed by joining the two parallel enterotomies with absorbable continuous suture.

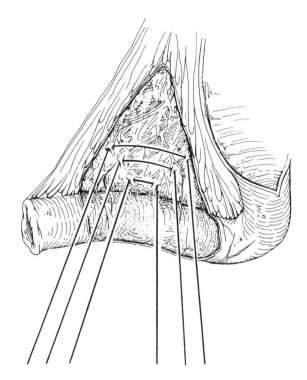

Figure 18–18. The denuded and defatted mesentery is brought together so as to maintain an intussusception by several silk sutures as illustrated. Note the defatting of the mesentery and the excision of the serosa from the portion of bowel to be intussuscepted. Sutures should be at the intestinal margin.

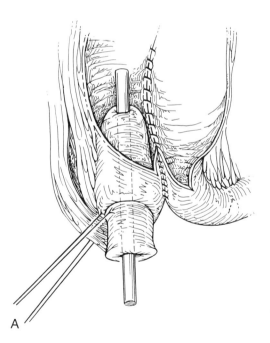

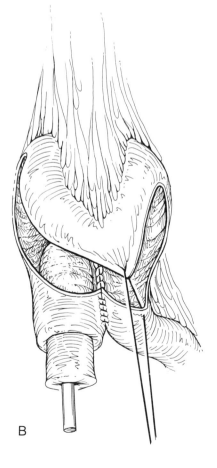

Figure 18–19. The ileum is intussuscepted by gentle traction into the pouch. The valve is stabilized by three rows of interrupted 3-0 silk sutures at the base of the valve to the surrounding pouch wall at its point of exit.

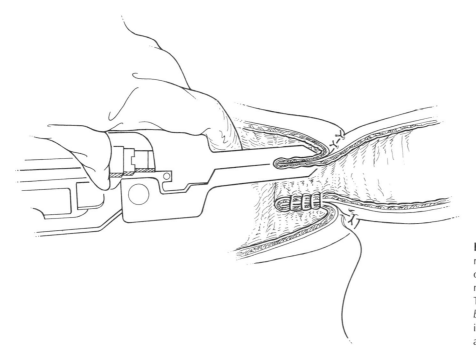

Figure 18–20. Alternate methods of maintaining intussusception. *Above,* Rows of staples are placed on either side of the mesenteric and the antimesenteric border. This is most easily applied with a *bladeless* linear stapler. *Below,* The intussusception is maintained by through-and-through silk sutures.

passed into the pouch via the outflow tract. Air is insufflated, and the catheter removed. The pouch should remain distended.

The stomal defect in the anterior abdominal wall is created as previously described. The marked site usually lies just above the pubic hair line, in the right lower quadrant. The pouch is anchored to the peritoneum at the stomal site with four 3–0 silk sutures. These are most easily placed before the outflow tract is brought through the abdominal wall. The pouch is rendered heart-shaped by pushing the lateral "ears" into the leaves of the mesentery. The outflow tract is passed through the abdominal wall defect, and the anchoring sutures are tied. A closed suction drain is placed in the right lateral gutter behind the pouch and is brought out through a separate abdominal wall stab wound.

The stoma is matured before the abdominal wound is closed. The exteriorized ileum is trimmed until the cut edge is flush with the skin. The ileal edge is anchored to the stomal dermis with interrupted 3–0 long-term absorbable sutures. A catheter introduced through the stoma should enter the pouch without difficulty. A 3-inch segment of 28-French rubber catheter is prepared as a crosspiece by cutting 1-cm holes in the middle of the opposing walls. The catheter is passed through the crosspiece and inserted into the pouch. The catheter's position within the pouch is ascertained by palpation. The catheter is held in this position, and the crosspiece is brought to skin level. The crosspiece is sutured to the abdominal wall skin. The abdominal wound is closed and dressed in standard fashion.

The catheter is attached to continuous gravity drainage. Drainage and periodic saline irrigations are continued for 2 weeks. The ileostomy tube *must* remain within the reservoir. The utmost care must be exercised during dressing changes to prevent its dislodgment.

Bowel function usually returns by the fourth or fifth postoperative day. Progressive refeeding can then resume. The regular diet should avoid undigestible fruit or vegetable materials in order to prevent plugging of the catheter. On the fifteenth postoperative day, continuous drainage is discontinued. A program of progressively longer intervals of catheter occlusion is begun. The catheter is returned to gravity drainage at night. After 3 weeks, the patient is instructed in intubation technique. Discharge instructions include

EDITORIAL COMMENT
The continent ileostomy (the abdominal Kock pouch) is infrequently constructed today, having been replaced by the pelvic pouch as part of the endorectal pull-through operation. For most surgeons, the Kock pouch for fecal elimination has been disappointing, and therefore abandoned, because of the high rate of revision required and the frequency of complications. However, variants of the Kock pouch for urinary diversion have met with success and universal acceptance as an alternative to the incontinent ileal-bladder.

The details of construction of the Kock pouch are included in this text for completeness, for reference when pouch construction is contemplated, and for the surgeon who will need to appreciate the details of construction when called on to repair or revise an established pouch.

intubation of the pouch every 2 hours during time awake and once during the night until the first postoperative office visit.

Ileostomy Closure

Ileostomy closure or reversal usually implies resumption of intestinal continuity by ileoileostomy or ileocolostomy. Although conversion of any type of ileostomy to an ileal reservoir–anal anastomosis or continent ileostomy also technically qualifies as a form of ileostomy closure, these procedures are generally regarded separately.

Typically, ileostomy closure is performed on the "temporary" stoma that served to provide proximal diversion while distal disease or surgery healed. The stoma is closed electively in appropriate candidates when their general health and nutritional and immunologic status are optimal. The surgeon must also ascertain that the problem that prompted creation of the stoma has resolved. This usually involves some form of endoscopic or radiographic evaluation of the distal bowel. In most patients, closure is deferred for at least 4 to 6 weeks from the initial surgery, so that stomal edema and inflammation can subside.

As closure is virtually always elective, antibiotic and mechanical bowel preparation is performed prior to surgery. Vigorous whole-gut lavage is generally not necessary. Clear liquid diet and a small dose of a saline cathartic are usually sufficient mechanical small bowel preparation for the ileostomate. If ileocolostomy is planned, defunctionalized colon should be mechanically prepared with antibiotic-containing solutions delivered via enema or mucous fistula. An abdominal wall scrub with iodophor or chlorhexidine is performed the night before surgery.[27]

In the operating room, the pouch and faceplate are removed. Residual adhesive is removed with acetone or adhesive remover. The abdominal wall scrub is repeated prior to the final antiseptic painting. The abdominal wall is dried, and an adhesive-backed sterile drape is applied over the entire operative field.

End-Ileostomy

The approach taken to close an end-ileostomy varies, depending on the disposition of the distal bowel. In most cases, the distal intestine has been matured at a separate location as a mucous fistula or closed as a Hartmann pouch. In these situations, formal laparotomy is usually necessary for purposes of retrieving the distal segment and bringing the proximal and distal ends together. If the ileostomy and a mucous fistula have been matured through the same abdominal wall opening, closure can be performed as described for a loop ileostomy (see further on).

OPERATIVE TECHNIQUE

Laparotomy is performed in standard fashion. The incision is planned so that the distal bowel will be accessible for mobilization, if necessary. A mucous fistula, if present, is liberated from the abdominal wall and returned to the abdominal cavity, as previously described. Otherwise the distal end is recovered and prepared for anastomosis.

The ileostomy is freed from its skin attachments via a circumstomal incision. Sharp and blunt dissection is used to free the serosal adhesions, and the stoma is unrolled, returning the mucosal surface to the interior of the bowel. Dissection is continued in the subcutaneous planes until the stoma is completely liberated from all layers of the abdominal wall. The stomal end is covered with a sterile glove or rubber dam and returned to the abdominal cavity.

Alternatively, traction is applied to the stomal limb, and the stomal mesentery is divided at its point of exit from the abdominal cavity. The stomal limb is transected with the linear cutter-stapler, flush with the peritoneal surface. The intramural portion of ileum is removed just before termination of the procedure. This technique sacrifices the portion of ileum that formed the stoma, usually no more than 5 or 6 cm. It offers the advantage of avoiding the open bowel end passing through the abdominal wall and lying free in the abdominal cavity.

When the ileum and distal ends have been recovered, they are brought into proximity to each other. Anastomosis is performed by a standard suture or staple technique. Any mesenteric defect is closed with absorbable sutures. In the case of ileoproctostomy, the transanal circular staple technique is often the fastest and easiest method.

The fascia of the stomal defect is closed with heavy long-term absorbable sutures before the main wound is closed. The subcutaneous tissues are lavaged, and the skin edges are packed open or loosely approximated with nylon sutures.

Loop and End-Loop Ileostomy

A loop or an end-loop ileostomy constructed in conjunction with restorative proctocolectomy is the stoma most often closed in our practice. Closure can almost always be performed without a formal laparotomy.

OPERATIVE TECHNIQUE

Both limbs of the stoma are freed from the abdominal wall by means of a circumstomal incision. The incision is placed 1 or 2 mm from the mucocutaneous junction.

The rim of skin is left adherent to the stomal limb. Dissection is continued in the subcutaneous tissues, liberating both stomal limbs completely into the peritoneal cavity. The stomal loop, once liberated from its adhesions, can often be delivered onto sterile towels on the abdominal wall.

Intestinal continuity is restored by anastomosis of proximal and distal limbs. This is accomplished by a suture or staple technique. We have found that creation of a functional end-to-end anastomosis with resection of the exteriorized ileum is the fastest and easiest method. Unrolling the stoma and excising the rim of resected skin are unnecessary.

Two 1-cm enterotomies are created with electrocautery on the antimesenteric borders of the proximal and distal limbs, just below the attached rim of skin. One blade of the 75-mm linear cutter-stapler is passed into the intestinal lumen through each enterotomy. The device is assembled, fired, and removed. A 60-mm linear stapler is placed across both ileal limbs, below the level of the enterotomies. This instrument is fired. The stomal end, including the rim of skin and the enterotomies, is resected above this staple line.

Alternatively, the stoma is unrolled by division of serosal adhesions after the rim of adherent skin is removed. The defect in the antimesenteric wall is closed transversely with sutures or staples. The last option involves complete resection of the stomal end and creation of an end-to-end ileoileostomy with sutures or staples.

The stomal defect in the anterior abdominal wall is closed with heavy long-term absorbable, fascial sutures. The subcutaneous tissues are lavaged, and the skin edges are either packed open or loosely approximated with nylon sutures.

Complications of Conventional Ileostomy

Complications of ileostomy parallel those encountered with colostomy. Unfortunately, problems requiring surgical revision have been reported in as many as 25% to 40% of cases.[67, 68] Complications can appear early in the postoperative period or many years later. As with complications of colostomy, closure, whenever possible, is the most effective long-term solution.

Early Complications

ISCHEMIA

Stomal ischemia usually becomes manifest within 24 hours of surgery.[9] The base of the ileostomy is actually the most distal portion of ileum, and it often shows ischemic changes before other portions. The mucosa becomes pale, cyanotic, and edematous. Progression to a dusky purple precedes frank necrosis. Stomal ischemia is usually caused by stomal tension or by overly vigorous "stripping" of the mesentery.

Ischemia of any portion of the stoma is an ominous sign. Ischemia extending below the level of the fascia is an indication for emergency exploration and stomal revision. The proximal extent of devascularization can be ascertained at the bedside by observation of the stomal mucosa. A plain glass test tube is gently inserted into the stoma, and the mucosa is visualized with the aid of a penlight.[9, 69] If the ischemic process is limited to the portion of intestine above fascial level, revisional surgery can be deferred, at least temporarily.[69]

Necrosis of any portion of the stoma is almost certain to cause problems. Loss of the most distal portion of ileum results in dissolution of the mucocutaneous junction with attendant separation and infection. This complication sets the stage for future stenosis. Even more proximal intestinal loss leads to stomal unrolling and exposure of the serosal surface. The resulting serositis, if extensive, causes obstruction and the "ileostomy dysfunction" described by Warren and McKittrick.[57] Necrosis of all exteriorized ileum results in a flush, stenotic, unpouchable stoma. For these reasons, revisional surgery should be planned at the earliest possible time.

SEPARATION AND INFECTION

Early postoperative separation of an otherwise viable stoma at the mucocutaneous junction is most often caused by infection.[9] It usually appears on the third to fifth postoperative day. This type of separation typically involves less than one half of the stomal circumference and rarely extends deeper than the level of Scarpa's fascia. More extensive separation usually presents earlier as an accompaniment of stomal ischemia.

Healing of a small separation is aided by scrupulous attention to pouching technique. The defect should be filled with a barrier paste or slurry before the faceplate is applied. A subcutaneous collection, if present, should be drained with a small mushroom catheter. Whenever possible, the catheter should emerge from the skin near the stoma, so that it may drain within the appliance. If this is not feasible, then the drain should exit the skin at a distance from the stoma that avoids interfering with the faceplate.

Circumferential separation, especially in conjunction with stomal ischemia, usually requires elective operative repair. This often involves creation of a new stoma at a different site.

Late Complications

PROLAPSE

Stomal prolapse involves a marked exaggeration of the intussusception created at the time of surgery. It usually results from inadequate fixation of the ileal mesentery or a too-large stomal aperture, or both. Prolapse is more commonly encountered some time after the initial surgery is performed.[70] The intussuscepting segment can be either fixed or mobile. Mobile or sliding prolapse can involve a considerable length of small bowel. Early fixed "prolapse" usually indicates that initially the stoma was made too long. Sudden prolapse with fixation of a formerly normal stoma or sudden fixation of a formerly mobile prolapse indicates incarceration with its attendant risk of strangulation.

Manual reduction of the prolapsed stoma should be attempted, unless there is clear evidence of strangulation. Compromise of the stomal blood supply is always an indication for emergency surgery. This involves formal laparotomy with reduction of the incarceration, resection of nonviable intestine, and recreation of the stoma, usually at a separate site.

The spout of most ileostomies should not protrude from the abdominal wall for more than 5 or 6 cm. Our patients are most comfortable with a spout of 3 or 4 cm. A stoma longer than 6 cm tends to pose cosmetic and pouching problems. Bleeding from mucosal irritation is common. Repair is undertaken on an elective basis when the patient has difficulty coping with these added burdens. Repair can usually be performed without a laparotomy.[71, 72]

Operative Technique. A circular, peristomal incision is made 1 or 2 mm from the mucocutaneous junction. Dissection in the subcutaneous tissues is limited to liberating the everted distal ileum. Once the serosa of the subcutaneous stomal limb is encountered, the stoma is unrolled by dividing any adhesions binding the opposing serosa. This is generally not difficult in the prolapsed stoma, as these adhesions will be few and filmy. Redundant ileum is resected at the distal end, leaving an 8- to 10-cm segment for maturation. Care is taken to avoid interference with the blood supply to the remainder of the ileum.

If the fascial defect is not snug against the ileum, the fascia is exposed and the aperture is narrowed with heavy, long-term absorbable sutures before the new stoma is matured. The ileostomy is matured with 3–0 absorbable sutures, as previously described.

Management of the mobile prolapse poses a greater problem. As inadequate mesenteric fixation is most often the cause, rectification usually requires some form of refixation, usually via laparotomy. We have found that simple suture fixation of the ileum and mesentery to the peritoneum and fascia does not offer satisfactory long-term results. Others have attained good results using natural and synthetic bolsters.[73] Our procedure of choice involves complete stomal revision with relocation.

RETRACTION

Stomal retraction is one of the most frequently encountered complications of ileostomy.[71, 72] The retracted stoma is too short to form an adequate spout, thereby making effective pouching difficult or impossible. The causes of retraction include inadequate initial stomal length, failure to maintain eversion due to inadequate stomal fixation, stomal ischemia, and dramatic postoperative weight gain.

A mild degree of retraction that does not completely efface the stomal spout can often be successfully managed by means of a convex faceplate. If leakage persists despite this measure, surgical revision is indicated.

Repair is frequently possible via a circumstomal incision.[71, 72] The stoma is freed completely from the abdominal wall by dividing subcutaneous, fascial, and peritoneal adhesions. Gentle traction should deliver the terminal 10 cm of ileum without tension. If this is not possible because of ileal or mesenteric tethering, conversion to formal laparotomy is indicated. Once sufficient length is obtained, the stoma is refashioned as previously described. Relocation of the stoma is usually not necessary.

STENOSIS

Narrowing of the stomal orifice can occur at the level of the fascia or the skin. This complication most often results from technical errors committed during initial creation of the stoma. The most commonly encountered problem is skin-level stenosis associated with stomal retraction.[72] Both problems are caused by stomal ischemia. Complete stomal revision, often requiring repeat laparotomy, is the best method of correcting stenoses.

Operative Technique. The scar is excised, and the stoma is dissected free of all subcutaneous, fascial, and peritoneal adhesions. Gentle traction may deliver enough ileum to permit maturation of a new stoma. Care must be exercised to avoid tearing the mesentery. Incising the fascia for 1 or 2 cm may facilitate delivery of the intestine. The exteriorized segment must have an adequate blood supply and must be free of tension. The fascial defect, if enlarged, should be sewn snugly against the ileum with a heavy absorbable suture. The subcutaneous tissues are lavaged, and the stoma matured in standard fashion.

Stricture at the fascial level, and occasionally at skin level, occurs if these apertures are not made large enough at the time of the initial surgery. Attempts at fascial dilatation are usually not effective and expose the patient to the risk of stomal perforation. Symptomatic fascial stenosis requires elective operative repair. The fascia is approached directly through a peristomal incision. If the abdominal wall is thin, the incision can be limited to one half the stomal circumference, and

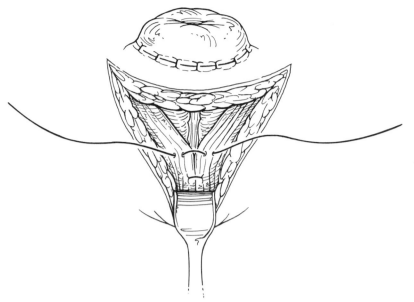

Figure 18–21. Repair of parastomal hernia. The sliding parastomal hernia sac has been excised, care being taken to maintain the mesentery of the stoma. Next the musculofascial defect is repaired with stout nonabsorbable suture material.

unrolling of the stoma can be avoided. The stoma is retracted away from the incision, and dissection proceeds to the fascia in the plane between the intestinal serosa and the subcutaneous fat. Once the fascia is exposed, the edge abutting the intestine is incised enough to permit a finger to slide next to the stomal limb. The wound is lavaged and the stoma rematured in the usual fashion.

A complete circumstomal incision or even laparotomy may be required for more obese patients. Extension of the peristomal incision into the skin at a distance from the stoma should be avoided whenever possible, as the resulting scar may interfere with pouching. If the fascia cannot be adequately exposed through a limited, peristomal incision, laparotomy is indicated. The ileum is returned to the abdominal cavity by completely liberating or excising the stoma. The existing stomal opening is enlarged by incising the fascia to the extent that two fingers will pass easily. The ileum is exteriorized, the laparotomy wound closed, and the stoma matured.

Isolated stenosis of the peristomal skin of a standard ileostomy is distinctly uncommon. Minor skin-level stenosis associated with an otherwise normal stoma can be repaired by the excision of a triangle of skin at the mucocutaneous junction. More pronounced stenosis requires revision by complete excision of the circumferential scar and reconstruction of the stoma. This does not usually require laparotomy.

Skin-level stenosis is more frequently encountered at the flush stoma of the continent ileostomy.[66] Revision by circumferential excision and reconstruction often leads to restenosis. We have found that revision by double Z-plasty avoids this problem. This technique

trades "length" of the outflow limb for increased stomal circumference at the skin level (see further on).

PARAILEOSTOMY HERNIA

Parastomal hernia is an uncommon complication of a properly placed transrectus ileostomy.[74] This complication becomes more frequent after stomal revision, particularly in patients with inflammatory bowel disease. Presenting symptoms include parastomal pain or bulging, difficulty fitting and maintaining the appliance, and bland or strangulated small bowel obstruction. The diagnosis can usually be established by careful peristomal palpation. Computed tomography is also useful.[75] In cases of intestinal obstruction, reduction of the hernia should be judiciously attempted. If this fails, or if strangulation is suspected, immediate laparotomy is indicated. Any nonviable bowel is resected, and a new stoma is created at an alternate site.

Nonoperative management of minimally symptomatic hernias should be attempted initially. This approach entails peristomal support by a fenestrated belt. If it does not relieve symptoms, elective repair is indicated.

Operative Technique. Bowel preparation and marking of a new site should precede elective surgery. The small hernia can initially be approached through a circumstomal incision. Dissection is continued to the level of the fascia. The defect is closed with heavy, long-term absorbable sutures, when possible. Larger hernias can be repaired with synthetic mesh, although this alternative is less desirable because of a higher incidence of infective complications (Figs. 18–21 and 18–22).[76]

For the large hernias, stomal revision by relocation

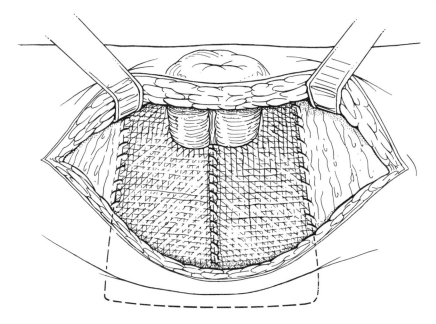

Figure 18–22. Repair of parastomal hernia defect utilizing synthetic mesh. After excision of the sliding sac, synthetic (Marlex) mesh is attached to transverse layer at all aspects of the defect. The stoma exits through the synthetic mesh, but no attempt is made to suture the mesh to the bowel wall, because of the possibility of fistula formation and catastrophic infection. The wound is closed with suction drainage in the potential dead space where the previous sac had resided.

is the recommended long-term solution. Transrectus stomal placement in the contralateral iliac fossa is preferred. Complete takedown or excision of the old ileostomy is required. This can occasionally be accomplished through the old stoma site but more often requires repeat laparotomy.

FISTULA

Fistula formation can occur anywhere along the full length of the ileostomy. Fistulas most commonly occur in patients with Crohn's disease.[77] Technical errors committed at the time of maturation and trauma associated with pouching are also causative. The patient with Crohn's disease often manifests symptoms and signs of active terminal ileal disease preceding fistula formation.

Transmural penetration of an inflammatory process below skin level causes a peristomal abscess. Surgical or spontaneous drainage results in an enterocutaneous fistula. Fistulas above skin level typically extend from mucosa to mucosa, through all layers of the inner noneverted and the outer everted ileal segments. An early postoperative, skin-level fistula often results from inadvertent transmural penetration of one of the everting sutures placed at the time of stomal maturation. Intestinal contents often leak through the fistula at or just above skin level. Effective pouching is virtually impossible, and peristomal skin breakdown is almost certain.

Operative Technique. Closure by placement of simple sutures at the fistula site is occasionally successful in the case of traumatic or suture-related stomal fistula. The mucocutaneous junction is divided, and the stoma unrolled. The serosal defects are proximally and dis-

tally débrided of granulation tissue and closed with fine absorbable sutures. Rematuration of the stoma is performed as usual.

In patients with recurrent Crohn's disease, stomal revision with resection of the involved ileum and relocation of the stoma is usually required.[77] This is virtually always performed at laparotomy, unless the segment of recurrent disease is prohibitively short.

INTESTINAL OBSTRUCTION

Adhesive small bowel obstruction requiring surgical intervention will complicate the postoperative course of 3% to 9% of all ileostomates.[74, 78] Obstruction is more common following colectomy for inflammatory bowel disease than for other conditions.[79] Restorative proctocolectomy renders the patient especially prone to obstruction, often related to complications of the temporary ileostomy.[80] Causes of obstruction include impaction of food, either proximally or at the level of the fascia, adhesion, internal herniation, recurrent Crohn's disease, and small bowel volvulus at a point of adhesive fixation or at the stomal limb.

The patient with intestinal obstruction presents with nausea, vomiting, abdominal cramping, and distention. Stomal output may cease entirely or become profuse, thin, and watery. Abdominal radiographs usually demonstrate dilated small bowel loops and differential air-fluid levels.

Management of small bowel obstruction in the ileostomate closely parallels that in any postsurgical patient. Initial efforts are directed toward correcting fluid and electrolyte disturbances. The subsequent course of therapy depends on careful assessment and monitoring of the clinical situation.

Clear evidence of peritonitis warrants emergent abdominal exploration after adequate resuscitation. In selected patients, generally those without peritoneal signs or evidence of sepsis, a trial of nonoperative management can be attempted. This course requires the surgeon to be even more diligent. Frequent assessments of the patient are mandatory. Early surgical intervention on the basis of minimal deterioration or lack of improvement can rarely be criticized.

Nonsurgical therapy usually includes tube decompression and parenteral hydration. Antibiotics are also recommended by some investigators.[81] We prefer small bowel intubation with a long, mercury-weighted tube.[82] The tube must leave the stomach for maximum benefit. Passage through the pylorus often occurs spontaneously if the patient remains in the right lateral decubitus position. Alternatively, the weight can be positioned at the pylorus fluoroscopically, or it can actually be passed through the pylorus endoscopically.

Some aspects of the management of small bowel obstruction are particular to the ileostomate.[77] Access to the small bowel by way of the stoma can be useful for both diagnostic and therapeutic purposes. For example, we have found that gentle irrigation of the stomal limb by means of a small, soft rubber catheter is often successful in dislodging an obstructing bolus of undigested food residue impacted at the level of the fascia. Fiberoptic ileoscopy and radiographic ileal enema are effective in establishing the cause of obstruction in selected patients.

PERISTOMAL SKIN COMPLICATIONS

Dermatitis. Peristomal dermatitis results from irritation, infection, or allergy. Skin irritation caused by chemical and/or mechanical trauma is the most commonly encountered of these three causes.[83] Many of these kinds of problems are related to improper pouching technique. Trauma resulting from an ill-fitting faceplate or from abrupt removal of the faceplate, application of adhesives or skin cleaners, and leakage of effluent are frequently at fault. Many of these problems can be solved by intensive enterostomal care and education. Application of any irritating skin products must also be discontinued.

Uncommonly, a patient develops allergic contact dermatitis from one of the components of the pouching system. Visual inspection does not differentiate an allergic dermatitis from the dermatitis caused by irritation. Patch testing is recommended in order to confirm allergy before abandoning a potentially helpful agent.[9]

Infection of the peristomal skin by *Candida albicans* is a common occurrence with both colostomies and ileostomies.[84] The patient notes a pruritic, papular eruption, typically appearing under the stomal faceplate. The rash may interfere with pouching. The diagnosis can usually be established by inspection and confirmed by microscopic evaluation of skin scrapings treated with 10% potassium hydroxide. As *C. albicans* is an organism commonly found on the skin and in the gastrointestinal tract, recurrent infection is common.

Treatment consists of nystatin powder topically applied three times daily until the rash clears.[84] Creams containing clotrimazole or ketoconazole are also effective topically, but the cream base may interfere with faceplate adhesion.

Bacterial infection of the peristomal skin is usually caused by *Staphylococcus aureus*. The resulting eruption has the typical appearance of impetigo. Culture of vesicular fluid confirms the diagnosis. Treatment consists of appropriate topical or systemic antibiotics.

Dermatoses. The peristomal skin may manifest the same dermatologic conditions affecting skin elsewhere. Psoriasis, pemphigus, and systemic lupus erythematosus have been reported.[85–87] Treatment is directed at the underlying cause. During treatment, alternate pouching techniques such as a two-piece system or a karaya-backed pouch may be beneficial.

Inflammatory bowel disease can be complicated by the development of pyoderma gangrenosum. This skin lesion may also appear in the peristomal region.[88] The typical lesion is an irregular ulcer with purple, overhanging edges. The base is formed by granulation tissue and fibrinopurulent exudate. The untreated ulcer enlarges by undermining the surrounding skin. Treatment consists of antibiotics and intralesional or systemic steroids.[89] Cyclosporin therapy has also been successful in managing difficult cases.[90]

Complications of the Continent Ileostomy

The patient with a continent ileostomy can experience a variety of early and late complications.[91, 92] Many of these problems, such as small bowel obstruction, are shared by patients with standard ileostomies and can be attributed to the proctocolectomy portion of the operation. Others are specific to the more complex reservoir stoma. Of these, hemorrhage, pouch leakage, and ischemic necrosis of the outflow tract or valve occur in the early postoperative period. Most late complications relate to the nipple valve and include slippage, fistula, and prolapse. The reservoir itself is prone to a form of mucosal ileitis termed "pouchitis."[66]

All researchers report complication rates that have lowered as experience with the procedure and technical modifications have evolved.[91–94] However, an overall reoperation rate of 12% to 25% is still common.[95] This is comparable to a reported reoperation rate of 18% to 23% for large series of standard ileostomies.[96, 97]

Early Complications

HEMORRHAGE

Hemorrhage from the reservoir usually occurs at the end of the first postoperative week. The indwelling ileostomy tube returns bloody fluid spontaneously or with irrigation. Bleeding is occasionally brisk, and transfusion may be required. The site of bleeding is usually one or more of the pouch suture lines.

It is imperative that the ileostomy catheter be kept free of clots by frequent saline irrigation. Addition of norepinephrine to the irrigation fluid often helps control bleeding. Systemic vasopressin has been used successfully in extreme cases. Fiberoptic ileoscopy is contraindicated because of the risk of perforation. Surgical exploration to control hemorrhage is almost never required, but when necessary, excision of the pouch and creation of a standard ileostomy are recommended.

SUTURE LINE DEHISCENCE

Suture line dehiscence is rare and usually can be avoided by scrupulous operative technique and careful postoperative management. This complication occurs with the symptoms and signs of localized or free visceral perforation.

Fluid resuscitation and systemic antibiotics are generally indicated. Leakage during the first postoperative week is often poorly contained and frequently leads to generalized peritonitis. Re-exploration for drainage and proximal diversion is necessary. Between the second and fourth weeks, localized abscess and enterocutaneous fistula are more common. Radiographically guided, percutaneous drainage of any collection and sump drainage of the reservoir usually lead to healing without further surgery. Total parenteral nutrition and octreotide are useful therapeutic adjuncts.

ISCHEMIA

Compromise of the blood supply to the most distal portion of the ileum causes ischemia of the stomal segment, or outflow tract, first. More extensive vascular insufficiency involves the intussuscepted, inner segment of the nipple valve. Compression or disruption of the ileal mesentery within the nipple is usually the cause of vascular insufficiency. A valve longer than 5 cm, excessive fattiness of the valve mesentery, and overly vigorous suturing or stapling of the valve at its mesenteric borders predispose the patient to this complication.[66]

Ischemia usually becomes manifest within 48 hours of surgery. Dusky discoloration of the stoma and bloody returns with irrigation are the hallmarks of poor distal vascularity. Fever and pain are also common. Frequent irrigation of the ileostomy catheter to maintain patency, systemic antibiotic therapy, and close observation are the best early approaches.[66]

Progression of the ischemic process results in necrosis of the outflow tract and, occasionally, the valve. Valve loss occurs in less than 2 percent of cases.[93] Loss of the valve leads to leakage of intestinal contents around the catheter. Blood clots, necrotic debris, and sutures or staples may return with irrigation. Sump suction of the reservoir should be instituted. Immediate operation is rarely indicated, as healing, albeit with incontinence, usually occurs spontaneously.

Valve Necrosis. Valve necrosis is an uncommon complication that is almost always accompanied by stomal incontinence. Revisional surgery can often be delayed until the pouch has healed completely.[66] Creation of a new valve involves "turning the pouch."[98]

Operative Technique. Valve recreation is usually possible through a circumstomal incision lengthened medially and laterally by a few centimeters. The remainder of the outflow tract and the reservoir are carefully removed from the abdominal wall. The pouch and 20 cm of proximal small bowel are delivered into the wound. Remnants of the outflow tract and valve are excised from the intact pouch with electrocautery. The pouch is opened from this point for another 10 cm along its antimesenteric aspect.

The new valve is created by orthograde intussusception of the proximal inflow tract. The afferent ileum is transected with electrocautery 15 cm from its junction with the reservoir. The proximal 10 cm of the inflow tract is prepared for intussusception by removing the mesenteric fat, abrading the serosal surface, and placing silk sutures as previously described. A Babcock clamp is passed into the inflow tract, and the ileum is grasped about 5 cm from the reservoir. The bowel is intussuscepted and fixed by sutures and staples, as done for the original procedure. The catheter is inserted into the pouch, and a collar of pouch is sewn to the new outflow limb with 3–0 silk sutures.

The reservoir is rotated 90 degrees about its axis, thereby bringing the new outflow tract to an anterolateral position. The cut end of the proximal ileum is anastomosed to the pouch at a convenient location by using the circular stapling instrument. The reservoir walls are reapproximated and closed with running, 2–0 long-term absorbable suture. The afferent limb is occluded with a noncrushing intestinal clamp, and the ileostomy tube is inserted through the new valve. The pouch is tested for continence by insufflating air and removing the catheter.

The outflow tract is brought through the old stomal opening in the abdominal wall. A closed suction drain is placed in the right gutter between the anterior abdominal wall and the reservoir. The drain end is brought out at a distance from the stoma. The pouch is secured to the anterior abdominal wall with 2–0 silk sutures. The fascia medial and lateral to the stomal opening is reapproximated with a heavy, long-term absorbable suture. The outflow tract is trimmed flush with the skin, and the stoma is matured with 3–0 long-term absorbable sutures. The ileostomy catheter is left in the reservoir and connected to dependent drainage.

Skin-Level Stricture. Ischemia of the outflow tract often leads to skin-level stenosis. Stenosis causing difficulty with catheter insertion, and any degree of incontinence unacceptable to the patient, requires surgical repair. It is preferable to plan elective revision 2 to 3 months after the initial surgery. This allows the reservoir enough time to heal completely. The catheter is left in place during this period. The tube is capped with a plastic button, and the reservoir emptied intermittently. If leakage around the catheter is a problem, the open catheter is incorporated into a standard ileostomy appliance. Stricture is most effectively repaired by the double Z-plasty technique (see further on).

Late Complications

VALVE SLIPPAGE

The most common late postoperative complication of the Kock ileostomy is "desusception," or slippage of the nipple valve.[91–93] This is most likely to occur within the first postoperative year.[92] This problem usually begins with dehiscence of the opposing mesenteries within the intussuscepted valve.[99] The nipple desuscepts asymmetrically, causing disproportionate "lengthening" of the mesenteric wall of the outflow tract. This change leads to angulation of the intact portion of the valve into the longer mesenteric wall.

Desusception with subsequent shortening of the valve may lead to stomal incontinence.[99] Most patients retain continence but are unable to intubate the pouch because of valve angulation.[92] Intestinal obstruction is therefore the common emergency presentation.[94]

Initial management is directed at relieving obstructive symptoms. Pouch intubation can be accomplished by fiberoptic or rigid ileoscopy by means of a pediatric gastroscope or an 11-mm rigid sigmoidoscope.[94, 100, 101] A guide wire or the shaft of a long cotton-tipped swab is left in the pouch, and the endoscope is removed. An ileostomy catheter is threaded over the guide and taped in place.

At the first episode of valve dysfunction, a trial of prolonged reservoir intubation is warranted. This often stabilizes the valve, allowing it to become fixed in the new position. The patient is instructed to leave the catheter taped in place for 2 to 3 weeks. The end of the catheter is occluded with a plastic button, which is removed to empty the pouch. At the end of this period intubation resumes as before. If difficulty in intubating persists, surgical revision is indicated.

Operative Technique. The pouch is approached through a circumstomal incision. Adequate visualization and mobilization are facilitated by extending the circumstomal incision 2 or 3 cm medially and laterally. The outflow tract and the reservoir are mobilized from the anterior abdominal wall and delivered into the operative wound.

The partially desuscepted valve can often be reduced into the reservoir by gentle inward pressure. If successful reduction can be achieved, it is not necessary to open the reservoir. The intussusception is maintained by suturing the pouch to the outflow tract, as done in a gastric fundoplication. The ileostomy catheter should be inserted into the reservoir before these sutures are placed, so that the outflow tract is not narrowed. Four or five sutures of 3–0 silk usually suffice. If there is any question about the adequacy of the valve, the pouch should be opened along its anterior wall. If recreation of the valve is necessary, pouch "turnaround," as previously described, is performed.

FISTULA

The reservoir ileostomy is prone to two distinct types of fistulas: internal and external. External fistulas cause an abnormal communication between the pouch and the skin. Internal fistulas traverse both limbs of the intussuscepted valve, causing communication between the lumen of the pouch and the lumen of the valve.

Most fistulas occur, on average, 2 years from the time of the initial surgery.[92] Nearly all fistulas are related to the presence of a foreign body, either a silk suture or plastic mesh.[91] The patient with Crohn's disease who has a reservoir ileostomy is five times more likely to develop a fistula than the patient with colitis or polyposis.[91]

The external fistula usually appears with evidence of cutaneous sepsis. Peristomal cellulitis or subcutaneous abscess usually precedes frank fistulization. Once the tract is established, leakage of intestinal contents will ensue. We have found the pouch-cutaneous fistula to be an uncommon complication. Fiberoptic ileoscopy is often helpful in establishing the diagnosis and in estimating the chance of nonoperative closure.[100] If the cause of the fistula is a foreign body, it must be removed, either operatively or endoscopically, before the pouch will heal. If the offending agent (usually a silk suture) can be endoscopically removed, 2 to 4 weeks of continuous pouch intubation and oral antibiotics are sufficient to close the defect. If the foreign body cannot be retrieved, operative removal by excision with primary closure of the pouch is indicated.

Internal fistulas of the nipple valve are more common and more troublesome than external fistulas.[91] Leakage of intestinal contents through the unintubated stoma is the common presentation of this complication. The size of the fistula and its location along the length of the valve determine the degree of incontinence. Leakage is generally greater when the fistula lies near the base of the valve.

Operative revision is indicated when the amount of leakage inconveniences the patient. Dozois and colleagues recommend complete nipple revision by pouch rotation in all patients with fistulas.[94] We have found this unnecessary, especially when the fistula lies at the base of the valve. However, we agree that if the fistula is not readily accessible or if the repaired valve is unsuitable for any reason, nipple recreation using the afferent ileum is indicated.

Operative Technique. The pouch is approached through a peristomal incision. The outflow tract is freed circumferentially. The wound is enlarged by medial and lateral incisions that are 2 to 3 cm long. The pouch is removed from the abdominal wall and delivered into the wound. A 5-cm incision is made with electrocautery on the antimesenteric pouch wall.

The nipple fistula is identified. The foreign body is removed, excising a small rim of normal ileum. The nipple is desuscepted to a point a few millimeters beyond the fistula. This is relatively easy if the fistula is at the base of the nipple. The edges of the fistula are freshened and then closed with 3–0 long-term absorbable sutures. The intussusception is restored, care taken to avoid overlapping the suture lines. The pouch is closed with a running 2–0 long-term absorbable suture. An ileostomy catheter is placed within the pouch, and valvular competence is ascertained.

The outflow tract is brought through the old stoma site. The medial and lateral incisions in the fascia are repaired with heavy, long-term absorbable sutures. The skin incisions medial and lateral to the stoma site are closed with fine nylon. The stoma is matured with 3–0, long-term absorbable sutures. The catheter is secured to the abdominal wall with a crosspiece arrangement, as previously described. Gravity drainage is instituted.

SKIN-LEVEL STENOSIS

Stenosis of the peristomal skin occurs in 8% of patients.[91] Patients suffering from this complication find insertion of the ileostomy catheter to be difficult, painful, and accompanied by modest bleeding. As previously mentioned, we have found that double Z-plasty of the peristomal skin offers the most satisfactory long-term results.

Operative Technique. The scar at the mucocutaneous junction is excised circumferentially. The subcutaneous outflow limb is mobilized completely to the level of the fascia. Slightly curved, 1.5-cm tangential skin incisions are made at opposite points on the stomal circumference. The skin edges are undermined, thereby creating two rotational flaps. The ileal walls opposing the skin incisions are divided longitudinally

for a distance of 1.5 cm on each side. The skin flaps are rotated into the groove cut on either side of the ileum. The two Z-plasties are completed by suturing the full thickness of the ileal wall to the dermis of the flaps. The revision is completed by fixing the remainder of the ileal circumference to the skin with 3–0 absorbable sutures (Fig. 18–23).

PROLAPSE

Prolapse of the intact nipple valve is uncommon, occurring in less than 3% of ileostomy patients.[91] There seems to be a greater tendency toward prolapse in patients who have undergone previous nipple revision.[66] Continence is maintained between episodes of prolapse.

We have found that prolapse is most often associated with an overly large fascial stomal defect. Increasing intra-abdominal pressure during exercise or late pregnancy can precipitate nipple extrusion. Reduction can usually be accomplished by gentle manual pressure. Iced hamamelis water (witch hazel) compresses may reduce stomal edema, thereby facilitating reduction after long-standing prolapse. Once reduced, the reservoir can usually be intubated without difficulty.

Recurring episodes of valvular prolapse generally require revisional surgery. Relocation of the reservoir and stoma to a new site, usually the midline or the left lower quadrant, yields superior results, in our experience, to attempts at fascial repair.

Operative Technique. The skin of the new stoma site is indelibly marked preoperatively. The stoma and outflow tract are mobilized through a peristomal incision. The incision is extended medially and laterally, and the abdominal cavity is entered. The pouch is carefully mobilized from the anterior abdominal wall. If doubt exists about the viability of the outflow tract, creation of a new valve by pouch rotation is warranted.

A circle of skin at the new site is excised. Dissection is continued into the abdominal cavity, as previously described. The outflow tract is brought through the new stoma site, and the reservoir is fixed to the anterior abdominal wall. The fascial defect at the old stoma site is closed with heavy, long-term absorbable sutures. The wound is covered with sterile towels, and the stoma is matured with 3–0 sutures.

Prolapse occurring during pregnancy can be managed nonoperatively.[102] After reduction, the patient is instructed to maintain constant indwelling reservoir catheterization. The tube is left in place throughout labor and delivery. If cesarean section is indicated, the extracorporeal portion of the catheter is draped laterally with a sterile, adhesive sheet. Midline incision is usually required. Operative delivery proceeds according to obstetric principles, care being exercised to avoid injury to the reservoir.

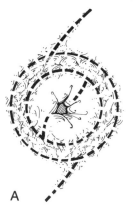

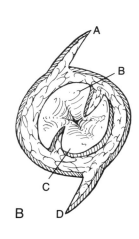

Figure 18–23. Repair of skin level stenosis by Z-plasty technique. *A,* The mucocutaneous junction of the stenotic stoma is incised, preferably with electrocautery. The subcutaneous outflow limb is mobilized completely to the level of the fascia. Slightly curved 1.5-cm skin incisions are made at opposite points on the stomal circumference. *B,* The skin edges are undermined, creating two rotational flaps, and the stomal walls opposing the skin incisions are divided longitudinally for a distance of 1.5 cm on each side. *C,* The skin flaps are rotated into the groove cut on either side of the stoma. *D,* The revision is completed by fixing the remainder of the stomal circumference to the skin with 3-0 absorbable sutures.

POUCHITIS

The syndrome of reservoir mucosal ileitis, or "pouchitis," has been reported to occur in 5% to 43% of reservoir ileostomates.[66, 91, 93, 94, 103, 104] It is manifest most characteristically as a change in the nature and quantity of the ileostomy effluent.[23] High-volume (more than 1,000 ml/day), thin, occasionally bloody returns are common. Intubation may become more difficult, and catheter-induced bleeding may ensue. The syndrome may also include abdominal cramps or pain, arthralgia, fever, and malaise.[105] Pouchitis appears to occur almost exclusively in patients whose initial diagnosis was mucosal ulcerative colitis.[66, 91, 94] More than one half of the patients who develop pouchitis present with the first episode within 6 months of surgery.[106]

The patient presenting with these symptoms for the first time warrants thorough investigation. A careful history and physical examination are performed. Assay of the ileostomy effluent for enteric pathogens and toxins, and fiberoptic ileoscopy are also indicated. Typically, ileoscopy reveals mucosal edema, friability, and granularity.[101] The presence of aphthous ulcerations strongly suggests the possibility of Crohn's disease.[105] Biopsy may establish an alternate diagnosis, or it may show only mild, nonspecific inflammation or even normal mucosal histologic findings.[107] Crohn's disease of the reservoir and infectious enteritis can mimic pouchitis. We have encountered subacute addisonian crisis and hyperthyroidism misdiagnosed as reservoir ileitis.[66]

The cause of pouchitis is unknown. Factors implicated as contributory or causative include pouch stasis, ischemia, altered bacterial flora, bacterial metabolites, and ileal mucosal metaplasia.[108] None is a proven cause. Resolution of the inflammatory process with treatment by antibiotics favors a bacterial etiology. It is intriguing to consider the possibility that pouchitis, "backwash ileitis," and ulcerative colitis share a common, albeit unknown, cause.

Pouchitis generally responds quickly to the oral administration of metronidazole.[109] Because pouchitis tends to recur in susceptible individuals, each subsequent episode does not require the same investigation as the first.[106] Rather, antibiotic therapy should be started empirically, on the basis of symptoms. The occasional patient fails to respond to antibiotic therapy. In these patients, steroids given by means of the catheter or by systemic administration may be of value.[104] Very rarely, unremitting pouchitis that is recalcitrant to all modes of medical therapy may prompt the patient to seek removal of the reservoir.[104]

EARLY POSTOPERATIVE PERIOD

Management for the ostomate during the immediate postoperative period is very similar to that for any patient undergoing intestinal surgery. Prophylactic systemic antibiotics are used during the perioperative period only.[110] Measures to prevent deep venous thrombosis are continued until the patient is fully ambulatory.[111] Early ambulation is encouraged. The urinary catheter is removed on the second postoperative day, unless the pelvic peritoneum has been opened. In that case it is removed on the fifth day. Pain is controlled with either narcotic infusion pump (patient-controlled analgesia) or indwelling epidural catheterization.[112, 113] We do not routinely employ nasogastric tubes.[114] Most patients experience a return of bowel function by the third to fifth postoperative day.

Immediately following surgery, conventional stomas should be pouched with a simple, one-piece, clear plastic, drainable appliance. A clear pouch permits frequent visual inspection of the stoma. The first postoperative appliance usually consists of a one-piece, combination skin barrier and pouch. The adherent faceplate should be cut to fit around the mucocutaneous junction, leaving only 1 to 2 mm of exposed skin. The adhesive backing secures the appliance in place, if the peristomal skin is clean and dry. Tincture of benzoin or other agents designed to promote adherence are not necessary. If undisturbed, this appliance can usually remain in place for 3 or 4 days.

The faceplate should avoid the main wound, if possible, for the first 24 to 48 hours. After that time, the wound will have sealed, and the faceplate can be placed over the wound and any staples or sutures closing it. Dependent drainage is promoted by positioning the appliance transversely until the patient is ambulatory.

A loop colostomy or ileostomy involving a plastic or glass support is somewhat more difficult to pouch. The opening in the faceplate needs to be cut slightly larger to accommodate the bulkier stoma. When possible, the barrier should be placed at the mucocutaneous junction. This means sliding the faceplate under the support. This maneuver is facilitated by dividing the remaining circumference of the faceplate after the opening has been cut. Once the faceplate is in position, the adhesive backing is removed, and the faceplate is applied to the peristomal skin.

The enterostomal therapist (ET) should begin or continue contact with the ostomate early in the postoperative period. The roles of the ET during this period are those of clinician and teacher. Inspection of the newly created stoma, wound assessment, pouching, patient education, and emotional support responsibilities are shared by the ET and the surgeon. At some centers, formal, staged teaching sessions are held for new ostomates.[115]

By the third to fifth postoperative day, most patients experience a return of bowel function. Rods or bridges, if present, are usually removed sometime during the seventh to tenth days. At these junctures, most patients are ready to switch to a more permanent pouching device. The ET should provide the patient with information about the various types of pouching systems available. The best option for the patient is chosen, and its use is explained. As soon as possible, the patient should begin managing the stoma under the supervision of the surgeon or ET. It is valuable to include the patient's family in these teaching sessions. Discharge is usually not planned until the patient or a family member is adept at caring for the stoma.

STOMAL MANAGEMENT

Once the perioperative period has ended, routine management of the new stoma begins. Most ostomates require a simple, yet reliable, pouching system capable of collecting the stomal effluent and protecting the peristomal skin. A wide variety of commercial products are available. The choice of pouching system should be tailored to the individual's needs.

Equipment

The most basic pouching equipment consists of a one- or two-piece disposable or semidisposable appliance.

The one-piece system consists of an integrated faceplate and reservoir. The faceplate usually fulfills skin barrier and adherence requirements by providing a pectin- or karaya-based disk and surrounding paper-backed adhesive. The attached reservoir is usually made of plastic, vinyl, or rubber. It can be clear or opaque, and it may be closed at the end or taper to an open spout for drainage. The two-piece system is essentially the same, except that the reservoir is separable from the faceplate or flange. The two pieces fit together by means of interlocking plastic O-rings. The reservoir can be removed from the flange and then emptied or discarded. The new or washed reservoir is reattached without disturbing the barrier or adhesive flange.

In addition to these basic components, other supplemental products are available. Barrier material of pectin or karaya can be obtained as separate wafers or rings. In powder, paste, or strip form, this substance is useful for filling gaps between the skin and the main barrier caused by irregularities in the peristomal topography. Adhesives for securing the faceplate are supplied as sprays, liquids, disks, and tapes. Adhesive removers, skin cleaners, and sealants are adjuncts available for maintenance of the peristomal skin. Belts and convex faceplates facilitate pouching of problem stomas.

Pouching

Most ostomates change the barrier-adhesive portion of the system every 4 to 5 days.[116] Pouch changes are easiest when the stoma is quiescent. The ostomate may prefer to stand or sit. The new pouch is first prepared by cutting an aperture in the barrier to conform to the patient's template. The template, usually provided by the ET, should hug the mucocutaneous junction, leaving a rim of no more than 1 or 2 mm of exposed skin.

The adhesive is moistened, and the old faceplate is slowly peeled from the peristomal skin with the aid of a moistened tissue or cotton ball. The peristomal skin is washed with warm water and dried thoroughly. Any peristomal hair is removed with scissors, an electric razor, or depilatory. A rim of barrier paste is placed around the stoma. The main barrier is brought to the base of the stoma, and the aperture is centered. The barrier is pressed onto the peristomal skin from bottom to top. The edges of the faceplate are secured with paper or waterproof tape.

Ascending and transverse colostomies as well as ileostomies generally have a liquid or semiliquid corrosive effluent. Except with the reservoir ileostomy, fecal output is variable, unpredictable, and nearly continuous. Most patients find a drainable, one-, or two-piece pouching system most convenient. The ap-

pliance is worn continuously and fills by "natural function." Descending or sigmoid colostomies produce a semiformed to solid noncorrosive stool. The stoma functions intermittently. For these reasons the stoma can be managed by natural function or by irrigation techniques. Ostomates choosing the former method generally find a drainable one-, or two-piece system to be the optimal selection.

Irrigation

An alternative to the continuously worn appliance exists for the management of mature end-colostomies or end-loop sigmoid or descending colostomies. Colostomy irrigation, essentially an enema delivered via the colostomy, can offer near-continence in selected patients. The irrigating fluid stimulates colonic evacuation in a predictable and reproducible fashion. In many patients, irrigation every second or third day is sufficient to keep the stoma free of leakage between irrigations.[117]

Only left-sided colostomies are amenable to control by this technique. Right or transverse stomas generally have an output that is too liquid to achieve adequate results. Other relative contraindications to irrigation include parastomal herniation, stomal prolapse, and a predisposition to diarrhea related to either the underlying disease process (e.g., inflammatory bowel disease) or ongoing treatment (e.g., chemotherapy or radiotherapy). Children and infants generally are not good candidates because of their increased risks of perforations and shorter attention spans.

Although the contraindications are few, irrigation is not for everybody. The patient must be generally healthy and possess the manual dexterity and motivation to learn and apply the technique. Uninterrupted access to the bathroom for at least 1 hour on irrigation days is also required. Even under ideal circumstances, not all patients achieve near-continence.

Patients thought to be good candidates should begin training with the ET or surgeon after their recovery from surgery is complete and the stoma has healed. This usually takes about 6 weeks. Necessary equipment includes a water bag with tubing and clamp, an irrigating cone, and an irrigating sleeve.

Irrigation Technique

Irrigations should be performed at approximately the same time of day on alternate days or every third day. The patient should be comfortable with the technique, relaxed, and unhurried. Many patients choose to irrigate seated in front of the toilet.

The water bag should be filled with no more than 1 quart of lukewarm tap water. The bag should be suspended at shoulder level and within the patient's view. After air is evacuated from the system, the tubing is clamped and the cone tip is attached.

The irrigating sleeve is placed around the stoma. The long end of the sleeve is placed in the toilet. The cone is lubricated and is inserted via the short arm of the sleeve into the stoma. Gentle pressure allows the tip to occlude the stoma. The clamp is opened and the water allowed to enter the colon slowly. The entire quart is instilled over 3 to 5 minutes. The infusion should be stopped momentarily if cramping occurs.

After infusion, the cone is removed and the short arm of the sleeve is clipped. The long arm is left in the toilet until the initial return of water and stool has ceased. This usually takes about 15 minutes. The sleeve is then rinsed clean but left in place. The patient can then leave the bathroom or perform other tasks if desired. Stool may continue to drain for the next 30 to 50 minutes. With time, the patient comes to know when the colon is empty.

When there is no further drainage of stool, the sleeve is rinsed and removed. The peristomal skin is cleaned, and a "security pouch," cap, or pad is applied. Although long-term results will vary, most patients can expect leakage of stool between irrigations for the first 2 to 6 weeks after beginning the irrigation regimen. A drainable pouching system is recommended during this transition period.

EDITORIAL COMMENT

The editors caution against the routine irrigation for end-colostomies. Serious and often lethal complications may occur with perforation of the stomal wall by the syringe tip or from extraordinarily high intraluminal pressures that may be generated by irrigation. From a practical standpoint, moreover, we have observed that this generally useless maneuver comes to occupy an increasingly important and time-consuming (often 1 hour per day) segment of the patient's life. Instead of being rehabilitated, the patient becomes fixed on enemas and the success or failure of evacuations. If the patient requires emptying of the distal colostomy for fear of embarrassment during social or business activities, this may be accomplished by dietary restrictions combined with a bisacodyl (Dulcolax) suppository inserted into the stoma in order to obtain evacuation.

REFERENCES

1. Hardy KJ. Surgical history. Evolution of the stoma. Aust N Z J Surg 1989;59:71–77.
2. Turnbull RW, Turnbull GB. The history and current status of paramedical support for the ostomy patient. Semin Colon Rectal Surg 1991;2:131–140.
3. Nichols RL, Broido P, Condon RE, et al. Effect of preoperative neomycin and erythromycin intestinal preparation on the incidence of infectious complications following colon surgery. Ann Surg 1973;178:453–459.
4. Watt RC. Stoma placement. In: Broadwell DC, Jackson BS, eds. Principles of Ostomy Care. St Louis: CV Mosby, 1982, pp 329–339.
5. Van Niel J, Spencer M, Hocevar B. Enterostomal therapy. In: Fazio VW, ed. Current Therapy in Colon and Rectal Surgery. Toronto: BC Decker, 1990, pp 426–431.
6. Corman ML. Intestinal stomas. In: Corman ML, ed. Colon and Rectal Surgery. 2nd ed. Philadelphia: JB Lippincott, 1989, pp 889–957.
7. Kodner IJ. Colostomy: Indications, techniques for construction, and management of complications. Semin Colon Rectal Surg 1991;2:73–85.
8. Goligher JC. Extraperitoneal colostomy or ileostomy. Br J Surg 1958;46:97–103.
9. Bubrick MP, Rolstad BS. Intestinal stomas. In: Gordon PH, Nivatvongs S, eds. Principles and Practice of Surgery for the Colon, Rectum, and Anus. St Louis: Quality Medical Publishing, 1992, pp 855–905.
10. Killingback M. Diverticulitis of the colon. In: Fazio VW, ed. Current Therapy in Colon and Rectal Surgery. Toronto: BC Decker, 1990, pp 222–231.
11. Gordon PH. Diverticular disease of the colon. In: Gordon PH, Nivatvongs S, eds. Principles and Practice of Surgery for the Colon, Rectum, and Anus. St Louis: Quality Medical Publishing, 1992, pp 739–797.
12. Rombeau JL, Wilk PJ, Turnbull RB Jr, Fazio VW. Total fecal diversion by the temporary skin-level loop transverse colostomy. Dis Colon Rectum 1978;21:223–226.
13. Morris DM, Rayburn D. Loop colostomies are totally diverting in adults. Am J Surg 1991;161:668–671.
14. Fielding LP, Stewart-Brown S, Hittinger R, et al. Covering stoma for elective anterior resection of the rectum: An outmoded operation? Am J Surg 1984;147:524–530.
15. Corman JM, Odenheimer DB. Securing the loop—historic review of the methods used for creating a loop colostomy. Dis Colon Rectum 1991;34:1014–1021.
16. Prasad ML, Pearl RK, Abcarian H. End-loop colostomy. Surg Gynecol Obstet 1984;158:381–382.
17. Unti JA, Abcarian H, Pearl RK. Rodless end-loop stomas. Seven year experience. Dis Colon Rectum 1991;34:999–1004.
18. Bauer JJ, Wertkin MG, Gelernt IM, Kreel I. A continent colostomy: The magnetic stoma cap. Am J Surg 1977;134:334–337.
19. Cerdan FJ, Diez M, Campo J, et al. Continent colostomy by means of a new one-piece disposable device. Preliminary report. Dis Colon Rectum 1991;34:886–890.
20. Heiblum M, Cordoba A. An artificial sphincter: A preliminary report. Dis Colon Rectum 1978;21:562–566.
21. Mercati U, Trancanelli V, Castagnoli P, et al. Use of the gracilis muscles for sphincteric construction after abdominoperineal resection. Technique and preliminary results. Dis Colon Rectum 1991;34:1085–1089.
22. Kock NG, Myrvold HE, Philipson BM, et al. Continent cecostomy. An account of 30 patients. Dis Colon Rectum 1985;28:705–708.
23. Parks SE, Hastings PR. Complications of colostomy closure. Am J Surg 1985;149:672–675.
24. Todd GJ, Kutcher LM, Markowitz AM. Factors influencing the complications of colostomy closure. Am J Surg 1979;139:749–751.
25. Demetriades D, Pezikis A, Melissas J, et al. Factors influencing the morbidity of colostomy closure. Am J Surg 1988;155:594–596.
26. Varnell J, Pemberton LB. Risk factors in colostomy closure. Surgery 1981;89:683–686.
27. Garibaldi RA. Prevention of intraoperative wound contamination with chlorhexidine shower and scrub. J Hosp Infect 1988;11(Suppl B):5–9.
28. Sloan MS, Krebs HB, Wheelock JB. A simplified technique for intestinal reanastomosis after the Hartmann procedure. Surg Gynecol Obstet 1985;161:390–391.
29. Buchmann P, Baumgartner D. A sigmoidoscope to facilitate

reanastomosis following a Hartmann procedure. Dis Colon Rectum 1987;30:145–146.

30. Ravitch MM. Varieties of stapled anastomoses in rectal resection. Surg Clin North Am 1984;64:543–554.

31. Minichan DP. Enlarging the bowel lumen for the EEA stapler. Dis Colon Rectum 1982;25:61.

32. Moseson MD, Hoexter B, Labow SB. Glucagon, a useful adjunct in anastomosis with a stapling device. Dis Colon Rectum 1980;23:25.

33. Shlasko E, Gorfine SR, Gelernt IM. Using lidocaine to ease the insertion of the circular stapler. Surg Gynecol Obstet 1992;174:70.

34. Mileski WJ, Rege RV, Joehl RJ, Nahrwold DL. Rates of morbidity and mortality after closure of loop and end colostomy. Surg Gynecol Obstet 1990;171:17–21.

35. Porter JA, Salvati EP, Rubin RJ, Eisenstat TE. Complications of colostomies. Dis Colon Rectum 1989;32:299–303.

36. Doberneck RC. Revision and closure of the colostomy. Surg Clin North Am 1991;71:193–201.

37. Leenen LP, Kuypers JH. Some factors influencing the outcome of stoma surgery. Dis Colon Rectum 1989;32:500–504.

38. Daly JM, DeCosse JJ. Complications in surgery of the colon and rectum. Surg Clin North Am 1983;63:1215–1231.

39. Finemore RG. Repeated haemorrhage from a terminal colostomy due to mucocutaneous varices with coexisting hepatic metastatic rectal adenocarcinoma: A case report. Br J Surg 1979;66:806.

40. Adson MA, Fulton RE. The ileal stoma and portal hypertension: An uncommon site of variceal bleeding. Arch Surg 1977;112:501–504.

41. Grundfest-Broniatowski S, Fazio V. Conservative treatment of bleeding stomal varices. Arch Surg 1983;118:981–985.

42. Hesterberg R, Stahlknecht CD, Roher HD. Sclerotherapy for massive enterostomy bleeding resulting from portal hypertension. Dis Colon Rectum 1986;29:275–277.

43. Fucini C, Wolff BG, Dozois RR. Bleeding from peristomal varices: Perspectives on prevention and treatment. Dis Colon Rectum 1991;34:1073–1078.

44. Beck DE, Fazio VW, Grundfest-Broniatowski S. Surgical management of bleeding stomal varices. Dis Colon Rectum 1988;31:343–346.

45. Holmes JWC, Nichols RL. Sepsis following colorectal surgery. In: Fazio VW, ed. Current Therapy in Colon and Rectal Surgery. Toronto: BC Decker, 1990, pp 396–408.

46. Leslie D. The parastomal hernia. Surg Clin North Am 1984;64:407–415.

47. Prian GW, Sawyer RB, Sawyer KC. Repair of peristomal colostomy hernias. Am J Surg 1975;130:694–696.

48. Sugarbaker PH. Prosthetic mesh repair of large hernias at the site of colonic stomas. Surg Gynecol Obstet 1980;150:577–578.

49. Chandler JG, Evans BP. Colostomy prolapse. Surgery 1978;84:577–582.

50. Mirelman D, Corman ML, Veidenheimer MC, Coller JA. Colostomies: Indications and contraindications: Lahey clinic experience 1963–1974. Dis Colon Rectum 1978;21:172–176.

51. Wara P, Sorensen K, Berg V. Proximal fecal diversion: Review of ten years' experience. Dis Colon Rectum 1981;24:114–119.

52. Brooke BN. Historical perspectives. In: Dozois RR, ed. Alternatives to Conventional Ileostomy. Chicago: Year Book, 1985, pp 19–28.

53. Brown JY. The value of complete physiological rest of the large bowel in the treatment of certain ulcerative and obstructive lesions of this organ. Surg Gynecol Obstet 1913;16:610–613.

54. Corbett RS. A review of the surgical treatment of chronic ulcerative colitis. Proc R Soc Med 1945;38:277–290.

55. Brooke BN. Ulcerative Colitis and Its Surgical Treatment. London: E & S Livingstone, 1954, p 75.

56. Strauss AA, Strauss SF. Surgical treatment of ulcerative colitis. Surg Clin North Am 1944;24:211–224.

57. Warren N, McKittrick LS. Ileostomy for ulcerative colitis. Surg Gynecol Obstet 1951;93:555–567.

58. Brooke BN. The management of an ileostomy including its complications. Lancet 1952;2:102–104.

59. Crile G Jr, Turnbull RB. Mechanism and prevention of ileostomy dysfunction. Ann Surg 1954;140:459–466.

60. Hill GL, Millward SF, King RFGJ, et al. Normal ileostomy output. Close relation to body size. Br Med J 1979;2:831–832.

61. Metcalf AM, Dozois RR, Beart RW Jr, et al. Temporary ileostomy for ileal pouch-anal anastomosis: Function and complications. Dis Colon Rectum 1986;29:300–303.

62. Slater G, Kreel I, Aufses AH Jr. Temporary loop ileostomy in the treatment of Crohn's disease. Ann Surg 1978;88:706–709.

63. Williams NS, Nasmyth DG, Jones D, et al. De-functioning stomas: A prospective controlled trial comparing loop ileostomy with loop transverse colostomy. Br J Surg 1986;73:566–570.

64. Kock NG. Historical perspective. In: Dozois RR, ed. Alternatives to Conventional Ileostomy. Chicago: Year Book, 1985, pp 133–145.

65. Schoetz DJ Jr, Coller JA, Veidenheimer MC. Alternatives to conventional ileostomy in chronic ulcerative colitis. Surg Clin North Am 1985;65:21–33.

66. Gelernt IM, Gorfine SR. Management of postsurgical problems. In: Gitnick G, ed. Inflammatory Bowel Disease: Diagnosis and Treatment. New York: Igaku-Shoin, 1991, pp 451–460.

67. Pearl RK, Prasad ML, Orsay CP, et al. Early local complications from intestinal stomas. Arch Surg 1985;120:1145–1147.

68. Bokey EL, Dent OF, Zubrzycki J, et al. Surgical morbidity after ileostomy in New South Wales. Med J Aust 1984;141:494–495.

69. Fry RD. End ileostomy: Techniques for construction and management of complications. Semin Colon Rectal Surg 1991;2:86–92.

70. Todd IP. Mechanical complications of ileostomy. Clin Gastroenterol 1982;11:268–273.

71. Weaver RM, Alexander-Williams J, Keighley MR. Indications and outcome of reoperation for ileostomy complications in inflammatory bowel disease. Int J Colorectal Dis 1988;3:38–42.

72. Carlstedt A, Fasth S, Hulten L, et al. Long-term ileostomy complications in patients with ulcerative colitis and Crohn's disease. Int J Colorectal Dis 1987;2:22–25.

73. Sohn N, Schulmann N, Weinstein MA, et al. Ileostomy prolapse repair utilizing bidirectional myotomy and a meshed split-thickness skin graft. Am J Surg 1983;145:807–808.

74. Watts JM, DeDombal FT, Goligher JC. Early results of surgery for ulcerative colitis. Br J Surg 1966;53:1005–1014.

75. Williams JG, Etherington R, Hayward MW, Hughes LE. Paraileostomy hernia: A clinical and radiological study. Br J Surg 1990;77:1355–1357.

76. Garnjobst W, Sullivan ES. Repair of paraileostomy hernia with polypropylene mesh reinforcement. Dis Colon Rectum 1984; 27:268–269.

77. Kodner IJ. Stoma complications. In: Fazio VW, ed. Current Therapy in Colon and Rectal Surgery. Toronto: BC Decker, 1990, pp 420–425.

78. Turnbull RB Jr. The surgical approach to the treatment of inflammatory bowel disease (IBD): A personal view of techniques and prognosis. In: Kirsner JB, Shorter RG, eds. Inflammatory Bowel Disease. Philadelphia: Lea & Febiger, 1975, pp 338–385.

79. Hughes ESR, McDermott FT, Masterton JP. Intestinal obstruction following operation for inflammatory disease of the bowel. Dis Colon Rectum 1979;22:469–471.

80. Francois Y, Dozois RR, Kelly KA, et al. Small intestinal obstruction complicating ileal pouch-anal anastomosis. Ann Surg 1989;209:46–50.

81. Laws HL. Management of small bowel obstruction. Am Surg 1978;44:313–317.

82. Wolfson PJ, Bauer JJ, Gelernt IM, et al. Use of the long tube in the management of patients with small intestinal obstruction due to adhesions. Arch Surg 1985;120:1001–1006.

83. Hellman J, Lago CP. Dermatologic complications in colostomy and ileostomy patients. Int J Dermatol 1990;29:129–133.

84. Martin AG, Leal-Khouri S. Principles of managing dermato-

logic and wound problems related to intestinal stomas. Semin Colon Rectal Surg 1991;2:161–167.

85. Storey VM. Persistent peristomal skin reaction: A case of psoriasis. J Enterostomal Ther 1982;9:63–64.

86. Rodriguez DB. Treatment for three ostomy patients with systemic skin disorders: Psoriasis, pemphigus, and dermatomyositis. J Enterostomal Ther 1981;8:31–32.

87. Williams SG, Halpin-Landry JE. Caring for the person with a stoma and systemic lupus erythematosus. J Enterostomal Ther 1990;17:128–130.

88. McGarity WC, Robertson DB, McKowen PP. Pyoderma gangrenosum at the peristomal site in patients with Crohn's disease. Arch Surg 1984;119:1186–1188.

89. Prystowsky JH, Kahn SN, Lazarus GS. Present status of pyoderma gangrenosum. Review of 21 cases. Arch Dermatol 1989;125:57–64.

90. Shelley ED, Shelley WB. Cyclosporine therapy for pyoderma gangrenosum associated with sclerosing cholangitis and ulcerative colitis. J Am Acad Dermatol 1988;18:1084–1088.

91. Kock NG, Myrvold HE, Nilsson LO, Philipson BM. Continent ileostomy: The Swedish experience. In: Dozois RR, ed. Alternatives to Conventional Ileostomy. Chicago: Year Book, 1985, pp 163–175.

92. Fazio VW, Church JM. Complications and function of the continent ileostomy at the Cleveland Clinic. World J Surg 12:148–154, 1988.

93. Jarvinen HJ, Makitie A, Sivula A. Long-term results of continent ileostomy. Int J Colorect Dis 1986;1:40–43.

94. Dozois RR, Kelly KA, Beart RW Jr, Beahrs OH. Continent ileostomy: The Mayo Clinic Experience. In: Dozois RR, ed. Alternatives to Conventional Ileostomy. Chicago: Year Book, 1985, pp 180–195.

95. Vernava AM, Goldberg SM. Is the Kock pouch still a viable option? Int J Colorectal Dis 1988;3:135–138.

96. Pemberton JH, Phillips SF, Dozois RR, Wendorf LJ. Current clinical results. In: Dozois RR, ed. Alternatives to Conventional Ileostomy. Chicago: Year Book, 1985, pp 40–50.

97. Morowitz DA, Kirsner JB. Ileostomy in ulcerative colitis: A questionnaire study of 1803 patients. Am J Surg 1981;141:370–375.

98. Kock NG, Brevinge H, Ojerskog B. Continent ileostomy. Perspect Colon Rectal Surg 1989;2:71–84.

99. Kock NG. Historical perspective. In: Dozois RR, ed. Alternatives to Conventional Ileostomy. Chicago: Year Book, 1985, pp 133–145.

100. Waye JD, Kreel I, Bauer J, Gelernt IM. The continent ileostomy: Diagnosis and treatment of problems by means of operative fiberoptic endoscopy. Gastrointest Endosc 1977;23:196–198.

101. Church JM, Fazio VW, Lavery IC. The role of fiberoptic endoscopy in the management of the continent ileostomy. Gastrointest Endosc 1987;33:203–209.

102. Ojerskog B, Kock NG, Philipson BM, Philipson M. Pregnancy and delivery in patients with a continent ileostomy. Surg Gynecol Obstet 1988;167:61–64.

103. Bonello JC, Thow GB, Manson RR. Mucosal enteritis: A complication of the continent ileostomy. Dis Colon Rectum 1981;24:37–41.

104. Zuccaro G, Fazio VW, Church JM, et al. Pouch ileitis. Dig Dis Sci 1989;34:1505–1510.

105. Phillips SF. Altered physiology. In: Dozois RR, ed. Alternatives to Conventional Ileostomy. Chicago: Year Book, 1985, pp 146–159.

106. Hulten L. Pouchitis—incidence and characteristics in the continent ileostomy. Int J Colorectal Dis 1989;4:208–210.

107. Kelly DG, Phillips SF, Kelly KA, et al. Dysfunction of the continent ileostomy: Clinical features and bacteriology. Gut 1983;24:193–201.

108. Nivatvongs S. Ulcerative colitis. In: Gordon PH, Nivatvongs S, eds. Principles and Practice of Surgery for the Colon, Rectum, and Anus. St Louis: Quality Medical Publishing, 1992, pp 667–715.

109. McLeod RS, Taylor DW, Cohen Z, Cullen JB. Single-patient randomized clinical trial: Use in determining optimum treatment for patients with inflammation of Kock continent ileostomy reservoir. Lancet 1986;1:726–728.

110. Jagelman DG, Fabian TC, Nichols RL, et al. Single-dose cefotetan versus multiple-dose cefoxitin as prophylaxis in colorectal surgery. Am J Surg 1988;155:71–76.

111. Persson AV, Davis RJ, Villavicenclo JL. Deep venous thrombosis and pulmonary embolism. Surg Clin North Am 1991;71:1195–1209.

112. Kreitzer JM, Reuben SS, Reed AP. Update on postoperative pain management. Mt Sinai J Med 1991;58:240–246.

113. Kilbride MJ, Senagore AJ, Mazier WP, et al. Epidural analgesia. Surg Gynecol Obstet 1992;174:137–140.

114. Bauer JJ, Gelernt IM, Salky BA, Kreel I. Is routine postoperative nasogastric decompression really necessary? Ann Surg 1985;201:233–236.

115. Gilley MT, Cassidy SM. Rehabilitation of the ostomy patient. Semin Colon Rectal Surg 1991;2:141–147.

116. Broadwell DC, Appleby CH, Bates MA, Jackson BS. Principles and techniques of pouching. In: Broadwell DC, Jackson BS, eds. Principles of Ostomy Care. St Louis: CV Mosby, 1982, pp 565–643.

117. Laucks SS, Mazier WP, Milsom JW, et al. An assessment of colostomy irrigation. Dis Colon Rectum 1988;31:279–282.

Lower Gastrointestinal Endoscopy: Diagnostic and Therapeutic Procedures

C H A P T E R 1 9

Thomas L. Dent

John S. Kukora

Steven G. Harper

Since ancient times, visual examination of the various cavities of the human body has been recognized as crucial in the evaluation of disease. Until 1970, however, endoscopic diagnosis and therapy of colorectal diseases were limited to the distal 25 cm because only rigid instruments were available. Flexible fiberoptic instruments now permit the direct visualization and the safe treatment of colonic lesions that previously could be seen only indirectly by contrast radiographs and could be treated only by abdominal exploration. In contrast to diagnosis and therapy of upper gastrointestinal disease, in which flexible instruments have rendered rigid ones obsolete, anoscopy and rigid proctoscopy are still important tools in the evaluation of anorectal and colon diseases.

DIAGNOSTIC ENDOSCOPY

Anoscopy

Indications

Anoscopic examination of the anal canal (the distal 2 to 4 cm of the alimentary tract) is integral to a complete evaluation of lower intestinal complaints. Unfortunately, the anal canal is often overlooked or examined only through a sigmoidoscope, which results in poor visualization and undetected pathology. The most common indications for anoscopy include rectal bleeding; anorectal pain; perianal mass, swelling, or protrusion; anal soiling or leakage; pruritus ani; and follow-up after surgical excision for benign or malignant conditions.

Preparation

Because anoscopy is usually performed in conjunction with sigmoidoscopy, preparation for both consists of the administration of one or two small-volume sodium biphosphate (Fleet) enemas 1 hour before the examination. If only an anoscopic examination is to be performed, enemas are not essential but do improve visualization of the anal canal.

Instrumentation

Anoscopes are available in several diameters, lengths, and designs. For example, anoscopes can be either end-viewing with an obturator to facilitate insertion, or side-viewing with a sliding, removable flange; some have a built-in light source and others require external lighting. Whichever size and type of anoscope is chosen, the endoscopist's goal is to gain the fullest visualization of the anal canal with the minimum of patient discomfort.

Technique

The patient is placed in the left lateral (Sims) position, although the knee-chest or the jackknife position can be used as well. The anal canal is lubricated with a water-soluble gel during digital rectal examination. The anoscope is inserted into the anal canal to its full length. Gentle rotation of the end-viewing anoscope during removal allows complete (360-degree) evaluation of the anal canal. With the side-viewing anoscope, the instrument should be removed after each quadrant of the anal canal is visualized and reinserted with the opening positioned in a different quadrant. This avoids stretching, cutting, or pinching the anal mucosa or skin. Unfortunately, three or four insertions of the anoscope are required, which increases patient discomfort.

Sometimes perianal pain makes anoscopic examination too uncomfortable. This discomfort may be reduced by the application of anesthetic cream, ointment, or gel to the sensitive anoderm several minutes before insertion of the anoscope. If topical anesthesia does not allow a complete and adequate examination and serious anal pathology is suspected, the patient may require examination using general, spinal, or local anesthesia.

Complications

Complications of anoscopy include lacerations and bleeding, both of which are uncommon and self-limited and require no specific therapy. However if bleeding originates from primary anal canal pathology, appropriate treatment measures for the underlying problem should be initiated.

Findings

Hemorrhoids are the most common pathologic finding in patients evaluated for rectal bleeding. Hemorrhoids are classified as internal (venous complexes existing above the dentate line), external (distal to the dentate line), or a combination of internal and external. Classically, the vascular cushions of internal hemorrhoids are located in the right anterior, right posterior, or left lateral position and appear as purple-red clusters of redundant mucosa that may prolapse beyond the anal canal. With chronic, enlarged, prolapsed internal hemorrhoids, the mucosal surface may appear ulcerated with bright red bleeding.

During anoscopy, anal fissures are identified as sharply demarcated elliptical tears, usually in the midline of the anal canal, that extend from the anal verge a variable distance above the dentate line. A chronic fissure may be associated with a "sentinel" skin tag at its distal margin and a hypertrophied anal papilla at its proximal margin. In deep fissures, the exposed underlying fibers of the internal sphincter may also be visible. Over 90% of anal fissures are located in the posterior midline. Fissures are painful and may require the topical application of an anesthetic cream before examination.

Anal fistulas are a common problem of the anal canal. Fistulas develop from infected anal glands located at the dentate line. Although the appearance of a small mound of inflammatory tissue in the perianal area and palpation of a fibrous cord of inflammatory tissue are diagnostic of an anal fistula, anoscopic evaluation may identify the internal opening and pus exuding from the infected anal crypt at the level of the dentate line.

Neoplasms of the anal canal are usually discovered by palpation of a firm irregular mass in the anal canal or by visualization of an irregularly shaped lesion that extends beyond the anal verge. Anoscopy can define the proximal limits of the lesion and facilitate exposure for obtaining a biopsy specimen. Although the gross appearance can vary, an anal neoplasm usually appears as a raised lesion with serrated edges, with or without an ulcerated central area. Bleeding may be present on the surface of the tumor. Rigid or flexible sigmoidoscopy complements anoscopy in evaluating anal neoplasms and excluding the possibility that the tumor originates from the rectum and prolapses into the anus.

Condylomata (venereal warts) are common sexually transmitted infections that affect the anal canal and perianal skin. The lesions appear as whitish, slightly raised plaques that may be solitary and discrete or conglomerated into a cauliflower-like configuration. Failure to locate and eradicate lesions located in the anal canal frequently leads to recurrence of the disease.

Sigmoidoscopy

Indications

The indications for sigmoidoscopy include rectal bleeding; iron-deficiency anemia; anorectal, lower abdominal, or pelvic pain; recent change in bowel habits; resolution and/or confirmation of abnormal findings on contrast radiographs; visualization of low-lying anastomoses for recurrent cancer; rectal or abdominal mass; monitoring of inflammatory bowel disease; and screening for rectosigmoid cancer. The American Cancer Society recommends screening sigmoidoscopy every 3 to 5 years after 50 years of age. Although flexible sigmoidoscopes have largely replaced rigid metal and disposable plastic sigmoidoscopes for both symptom evaluation and screening, rigid sigmoidoscopy allows a more accurate measurement of the distance of a lesion from the anal verge and larger biopsy specimens.

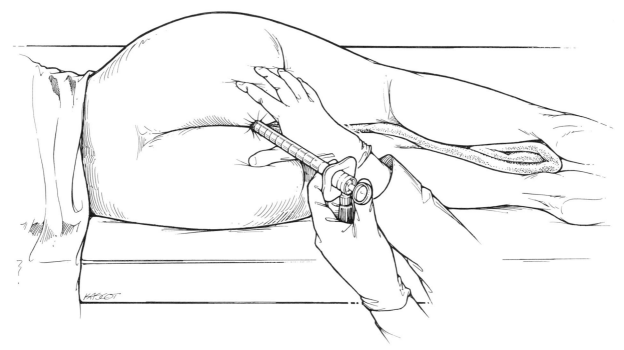

Figure 19–1. Insertion of rigid proctoscope with patient in Sims' position.

Because the rectosigmoid is the most difficult region of the colon to assess radiographically, an evaluation of colonic symptoms by barium radiograph is incomplete unless a sigmoidoscopic examination is also performed.

Preparation

Preparation consists of the administration of two low-volume sodium biphosphate enemas approximately 1 hour before examination. No dietary restrictions or laxatives are necessary. For endoscopists who wish to examine the anorectum before any trauma from enema instillation occurs, the enemas may be given after anoscopy and immediately before the flexible sigmoidoscopic portion of the examination.

Instrumentation

For rigid sigmoidoscopy, a 25-cm reusable metal or a disposable plastic sigmoidoscope with attached light source, bulb insufflator, and magnifying lens is used. For children or for adults with painful or narrow anorectal openings, smaller-diameter rigid sigmoidoscopes are available. A common misconception is that children should be examined only with a pediatric instrument. In fact, young patients tolerate examination with the standard-sized rigid sigmoidoscope quite well, thereby allowing better visualization of the rectum than would be possible with the narrower pediatric sigmoidoscope. For flexible sigmoidoscopy, a 60-cm

flexible sigmoidoscope, light and air source, suction apparatus, and biopsy forceps are necessary.

Technique

Rigid Sigmoidoscopy. The rigid sigmoidoscopic examination is performed with the patient in either the left lateral (Sims) (Fig. 19–1) or the knee-chest position. After insertion of the well-lubricated sigmoidoscope and obturator, the obturator is withdrawn and the magnifying lens is secured in place. With constant direct visualization of the rectal lumen, the instrument is gently advanced by using up-and-down, left-and-right, and circular motions, which keep the instrument tip directed away from the mucosal folds. When needed, air is insufflated to visualize the mucosa more clearly and to determine the direction of the bowel lumen to facilitate further advancement. Residual mucus and feces are aspirated with a suction catheter. Another important maneuver involves depressing the valves of Houston and redundant mucosal folds in the sigmoid colon to visualize the "blind" spaces behind them. The examination is complete at insertion of the full 25 cm of the instrument or when the patient's discomfort dictates—often at the flexure of the rectosigmoid colon (15 to 17 cm from the anal verge). During withdrawal, the sigmoidoscope is rotated in wide circular arcs to ensure full visualization of the mucosal surface of the rectum and lower sigmoid colon.

Flexible Fiberoptic Sigmoidoscopy. The patient undergoing flexible fiberoptic sigmoidoscopy (FFS) is usually examined in the left lateral decubitus position. The examiner talks to the patient about what to expect and repeats these points as the sigmoidoscopy progresses. Specifically, the patient may experience abdominal bloating, occasional cramping, and urge to defecate that may be embarrassing. Employing this form of "verbal anesthesia" greatly increases the patient's tolerance of the procedure.

The assistant plays a vital role in all flexible endoscopic procedures. In addition to reassuring the patient during the procedure, the assistant must be familiar with the equipment and know how to handle mechanical problems as they arise. The assistant may be called on to hold the instrument if the endoscopist needs both hands to maneuver the deflection controls or to assist with biopsies or cytologic brushings. With the patient in the left lateral position and the assistant on the side of the table opposite the physician, the patient and the assistant can see each other and the assistant can report to the physician how well the patient is tolerating the procedure.

Before undertaking FFS, it is essential that the physician be completely knowledgeable about the equipment (including not only the sigmoidoscope but also the light source, suction apparatus, biopsy forceps, and brushes), the technique required to advance the instrument through the various portions of the distal large bowel, the events that may occur during the examination, and the common gross findings of normal anatomy and large bowel pathology.

Before the procedure is performed, a digital rectal examination is done to evaluate the caliber of the anal canal, rule out anal or low rectal masses, and lubricate the anal canal. With the lubricated tip of the sigmoidoscope held parallel to the right index finger, lateral pressure is applied as the instrument is advanced into the rectum to overcome the resistance of the anal sphincter. Inspection of the rectum through the eyepiece usually reveals a "red-out" or "white-out," which indicates that the end of the sigmoidoscope is flush against the bowel wall. Retracting the instrument several centimeters should remove the lens from the bowel wall and reveal the rectal lumen. The general principles of performing FFS are to keep the lumen in view; avoid the forceful advancement of the sigmoidoscope; minimize the amount of air insufflation; and, above all, avoid hurting the patient.

There are two ways to perform FFS. In the one-person technique, the physician holds the control head of the instrument in the left hand so that the index finger and middle finger control the suction and insufflation valves and the thumb controls the tip deflection dials (Fig. 19–2). The right hand feeds the shaft of the instrument into the anus with the necessary clockwise and counterclockwise torque as the sigmoidoscope is advanced. In the two-person method, the assistant advances the shaft under the direction of the physician, who uses both hands on the control head of the sigmoidoscope. The right hand controls the tip deflection dials while the left hand supports the weight of the instrument and controls the insufflation and suction valves.

As the lumen is visualized, the instrument should be advanced slowly by means of clockwise or counterclockwise torque to keep the tip of the sigmoidoscope in the center of the lumen. As semilunar valves of the colon and rectum are identified, the tip of the sigmoidoscope should be rotated over the fold by torquing the instrument or by deflecting the tip in the appropriate direction so that the instrument flattens the fold and reveals the lumen beyond. This can be accomplished either by torquing the instrument or by dialing the tip in the appropriate direction. If this maneuver proves difficult, the instrument should be withdrawn and rotated, which straightens the colon and telescopes the bowel onto the shaft of the sigmoidoscope. A constant advancement and withdrawal technique and twisting the sigmoidoscope both clockwise and counterclockwise facilitate progression of the instrument through the sigmoid colon. If the instrument is advanced *only* (and not withdrawn), a large loop will be created in the sigmoid colon, further advancement of the instrument will be hindered, and a significant amount of patient discomfort will result. If this occurs, withdrawal of the sigmoidoscope and clockwise rotation will straighten the sigmoid colon and remove the loop.

Previous disease or individual anatomy may prevent complete insertion. The endoscopist should not consider a less-than-60-cm examination as a failure. As the sigmoidoscope is removed, the lumen should be kept in full view by rotating the sigmoidoscope back and forth. As the instrument is withdrawn, distending luminal gas should be aspirated, thereby minimizing patient discomfort following the procedure. Although some inspection is performed during insertion of the sigmoidoscope, most visualization is performed during the withdrawal phase, especially the inspection of "blind" spots proximal to each semilunar valve.

Complications

The two most serious complications of diagnostic sigmoidoscopy are bleeding and bowel perforation. Both are extremely uncommon and should become increasingly rarer as the endoscopist's experience increases.

Bleeding from instrument trauma is usually minor and self-limited, even in patients taking anticoagulant or antiplatelet drugs. Bleeding following mucosal biopsy can be more brisk but usually is either self-limited or responds to local pressure. A thorough medication history should be taken and large-forceps biopsy

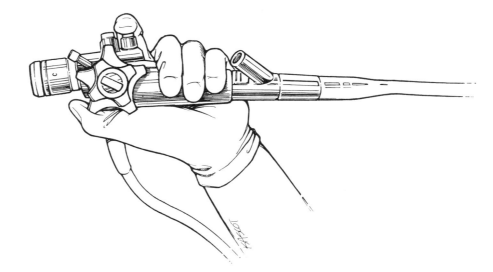

Figure 19–2. Proper hand position on controls of colonoscope.

avoided for patients taking anticoagulant or antiplatelet medications, including aspirin. Small-forceps (2-mm) biopsy can usually be performed safely even in fully anticoagulated cases.

Perforation during diagnostic sigmoidoscopy can result from excessively forceful advancement or torquing of the sigmoidoscope or from the vigorous application of the biopsy forceps. The tip or side of the sigmoidoscope can be pushed through the bowel wall during bowing and stretching of the sigmoid colon. These kinds of perforation can be minimized by terminating the examination when the patient develops significant abdominal pain during sigmoidoscope insertion. Sedation and analgesia during diagnostic sigmoidoscopy are rarely necessary and have the serious disadvantage of blunting pain sensation, thus increasing the possibility of perforation. Care should be taken to perform only mucosal biopsies. Deep and forceful penetration of the biopsy forceps should be avoided. Use of electrocautery snare or "hot" biopsy forceps must be avoided when the colon has been prepared only with enemas, because combustible gases may be present and cause a disastrous explosion. If a perforation is identified by physical or radiographic examination either during or following diagnostic sigmoidoscopy, urgent celiotomy and repair are indicated. Occasionally, mild to moderate lower abdominal pain and cramps follow sigmoidoscopy, presumably resulting from air insufflation or stretching of the bowel. These symptoms usually disappear within a few hours.

Findings

Generally, examination of the most distal part of the large bowel up to the rectosigmoid junction is accomplished easily. Special care should be taken to visualize the portion of the bowel above and adjacent to the valves of Houston to avoid missing small abnormalities (i.e., polyps or small malignancies). Full visualization of the rectum and sigmoid colon permits inspection of the portion of the bowel that harbors most of the significant colonic pathology. Common findings include polyps, carcinomas, and diverticulosis and inflammatory changes, such as diverticulitis, ulcerative proctitis or colitis, and Crohn's disease. Less common pathologic findings include arteriovenous malformations and colorectal strictures.

Colonoscopy

Indications

Compared with barium enema examination, diagnostic colonoscopy has advantages (e.g., greater diagnostic accuracy and specificity, biopsy and therapeutic capabilities) and disadvantages (e.g., slightly greater risk, need for sedation or analgesia, inability to examine the entire colon in a few patients, higher cost). The indications for diagnostic colonoscopy include signs or symptoms suggestive of disease of the lower gastrointestinal tract, gastrointestinal bleeding, need to monitor known colorectal disease, need to evaluate the entire colon preoperatively for coexisting lesions, and need to clarify a roentgenographic finding.

Signs or Symptoms Suggestive of Disease of the Lower Gastrointestinal Tract. Persistent diarrhea, obstipation, abdominal mass, and altered bowel habits are common signs and symptoms of inflammatory bowel disease and colorectal cancer.

Gastrointestinal Bleeding. The evaluation of a patient with occult fecal blood loss or hematochezia should include evaluation of the entire colon either by total colonoscopy or by the combination of flexible sigmoidoscopy and air-contrast barium enema. Similarly, an adult with iron-deficiency anemia and no identified source of blood loss requires the same evaluation, even in the absence of fecal occult blood. A patient with bright red rectal bleeding that is not mixed with feces and an identified anorectal source of bleeding need not undergo total colonoscopy for adequate evaluation, although flexible sigmoidoscopy is still recommended.

Need to Monitor Known Colorectal Disease. In patients with granulomatous or ulcerative colitis, colonoscopy can assess the extent of disease, clarify the diagnosis, assess the severity of mucosal changes, modify the extent of surgical resection, and monitor for dysplasia or carcinoma. In patients with polyps or carcinomas, colonoscopy is also indicated to detect synchronous or metachronous neoplastic lesions.

Need to Evaluate the Entire Colon Preoperatively for Coexisting Lesions. "Clearing" colonoscopy excludes other significant lesions of the colorectum, such as carcinomas and large sessile polyps, or segments with stricture or extensive diverticulosis that might affect the type and extent of operative intervention for a target or an index lesion.

Need to Clarify a Roentgenographic Finding. Diagnostic colonoscopy can be used to observe directly and, when indicated, to obtain a biopsy specimen of colorectal abnormalities, such as filling defects, strictures, mucosal irregularities, or colonic dilatation, that have been identified or suggested by a barium contrast radiograph.

Contraindications

Contraindications to diagnostic colonoscopy include recent myocardial infarction, pulmonary embolus, or cerebrovascular infarction; severe cardiovascular instability; and acute abdominal inflammation with peritonitis. Relative contraindications include late-stage pregnancy, massive splenomegaly, abdominal aortic aneurysm, poor bowel preparation, recent bowel or pelvic operation, and other medical conditions in which the risk-to-benefit ratio may be predicted to be excessive.

Preprocedure History and Physical Examination

A thorough history and physical examination are necessary for safe and effective colonoscopy. Awareness of the nature of the patient's symptoms, physical findings, prior relevant operations, and prior roentgenographic and laboratory studies is necessary for optimal interpretation of endoscopic observations.

The endoscopist should determine whether there are any coexisting medical conditions that may increase the risk of colonoscopy or sedation. Common examples include uncontrolled hypertension, coronary atherosclerosis, cirrhosis or other significant hepatic disease, pulmonary insufficiency, bleeding tendency, cerebrovascular disease, abdominal aortic aneurysm, and drug allergy or intolerance. The patient's overall strength and ability to cooperate during the procedure are also considered. Anticoagulant and antiplatelet medications should be discontinued before the procedure is performed.

Preoperative Studies

Although routine laboratory studies are unnecessary before diagnostic colonoscopy, appropriate laboratory studies are indicated in the preprocedure clarification of any abnormality suggested by history or physical examination (e.g., history of heart disease, bleeding tendency).

Informed Consent

The colonoscopic procedure, including its risks and alternatives, should be explained to the patient. Its significant advantages of detection and immediate biopsy or removal of colonic lesions, compared with roentgenographic studies, should be stressed. In addition, the patient should be informed of the complicating risks of perforation, bleeding, and drug reactions and of the disadvantage that in 5% to 10% of cases the colonoscope cannot be fully advanced to the cecum.

Mechanical Preparation

Good mechanical preparation of the colon is essential to a safe and accurate colonoscopic procedure. An extra moment spent to explain the instructions for mechanical bowel preparation can avert time-consuming frustration and potential hazard at the time of the procedure. Preparation consists of a diet of only clear liquids for 24 hours, which is extended to 48 hours in the patient with a history of constipation or cathartic use. Oral polyethylene glycol (GoLYTELY or CoLyte) is begun 8 to 12 hours before the procedure. The cathartic and accompanying electrolytes are reconstituted in 1 gallon of water according to the manufacturer's instructions and drunk in a volume of 8 ounces every 10 minutes until the entire gallon is consumed. At the termination of the preparation, feces should be clear or slightly bile-colored with no particulate matter. The advantages of this regimen are good patient tolerance, avoidance of cleansing enemas, rapidity and thoroughness of evacuation, and avoidance of systemic fluid and electrolyte imbalance.

Prophylactic Antibiotics

Although bacteremia may occur during endoscopic procedures, prophylactic antibiotics are not routinely recommended before diagnostic or therapeutic colonoscopy. They should be considered for patients with an artificial heart valve or a previous history of endocarditis.

Endoscopy Suite

On the day of the procedure, vital signs should be recorded and a nursing assessment performed to ensure that the preparation has been completed and that the latest stools were liquid and clear. Any last-minute questions should be answered, and an individual who will accompany the patient home after outpatient colonoscopy should be identified. The patient should be completely unclothed, except for an examination gown.

A fully equipped endoscopy suite is described in Table 19–1. The colonoscope should have been cleaned and disinfected and should be in proper working order with a suitable light source, an air-feed, suction, and accessories available. Blood pressure monitors (manual or automatic), electrocardiographic monitors, and pulse oximeter monitors (depending on the perceived risks from coexisting disease, age, or debility) should be available, in working order, and properly attached to the patient. Many endoscopists consider fluoroscopy to be a routine adjunct to colonoscopy, whereas others use it selectively. Fluoroscopy can assist maximum insertion of the colonoscope and can confirm the precise colon segment seen and the location of identified lesions, such as polyps.

Intravenous access should be obtained before colonoscopy is performed. Although other regimens are available, the intravenous combination of meperidine (25 to 75 mg) or morphine sulfate (5 to 10 mg) with diazepam (5 to 20 mg) is our preference. These should be administered in a deliberately slow manner (over

Table 19–1. EQUIPMENT FOR THE ENDOSCOPY UNIT

Examination table or gurney
Intravenous solutions and administration sets
Suction capabilities for endoscope and oropharynx
Medications: sedatives, narcotics, narcotic antagonists, cardiac drugs, antiarrhythmics, and anticholinergics
Cardiopulmonary resuscitation equipment: oxygen; blood pressure monitor; laryngoscope, endotracheal airway, Ambu bag; access to oximetry, electrocardiographic machine or cardiac monitor; and defibrillation equipment
Storage and disinfection capabilities, including gas sterilization
Endoscopes, light sources, accessories, and electrocautery
Washstand and proximity to toilet

several minutes) to achieve the desired level of sedation, usually manifested by slurring of speech. The amount of medication required varies according to the patient's level of anxiety, body size, and age. An ever-present danger in their use is the possibility of apnea, which may require narcotic antagonists or even urgent mechanical ventilation.

Technique

Colonoscopy is performed with the patient in the left lateral decubitus position (Fig. 19–3). Gowns, gloves, and eye protection are recommended for both endoscopist and assistant. The procedure begins with a careful digital rectal examination in which abundant water-soluble lubricant is used. The tip of the 180-cm colonoscope is inserted into the anus.

The proper position of the left hand on the endoscope control handle is shown in Figure 19–2. With gentle air insufflation to distend the bowel, the tip of the colonoscope is advanced through the rectum and then through the colon. Safe advancement of the colonoscope to the cecum depends on a combination of advancement and withdrawal of the colonoscope, tip deflection, and torquing the insertion tube along its long axis. These maneuvers should be accomplished with minimal air insufflation (just enough to distend the lumen slightly), as excessive insufflation causes patient discomfort and hampers insertion of the colonoscope. Ideally, the colonoscope is advanced only when the lumen is clearly visible. Blind "slide-by" techniques increase the risk of perforation, and although they are sometimes necessary to negotiate the sigmoid colon and flexures, the forward advancement of the colonoscope must be stopped if the patient complains of pain or if a red-out or white-out (indicating the tip of the scope is impacted against the bowel wall) occurs. The observation of mucosal folds easily passing by the field of view ensures that the slide-by maneuver is progressing satisfactorily. If feces preclude adequate visualization of the mucosa or the direction of the luminal channel, the procedure should be terminated until the patient has been better prepared.

The process of advancement and withdrawal of the colonoscope or the "hook-and-pull" technique (Fig. 19–4) causes the redundant sigmoid colon or flexures to "telescope" onto the insertion tube, thus eliminating the tendency of the colonoscope to form a loop (without forward advancement of the tip), as the insertion tube is advanced through the anus (Fig. 19–5). The importance of periodic withdrawal of the colonoscope to achieve this telescoping (Fig. 19–6) cannot be overemphasized. Although this maneuver might appear to be counterproductive, it is essential to efficient insertion of the colonoscope up to the cecum in most patients. Suction for deflation and colonic shortening

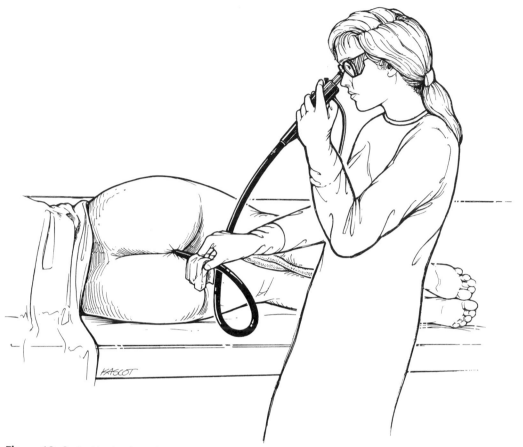

Figure 19–3. Positioning for colonoscopy.

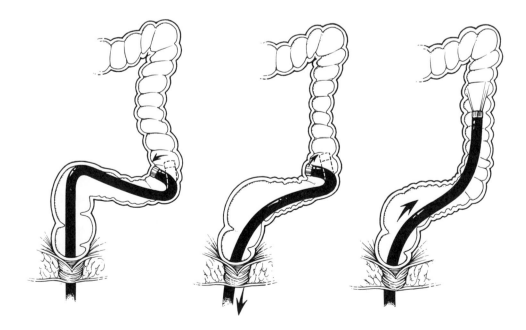

Figure 19–4. "Hook-and-pull" technique.

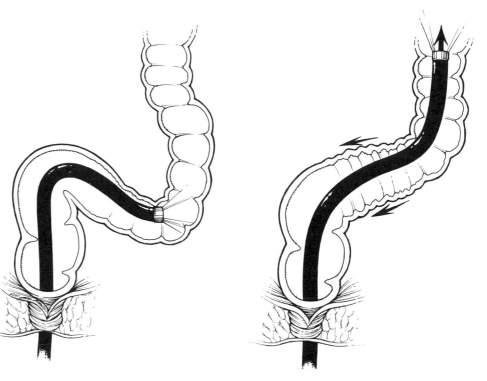

Figure 19–5. Telescoping of sigmoid colon onto scope.

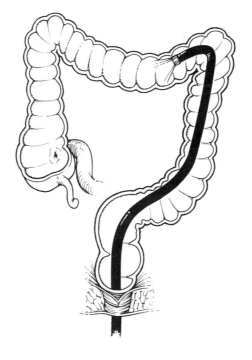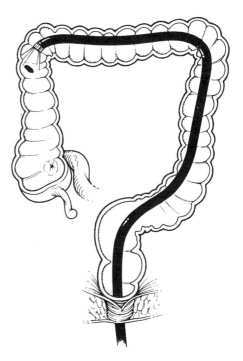

Figure 19–6. Scope advancement through splenic and hepatic flexures.

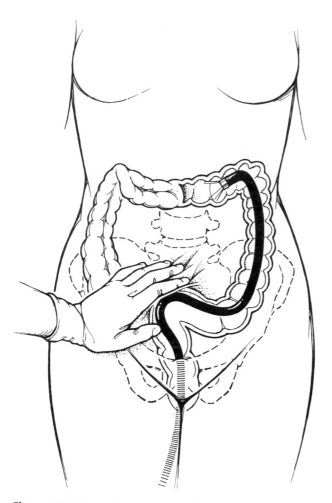

Figure 19–7. External pressure on abdomen.

can often facilitate advancement into the proximal transverse colon and ascending colon when insertion and withdrawal or the hook-and-pull technique fails to advance the tip.

The location of the tip of the colonoscope is usually identified by the distance of insertion, the internal landmarks, and the observation of the tip as it transilluminates the abdominal wall; less commonly, it is identified by fluoroscopy. Recognizable internal landmarks of the colon segments include the following: rectum (immediate proximity to anus, valves of Houston), sigmoid colon (multiple serpentine curves, proximity to rectum), descending colon (straight segment after traversing sigmoid colon), splenic flexure (abrupt angulation, blue shadow of spleen may be visible through bowel wall), transverse colon (triangular lumen after traversing splenic flexure), hepatic flexure (abrupt bend after traversing transverse colon, blue shadow of liver may be visible before the flexure), and ascending colon and cecum (large-diameter lumen, confluence of teniae in cecum, appendiceal orifice, ileocecal valve, liquid stool in blind sac). Full insertion of the endoscope to the cecum can be further confirmed by observing indentation of the cecal wall by finger pressure over McBurney's point or lower and noting transillumination of the abdominal wall in the right lower quadrant or the inguinal area.

In about 5% to 10% of patients, full advancement to the cecum is impossible. Having the patient roll to a supine position or manipulating the colonoscope by deeply indenting the abdominal wall and compressing the viscera by the hands of the assistant may facilitate further insertion (Fig. 19–7). Judgment must be exercised in deciding how much maneuvering and effort to expend in attempting to reach the cecum without subjecting the patient to excessive discomfort or risk.

If appropriate, the endoscope can be maneuvered into the terminal ileum in many patients. This is most effectively accomplished by moving the tip of the colonoscope beyond the ileocecal valve and its prominent mucosal fold and by angling the tip acutely backward toward the fold. Then, while the endoscope is withdrawn and the tip "jiggled," the ileocecal valve can be hooked and cannulated to allow visualization of 10 to 30 cm of terminal ileum.

The initial efforts of the endoscopist should be directed primarily toward safe and efficient insertion of the colonoscope; careful scrutiny of the entire mucosal surface is the main objective on withdrawal of the colonoscope. Examination is best accomplished by very gradual withdrawal and by torquing the colonoscope with a slight deflection of the tip as needed to survey the entire colon circumference.

In the patient with a colostomy, colonoscopic examination is performed through the stoma, usually while the patient is in the supine position. Initial insertion of the endoscope should be done carefully, as peristomal herniation and tightness of the abdominal fascial opening can predispose the patient to colon perforation.

Postprocedure Care

The patient is kept under observation until the effects of the sedation have begun to disappear. The patient should not drive home and should be accompanied by a responsible adult. The patient and responsible adult should be instructed to notify the endoscopist if severe abdominal pain, significant rectal bleeding, or fever occurs.

Findings

Abnormalities that can be identified during colonoscopic examination are usually obvious and include carcinomas; pedunculated and sessile polyps; inflammatory changes including erythema, ulceration, and stricture; diverticulosis with or without muscular hypertrophy; and arteriovenous malformations. Submucosal lesions, such as lipomas, can be subtle, but they are usually identified visually as mass lesions covered by normal mucosa and tactilely as being indentable with the biopsy forceps.

Complications

Complications of diagnostic colonoscopy occur in less than 2% of examinations and include apnea, cardiovascular instability, perforation, and bleeding. There is also a possibility of transmission of infectious diseases.

Apnea is due to analgesics and sedatives and although usually dose-related can be unpredictable. Vigilant monitoring of respiration by the endoscopist and assistant is required. The incidence of apnea is reduced by titrating the amount of sedation or narcotic given to the individual patient and by administering medication slowly. Treatment consists of narcotic antagonists and mechanical ventilation by mask with oxygen. Although not necessarily drug-related, cardiac arrhythmias, hypertension, or hypotension may develop during colonoscopy, possibly from stress, discomfort, or the vagal effects of colonic distention. If these complications are severe or persistent, the colonoscopic procedure should be stopped and specific pharmacologic or other resuscitative interventions implemented.

Perforation is the most serious complication of colonoscopy. It occurs about once or twice per thousand diagnostic colonoscopies and may result from either a pneumatic insufflation injury or a tearing injury from forces transmitted by the endoscope. Pneumatic perforation is less common than direct injury and usually

is a cecal "blow-out" tear. Pneumatosis of the colon with or without pneumoperitoneum is often asymptomatic and presumably results from slow dissection of insufflated gas through the layers of the colon wall. Pneumatosis does not necessarily progress to a significant transmural tear with resultant fecal spillage and peritonitis. Minimally symptomatic pneumatosis or pneumoperitoneum can be treated expectantly with intravenous broad-spectrum antibiotics, bowel rest, and in-hospital observation. Mechanical tears usually occur at points of colon angulation and fixation, most commonly in the sigmoid colon. Perforation can result in fecal spillage and progressive peritonitis that requires operative repair or resection, with or without a colostomy.

Bleeding following diagnostic colonoscopy usually results from mechanical irritation of either hemorrhoids or anal fissures or follows tissue biopsy. Such bleeding is usually minimal and self-limited, rarely requiring any treatment.

Transmission of bacterial, protozoal, or viral disease by contaminated endoscopic equipment remains more theoretical and anecdotal than significant. Proper adherence to the manufacturer's recommendations for mechanical cleaning, disinfection, gas sterilization, and dry storage of the endoscope and accessories should all but eliminate this potential hazard.

THERAPEUTIC LOWER GASTROINTESTINAL ENDOSCOPY

Polypectomy

Colonoscopic snaring has replaced colotomy and polypectomy in the treatment of colon polyps. Instead of weighing the risk of malignancy present in a polyp against the operative mortality of its open removal, excision of all polyps is recommended. This not only removes small polypoid cancers but prevents the removed benign polyp from becoming malignant.

Indications

Generally the presence of any colon polyp is an indication for its removal, regardless of whether symptoms are present. Polyps may be identified by digital rectal examination, barium radiography, sigmoidoscopy, or colonoscopy. In adults, most colon polyps larger than 1 cm in diameter are neoplastic (adenomas or carcinomas) and are frequently associated with synchronous polyps. Any colon polyp should be considered a premalignant lesion and should be removed. Because neoplastic polyps are visually indistinguishable from non-neoplastic polyps, all polypoid lesions should have endoscopic verification of their presence, location, and configuration; removal and histologic examination; and complete search of the entire colon for synchronous polyps or cancers. Total colonoscopy and snare polypectomy, therefore, are indicated whenever a polyp (or possible polyp) is identified in an adult patient.

Size Considerations

Although any neoplastic polyp has a malignant potential, the transformation to invasive carcinoma increases in direct proportion to the size of the polyp and to the amount of villous (compared with tubular) tissue within it. Diminutive polyps are very common, are less than 1 cm in diameter, and are usually discovered at sigmoidoscopy. The majority are histologically hyperplastic with no malignant potential.

The treatment of diminutive polyps is controversial, but our practice is to perform a biopsy when they are discovered during sigmoidoscopy and to recommend colonoscopy and polypectomy only if the histologic examination reveals an adenoma or carcinoma. Forceps biopsy of polyps larger than 1 cm is unnecessary and frequently misleading, because the tiny 2-mm fraction of tissue may not be representative of the rest of the polyp and a malignant focus might be missed.

The optimal strategy for polyps larger than 1 cm is colonoscopic excisional biopsy and histologic examination of the entire lesion. Very large and/or sessile polyps are more frequently malignant and can be difficult to remove endoscopically, but colonoscopic polypectomy should still be attempted before considering celiotomy, because many large polyps are removable with snare techniques. A stalk that facilitates polypectomy may be obscured by a large polyp during barium enema examination. If colonoscopy confirms the presence of a polyp too large or too sessile for snare excision, *total* colonoscopy should still precede celiotomy because it will "clear" the colon of other synchronous lesions.

For polyps that cannot be removed colonoscopically, a colectomy appropriate for carcinoma at that location (e.g., right or left radical hemicolectomy), rather than just a colotomy and polypectomy, is recommended, because frozen-section diagnosis of colon polyps is notoriously inaccurate and because a second operation can thus be avoided if the polyp proves to be an invasive malignancy.

Age Considerations

Polyps in children are usually non-neoplastic juvenile polyps (hamartomas) that have little or no malignant potential, are frequently multiple, and spontaneously amputate or regress during puberty. Polypectomy is indicated only if the polyp becomes symptomatic with bleeding or prolapse or if the histology of the lesion is in doubt.

For the elderly patient, colonoscopic polypectomy usually is a safe procedure, but the individual must be in suitable medical condition to tolerate celiotomy if a complication, such as perforation, occurs. The surgeon should always weigh the risk of allowing a small polyp to remain (usually a small risk in an elderly patient) against the risk of snare excision and possible complications.

Contraindications

Contraindications to colonoscopic polypectomy include recent myocardial infarction, peritonitis, severe colitis, diverticulitis, and bleeding diathesis. Any medical condition that contraindicates celiotomy should a complication, such as perforation or bleeding, occur should also contraindicate colonoscopic polypectomy. Relative contraindications include inadequate visualization of the polyp or stalk (feces from suboptimal preparation, large size of the polyp) and anatomic factors that hinder safe positioning of the snare.

Preparation

The colon is prepared exactly as that for diagnostic colonoscopy. Enemas alone are inadequate. Complete evacuation of all fecal material is especially important before polypectomy, because electrocautery may cause combustible colonic gases to explode. Polypectomy should not be attempted if the colon is incompletely prepared. Conscious sedation and analgesia with diazepam and either meperidine or morphine, as in diagnostic colonoscopy, produce a comfortable, cooperative patient and improve the safety of the procedure.

Instrumentation

In addition to the equipment described for colonoscopy, a supply of electrocautery snares, regular biopsy forceps, insulated hot biopsy forceps, and an electrosurgical generating unit that provides cutting, coagulating, and blended current are needed.

Technique

When one plans to resect an identified polyp, the *entire* colon should be visualized because of the 30% to 50% incidence of synchronous neoplasms of the colon. Theoretically, the colon should be surveyed first and then the polyps resected so that all lesions are identified before the colon wall potentially damaged by electrocautery is exposed to endoscopic manipulation. Practically speaking, however, polyps less than 1 cm in

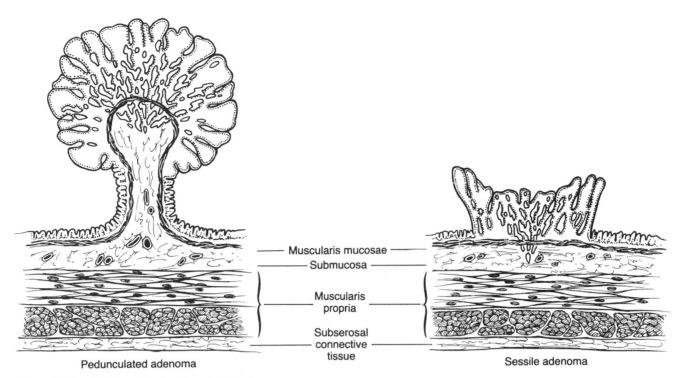

Figure 19–8. *(A)* Pedunculated and sessile *(B)* polyps.

diameter should be resected immediately, because they may be difficult to find later and colon damage is unlikely after resection of small or pedunculated polyps. Conversely, a suboptimal position for removal of the polyp during intubation frequently improves during withdrawal. Proper positioning of the polyp for safe removal is necessary, and a combination of patient positioning, abdominal counterpressure by an assistant, and advancement and withdrawal of the colonoscope usually provide an adequate view of the lesion. Excisional biopsy of the entire intact polyp facilitates accurately orienting the specimen and identifying the extent of penetration by malignant cells of the various layers of the head and stalk.

Pedunculated Polyps. Most adenomatous polyps appear as a "head" of adenomatous tissue on a "stalk" of normal colon mucosa and submucosa (Fig. 19–8*A*). After a complete view of the polyp and surrounding colon lumen is obtained, it is usually possible to maneuver the fully opened snare over the head of the polyp (Fig. 19–9). The plastic sheath of the snare should be placed adjacent to the point on the stalk to be transected before the wire snare is tightened. Transection near the head of a polyp reduces the possibility of coagulation injury to the adjacent colon, and because the stalk extends into the center of the polyp, the excised specimen permits adequate histologic evaluation of stalk invasion by malignant cells. Taking care always to see the snare in relation to the stalk and the

colon wall, the snare is slowly closed until resistance is felt. At this point, the endoscopist should check that the amount of snare wire still extending beyond the sheath corresponds to the estimated thickness of the stalk. If there seems to be more wire than expected, a knuckled portion of the colon wall may also have been ensnared, and the snare should be loosened and repositioned before the electrosurgical current is applied. As the snare is tightened, the coagulating current is applied in several 1- to 2-second bursts, and the stalk is slowly divided. A small amount of cutting current may be necessary to divide a thick stalk, but coagulation current is preferred because it reduces the incidence of bleeding from the stalk.

A short or thick stalk presents greater technical difficulty and increases the danger of bleeding or colon perforation. If more than a few bursts of current are needed to transect the stalk, the polyp should be repositioned using the snare and directional dials of the colonoscope so that the head of the polyp touches several different areas of the colon wall in order to prevent coagulation necrosis of a single area (see Fig. 19–11*A*). The polyp is retrieved for histologic examination by regrasping the transected stalk with the snare or by suctioning the polyp up against the colonoscope tip and withdrawing the colonoscope.

Small Sessile Polyps. Small sessile polyps (Fig. 19–8*B*) can usually be removed by using the snare technique as described previously or by using the hot biopsy

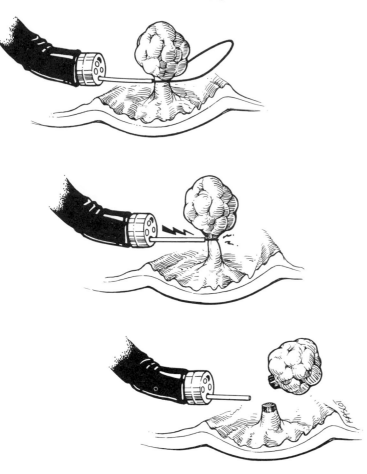

Figure 19–9. Snare around pedunculated polyp.

forceps. If the snare technique is used, colon injury can be minimized by elevating the firmly ensnared polyp off the underlying muscularis propria with the control knobs of the endoscope or by slightly withdrawing the snare prior to transection. Tiny polyps can be retrieved as described, or can be suctioned and retrieved from a tissue trap in the suction line. Hot biopsy forceps can be used to completely ablate a small polyp while at the same time recovering a small tissue sample for histologic examination. The polyp is grasped with the jaws of the insulated forceps and lifted away from the underlying colon wall. Coagulation current is applied until a small burn surrounds the forceps and the polyp separates. Care must be taken to avoid excessive current or pushing the forceps against the colon wall, which can result in a deep colon burn and perforation. The tissue remaining in the forceps is sent for histologic examination.

Large Sessile Polyps. Large sessile polyps generally exhibit more aggressive growth, are more likely to contain malignancy, are more difficult to remove with snare techniques, and are more prone to recur than are smaller pedunculated ones. Although piecemeal electrocautery snare excision (Fig. 19–10) can remove many of these lesions, it leads to a higher incidence of

complications and should be used with great caution and only by an experienced colonoscopist. The snare is tightened around the most convenient part of the polyp, and the piece is transected carefully. The snare is then repositioned and another piece is transected. The process is continued until the entire polyp is removed or until there is concern about colon damage or excessive hemorrhage. The polypectomy can be completed 2 to 3 months later. The endoscopist should always lift the polypoid tissue off the underlying muscularis propria to minimize colon damage.

All transected tissue should be removed from the colon by either suctioning the pieces up against the tip of the colonoscope or grasping them with the snare and then withdrawing the instrument. Several reintubations of the colon are required for these large lesions, and some tissue may be lost. The transected tissue should be sent for histologic examination.

Results

Colonoscopic polypectomy has improved the management of colon polyps significantly. Over 95% of colon polyps can be removed safely, without the risks and complications of general anesthesia, celiotomy, and colotomy. Complete removal of a benign polyp eliminates subsequent malignant transformation. If histologic examination of the polyp reveals a focus of invasive cancer, as it will in up to 5% of patients, the excision will still have been curative in most patients. For those few polyps with histologic evidence of a greater likelihood of regional lymphatic metastasis or local recurrence (incomplete excision, lymphatic invasion, poor histologic differentiation), an appropriate radical colectomy can be performed electively.

Complications

Bleeding has been reported in up to 2% of patients following polypectomy. Bleeding is usually immediate, minimal, and self-limited, but delayed hemorrhage has been reported. If active bleeding occurs immediately after transection of a stalked polyp, the stalk should be regrasped with the snare and held for 10 to 15 minutes to encourage vessel thrombosis. The stalk should not be retransected, because if bleeding recurs there may be little or nothing to regrasp to achieve hemostasis. If the stalk cannot be regrasped or if the bleeding recurs, the patient should be carefully observed and evaluated for transfusion or celiotomy.

Electrothermal injury to the colon wall occurs in 1% to 2% of patients. The greatest amount of tissue damage is at the point of least surface contact in the electrical circuit, ideally at the snare wire itself around the stalk of the polyp. This complication usually results from using excessive current, including a portion of the colon wall within the snare (Fig. 19–11*A*), or allowing the tip of the polyp to touch only one small area of the opposite colon wall during stalk transection (Fig. 19–11*B*). The damaged colon wall may then progress to immediate or delayed perforation with generalized peritonitis, thereby requiring celiotomy. More commonly, however, the patient may exhibit only localized abdominal pain and tenderness signifying a transmural coagulation burn without frank perforation that frequently responds to nonoperative therapy, including nasogastric suction and antibiotics. Perforation following polypectomy has been reported in up to 0.3% of patients. Coagulation injury is most common following removal of large sessile polyps.

As with any operative procedure, hypertension, hypotension, myocardial infarction, respiratory depression due to oversedation, and allergic and idiosyncratic reactions to medications can occur.

Decompression

Acute Pseudo-obstruction of the Colon (Ogilvie's Syndrome)

A massive abdominal distention and typical abdominal radiograph (Fig. 19–12*A*), in the absence of a mechan-

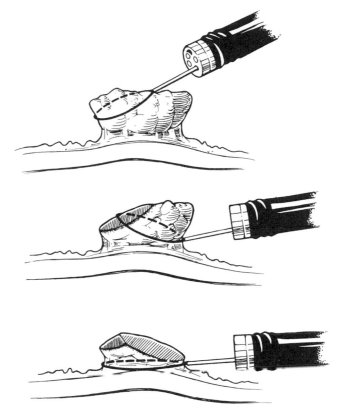

Figure 19–10. Piecemeal excision.

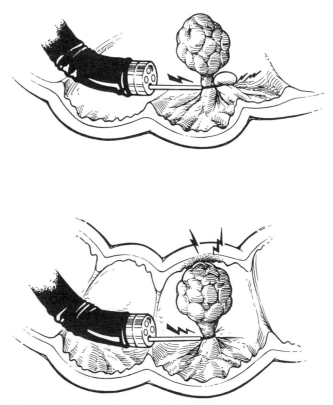

Figure 19–11. Complications of polypectomy.

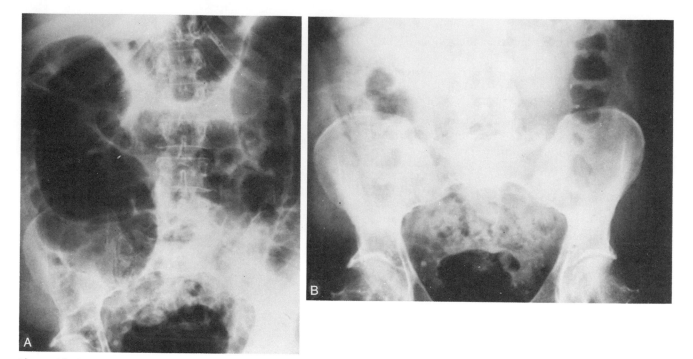

Figure 19–12. *A* and *B*. Before and after colonoscopic decompression of Ogilvie's syndrome.

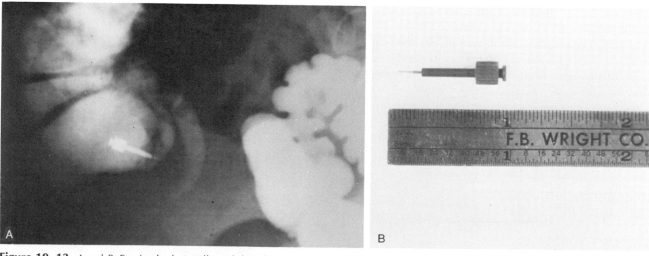

Figure 19–13. *A* and *B*. Foreign body (swallowed dental instrument).

ical obstruction, are occasionally seen in a critically ill or postoperative patient. If untreated, this colon dilatation may progress to perforation with a high patient mortality rate. Operative treatment by tube cecostomy is also accompanied by a high mortality rate. Colonoscopy for suspected Ogilvie's syndrome is both diagnostic and therapeutic: it can exclude the presence of a causative organic obstructing or ischemic lesion, and if these are absent, the colon can be decompressed in up to 80% of patients by aspiration. Perforation of the colon is a potential complication of colonoscopic decompression, but it has been reported only rarely.

Colonoscopic examination and decompression of an unprepared colon should be attempted only by an experienced endoscopist. Several careful enemas should be administered before the procedure to evacuate as much stool as possible from the rectosigmoid colon. The patient's vital signs, electrocardiogram, and oxygenation should be carefully monitored. If an obstructing lesion or ischemic bowel is visualized, the procedure should be terminated immediately. It is most effective to advance the colonoscope all the way into the cecum for optimal decompression (Fig. 19–12B), although aspiration from the proximal transverse colon may partially reduce the massive distention. A second, or occasionally even a third, colonoscopy may be required to treat a recurrence of colon dilatation, and in the 20% of patients for whom colonoscopic decompression is unsuccessful, operative tube cecostomy, colectomy, or colostomy is usually required.

Sigmoid Volvulus

For patients with the characteristic history, physical, and roentgenologic findings of sigmoid volvulus, the initial therapy should be decompression by either rigid or flexible sigmoidoscopy. Successful intubation of the sigmoid colon frequently reduces the volvulus and allows elective sigmoid colon resection or at least corrects this life-threatening condition in poor operative candidates.

If a rigid sigmoidoscope is used, a rectal tube is usually fed carefully through it into the dilated sigmoid colon and left in place for 24 to 48 hours following decompression. The flexible sigmoidoscope has the theoretical advantage of direct visualization of the dilated segment and avoids the need for blind passage of a rectal tube. Because the sigmoidoscope is passed through unprepared rectosigmoid colon, great care must be taken to avoid perforation, and if ischemic bowel is seen, the procedure should be terminated.

Arteriovenous Malformations

Angiodysplasia (arteriovenous malformation) and diverticulosis of the colon are each responsible for ap-

proximately 50% of cases of acute massive colon hemorrhage. In our experience, angiodysplastic lesions are best identified through arteriography. Identifying such lesions endoscopically in the acutely bleeding patient or even following cessation of the hemorrhagic episode is difficult, probably because of their location deep in the submucosa. Conversely, incidental angiodysplastic lesions can be identified in patients who have never bled. Therefore unless such a lesion is demonstrated to be actively bleeding, it may not have been the bleeding source. Successful results of endoscopic treatment (argon laser, heater probe, alcohol injection, and electrocoagulation) have been reported anecdotally, but the detection and optimal management (operative versus endoscopic) of these lesions remain controversial.

Foreign Body Retrieval

Most foreign bodies that pass into the colon from the upper gastrointestinal tract are easily eliminated with the feces. Most foreign bodies that are inserted into the colon through the anus require forms of instrumentation other than endoscopes to effect removal. On rare occasions, colonoscopy has been employed to retrieve foreign bodies that have not passed spontaneously, such as nasointestinal tubes, coins, pins, displaced wire sutures, and even swallowed dental instruments (Fig. 19–13A and B).

BIBLIOGRAPHY

Brostrom O, Lofberg R, Ost A, Reichard H. Cancer surveillance of patients with longstanding ulcerative colitis: A clinical, endoscopical, and histological study. Gut 1986;27:1408–1413.

Carlsson G, Petrelli NJ, Nava H, et al. The value of colonoscopic surveillance after curative resection for colorectal cancer of synchronous adenomatous polyps. Arch Surg 1987;122:1261–1263.

Christie JP. Colonoscopic excision of sessile polyps. Am J Gastroenterol 1976;66:23–28.

Cotton PB, Williams CB. Practical Gastrointestinal Endoscopy. 2nd ed. London: Blackwell Scientific Publications, 1982.

Dajani AS, Bisno AL, Chung KJ, et al. Prevention of bacterial endocarditis: Recommendations by the American Heart Association. JAMA 1990;264:2919–2922.

Dent TL, Kukora JS, Buinewicz BR. Endoscopic screening and surveillance for gastrointestinal malignancy. Surg Clin North Am 1989;69:1205–1225.

Dent TL, Kukora JS, Nejman JH. Colon, rectum, and anus. In: Hardy JD, ed. Hardy's Textbook of Surgery. 2nd ed. Philadelphia: JB Lippincott, 1988.

Dent TL, Strodel WE, Turcotte JG, eds. Surgical Endoscopy. Chicago: Year Book Medical Publishers, 1985.

Ernstoff JJ, Howard DA, Marshall JB, et al. A randomized blinded clinical trial of a rapid colonic lavage solution (Golytely) compared with standard preparation for colonoscopy and barium enema. Gastroenterology 1983;84:1512–1516.

Fenoglio-Preiser CM, Hutter RVP. Colorectal Polyps: Pathologic Diagnosis and Clinical Significance. New York: American Cancer Society, 1986.

Finian PJ, Ritchie JK, Hawley PR. Synchronous and "early" metachronous carcinomas of the colon and rectum. Br J Surg 1987;74:945–947.

Gilbertson VA, Nelms JM. The prevention of invasive cancer of the rectum. Cancer 1978;41:1137–1139.

Holt RW, Wherry DC. Flexible fiberoptic sigmoidoscopy in a surgeon's office. Am J Surg 1980;139:708–710.

Hunt RH. Colonoscopy intubation techniques with fluoroscopy. In: Hunt RH, Waye JD, eds. Colonoscopy: Techniques, Clinical Practice, and Colour Atlas. London: Chapman and Hall, 1981.

Kiefer PJ, Thorson AG, Christensen MA. Metachronous colorectal cancer: Time interval to presentation of a metachronous cancer. Dis Colon Rectum 1986;29:378–382.

Langevin JM, Nivatvongs S. The true incidence of synchronous cancer of the large bowel. A prospective study. Am J Surg 1984;147:330–333.

Macrae FA, Tan KG, Williams CB. Towards safer colonoscopy: A report on the complications of 5000 diagnostic or therapeutic colonoscopies. Gut 1983;24:376–383.

Marks G, Boggs HW, Castro F, et al. Sigmoidoscopic examinations with rigid and flexible fiberoptic sigmoidoscopes in the surgeon's office. Dis Colon Rectum 1979;22:162–168.

Maxfield RG. Colonoscopy as a routine preoperative procedure for carcinoma of the colon. Am J Surg 1984;147:477–480.

McCallum RW, Meyer CT, Marignani P, et al. Flexible sigmoidoscopy: Diagnostic yield in 1015 patients. Am J Gastroenterol 1984;79:433–437.

Morson BC, Bussey HJR. Magnitude of risk for cancer in patients with colorectal adenomas. Br J Surg 1985;72:S23–S28.

Nivatvongs S. Complications in colonoscopic polypectomy: An experience with 1555 polypectomies. Dis Colon Rectum 1986;29:825–830.

Nivatvongs S, Vermeulen FD, Fang DT. Colonoscopic decompression of acute pseudoobstruction of the colon. Ann Surg 1982;196:598–600.

Previti FW, Holt RW. Detorsion of sigmoid volvulus by flexible fiberoptic sigmoidoscopy. J Med Soc NJ 1981;78:288–290.

Reeve T, Kukora JS. Pneumatic perforation of the colon during colonoscopy: Is the hypermobile right colon a risk factor? Dis Colon Rectum 1984;27:751–753.

Rogers BHG. Complications and hazards of colonoscopy. In: Hunt RH, Waye JD, eds. Colonoscopy: Techniques, Clinical Practice, and Colour Atlas. London: Chapman and Hall, 1981.

Rosenstock E, Farmer RG, Petras R, et al. Surveillance for colonic carcinoma in ulcerative colitis. Gastroenterology 1985;89:1342–1346.

Schwesinger WH, Levine BA, Ramos R. Complications in colonoscopy. Surg Gynecol Obstet 1979;148:270–281.

Silverstein FE, Tytgat GNJ. Atlas of Gastrointestinal Endoscopy. Philadelphia: WB Saunders, 1987.

Silvis SE, ed. Therapeutic Gastrointestinal Endoscopy. 2nd ed. New York: Igaku-Shoin, 1989.

Sivak MV Jr, ed. Gastroenterologic Endoscopy. Philadelphia: WB Saunders, 1987.

Strodel WE, Nostrant TT, Eckhauser FE, et al. Therapeutic and diagnostic colonoscopy in nonobstructive colonic dilatation. Ann Surg 1983;197:416–421.

Stulc JP, Petrelli NJ, Herrera L, et al. Anastomotic recurrence of adenocarcinoma of the colon. Arch Surg 1986;121:1077–1080.

Tedesco FJ. Differential diagnosis of ulcerative colitis and Crohn's ileocolitis and other specific inflammatory diseases of the bowel. Med Clin North Am 1980;64:1173–1183.

Waye JD, Geenen JE, Fleischer D, Venu RP. Techniques in Therapeutic Endoscopy. Philadelphia: WB Saunders, 1987.

Williams CB. Diathermy-biopsy—a technique for the endoscopic management of small polyps. Endoscopy 1973;5:215–218.

Williams CB, Macrae FA, Bartram CI. A prospective study of diagnostic methods in adenoma follow-up. Endoscopy 1982;14:74–78.

Winnan G, Berci G, Panish J, et al. Superiority of the flexible to the rigid sigmoidoscope in routine proctosigmoidoscopy. N Engl J Med 1980;302:1011–1012.

Complications of Colorectal Operations

CHAPTER 20

A. R. Moossa
George E. Block
Jonathan M. Sackier

All complications are made in the operating room.

Many complications can occur after any abdominal operation. These include wound infection or dehiscence, thromboembolic disorders, cardiopulmonary failure, urinary tract dysfunction, metabolic disorders, and neurologic-type psychological problems. We confine ourselves to intra-abdominal and pelvic complications that are directly related to operations on the colon and rectum. Postoperative complications (judgmental, technical, or incidental) increase morbidity, prolong hospital stay, increase cost of health care delivery, and are sometimes fatal.

In a series of 10,000 intestinal operations reported by McGuire,[1] the causes of 600 resulting complications were estimated as follows: (1) technical or judgmental error, 60%; (2) progression of disease despite hope of cure or palliation by a correctly performed operation, 15%; (3) inherent risk of necessary and correctly performed operation (e.g., for pulmonary embolus), 10%; (4) deficient equipment or nursing support, 3%; (5) unrelated coincidence, 7%.

ALIMENTARY TRACT DYSFUNCTION AFTER COLORECTAL OPERATIONS

Numerous complications involving the alimentary tract may occur after operations on the colon and rectum. These include acute gastric dilatation, paralytic ileus, gastroduodenal mucosal hemorrhage, intestinal obstruction, fecal impaction, suture line hemorrhage, and dysfunction of the hepatobiliary system. Most of these complications may also occur after any prolonged abdominal operation. However, anastomotic leakage and/or disruption is most common after resection of the colon or rectum.

Paralytic Ileus

After any laparotomy, probably as a result of surgical manipulation of the viscera, reflex inhibition occurs. This is mediated by excitation of the sympathetic nerves and affects the entire gastrointestinal tract. The stomach usually recovers in a few hours and the small bowel within a day or two, but the colon may take 2 or 3 days or longer. Clinical experience suggests that the duration and the severity of paralytic ileus are directly proportional to the extent and duration of the abdominal operation with its inherent visceral and retroperitoneal dissection and manipulation. It is also generally accepted that a paralytic ileus lasting longer than 3 or 4 days is indicative of continuing splanchnic stimulation and may be the first clue to a complication such as hemoperitoneum, retroperitoneal or mesenteric hematoma, or peritonitis.

The paralyzed bowel should be kept empty by continuous nasogastric suction; otherwise, gaseous distention delays the effective resumption of normal bowel muscular activity. In addition, the distended gut loses rather than absorbs potassium, and the resulting hypokalemia further prolongs the ileus, thus creating a vicious circle. Overmedication with opiates may also contribute to the prolongation of ileus. The resolution of paralytic ileus is heralded by the appearance of audible peristalsis on auscultation and by the return of the patient's appetite. However, the only reliable evidence of resumption of colonic motility is the passage of flatus.

Prolonged ileus may be prevented by paying meticulous attention to surgical principles of operative technique. Such preventive measures include washing powder off surgical gloves, gentle and careful handling of all viscera, covering the peritoneal surfaces with moist pads to prevent tissue drying, avoiding unnecessary trauma with instruments, carefully controlling spillage of gastrointestinal content, applying meticulous hemostasis, and performing bowel exteriorization whenever a primary anastomosis cannot be safely performed.

Paralytic Ileus Versus Mechanical Bowel Obstruction

In theory, prolonged or recurrent paralytic ileus is characterized by painless abdominal distention, whereas mechanical obstruction declares itself by the presence of colicky abdominal pain. In practice, both conditions may coexist during the first 2 or 3 postoperative weeks, and it may be virtually impossible to distinguish the relative contributions of each entity. Complete mechanical bowel obstruction clearly requires a re-exploration of the abdomen, whereas a prolonged ileus can be treated conservatively for a period of time until the source of the ileus is identified. If the ileus is due to a localized abdominal abscess, percutaneous drainage of the abscess may be appropriate. However, if the ileus is due to a generalized peritonitis, reoperation becomes mandatory. Judicious use of meglumine diatrizoate (Gastrografin) injected via a nasogastric tube and followed by serial abdominal radiographs is often helpful. A computed tomography (CT) scan of the abdomen may also be of diagnostic value, especially when an abscess is suspected. The gallium scan is largely outdated in this setting, and ultrasonography is inappropriate because gaseous distention of the bowel limits its efficacy.

Mechanical Intestinal Obstruction

Any patient who fails to pass flatus within the first postoperative week should be suspected of having a mechanical bowel obstruction until the condition is proven to be otherwise. Goligher et al. estimate an incidence of mechanical obstruction of 3% in over 1,300 patients who underwent an abdominoperineal resection.[2] The obstruction is most commonly due to adhesions between loops of bowel or between a loop of bowel and the anterior abdominal wall. Although this can occur after any abdominal operation for any cause, two specific clinical entities must be considered after an abdominoperineal resection or after a total proctocolectomy with an ileostomy; these are now described.

Herniation of a Loop of Bowel Through the Lateral Paracolostomy or Paraileostomy Gutter. This herniation occurs most frequently if the gutter has been partially or inadequately closed when a loop of bowel can easily get caught in the gap. As a preventive measure, all colostomies or ileostomies are best constructed by using the extraperitoneal approach of Goligher. Alternatively, if the lateral gutter cannot be adequately closed, it should be left wide open to create a large defect rather than a small one. At reoperation the internal hernia can be reduced and the defect of the lateral gutter repaired.

Herniation of a Loop of Bowel Through the Pelvic Floor. This usually occurs following closure of the peritoneum of the pelvic floor after proctectomy for inflammatory bowel disease. A suture may pull out of this peritoneal closure, leaving a gap through which a loop of bowel can protrude and become entrapped. Gangrene in the bowel due to resulting ischemia can occur but is rare. The proper treatment is a laparotomy, liberation of the bowel through the internal hernial defect and reclosure of the peritoneum. Some surgeons prefer to leave the peritoneal surface of the pelvic floor open after performing proctectomy for inflammatory bowel disease and believe that this prevents any obstructive complication. In cases of rectal excision for cancer, there is usually no residual peritoneum to close, and small bowel is allowed to fill the pelvis. In this setting, the lesser pelvis can be filled with a pedicle graft of omentum as previously described (see subchapter Proctocolectomy in Chapter 8); this keeps the small bowel out of the pelvis and is a useful maneuver if postoperative radiotherapy is anticipated.

ABDOMINAL WOUND INFECTION

Abdominal wound infection is not an uncommon complication of colon and rectal surgery and invariably prolongs the hospital stay. With any of the many current protocols of preoperative bowel preparation, prophylactic systemic antibiotics, and careful operative technique, the overall incidence of wound infection is 5% or less.

Because the colon and rectum can never be rendered totally free of bacteria, some degree of wound contamination with pathogenic organisms invariably occurs during the operation. Several host factors are statistically known to increase the incidence of wound infection after colorectal surgery. These include (1) the presence of preoperative stoma, (2) inadequate bowel preparation, (3) a low serum albumin (less than 2.9 g/dl), (4) preoperative irradiation, (5) excessive blood loss (more than 2 units), (6) lengthy operation (operating time longer than 2 hours), (7) Crohn's disease.

To these may be added three other predisposing factors, namely, (1) incidental splenic trauma necessitating splenectomy during a colon operation, (2) obesity, and (3) chronic use of immunosuppressive drugs.

If there is unavoidable gross fecal contamination of the wound (the authors *do not* routinely use abdominal wound protectors), the skin and subcutaneous tissues should be left open and closed secondarily later. Minimal contamination can be handled by standard surgical techniques of careful hemostasis, gentle handling of tissues, copious irrigation with saline solution, reduction of operating time, and, sometimes, instillation of broad-spectrum antibiotics into the wound before primary closure is performed.

ABDOMINAL WOUND DEHISCENCE

Abdominal wound disruption may be partial or complete. When it is partial, one or more layers of the abdominal wall have separated, but the skin or the peritoneum has remained intact. This later declares itself as an incisional hernia.

When the abdominal wound disruption is complete, all layers of the abdominal wall have burst open. This is often associated with protrusion of small bowel and/or omentum and referred to as "evisceration." The incidence of abdominal wound dehiscence in the postoperative period is difficult to estimate, and figures of 0.5% to 3.5% of all laparotomy incisions are usually quoted. The incidence is clearly higher in emergency cases, and it is generally accepted that the following factors are associated with abdominal wound disruption: (1) faulty technique in closure; (2) increased intraabdominal pressure resulting from factors such as chronic cough, increasing ascites, and prolonged ileus due to any cause; (3) operations for malignant disease in elderly patients with associated severe malnutrition, hypoproteinemia, anemia, and vitamin deficiencies. Bucknall et al.[3] reported 341 major abdominal wounds performed between 1975 and 1977 with a wound dehiscence rate of 3.8%. These results were compared with those of 788 subsequent patients with a dehiscence rate of 0.8%. The authors attributed the improvement

to the introduction of a mass closure technique in which nonabsorbable suture material was used.

As soon as an abdominal wound dehiscence is recognized, the wound and any protruding viscera are covered with sterile towels soaked in normal saline, and the patient is given some intravenous sedation and broad-spectrum antibiotics. Intravenous fluids are administered as needed, and a nasogastric tube is passed and connected to suction to aspirate the gastric contents. While the patient is under general endotracheal anesthesia, the wound is closed with retention sutures after the viscera and the rest of the abdominal cavity are gently explored and washed copiously with normal saline. The sutures are left for 3 weeks in the postoperative period. Active standard postoperative measures are taken to combat any infection and postoperative ileus.

INCISIONAL HERNIA

Incisional hernia must be considered to be iatrogenic in origin. In view of the enormous number of laparotomies being performed each day, it is virtually impossible to determine the true incidence of incisional hernias. As early as 1887, Homans[4] estimated that about 10% of abdominal operations were complicated by the later development of an incisional hernia. More recent reports give an incidence of 7.9% to 8.4%.[5, 6]

Several important etiologic factors are recognized in the development of an incisional hernia. These include the following:

1. *Sepsis.* Over 60% of patients who develop an incisional hernia have a history of significant wound infection.
2. *The placement of drains through the abdominal incision.* In a series of 126 patients with incisional hernia through a Kocher subcostal incision for biliary tract surgery, Ponka reports that all had had drains brought out through the main incision at the time of the operation.[5]
3. *The placement of a stoma through the abdominal incision.* This leads to inevitable continuous wound contamination, sepsis, and eventual breakdown.
4. *Long-term immunosuppressive therapy with drugs such as steroids and azathioprine (Imuran).*
5. *Inflammatory bowel disease.*

There is a distinct clinical impression that other factors, such as increasing age, malnutrition, hypoproteinemia, anemia, obesity, diabetes, and postoperative pulmonary infection, may contribute to the development of incisional hernias. The type of incision appears to be important. Transverse incisions have a lower incidence of wound dehiscence and incisional hernias than do vertical ones. Lower midline incisions are at greater risk than upper midline incisions.

The technical aspects of incisional hernia repair are beyond the scope of this book, but the principles should be reiterated:

1. General surgical principles of asepsis, hemostasis, and gentle handling of tissues must be adhered to.
2. The normal abdominal wall anatomy should be reconstituted as far as possible, and only aponeurotic-fascial layers should be sutured together. If the abdominal wall defect is large with extensive attenuation or loss of musculofascial layers, a synthetic mesh should be used to close the defect.
3. Strong, nonabsorbable suture material should be used.
4. When viscera are returned to the confines of the peritoneal cavity, every precaution should be taken to handle the viscera minimally in order to prevent postoperative ileus and abdominal distention, which cause additional stress on closure. The protective role of abdominal binders in the early postoperative period is uncertain.
5. Postoperative coughing is a problem in patients with chronic pulmonary disease. Preoperative cessation of smoking, breathing exercises, and weight reduction are important to facilitate the repair and to increase chances of success.

UNHEALED PERINEAL WOUND OR PERSISTENT PERINEAL SINUS

Delayed healing of the perineal wound after proctectomy for cancer is uncommon. However, since the advent of pre- and postoperative radiotherapy for rectal cancer, the incidence of this problem appears to be increasing.

It is estimated that 25% to 60% of patients undergoing total proctocolectomy for inflammatory bowel disease suffer from an unhealed perineal wound at 6 months. The terms "unhealed perineal wound" and "persistent perineal sinus" are deceptively innocuous. The wound is often malodorous, draining, and painful. It is difficult to keep clean, necessitating frequent showers, irrigation, and protective pads. Many factors have been postulated to explain the poor wound healing in inflammatory bowel disease. De Dombal et al. proposed that pre-existing perianal disease in many of these patients leads to gross and subclinical wound infection that slows down the rate of healing.[7] Others attribute the wound contamination to increased friability of the bowel, which leads to microscopic perfo-

rations of the rectal wall. Long-term use of corticosteroids and malnutrition have been thought to have a role. More recently, Ferrari and DenBesten[8] as well as Warshaw et al.[9] have implicated the creation of dead spaces in the lesser pelvis and their secondary infection as the explanation for the persistent perineal sinus.

The interpretation of many published series and their recommendations for the unhealed perineal sinus poses several difficulties to the discerning reader. The series involves too many surgeons, thus guaranteeing no uniformity of surgical technique. The patients often include those with cancer, inflammatory bowel disease, and other diseases of the rectum. There is often an insufficient length of follow-up. A few perineal wounds break down long after they were thought to be completely healed.

The least-acknowledged difficulty encountered in the literature concerns definition. The persistent perineal sinus is traditionally defined as "a perineal wound unhealed for about 6 months after operation." This arbitrary definition does not distinguish between deep wounds in the presacral space and wounds that are closed except for small unepithelialized areas. The surgeon wishes to understand the aspects of perineal wound healing that are amenable to surgical manipulation in order to achieve more rapid healing; unfortunately, epithelialization is not one of those aspects. Thus, the statistical correlations between various factors and the incidence of persistent perineal sinus calculated on the basis of the conventional definition are difficult to interpret.

We propose a more functional definition of the true persistent perineal sinus[10]: a perineal wound deeper than the subcutaneous tissues unhealed for over 6 months, often draining seropurulent material and requiring reoperation (curettage or excision) to achieve healing. This definition more accurately captures the clinical essence of a "difficult" perineal wound.

It is important to understand the state of the pelvic cavity after proctectomy. The perineum becomes a gaping defect bounded anteriorly, posteriorly, and laterally by the bony pelvis. The cavity is dumbbell-shaped with large defects above and below a narrowing caused by the remnants of the levator ani muscles. Initially, the wound cavity is filled with serous fluid and, if hemostasis is incomplete, serosanguineous fluid. This is an excellent culture medium for bacteria implanted during the operation. Thus, adequate drainage must be provided to prevent abscess formation and eventual sinus formation. If this is accomplished, healing progresses by obliteration of the large remaining cavity. How this obliteration occurs depends on several factors, including granulation tissue formation, posterior migration of the urogenital structures, and upward migration of the buttocks. Downward migration of the small bowel is limited when the pelvic peritoneum has been reapproximated, as is our custom in treatment for inflammatory bowel disease.

We have found that the open technique, gross bacterial contamination, and persistence of a supralevator dead space are prime factors contributing to a nonhealing perineal wound.[10]

Traditionally, we have employed wound packing for two reasons: (1) to ensure hemostasis and (2) to exteriorize the potential abscess cavity. However, wound management by the open method with slow daily advancement of the pack can be painful, requires much more nursing care, and is slower to heal than management by the closed method. We recommend meticulous surgical technique to achieve hemostasis and judicious administration of perioperative antibiotics. We employ suction drainage to help hold the pelvic tissues in approximation and to obliterate the dead space.

BLADDER DYSFUNCTION: URINARY RETENTION AND INFECTION

Urinary retention and urinary tract infection are common complications of abdominoperineal resection or low anterior resection. The incidence is from 22% to 41%, and there are multifactorial predisposing or causative factors.[11, 12] These include male gender, wide lymphadenectomy, injury to the sympathetic and parasympathetic innervation to the bladder, local trauma, prostatic hypertrophy, prolapse of the bladder into the posterior pelvis, and postoperative bladder distention. Some have advocated thorough urologic evaluation of elderly male patients before any operation on the rectum and selective performance of a concomitant prostatectomy under the same anesthetic. Such a combined operation increases the risk of urinary tract infection, pelvic sepsis, and urinary tract–perineal fistula formation.

Probably the most critical postoperative preventive measure is to leave the Foley catheter in place for a minimum of 6 to 7 days. Urodynamic studies are recommended only if the patient is unable to void after the catheter is removed. Some advocate prophylactic medication with bethanecol chloride (Urecholine) to improve the detrusor tone before the catheter is removed. Prevalent urologic opinion discourages the old practice of clamping and unclamping the catheter to strengthen detrusor muscle tone. It is generally believed that detrusor tone will ultimately return if the bladder is kept empty by catheter drainage. If the patient fails to void after the catheter is removed, an additional period of catheter drainage for about 1 week combined with bethanecol chloride medication is generally recommended. Intermittent self-catheterization is an alternative while the patient undergoes the full range of urodynamic studies.

ANASTOMOTIC LEAK AND DEHISCENCE

An anastomosis that is not made will not leak.

Formation of a safe colonic or colorectal anastomosis continues to challenge surgeons. This is especially true for anterior resection of the rectum, which since its acceptance as a treatment modality, has been associated with a significant rate of anastomotic dehiscence.[13] Colonic anastomoses are more prone to leakage because of various inherent factors such as (1) the high intraluminal bacterial concentration, (2) the thin, single, circular, muscular layer of the colon, (3) the tendency of the colon to distend, (4) the slow recovery of the colon from ileus, (5) the more segmental rather than directional nature of colonic contractions.

The more distal the anastomosis, the greater is its tendency to leak. If routine meglumine diatrizoate enemas are done in the postoperative period following a low colorectal anastomosis, the incidence of radiologic leak may be as high as 20%, but a clinically significant leak is estimated to be only about 5% or less when managed by an expert surgeon.

Leakage following colonic anastomosis does not appear to depend on the choice of anastomotic technique. Sutured anastomoses have a reported clinical leakage rate of between 3.3% and 28.0%,[14–18] and surgical stapling is attributed a rate of 2.0% to 10.3%.[19–24] A prospective randomized clinical trial suggested that there is no difference in leakage rate between the two techniques.[25–27] A wide variety of general factors may contribute somewhat to the development of an anastomotic dehiscence but are sometimes used as a "scapegoat" for imperfect surgical techniques. Age, nutritional status, and general physical condition, previous irradiation, anesthetic drugs, severe blood loss, diabetes mellitus, Crohn's disease, jaundice, long-term corticosteroid therapy, and obesity all have been implicated.[28–32]

Experimental work in animals has shown conclusively that anastomotic dehiscence is more likely to occur in the presence of fecal soiling.[33] Clinical trials of both preoperative bowel preparation and on-table colonic lavage confirmed the value of creating an anastomosis in an environment free of feces.[14, 15, 34–38] Thus, it is generally accepted that the local technical factors in the creation of the anastomosis, discussed in Chapter 5, are of greater practical importance than the systemic factors mentioned.

Clinical Manifestation of Anastomotic Leaks

Anastomotic leaks usually become clinically manifest during the second postoperative week. Breakdown of the suture line can present in multiple ways that can generally be categorized into five clinically distinct groups.

Subclinical Group. Unless the surgeon routinely performs a contrast study using a water-soluble medium such as a meglumine diatrizoate enema in the postoperative period, it can well be argued that such small or microscopic dehiscence is of no practical importance and does not affect the postoperative course of the patient.

Clinical Evidence of Sepsis. Sepsis can be manifested in several ways. The patient feels generally unwell and has a fever, leukocytosis, and/or tachycardia. There is often an associated paralytic ileus with minimal, if any, abdominal tenderness or guarding. At first, the patient is in a good general condition.

Localized Peritonitis. In localized peritonitis, the patient's postoperative course is usually uneventful for a few days until the patient develops some increasing pain and tenderness in the abdomen. The temperature is elevated and there is leukocytosis. There are often associated paralytic ileus and abdominal distention.

External Fecal Fistula. Often, after an insidious deterioration of the patient in the postoperative period suggestive of localized peritonitis, an area of the abdominal wound or of the drainage site (if an external drain was left in) becomes more swollen and tender. A discharge of pus and, invariably, a later discharge of fecal material may occur along with considerable improvement in the patient's general condition. Such a discharge may be delayed for several days, even when a definite leak has occurred from the anastomosis, and this may lead to a delay in diagnosis.

Generalized Peritonitis. Diffuse peritonitis may be insidious, and the patient may have a sepsis-type picture including a rising pulse rate, fever, and leukocytosis as well as a prolonged ileus; alternatively, it may evolve in a patient who is already suspected of having an anastomotic leak and localized peritonitis. Occasionally, the patient may develop a sudden cardiovascular collapse with septic shock and rapid deterioration.

Management of Anastomotic Leak

The general recommendations for breakdown of a colonic suture line are as follows.

General measures such as nasogastric suction and administration of intravenous fluids and antibiotics should immediately be instituted. If one is in doubt, the presence and extent of a leak should be radiologically confirmed. Contrast studies with meglumine diatrizoate and CT scans are most valuable. The worst time to reoperate on the abdomen is during the second and third postoperative weeks.

If a patient has localized peritonitis as a result of breakdown of a colon or colorectal suture line, it is most important to ensure adequate local external drainage. This is quite successfully performed by the percutaneous, radiologic approach in which CT or ultrasound is used for guidance. If the expertise is not available, the old-fashioned surgical approach should be considered; preferably, the perianastomotic collection is drained through the extraperitoneal route without disturbing the peritoneal cavity. At this early stage of the treatment, the surgeon should seriously consider the need for a proximal fecal diversion.

By definition, external drainage of a localized anastomotic leak results in the development of an external fecal fistula. Supportive treatment, such as total parenteral nutrition, appropriate antibiotics, and cessation of oral intake, helps a small fistula to close spontaneously, provided that the bowel lumen distal to the anastomosis is widely patent.

Immediate reoperation in the early postoperative period is mandatory for all cases of generalized peritonitis. After adequate resuscitation, the entire abdomen is re-explored. The patient is often in poor general condition with septic shock. Hence, active resuscitation with both crystalloid and colloid infusion may have to be supplemented with pressor agents and hydrocortisone while the patient is prepared for laparotomy. Thorough peritoneal débridement and lavage with several liters of saline are recommended. The value of supplemental irrigation with antibiotic solution is debatable. It is essential to provide the patient with appropriate broad-spectrum antibiotic therapy intravenously. The removal of fibrinous deposits (septic peel) off the peritoneal surfaces is essential. The suture line should be excised, and, if at all possible, both ends of the bowel should be exteriorized. If the distal end of the anastomosis cannot be exteriorized, it can be stapled shut and the proximal active end brought out as an ileostomy or a colostomy. External drainage of the peritoneal cavity is not recommended unless there is a localized abscess (i.e., in the presacral space) that may need to be drained. The abdominal wound is carefully closed with nonabsorbable sutures, and the skin and subcutaneous tissues are left open.

Depending on the state of the peritoneal cavity at the end of the procedure and on the clinical course of the patient, a second-look laparotomy for further peritoneal irrigation and débridement may be indicated 48 to 72 hours later.

Prevention of Anastomotic Leak

It is widely accepted that it is preferable to prevent an anastomotic leak than to treat it. If we assume that all anastomotic leaks are technical or judgmental errors, then attending to the technical details outlined in Chapter 5 is of paramount importance. The criteria for a successful anastomosis include (1) adequate blood supply, (2) good mechanical apposition of the bowel ends, (3) no gross contamination, (4) no tension on the suture line, and (5) no obstruction distal to the suture line. If these criteria are satisfied, *ipso facto,* the anastomosis will not leak. Some anastomoses are done under less than perfect circumstances, and some of the above criteria are not totally satisfied. For such situations, several additional maneuvers have been recommended to increase the security of the colonic anastomosis.

Value of a Protective Omental Wrap. The omentum is a useful structure for avoiding or restraining leakage from an anastomosis. It is also valuable for closing a dead space (i.e., the presacral space) as described for a low anterior resection or for an abdominoperineal resection. However, the omental wrap must not be an adjunct to a poorly constructed anastomosis.

Value of a Temporary Protective Ileostomy or Colostomy. Generally, it is probably wise to accept the adage that "an anastomosis that needs protecting is probably not well done." However, sometimes a proximal temporary colostomy or ileostomy to divert the fecal stream is justifiable. Such situations include ileoanal anastomosis or coloanal anastomosis, low anterior resection of the rectum following radiotherapy, in the repair of severely destroyed anal sphincters, as part of the management of high anorectal fistulas and, finally, in the management of severe anorectal injuries associated with multiple displaced pelvic fractures. If total fecal diversion is needed, a loop stoma does not provide complete safety; as a result, some form of double-barrel stoma is necessary. Alternatively, the distal end of the bowel at the site of the stoma can be stapled and the proximal active end brought out as a functional end-colostomy.[39, 40]

Exteriorized Closure or Anastomosis. Exteriorized closure or anastomosis has been advocated for some cases of relatively minor injury to the colon. The closure or anastomosis is performed, and that area of the bowel is left exposed through the abdominal wall musculature and fascia with the skin and subcutaneous tissues left open for a few days, before the colonic anastomosis is returned back into the peritoneal cavity. The concept does not make sense and is akin to "sitting on the fence." The best place for an anastomosis or colonic closure to heal is in the peritoneal cavity; as the adage says, "serosa hates fresh air while mucosa does not care."

Use of Drains. We condemn the use of drains around any type of bowel anastomosis. Theoretically, drains are indicated whenever there is a suspicion that fluid might leak into the peritoneal cavity. Thus, drains function well for bile, urine, lymph, ascitic fluid, and pancreatic juice. Drains should *not* be used as a protective mechanism for inadequate hemostasis or for a poorly performed bowel anastomosis.

Use of the Intraluminal Bypass Tube (Coloshield). As mentioned, in some situations, such as large bowel obstruction, peritoneal soiling, and suspected faulty colon anastomosis, many surgeons have advocated a proximal loop colostomy or a cecostomy to protect the anastomosis. The addition of such a temporary stoma increases morbidity, and the subsequent closure of a colostomy may carry a mortality rate of up to 4.2%.[39, 40]

The concept of using an intraluminal bypass tube for bowel surgery to avoid a temporary protecting colostomy is not new and dates back to Ruggiero Frugardi in 1180.[41] He reported the use of animal trachea as a stent across an intestinal anastomosis. While working as a resident surgical officer in Leeds, Mr. (Later Lord) Moynihan assisted Littlewood with an intraluminal stent and colonic anastomosis utilizing Senn bone plates.[42] These surgical pioneers were striving to achieve a safer colonic anastomosis and overcome the problem of dehiscence. Although bowel preparation, safer anesthesia, and excellent antibiotics have done much to reduce the leakage rate, it remains a problem today, particularly with emergency colonic surgery and low anterior resection of the rectum.

Preliminary experimental work demonstrated that an intraluminal bypass tube is a safe, uncomplicated procedure to prevent anastomotic dehiscence in esophageal surgery.[43] This led to an assessment of the intraluminal bypass tube with colonic anastomoses, and experimental work confirmed that the tube prevented leakage, even from gross dehiscence, and that these dehiscences progressed to complete healing.[44]

Technique. Having decided to utilize the intraluminal bypass (Coloshield, Deknatel (Fall River, MA)) an appropriate size is chosen. The device is available in four diameters: 25 mm, 32 mm, 38 mm, and 44 mm, but all are 75 cm long and are folded in parachute fashion to aid insertion (Fig. 20–1).

Having completed the colonic resection, the proximal colon is cleaned with povidone-iodine, and a 4-cm cuff is everted by four intraluminal stay sutures. Alternatively, Babcock clamps are placed at the edge of the bowel to produce the eversion. An appropriately sized device is lubricated with water-soluble jelly and inserted into the proximal colon lining the four dots with the stay sutures (Fig. 20–2). A continuous locking suture of 2.0 polyglycolic acid is used to secure the reinforced proximal end of the tube to the bowel,

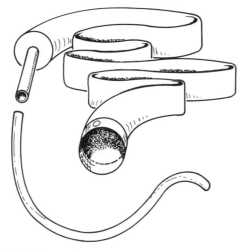

Figure 20–1. The intraluminal bypass tube. The radiopaque stripe, reinforced polyester cuff, and rubber nipple to accommodate the rectal probe or staple gun are shown.

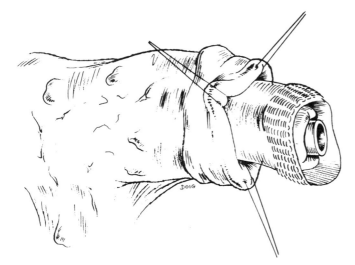

Figure 20–2. Cuff of proximal colon everted by four stay sutures and tube has been inserted.

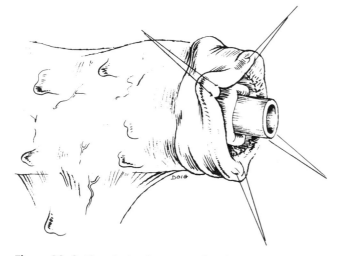

Figure 20–3. The tube has been sutured to the mucosa and submucosa of the proximal colon by using the locking running stitch of 2/0 polyglycolic acid.

ensuring that the sutures pick up only mucosa and submucosa (Fig. 20–3). Earlier work has demonstrated that the suture that does not incorporate the submucosa will lead to early expulsion of the device.[45] One must ensure that the colotubal anastomosis is secure, and small mosquito forceps are used to probe for gaps that, if present, are closed with interrupted suture. The proximal colon is reverted, and the posterior layer of the anastomosis is completed. The rectal probe is attached and passed into the distal bowel, where it is retrieved at the anus (Fig. 20–4). Once the anterior layer of the anastomosis has been sutured, gentle traction on the rectal probe unfolds the tube.

For a stapled anastomosis, the procedure is identical until reversion of the cuff of proximal bowel. At this stage, pursestring sutures are placed, the end-to-end stapling instrument is inserted, and the tube is attached to the nut on the anvil (Fig. 20–5). When the gun is fired and removed, it unfolds the tube and draws it out of the anus. The tube is then cut at the anus, or, for coloanal or low rectal anastomosis, it is placed inside a perineal incontinence bag (Fig. 20–6). Thus, the tube comes to lie across the anastomosis, preventing fecal contamination of the anastomosis but not disturbing intraluminal continuity. The presence of the tube within the rectal ampulla causes no symptom to the patient. If it is brought out across the anus, the patient suffers only minor tenesmus until the tube is cut a few days later.

The tube passes spontaneously at an average of 15 days postoperatively, when the suture works its way through from submucosa to mucosa. Experience has demonstrated that the tube does not fall out from degradation of the suture material since tubes have been retrieved with sutures still intact.[40]

Indication for the Intraluminal Bypass Tube

The intracolonic bypass tube is merely an *added insurance* for sound anastomotic healing in special situations in which there is cause to worry about the security of the anastomosis. It is not an excuse for poor surgical technique, and it merely protects the anastomosis from a minor dehiscence (which probably occurs commonly) developing into a clinically significant leak.

In general, the tube should be used only in situations in which the surgeon has some concern about the integrity of the anastomosis. This includes situations such as low anterior resection (especially if the patient has had preoperative radiotherapy), obstructed colon, perforated diverticulitis and trauma, and as an alternative to a defunctioning ileostomy to protect an ileal pouch–anal anastomosis.[46–50]

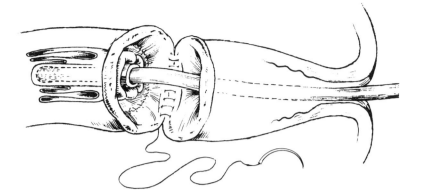

Figure 20–4. The rectal probe has been placed in the nipple of the tube and passed into the distal bowel.

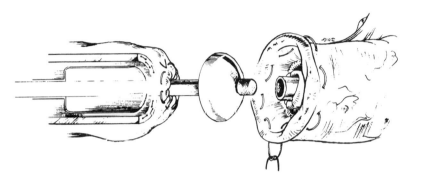

Figure 20–5. The end-to-end staple gun has been inserted into the anus, and the tube has been attached to the nut on the anvil.

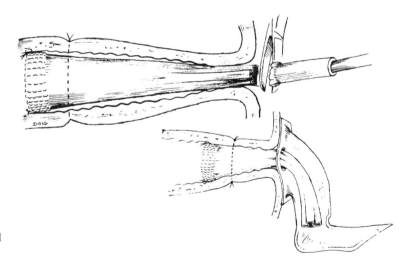

Figure 20–6. The intracolonic bypass tube is seen to traverse the anastomosis and is being placed by a perineal incontinence bag.

Special Technical Problems with the Intracolonic Bypass Tube

Small-diameter Colon. If it proves problematic to insert the parachute-folded intracolonic bypass tube, there are a number of alternatives. The proximal colon may be enlarged by using Hagar dilators and staple-sizing devices, by wrapping the bowel in warm saline gauze, or by administering intravenous glucagon. The anesthesiologist should refrain from using a spinal anesthetic in this setting.

Unfolding the Tube. Some surgeons choose to draw the tube out when the anterior layer of the colorectal or colocolonic anastomosis has been completed. However, this approach carries the risk of injuring the tube during insertion of the anterior layer of sutures. The advantage of this technique is that the surgeon is assured that the tube will unravel. If, on drawing the rectal probe or stapling gun from the anus, the tube fails to unfold, gentle pressure from above and the application of ring forceps from below are always useful.

Checking the Anastomosis. With the unfolded tube at the anus, an irrigation syringe is attached to the nipple, and povidone-iodine solution is instilled. This should fill the proximal colon above the colotubal anastomosis and no leakage should be seen. The side of the colotubal anastomosis should be checked for serosal penetration. If this is seen, a serosal-serosal mattress stitch should be placed. If the surgeon wishes to instill povidone-iodine or saline around the tube to check the colocolonic anastomosis, this should be done in the usual fashion.

LATE SEQUELAE OF COLORECTAL OPERATIONS

Stricture Formation

The most important consequence of an anastomotic leak is a benign colorectal stricture. This is most common after an anastomotic leak and subsequent healing with fibrosis. Stricture formation is inevitable if the anastomotic dehiscence occupies 50% or more of the circumference. It is usually more significant after a low anterior resection, especially if it is combined with preoperative or postoperative radiotherapy. The development of an anastomotic stricture appears to be more frequent if there has been a protecting proximal temporary colostomy, especially if the colorectal anastomosis was performed with staples. Other risk factors appear to be obesity, incomplete tissue doughnut, pelvic abscess, and male gender.[51, 52]

Treatment is by repeated dilatation with Hagar dilators or, if the stricture is very narrow, with an endoscopic balloon technique after passage of a guide wire. If a symptomatic stricture persists, consideration should be given to progressively more extensive procedures. These include transanal stricturoplasty and excision of the stricture by using the transanal circular stapling device; occasionally, even an abdominoperineal resection with a terminal colostomy may be needed. Fortunately, most strictures respond to periodic dilatation, and the lumen is further dilated by the regular passage of stools. The stricture may be a manifestation of recurrent cancer in the pelvis. Appropriate CT scans of the pelvis and deep biopsies may be necessary to confirm the suspicion.

Incontinence

Most patients who undergo a low anterior resection have difficulties with irregular and frequent bowel movements for several months. Soiling and frank incontinence are also common, especially in elderly patients and in those whose anal sphincter musculature has been dilated. Diminution of rectal reservoir capacity, loss of rectal compliance, colorectal denervation, narrowing of the anastomosis, postsurgical inflammatory reactions, and abnormal anorectal reflexes all have been implicated.[13, 53, 54] These symptoms improve over time and return to nearly normal in about 12 months in most instances. Meanwhile, patients should pay special attention to diet and perform regular pelvic floor and anal sphincter exercises. It is unwise to resort to constipating medications early in these situations.

Sexual Impotence in the Male Patient

In a standard operation for rectal cancer, the afferent pudendal nerves, which are essential for penile erection, and the pelvic sympathetic nerves, which control ejaculation, are often sacrificed in an attempted curative procedure (see subchapter Operative Treatment for Carcinoma of the Rectum in Chapter 9). During proctectomy for inflammatory bowel disease, neither erection nor ejaculation should be affected. As mentioned, the dissection stays close to the rectal wall, and autonomic nerves are spared (see subchapter Proctocolectomy in Chapter 8). If erectile capacity is lost, the patient should be given the option of having a penile prosthesis.

The issue of "informed consent" sometimes looms large in the medicolegal arena when a male patient experiences postoperative sexual difficulties. It is important to discuss this risk with relatively young men who are about to undergo abdominoperineal resection or low anterior resection for rectal cancer. The individual patient may then elect to choose a less extensive form of therapy (e.g., local fulguration, primary radiotherapy) or may chose to "bank" his sperm before the operation.

Dyspareunia in the Female Patient

It is not uncommon for women to have gynecologic complaints, such as irregular menstrual cycles, menstrual cramps, and/or vaginal discharge, after an abdominoperineal resection. These usually subside with reassurance and time, if primary gynecologic ailments are excluded. The most distressing symptom for the relatively young female is dyspareunia: In one study, the incidence after abdominoperineal resection was 50%. Dorsocaudal dislocation of the vagina (horizontal vagina syndrome) has been offered as an explanation, and an extensive operation has been proposed to correct the anatomic problem.[55] This entails excision of the coccyx, separation of the posterior vaginal wall from the sacral curve, and interposition of muscle flaps from the gluteus maximus muscles on both sides (Kylberg operation).

Perineal Symptoms Following Abdominoperineal Resection

Several *phantom sensations,* akin to those reported after extremity amputations, can occur after proctectomy. These include the urge to defecate or pass flatus and invariably resolve with time. No treatment, except reassurance, is indicated. *Perineal pain,* if severe or intractable, is a major problem and may be the first indication of recurrent cancer. Full evaluation, including pelvic CT scan, is essential to exclude this possibility, especially if the pain is persistent. However, intermittent sharp, severe, deep-seated pain is sometimes encountered and is analogous to proctalgia fugax (levator ani muscle spasm). Treatment is unsatisfactory. Steroid or sclerosant injections are fraught with danger. An electrogalvanic stimulating device inserted in the vagina sometimes helps the female patient.

Perineal hernia is rare. The affected patient may be asymptomatic or may complain of "sitting on a lump," perineal pressure, or discomfort. Partial small bowel obstruction may occur. Skin wound breakdown and evisceration via the perineal route have also been reported. The generally recommended treatment is a combined abdominoperineal approach, removal of the small bowel from the pelvis, and repair of the pelvic floor by using Marlex mesh.

REFERENCES

1. McGuire HH Jr. Complications of intestinal surgery. In: Greenfield LJ, ed. Complications in Surgery and Trauma. Philadelphia: JB Lippincott, 1984, pp 447–465.
2. Goligher JC, Lloyd-Davies OV, Robertson CT. Small gut obstructions following combined excision of rectum, with special reference to strangulation around the colostomy. Br J Surg 1951;38:467–470.
3. Bucknall TE, Cox PJ, Ellis H, et al. Burst abdomen and incisional hernia: A prospective study of 1129 major laparotomies. Br Med J 1982;284:931–934.
4. Homans J. Three hundred and eighty-four laparotomies for various diseases with tables showing the results of the operations and the subsequent history of the patients. Boston: N. Sawyer, 1887.
5. Ponka JL. Hernias of the Abdominal Wall. Philadelphia: WB Saunders, 1980.
6. Harding KG, Leister SJ, Mudge M, et al. Aetiology of incisional hernia—a prospective follow-up of 564 patients undergoing major abdominal surgery. Presented to the surgical section of the Royal Society of Medicine in London, June 10, 1981.
7. De Dombal FT, Burton L, Goligher JC. The early and late results of surgical treatment for Crohn's disease. Br J Surg 1971;58:805–811.
8. Ferrari BT, DenBesten L. The prevention and treatment of persistent perineal sinus. World J Surg 1980;4:167–172.
9. Warshaw AL, Ottinger LW, Bartlett HW. Primary perineal closure after proctocolectomy for inflammatory bowel disease. Am J Surg 1977;133:414–419.
10. Eisenbud DE, Block GE, Moossa AR. Management of the perineal wound following abdomino-perineal resection of the rectum for inflammatory bowel disease. Surg Gastroenterol 1982;1:115–121.
11. Janu Nc, Bokey EL, Chapuis PH, et al. Bladder dysfunction following anterior resection for carcinoma of the rectum. Dis Colon Rectum 1980;29:182–185.
12. Cunsulo A, Bragaglia RB, Manura G, et al. Urogenital dysfunction after abdominoperineal resection for carcinoma of the rectum. Dis Colon Rectum 1990;33:918–922.
13. Goligher JC. Further reflections on sphincter conservation in the radical treatment of rectal cancer. Proc R Soc Med 1962;55:341.
14. Goligher JC, Graham NG, De Dombal FT. Anastomotic dehiscence after anterior resection of rectum and sigmoid. Br J Surg 1970;57(20):109–118.
15. Irvin TT, Goligher JC. Aetiology of disruption of intestinal anastomosis. Br J Surg 1973;60:461–464.
16. Morgenstern L, Yamakawa T, Ben-Slosham M. Anastomotic leakage after low colonic anastomosis. Am J Surg 1972;123:104–109.
17. Mc Ginn FP, Gartell PC, Clifford PC, Brunton FJ. Staples or sutures for low colorectal anastomosis: A prospective randomized trial. Br J Surg 1985;7(8):603–605.
18. Matheson NA, McIntosh CA, Krukowski ZH. Continuing experience with single layer appositional anastomosis in the large bowel. Br J Surg 1985;72(Suppl):S104–106.
19. Goligher JC. Bradshaw lecture, 1978. Recent trends in the practice of sphincter saving excision for rectal cancer. Ann R Coll Surg Engl 1978;61:169–176.
20. Shahinian TK, Bowen JR, Dorman BA, et al. Experience with the EEA stapling device. Am J Surg 1980;139:549–553.
21. Cade D, Gallagher P, Schofield PF, et al. Complications of anterior resection using the EEA stapling device. Br J Surg 1981;68:339–340.
22. Heald KRJ, Leicester RJ. The low stapled anastomosis. Br J Surg 1981;68:333–337.
23. Goldberg SM, Gordon PH, Nivatjongs S. In: Essentials of Anorectal Surgery, Philadelphia: JB Lippincott, pp. 181–182.
24. Blamey SL, Lee PWR. A comparison of circular stapling devices in colorectal anastomoses. Br J Surg 1982;69:18–22.

25. McGregor JR, Galloway DJ, Bel G, et al. Sutures or staples in colonic surgery. Br J Surg, 1987;74:601–606.
26. Everett WG, Friend PJ, Forty J. Comparison of stapling and hand-suture for left-sided large bowel anastomosis. Br J Surg 1986;73:345–348.
27. Waxman BP. Large bowel anastomoses, II. The circular staplers. Br J Surg 1983;70:64–67.
28. Chvapil M, Koopman CF. Age and other factors regulating wound healing. Otolaryngol Clin North Am 1982;15(2):259–270.
29. Daly JM, Vars HM, Dudrick SJ. Effects of protein depletion on strength of colonic anastomoses. Surg Gynecol Obstet 1972;134:15–21.
30. Morgenstern L, Sandes G, Wahlstrom E, et al. Effect of preoperative irradiation on healing of low colorectal anastomoses. Am J Surg 1984;147:245–249.
31. Bell CM, Lewis CB. Effect of neostigmine on integrity of ileorectal anastomoses. Br Med J 1968;3:578–588.
32. Whitaker BL, Dixon RA. Anastomotic failure in relation to blood transfusion and blood loss. Proc R Soc Med 1970;63:751–752.
33. Hawley PR. Infection—the cause of anastomotic breakdown: An experimental study. Proc R Soc Med 1970;60:152.
34. Jagelman G, Fazio VW, Lavery IC, Weakley FL. A prospective randomized double-blind study of 10% mannitol mechanical bowel preparation combined with oral neomycin and short-term peri-operative, intravenous Flagyl as prophylaxis in elective colorectal resection. Surgery 1985;98(5):861–865.
35. Minervinis S, Young D, Alexander-Williams J, et al. Prophylactic saline peritoneal lavage in elective colorectal operations. Dis Colon Rectum 1980;23:392–394.
36. Dudley HAF, Radcliffe AG, McGeehan D. Intraoperative irrigation of the colon to permit primary anastomosis. Br J Surg 1980;67:80–81.
37. Korath NM, Krukowski ZH, Youngson GG, et al. Intraoperative colonic irrigation in the management of left-sided bowel emergencies. Br J Surg 1985;72:708–711.
38. Thomson WHF, St C Carter. On-table lavage to achieve safe restorative rectal and emergency left colonic resection without covering colostomy. Br J Surg 1986;73:61–63.
39. Mirelman D, Corman ML, Veidenheimer MC, Coller JA. Colostomies and contra-indications: Lahey clinic experience, 1963–70. Dis Colon Rectum 1978;21:172–176.
40. Ravo B, Ger R. Temporary colostomy—an outmoded procedure? Dis Colon Rectum 1985;28(12):904–907.
41. Garrison FH. In: History of Medicine. Philadelphia: WB Saunders, 1929, p. 152.
42. Littlewood H. Ileosigmoidostomy (Senn's method) for intestinal obstruction due to malignant disease of the hepatic flexure of the colon. Lancet 1892;142:864–866.
43. Ravo B, Ger R. Management of oesophageal dehiscence by an intraluminal bypass tube—an experimental study. Am J Surg 1985;149:733–738.
44. Ravo B, Ger R. Intracolonic bypass by an intraluminal tube. Dis Colon Rectum 1984;27(6):360–365.
45. Ger R, Ravo B. Prevention and treatment of intestinal dehiscence by an intraluminal bypass graft. Br J Surg 1984;71:726–729.
46. Sackier JM, Wood CB. Low anterior resection and the intraluminal bypass tube. Br J Surg 1988;75:1232.
47. Ravo B, Mishrick A, Addeik, et al. The treatment of perforated diverticulitis by one-stage intracolonic bypass procedure. Surgery 1987;102(5):771–776.
48. Carpenter D, Bello J, Sokol TP, et al. The intracolonic bypass tube for left colon and rectal trauma. Am Surg 1987;56(12):769–773.
49. Keane PF, Ohri Sk, Wood CB, Sackier JM. Management of the obstructed left colon using the intraluminal bypass procedure. Dis Colon Rectum 1988;31(12):948–951.
50. Launer DP, Sackier JM. Pouch anal anastomosis without diverting ileostomy. Dis Colon Rectum 1991;34(11):993–998.
51. Graffner H, Freidlund P, Olsson SA, et al. Protective colostomy in low anterior resection of the rectum using EEA stapling instrument—a randomized study. Dis Colon Rectum 1983;26:87–91.
52. Luchtefeld MA, Milson JW, Senagore A, et al. Colorectal anastomotic stenosis. Results of a survey of the ASCRS membership. Dis Colon Rectum 1989;32:733–735.
53. Nakahama S, Itoh H, Mibu R, et al. Clinical and manometric evaluation of anorectal function following low anterior resection with low anastomotic line using EEATM stapler for rectal cancer. Dis Colon Rectum 1988;31:762–765.
54. Pedersen IK, Hint K, Olsen J, et al. Anorectal function after low anterior resection for carcinoma. Ann Surg 1986;204:802–806.
55. Sjodahl R, Nystrom PO, Olaison G. Surgical treatment of dorsocaudal dislocation of the vagina after excision of the rectum. The Kylberg operation. Dis Colon Rectum 1990;33:762–766.

DISEASES OF THE COLON, RECTUM, AND ANUS IN THE PEDIATRIC PATIENT

Anorectal Malformations in Infants and Children

CHAPTER 21

Neill Freeman

The surgeon must be familiar with the various types of congenital anorectal anomalies and must precisely delineate the anatomy before undertaking operative correction. Willis Potts cautioned:

> In general, atresia of the rectum is more poorly handled than any other congenital anomaly of the newborn. A properly functioning rectum is an unappreciated gift of the greatest price. The child who is so unfortunate to be born with an imperforate anus may be saved a lifetime of misery and social seclusion by the surgeon who with skill, diligence and judgment performs the first operation on the rectum.[1]

Realistically, there is no second chance to rectify the mistakes of an improper operation, in the hope of achieving adequate fecal control. Even for the most experienced surgeon, performing this type of surgery is always a formidable challenge.

There is rarely an urgent situation or emergency in which definitive surgery must be performed immediately. A colostomy is the proper operation for the inexperienced surgeon, even in infants in whom the diagnosis of an anorectal malformation has been overlooked and who presents with gross distention and intestinal obstruction. Appropriate advice about the timing and type of the definitive operation can then be sought at leisure.

Congenital anorectal anomalies demand special knowledge and operative experience, and there is a cogent argument that children suffering from these anomalies should be treated exclusively in highly specialized units by experienced surgeons. The incidence of anorectal anomalies is approximately 1 in 5,000 live births; therefore the experience gained by any one surgeon is necessarily limited.

In a review of a collective series of 5,454 patients from the literature, the male-to-female ratio was 55:44. It is impossible to compare the various types of anomalies on the basis of a review of the many publications, mainly because of the lack of an accepted international classification.[2-4] An analysis of 2,376 patients with anorectal anomalies from the world literature showed that in males 740 were "rectal" and 659 were "anal." In females the figures were 330 rectal and 171 anal. The division into rectal and anal cases is roughly equivalent to the "high" and "low" anomalies in the current Wingspread Classification. In 15% of the anorectal anomalies in males and in 8% in females, the bowel did not communicate with either the urinary tract or the perineum.

Several reports have shown more than one sibling being affected or a parent and child being affected, but these occurrences are rare. It has been concluded, following studies of all the families reported in the literature, that heredity plays only a minor and insignificant role in etiology.[2]

ASSESSMENT OF OTHER VISCERAL ANOMALIES

Syndromes Associated with Anorectal Anomaly

The acronym VATER or the expanded version VACTERL is a reminder of the other systems that are most likely to be involved in anorectal anomalies and need careful examination. The acronym VACTERL consists of the first letters of the involved systems: *v*ertebral, *a*nal, *c*ardiac, *t*racheo-*e*sophageal, *r*enal, and *l*imb anomalies. If three or more of the anomalies are present, the child is said to suffer from the VATER or VACTERL syndrome. Of patients with anorectal anomalies, 10% have concomitant esophageal atresia. Therefore, an 8-French or a 10-French gauge nasogastric tube should always be passed if there is any doubt about the presence of esophageal atresia or if the baby has symptoms suggestive of the disorder.

At the earliest convenient time, all children should have sonographic or excretory urographic (IVP) assessment of the urinary tract to exclude an anomaly of the renal tract, the incidence of which is high, varying from approximately 20% in low lesions to 50% in the high lesions.

Currarino Triad

The Currarino triad is an eponym for an autosomal-dominant, non–sex-linked condition of variable expression. The triad consists of an anorectal stenosis, a sacral bony anomaly, and a presacral mass. A bony defect of a scimitar or crescent shape is pathognomonic. The name commonly describes the triad, although the association of the three entities was recognized many years before the series reported by Currarino.[5] The constipation associated with the anal canal stenosis is intractable to treatment, and the surgeon caring for these children needs to be aware of the possible communication of the presacral mass with the spinal canal and the risk of meningitis. A strong familial association warrants screening of the siblings and immediate relatives, especially those with symptoms of constipation.

Syndromes Involving Both a Chromosomal and an Anorectal Anomaly

Several other syndromes, besides the VATER or VACTERL association, involve multiple congenital anomalies one feature of which is an anorectal anomaly.

Cat-Eye Syndrome

In the cat-eye syndrome, there is an acrocentric chromosome of the G group together with coloboma of the iris and choroid, microphthalmia, hypertelorism, and imperforate anus. It was first described by Haab in 1878.[6]

Townes-Brocks Syndrome

The Townes-Brocks syndrome is an autosomal-dominant syndrome of imperforate anus, triphalangeal thumbs, other bony anomalies of the hands and feet, and sensorineural deafness.

FG Syndrome

The features of the FG syndrome are imperforate anus with dolichocephaly, frontal bossing, down-slanting palpebral fissures, hypertelorism, long philtrum, micrognathia, cleft palate, and mental retardation.[6a]

Other Syndromes

The anal lesion may be part of other genetic syndromes such as trisomy 8 mosaicism. A correlation between imperforate anus and maternal ingestion of thalidomide has been reported.[7]

DIAGNOSIS

It is surprising that an anomaly that is not occult and is usually obvious on inspection should so often be overlooked. Both the obstetrician and the pediatrician who examine the child at birth have an obligation to determine whether the infant has a patent anus.

Normal Size and Position of the Anus

Physicians often subjectively diagnose patients as having anal stenosis or anterior displacement of the anus without understanding the variation of normal anatomy in this region. A formula for gauging the appropriate size of the neonatal anus is as follows: 1.3 + (birth weight in kilograms × 3) expressed as millimeters or a Hegar dilator size.[8]

The normal position of the anus must be defined and determined. Leape and Ramenofsky defined the position of the normal anal site as the midpoint between the fourchette and the tip of the coccyx.[9] Reisner and associates defined normal values by calculating a ratio of these distances: midanus to fourchette and midanus to coccyx in the female, and midanus to scrotum and midanus to coccyx in the male.[10] If the ratio is less than 0.34 in females (the range varies from 0.44 in newborns to 0.40 in infants from 4 to 18 months of age) and less than 0.46 in males (the range being 0.58 in newborns and 0.56 in infants from 4 to 18 months of age), the anal position can be regarded as abnormal.

Therefore in practical terms, the anus must lie less than two thirds of the distance between the coccyx and fourchette or between the coccyx and scrotum, before the diagnosis of ectopia can be entertained.

If there is any doubt about the normality of the anus following inspection of the perineum, a thermometer or similar instrument should be passed into the anal canal for not more than 2 cm to establish patency. One must record whether meconium has been passed and the time interval following delivery.

Clinical Examination in Males

One must search carefully for any communication of the bowel with skin. This tract may be filled with air, white epithelial pearls, or black meconium, and it may be anywhere from the normal anal site to the tip of the penis.

The urethral opening is inspected and urine collected to establish whether meconium is present in the urine. The meconium may be visible on macroscopic examination or as squamous or epithelial cells in the urine on microscopic examination. If meconium is found in the urine, it always indicates the presence of a fistula between the bowel and urinary tract.

Clinical Examination in Females

The perineum is inspected and a determination made of whether the anus is in the normal or "ectopic" site. It is determined whether one, two, or three orifices are present. In the newborn, this is not always easy to do. If the anus is not in the normal site, it should be ascertained whether the opening is on the perineal skin or within the mucosa of the vulva.

The infant's back is examined to exclude spina bifida or vertebral anomaly. The tip of the coccyx is palpated and note is made of whether the buttocks are flat with little or no natal cleft suggestive of sacral agenesis. These bony anomalies are visible on plain radiographs. Perineal sensation and sphincter function are assessed by pinprick or nerve stimulation of the perineum.

Supplementary Diagnostic Aids

The surgeon should not embark on an operation until certain of the exact anatomy of the malformation. Some, or all, of the following investigations may be performed in cases of anorectal anomalies, depending on local circumstances and available facilities.

Inspection and Probing

Careful inspection of the perineum in a good light supplemented by a malleable probe helps in the examination of various fistulas and orifices.

Radiology

PLAIN RADIOGRAPHS

The most commonly implemented radiograph remains the classic "invertogram" described by Wangensteen and Rice in 1930.[11] A lateral prone decubitus view with the buttocks raised has since proved to be equally diagnostic and does not require the baby to be held upside down for 3 minutes.[12]

The purpose of the radiographic examination is to try to determine the distance of the blind pouch or the fistula from the perineum and to judge the relationship of the blind pouch to the pelvic diaphragm and striated muscle complex.

The radiographic view must be a true lateral one, centered over the greater trochanter, and it should include the pubis, sacrum, coccyx, and perineum. The anal site should be marked with a radiopaque object.

Various lines or landmarks can be drawn on the film as guides (Fig. 21–1).

Pubococcygeal Line. The pubococcygeal (PC) line passes from the upper border of symphysis, which is taken as the center of bony shadow of the os pubis, to the sacrococcygeal articulation. This point is just distal to the fifth sacral segment, as the coccyx does not ossify until 2 to 5 years of age. The soft tissue structures lying on the PC line are the bladder neck, the verumontanum, the peritoneal reflection, and the external os of the cervix.

Ischial Line. The ischial line (I line) lies parallel to the PC line at the lowermost point of the ossified ischial bone. The important soft tissue structures at this level are the upper surface of the bulb of the urethra in the male and the upper level of the perineal body and triangular ligament in the female.

Anal Pit Line. The anal pit line lies 1 to 2 cm below the I line and passes through the site of the normal anal pit.

Gas in Other Viscera. Gas may be seen in the bladder or urethra or in a subcutaneous tract, indicating a connection with the bowel.

CONTRAST RADIOGRAPHY

If a fistula is present, dye can be injected into its orifice to delineate the anatomy accurately.

If a colostomy is present, a distal loopogram should be performed prior to any definitive surgery.

If no fistula is present and the lesion is thought to be low or intermediate on the basis of radiography, needle aspiration of the midline of the perineum is a worthwhile procedure. If meconium or gas is encountered, contrast material may be injected.[13]

Micturition cystography, either by means of a catheter inserted into the bladder or a retrograde injection

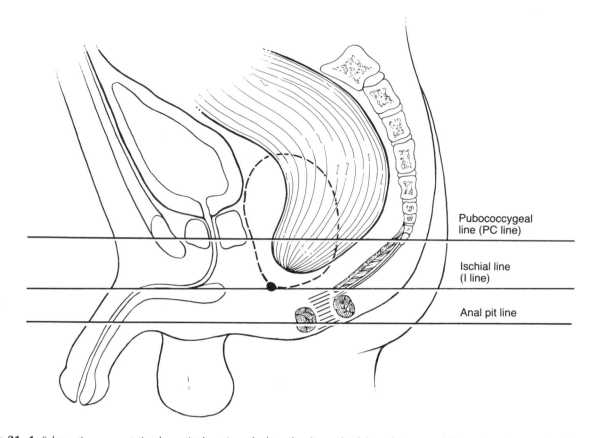

Figure 21–1. Schematic representation by sagittal section of a lateral radiograph of the pelvis onto which various lines can be drawn to judge the relationship of the blind pouch to the pelvic diaphragm and striated muscle complex. The radiograph must be in the true lateral position centered over the greater trochanter, and the film should include the pubis, the sacrum, the coccyx, and the perineum. The anal site should be marked with a small radiopaque marker. The pubococcygeal line (PC line) extends from the upper border of the symphysis (center of bony shadow of os pubis) to sacrococcygeal articulation (just distal to the fifth sacral segment. The coccyx does not ossify until 2 to 5 years). The soft tissue structures lying on this line are bladder neck, verumontanum, peritoneal reflection, and the external os of the cervix. The ischial line (I line) lies parallel to the PC line at the lowermost point of the ossified ischial bone. Soft tissues at this level are the upper surface of the bulb of the urethra in the male and the upper level of the perineal body and triangular ligament in the female. The anal pit line is 1 to 2 cm below the I line passing through the normal anal pit.

of contrast material into the urethra, may demonstrate the fistula. A combination of procedures is even more helpful.

OTHER DIAGNOSTIC AIDS

Ultrasonography of the pelvis by way of the perineum may demonstrate the type and level of the anomaly.[14] This technique has not received wide application and requires an experienced ultrasonographer for interpretation.

Computed tomography (CT) and magnetic resonance imaging (MRI)[15] are now often utilized to demonstrate the anorectal anatomy and striated muscle complex. The baby is small enough to be placed sagittally on the gantry of the scanner to obtain a midline, rather than a transverse, view.[16]

Electromyography of the external sphincter by bipolar needle electrodes inserted into the perineum may also be employed to determine the presence of the striated muscle complex.[17]

Endoscopy of the urethra or vagina provides further information about the size and site of the fistula, but it is best done at the beginning of the definitive operative procedure.

Diagnostic Pitfalls

The gas shadow of the atretic bowel must be smooth and rounded. This feature indicates complete filling and that all the distal meconium has been displaced. The radiograph should be taken preferably more than 24 hours after birth, because gas does not reach the rectum before this time. Sticky meconium occupying the distal bowel may lead to errors in interpretation as to the level of the lesion. Gas may escape through a fistula to skin, urethra, or vagina, thereby preventing full distention of the rectum. Misleading levels of the gas shadow are seen when the baby cries, as the rectal gas shadow is pushed beyond the ischial point by the increased intra-abdominal pressure. A strong contraction of the levator complex at the moment of radiograph exposure gives an erroneous impression of the length of a fistula or the anal canal.

In the classic invertogram, the rectum may be displaced cranially by gravity, depicting a higher level of the gas shadow in relation to the bony landmarks—especially if the rectum is not fully distended.

DETERMINATION OF TYPE AND LEVEL OF ANOMALY AND APPROPRIATE SURGICAL APPROACH

There is no universally accepted classification of anorectal anomalies. An accepted classification developed from a workshop held at Wingspread in 1984. An attempt was made to update the previous International Classification devised in Melbourne in 1971.[18] A classification is necessary to ensure that surgeons have defined criteria against which to compare their results. The clinical outcome in patients must be based on a classification, as the prognoses for subsequent normal fecal control with the high, intermediate, and low anomalies vary considerably. Such a classification is a valuable guide to management of the patient. It is also useful in counseling parents preoperatively about long-term prognosis. The anomalies are classified as high, intermediate, or low, depending on the relationship of the terminal bowel or fistula to the pelvic diaphragm, and annotated for the male and female anatomies (Table 21–1). The criticism remains, however, that although the Wingspread classification is a simplified

Table 21–1. WINGSPREAD CLASSIFICATION OF ANORECTAL ANOMALIES

Female	Male
High	
Anorectal agenesis with a rectovaginal fistula without fistula	Anorectal agenesis with a rectoprostatic fistula without fistula
Rectal atresia	Rectal atresia
Intermediate	
Rectovestibular fistula	Rectobulbar urethral fistula
Rectovaginal fistula	
Agenesis without fistula	Agenesis without fistula
Low	
Anovestibular fistula	
Anocutaneous fistula	Anocutaneous fistula
Anal stenosis	Anal stenosis
Cloacae	
Rare malformations	Rare malformations

version of the 1971 International Classification, it is still too cumbersome for most surgeons to remember. It is also argued that because the posterior sagittal anorectoplasty is now the operation of choice, the level of the lesion does not matter; the operations are similar for high, intermediate, and low anomalies.

Colostomy

Because complications and even deaths are associated with colostomy, the operation should not be performed unless absolutely indicated. A colostomy is required for all high lesions. Aluwihare, however, performs pull-through operations by way of an anterior perineal approach in the neonatal period for high lesions without a colostomy.[19] Opinions differ regarding colostomy for intermediate lesions. A colostomy is not required in the low lesions. Several precautions are necessary in the establishment of a colostomy.

The colostomy should be defunctioning. A simple loop sigmoid colostomy in the left iliac fossa is satisfactory; enough distal sigmoid colon should be left for the subsequent definitive pull-through operation. Because most of these patients are still in diapers, the site of the colostomy on the abdominal wall is of less consequence than that of a permanent colostomy, in which the colostomy appliance must fit accurately in order not to leak. Many parents prefer not to use colostomy bags, as the feces are easily managed in the diapers. Some surgeons insist on complete division of the colon with separation of the loops by a skin bridge. In most patients this is not necessary, especially if the definitive operation is performed early in the neonatal period. The site of the colostomy depends on the marginal blood supply, which must be carefully inspected and preserved so as not to compromise the distal bowel on subsequent closure of the colostomy. The distal loop must be washed out until completely emptied of meconium at the time of colostomy. Normal saline or 1% aqueous povidone-iodine can be utilized for the washout.

Optimal Age for the Definitive Operation

In the low anomalies in both male and female infants, a simple dilatation or an anoplasty to widen the orifice can be performed in the immediate neonatal period.

In the high anomalies, because of intestinal obstruction, a colostomy is necessary, usually within the first 24 to 48 hours of life. Once the obstruction has been relieved, the timing of the definitive pull-through operation is optional and somewhat controversial. Most surgeons believe that the operation is safer and the anatomic structures more clearly defined at 9 to 12 months of age. However there is physiologic evidence

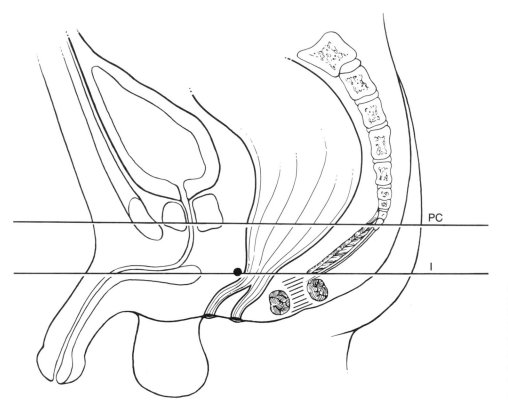

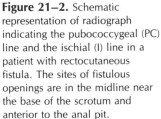

Figure 21–2. Schematic representation of radiograph indicating the pubococcygeal (PC) line and the ischial (I) line in a patient with rectocutaneous fistula. The sites of fistulous openings are in the midline near the base of the scrotum and anterior to the anal pit.

that early operation within the first 3 months of life may have definite advantages. Because the brain is immature at birth, the appropriate cortical connections, as measured by evoked anal potentials, are made in the early weeks or months of postnatal life.[20] If the bowel is placed in the correct site before 3 months of age, appropriate cortical connections may be made and the eventual outcome improved.[21]

Once a colostomy has been performed in the intermediate anomalies, the definitive operation can be delayed to suit the surgeon's preference. If colostomy is not elected, a definitive operation in the neonatal period is needed to relieve the intestinal obstruction.

Males with "Low" Anomalies

In males with low anomalies, the two lesions most often seen are anocutaneous fistula and anal stenosis.

Anocutaneous Fistula. The anocutaneous fistula was known as the "covered anus—complete" according to the 1970 classification. The anus is in the normal site and is covered by a hypertrophied raphe or triangular fold, with a fistulous tract in the midline, opening near the base of the scrotum (Fig. 21–2).

Anal Stenosis. Anal stenosis was called "covered anus" according to the earlier classification. A hypertrophied bar that resembles a bucket handle covers the anus anteriorly and posteriorly, but not completely.

Under the so-called bucket handle, in the midline or on either side, one or two tiny orifices containing meconium are usually found.

Management. A cutback operation or a Y-V plasty can correct either anocutaneous fistula or anal stenosis. All procedures must be followed by regular dilatation, commencing on the seventh postoperative day and continuing for several weeks or months until the anus is soft and supple.

Males with "Intermediate" Anomalies

In males with intermediate anomalies, the anal canal is agenetic, and the distended bowel is on or above the pelvic diaphragm; however if a fistula is present, it passes through the puborectal sling. Cases of intermediate anomalies generate the most controversy about the correct operative approach.

RECTOBULBAR URETHRAL FISTULA

The rectum ends at the upper border of bulbocavernous muscle. From here the fistula enters the bulb of the urethra below the membranous urethra. In the perineum there may be no anal pit. Sometimes the lesion is associated with a groove or double raphe. Frequently, hypospadias is present together with a cleft scrotum or flimsy membrane representing the urethra.

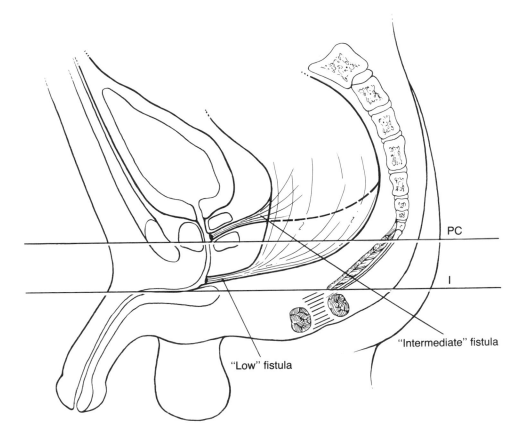

Figure 21–3. Schematic representation of rectourethral fistulas lying above and below the pubococcygeal (PC) line representing both high and intermediate anomalies. (I indicates ischial line.)

"Intermediate" fistula

"Low" fistula

Management. It is safer for an inexperienced surgeon to perform an initial sigmoid colostomy. In experienced hands a posterior sagittal anoplasty can be accomplished in the neonate without need of a preliminary colostomy.

ANAL AGENESIS WITHOUT FISTULA

Anal agenesis without fistula occurs almost exclusively in males. The rectum ends at the upper border of the bulbocavernosus muscle, in close proximity to the urethra but without a fistula. The rectum may exhibit an anterior protrusion suggestive of a preexisting fistula.

Management. If there is doubt regarding the experience of the surgeon, a colostomy should be performed in the first instance to be followed later by definitive operation. Alternatively, a perineal approach without diverting colostomy can be carried out in the newborn period.

Males with "High" Anomalies

In males with high anomalies, the rectum with its fistulous connection lies above the levator diaphragm (Fig. 21–3). The most common variety is anorectal agenesis with a rectoprostatic-urethral fistula. The perineum has no distinctive pattern, and the natal cleft may be obliterated. A dimple, raphe, or pigmented patch may lie over the anal site. The internal anatomy cannot be predicted from the external appearance. The perineum may bulge on crying, especially in the presence of sacral agenesis. Preliminary colostomy is always indicated.

Management. The surgical approach and the age at which the definitive operation should be carried out remain controversial. I prefer a preliminary colostomy followed by an early neonatal pull-through operation.[21] Most pediatric surgeons, however, still prefer to wait until the patient is 12 to 15 months old before performing the definitive procedure.

Females with "Low" Anomalies

ANOVESTIBULAR FISTULA

The most common of the low anomalies is the anovestibular fistula. There is no opening on the perineal skin. The "anus" or "fistula" opens into the vestibule between the hymen and skin of the fourchette and is surrounded by moist mucous membrane rather than dry skin. The difficulty is in deciding whether this is an anus or a long nonsupple fistula. Radiography can be misleading because occasionally the fistula or anal canal is not distended and appears deceptively long. Inserting a Foley catheter into the opening, inflating the balloon, and pulling down on the catheter will give a more accurate measurement of the anal canal or the length of the fistula (Fig. 21–4).

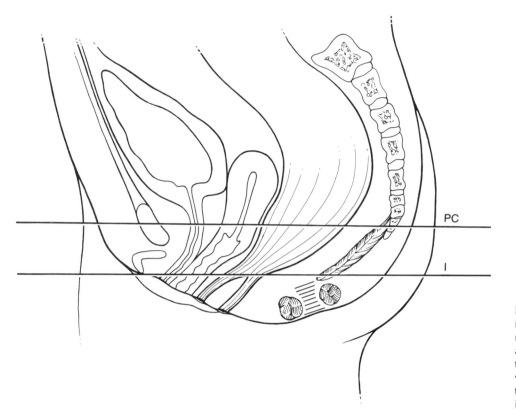

Figure 21–4. Schematic representation of lateral radiograph of a female with low anomaly below the (I) line with the fistula opening into the vestibule between the hymen and the skin of the fourchette. (PC indicates pubococcygeal line.)

Management. Controversy about the appropriate surgical treatment for anovestibular fistula continues. The surgeon's decision may be influenced by the attitude of the local culture and may be different in occidental and oriental countries. Satisfactory defecation can be obtained by a simple dilatation or a cutback operation. This leaves the opening of the anus anteriorly placed in the vulva with no perineal body, which is unacceptable in many societies. Transplantation of the anus posteriorly by using a limited midline sagittal approach without a colostomy, either in the neonatal period or later, is preferable. A perineal body is created with separation of the rectum and vagina by this approach.

It is a grave error to mistake the "intermediate" anomaly of a rectovestibular fistula, which has an identical opening in the same position (vestibular), for a low anovestibular fistula, because the types of management of the two lesions are different. Intermediate rectovestibular fistula is diagnosed by inserting a probe into the fistula and noting the direction, that is, parallel to the vagina rather than parallel to the perineal skin, or by injecting contrast medium into the fistula. The high rectovestibular fistula anomaly requires a colostomy and an extensive posterior sagittal rectoplasty.

ANOCUTANEOUS FISTULA

Here the anus is anteriorly placed between the posterior limit of the vulva and the normal anal site. It is skin-lined and surrounded by dry skin, not by mucous membrane. The opening may be stenotic as well as ectopic.

Management. Controversy remains as to the optimal treatment. Simple dilatation, cutback, Y-V plasty, or transplantation posteriorly are all recommended methods. I now favor a limited sagittal anoplasty to transpose the anus into a more normal position. If an anus rather than a fistula is present, this can be performed without a colostomy.

Females with "Intermediate" Anomalies

Rectovestibular fistula, rectovaginal fistula (low), and anal agenesis without fistula are the three intermediate anomalies in the female. The distinction must be made between the rectovestibular and anovestibular anomalies as already discussed (Fig. 21–5).

Management. Colostomy followed by a posterior sagittal rectoplasty is recommended for rectovestibular fistula, low rectovaginal fistula, and anal agenesis.

Females with "High" Anomalies

Anorectal agenesis with a rectovaginal fistula, a normal vagina and urethra, and a rectal opening (usually large) into the posterior fornix is rare in the female. The rectovaginal fistula is more likely to be associated with the single perineal opening typical of the "cloacal"

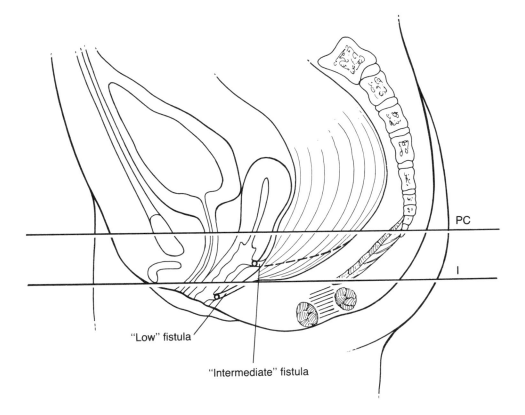

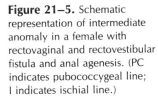

Figure 21–5. Schematic representation of intermediate anomaly in a female with rectovaginal and rectovestibular fistula and anal agenesis. (PC indicates pubococcygeal line; I indicates ischial line.)

anomalies, which account for less than 15% of high anomalies in the female.

Management. A colostomy followed by an extensive posterior sagittal rectoplasty is required. The management of rectal atresia without fistula is similar. The cloacal anomalies need individualization.

PERIOPERATIVE AIDS IN ANORECTAL ANOMALIES

The following principles apply to all anorectal operations. Skilled administration of anesthesia and complete facilities for intensive monitoring are necessary, because many of these operations are prolonged. The monitoring should include two probes for core and skin temperatures, pulse oximetry, and measurement of blood loss, blood gases, and pH. Venous access by means of peripheral or central veins is usual, although in most instances the blood loss should be minimal as the surgeon tries to operate in a virtually bloodless field. Diathermy throughout the procedure, even for cutting the skin, is helpful in this respect.

The theater should be designed to keep the baby warm. This should include the ability to control the ambient air temperature individually in each theater.

As the baby is exposed to the ambient temperature during induction and insertion of intravenous lines, an overhead radiant heater in the anesthetic room and theater and a circulating water mattress on the operating table help to prevent further heat loss. The baby's arms, legs, and head should be wrapped in cotton wool or absorbent tissue (Gamgee) before the skin is prepared. At operation a large sheet of plastic drape covers the whole baby. If the baby is well positioned on the water blanket, the heat from the blanket is entrapped.

Position of Patient on Operating Table

Three basic patient positions can be used: the jackknife, the lithotomy, or the modified lithotomy.

Jackknife Position. Here the baby is placed prone with the buttocks raised by means of a sandbag under the pelvis. The sandbag is best placed under the water blanket, rather than under the patient, to preserve patient contact with the circulating water.

Lithotomy Position. Unfortunately, even with small stirrups, only the older children can be placed comfortably in the lithotomy position.

Modified Lithotomy Position. The modified lithotomy position can be utilized if the baby's legs are too short for the conventional lithotomy position. In the neonate it is not feasible to place the legs in stirrups, but strapping the feet and legs together across the lower abdomen is satisfactory. If a laparotomy is anticipated as part of the procedure, the legs can be kept clear of the lower abdomen by strapping them laterally over a sandbag.

Position of the Surgeon

Ideal placement of the anaesthetist, surgeon, assistant, and scrub nurse around a small baby, each having a reasonable view and access, can be difficult to achieve. The surgeon may sit at the foot of the table; the baby is in either the jackknife or the lithotomy position and is directly in front of the surgeon. Standing on the right side of the operating table is also suitable, but it involves bending over the baby, causing more strain on the surgeon's back. A Mayo table should be fixed to the upper part of the operating table, with the lower edge at about the level of the patient's xiphisternum and the bottom of the table raised to about 6 inches from the baby's face. This arrangement provides a space under the drapes in which the anesthetist can work and monitor the baby during the operation.

The baby is further protected with Gamgee or a large gauze swab, which is stuck onto the skin after preparation with a dressing (Op-Site) before the entire baby is covered by a large plastic drape film. The bottom and side drapes are applied first, and then a large drape is placed over the Mayo table. The leading edge of this drape is raised and folded upward for approximately 12 inches at the upper edge of the Mayo table and attached to a drip stand or suitable upright structure, thereby creating "wings." The lower operative field is kept sterile and separate from the anesthetist, who can work undisturbed from the other side of the drape and under the Mayo table. The drapes should be sutured to the patient, or the adherent Gamgee, to prevent slippage and contamination of the operative field. The back of the surgeon, who is seated, should be covered in a sterile manner, as the scrub nurse may need to work from behind the back or the right side.

Bowel Washout on the Table

Even if preoperative bowel washouts have been performed, a further liberal application of 1% to 2% aqueous povidone-iodine is recommended for the final mechanical cleansing of the bowel just before operation. This should be done either in the anesthetic room or on the table before preparation, and it may be repeated during the procedure. Warm solutions should be available at all times to prevent heat loss.

Antibiotics

Metronidazole, gentamicin, and ampicillin, or a similar combination, given systemically with the premedication or started with the induction of anesthesia and continued postoperatively, usually suffice as "prophylaxis."

Operating with magnification by means of a loupe or a dissecting microscope is recommended. A loupe is more practical because the microscope is cumbersome, especially if there is any movement in the field, either from retraction or respiratory movements.

Electrostimulation during operation is essential in order to identify functioning bands of muscle. Specific powerful electrostimulators are commercially available. A simple probe can easily be made in most hospital workshops and connected to the peripheral nerve stimulator. The peripheral nerve stimulator is capable of delivering 60 mA, which is adequate.

Postoperative Management

The success of most anorectal operations depends on a careful and meticulous personal follow-up by the surgeon. Primary healing without breakdown of wounds, leakage, or sepsis is the ideal goal. If sepsis occurs, a fibrotic stricture at the mucocutaneous junction or behind the anus may develop.

Fecal contamination of the area can be prevented by a diverting colostomy. As stated previously, a colostomy is not always necessary, and careful bowel preparation and a low-residue preoperative diet may suffice. When the bowel starts to function postoperatively and fecal soiling occurs, the operative area should immediately be irrigated with normal saline or washed with water, preferably from a shower if the patient can be transported to the appropriate room.

Pressure on the perineum as occurs during sitting, which is particularly harmful, should be avoided. Sitting on the perineum exerts tremendous lateral forces on the midline suture lines and should be avoided for at least the first week or 10 days after operation. The patient should be permitted to stand or lie on the back or on one side, although this may be difficult to accomplish.

Nylon skin sutures, rather than subcutaneous absorbable sutures, are recommended and should be left in place for at least 10 days. Catheterization of the patient for 3 to 4 days postoperatively limits movement and helps protect the suture line from excessive forces, thereby facilitating primary healing.

When healing has occurred, at approximately 10 days, dilatations are started. The dilatations must be gentle and graduated. Increasing the size too rapidly, thereby causing bleeding and tearing, is to be avoided because scarring and fibrosis will occur. Initially, the dilatations must be done by the surgeon who performed the operation; the surgeon will know the direction, the size, and the force to be applied to avoid creating a false passage, perforating the rectum, or disrupting a suture line that tapers the bowel. As soon as is practical parents should be involved in the dilatations. Most are initially horrified, but once shown and encouraged, they become confident and proficient. This means that the dilatations are done daily. A 5% lidocaine (Xylocaine) ointment should be applied as the lubricant to minimize any pain or discomfort.

SPECIFIC OPERATIONS FOR ANORECTAL ANOMALIES

Cutback Operation

The "cutback" operation, first described by Browne, has been widely followed and is favored by most British surgeons (Fig. 21–6).[22] The operation is simple and is recommended by some as the procedure of choice in all "low" anomalies, especially in females, in the neonatal period.[23]

The patient is placed in the supine position with the legs held or strapped. The bowel is cleansed by several irrigations of 1% aqueous providone-iodine. One blade of a pair of straight, blunt-tipped scissors is placed in the ectopic bowel orifice and directed posteriorly in the midline under the skin approximately to the position of a normal anus. The inner blade of the scissors must not be advanced too deeply into the rectum, as the encircling fibers of the puborectal muscle will be divided and subsequent continence affected. Closing the blades and cutting the intervening tissue between the skin and posterior rectal wall complete the operation. The cut surfaces can be apposed with a 4-0 Vicryl or a similar suture or the raw edges left open, because healing is usually rapid. The enlarged orifice should admit an 8- to 10-mm dilator. Excess skin tags should be trimmed, because they do not regress and may later cause excoriation and soreness (Fig. 21–7).

The cosmetic result with no perineal body is unacceptable to many cultures. Patients from these cultures return for a secondary transplant of the anus into a more normal position.

The functional outcome of the cutback operation should be satisfactory, but in many patients it is not. The ectopic opening forces the patient to strain unduly. As a result, the perineum and posterior rectal wall descend excessively, producing mechanical constipation. Intractable constipation due to the mechanical disadvantage produced by the cutback operation is another factor avoided with an anal transplant opera-

tion. As in all anal surgery, regular dilatations must start early (about 7 to 10 days after operation) and continue for at least 3 to 6 months or until healing is complete and the anus is soft and supple. Initially the dilatations are performed with a dilator, candle, or similar smoothly shaped object. Later, the parents should be encouraged to insert the small finger, and eventually the index finger, as indicated.

Y-V Plasty

This procedure is more precise than the cutback operation for enlarging and transposing the posterior wall of the abnormal orifice to a more normal site. The disadvantage of this operation is that the anterior wall remains in close contact with the vagina, and it is not possible to construct a perineal body.

The position on the operating table and preparation are similar to those for the cutback operation. The exact position of the anus, as shown by contraction of the external sphincter, is identified with an electrostimulator. An inverted V- or U-incision is made over the proposed site of the anus, and a subcutaneous flap is raised, identifying and leaving behind the obvious muscle fibers of the contracting external sphincter. A midline skin incision is made from the opening of the fistula on the perineum to the apex of the inverted V-incision. The posterior wall of the rectum is defined and cleared of any muscle fibers upward in the median plane, for a distance of about 2 cm. When the posterior wall is free, an incision is made exactly in the midline to enlarge the orifice. The apex of the V-skin flap is now turned into the gap in the posterior rectal wall and sutured into position with 4-0 Vicryl or similar sutures. The base of the V-flap must be broad and posterior enough to widen the anal opening to a diameter of 10 to 12 mm. Any excess anal tag tissue may be trimmed. Regular dilatations with Hegar dilators are initiated after 7 days and continued until the orifice is large enough for the parent to follow with daily digital dilatation. The dilatations are continued, and supervised, until there is no tendency for stricture or stenosis to form (Fig. 21–8A to D).

The Y-V anoplasty is applicable to both male and female infants, and I am convinced that it is a more satisfactory operation than the simple cutback procedure.

Templeton describes the Y-V plasty operation in which a noninverted Y incision is made.[24] The incised posterior wall of the rectum is sutured directly to the perineal skin. The disadvantage of this technique is that the perineal skin is not turned into the anal canal, and therefore subsequent development of anal sensation may be jeopardized.

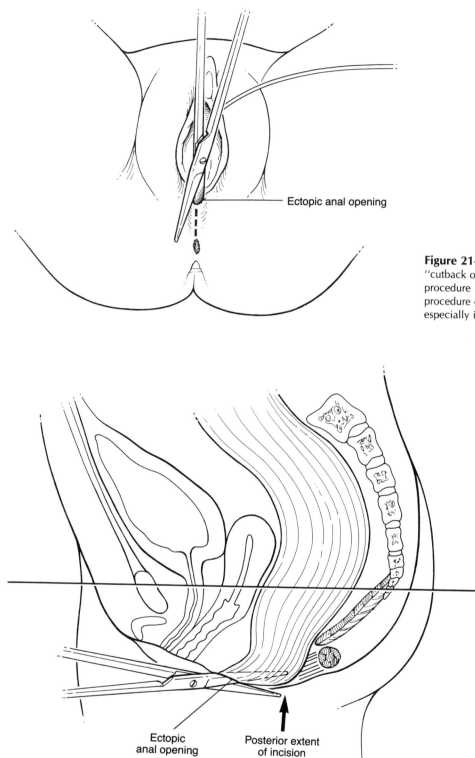

Ectopic anal opening

Figure 21–6. Schematic representation of the "cutback operation" from the perineal view. This procedure is recommended by some authors as the procedure of choice in all "low" anomalies, especially in females.

Ectopic anal opening

Posterior extent of incision

Figure 21–7. Sagittal view of cutback operation. One blade of the straight scissors is placed in the midline of the ectopic bowel orifice and directed posteriorly in the midline to approximately the position of a normal anus. The inner blade of the scissors must not be advanced too deeply into the rectum.

Anal Transplant

This operation is reserved for the female infant with a low lesion, either an anovestibular or an anocutaneous fistula. It is not chosen for the anocutaneous fistula of the male. The operation can be carried out in the newborn period without a diverting colostomy. Cosmetically, it is preferable to the cutback operation. A controversial issue is whether the operation should be carried out with the patient in the prone or the supine position. Although performing all the operations with patients in the prone position and varying the extent of the operations only to produce a "minimal," "limited," or "extended" posterior sagittal anoplasty have obvious attractions, I prefer the supine position for this operation.

The operation is more successful if the lesion resembles an anus, which is ectopic, rather than a long narrow fistula. In the ectopic anus there are good tissue planes that can be differentiated, and the rectum and vagina can be separated without damage to either structure. Before starting the operation one must confirm that the diagnosis is correct and that a high lesion with an opening on the perineum does not occur at the same site.

The patient is placed supine on a water blanket with a small sandbag under the blanket, rather than under the patient, to raise the buttocks. The legs are supported on sponge pads, and the feet are strapped together. A Mayo table is fixed to the upper half of the operating table, as previously described.

After the bowel is further cleansed with 1% aqueous povidone-iodine, a Foley catheter is placed in the fistula and inflated. By placing gentle traction on the catheter, the wall of the rectum can be pulled down, more clearly defined, and dissected off the vagina.

The opening or fistula is identified, and four to eight stay sutures are placed around the orifice. These are held in a single clamp, which creates traction throughout the operation. An error of opening the vagina is preferable to that of opening the rectum, as the vaginal injuries will heal spontaneously, whereas damage to the rectum may also injure the rudimentary internal sphincter at the tip of the rectum. The dissection is facilitated if the posterior aspect is freed first, leaving the more difficult separation of the vagina from the rectum for last. The striated muscle complex is divided only as far as is necessary, and the rectum is freed just enough to reach the perineum. Too much mobilization may lead to subsequent prolapse of the rectum. Once mobilization is complete, the anterior aspect of the wound, between the vagina and the striated muscle, can be repaired with 3-0 Vicryl sutures. The rectum is placed accurately within the divided muscle complex, employing electrostimulation. Tapering of the bowel is usually not necessary. If tapering is necessary, a temporary diverting colostomy is required. Without tapering, the procedure can be done safely without the aid of a colostomy (Fig. 21–9A to F).

Abdominoperineal Pull-Through

Although this was the first one-stage operation described in neonates in 1944,[25] the abdominoperineal operation is not often performed by pediatric surgeons today. The operation is carried out as an emergency in the neonatal period. The patient is placed on the operating table with the legs abducted over sandbags. The abdomen and perineum are exposed. A lower paramedian or midline incision can be made in order to enter the abdomen. The distended rectum is identified and deflated by aspiration within a pursestring suture. The rectosigmoid is freed by dividing the lateral attachments of peritoneum on either side and joining the incisions anteriorly across the rectum. Care must be taken to identify the ureters and vas deferens at this stage. The rectum is freed by sharp dissection laterally and posteriorly. Anteriorly, as the dissection proceeds and the bladder and prostate are reached, the bowel is seen to narrow in the region of the fistula. The fistula is cleared on all sides and ligated after the rectal end is clamped.

A firm catheter should always be placed in the bladder prior to operation. This maneuver can be frustratingly difficult, because the catheter tends to follow the course of the fistula rather than that of the urethra. The catheter must be palpated in the urethra before the fistula is divided, because occasionally the urethra has been mistaken for the fistula, resulting in its complete division. Leaving a portion of the fistula is preferable to the risk of narrowing the urethra by excision or suture. The puborectal muscle is not visible from within the abdominal cavity, and although the surgeon attempts to stay close to the urethra in developing the tunnel for the pull-through, the major problem with the operation has been poor placement of the bowel in relation to the striated muscle complex. The rectosigmoid mesentery is freed, and one or two vessels—or sometimes the origin of the inferior mesenteric artery—are divided in order to obtain enough length to pull the bowel down without tension.

Previously, the anal site was chosen at random, and the tunnel developed forward and upward in the perineal fat toward the fistula. The upper end of the tunnel was developed by the abdominal operator, beginning at the site of the fistula and working downward to meet the perineal operator. Once the tract was complete, a tape was passed through the opening and lifted forward. The tunnel was dilated with sounds until it was

Text continued on page 539

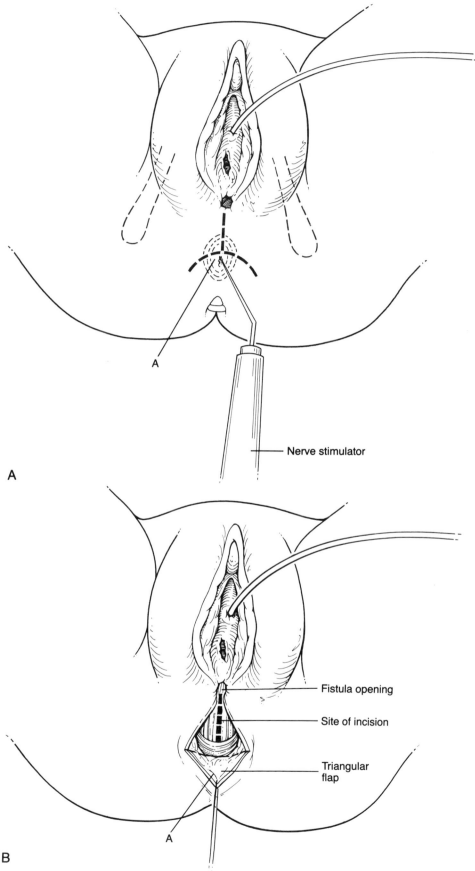

— Nerve stimulator

A

Fistula opening

Site of incision

Triangular
flap

B

Figure 21–8. Y-V plasty for
correction of low ectopic bowel
orifice. *A,* Using an
electrostimulator the exact
position of the anus as shown by
contraction of the external
sphincter is identified. An
inverted V or U incision is made
over the proposed site of the
anus, and a subcutaneous flap is
raised. *B,* The fibers of the
contracting external sphincter are
visualized, and a midline incision
is made from the opening of the
fistula on the perineum to the
apex of the inverted V incision.
The posterior wall of the rectum
is defined and incised exactly in
the midline.

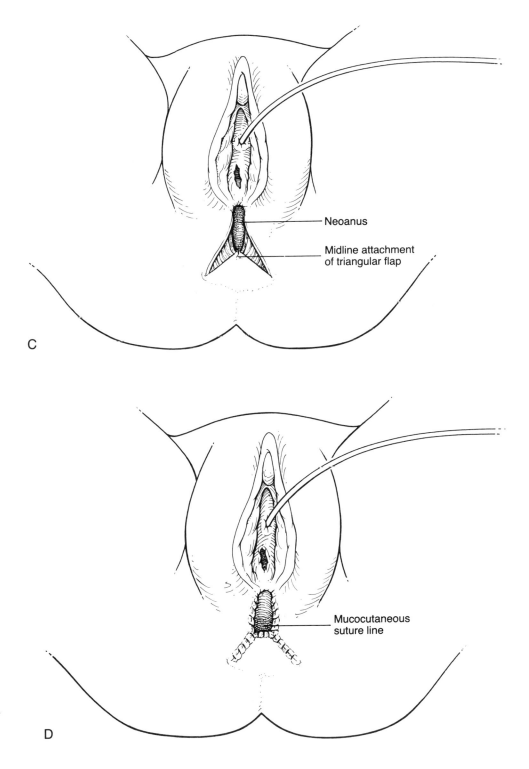

C

Neoanus

Midline attachment
of triangular flap

D

Mucocutaneous
suture line

Figure 21–8 *Continued C,* The apex of the V skin flap is now turned into the gap in the posterior rectal wall and sutured into position. *D,* The mucocutaneous junction is then closed, completing the anoplasty. This procedure is applicable to both male and female infants.

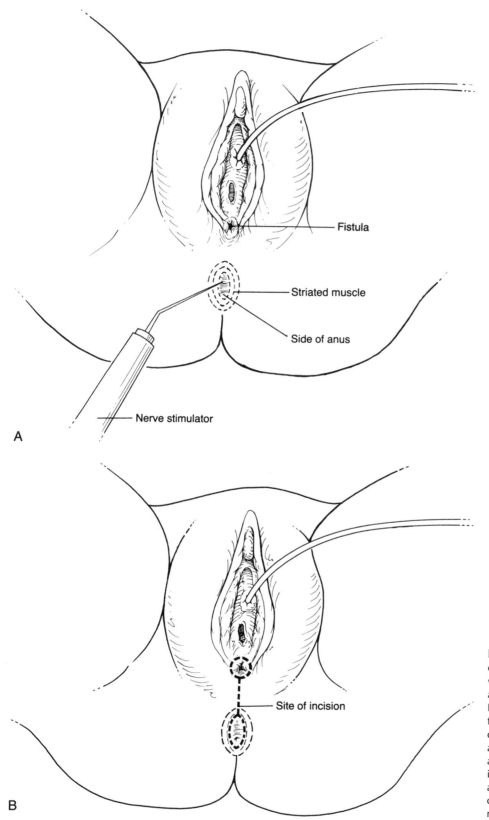

Fistula

Striated muscle

Side of anus

Nerve stimulator

A

Site of incision

B

Figure 21–9. Anal transplant. This operation is reserved for female infants with a low lesion in either anovestibular or anocutaneous fistula. It is not used for the anocutaneous fistula of the male. *A*, The fistulous orifice is identified, and with the aid of a nerve stimulator the voluntary anorectal sphincter is identified. *B*, An incision is made encircling both the anal complex and fistula, and the two circular incisions are connected in the midline.

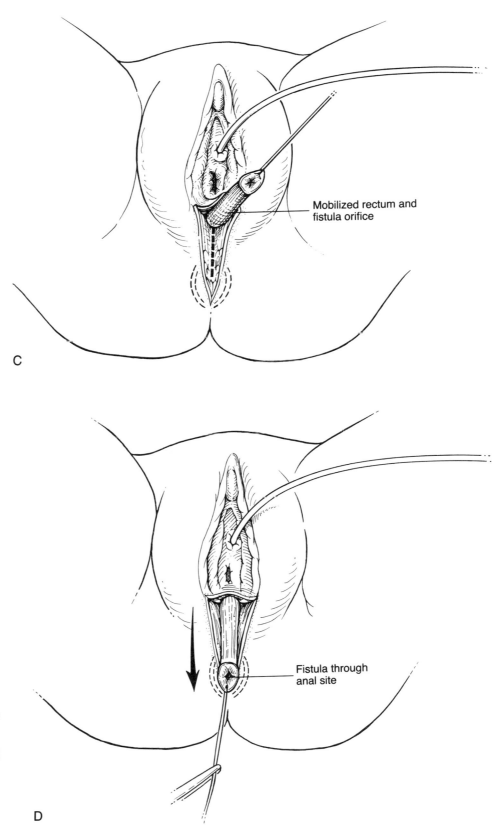

Mobilized rectum and
fistula orifice

Fistula through
anal site

Figure 21–9 *Continued C,* The
rectum is dissected free beginning
at the posterior aspect, leaving the
separation of the vagina from the
rectum until the posterior dissection
is complete. *D,* The rectum is
mobilized just enough to reach the
perineum, and the rectum is placed
accurately within the divided
muscle complex using
electrostimulation.
*Illustration continued
on following page*

C

D

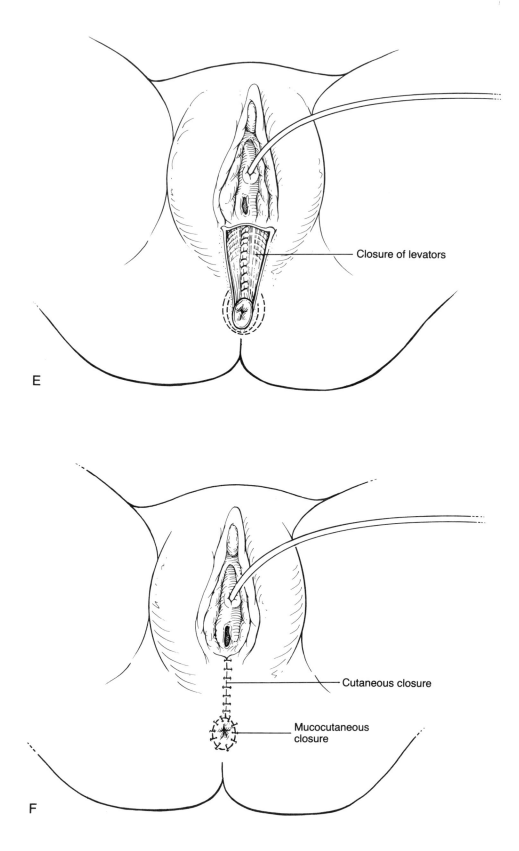

E

Closure of levators

F

Cutaneous closure

Mucocutaneous closure

Figure 21–9 *Continued E,* The anterior aspect of the wound between the vagina and the striated muscle is repaired, and the striated muscle is approximated in the midline. The rectum is sutured to the cutaneous junction, and the wound is closed in layers. *F,* The anal transplant operation is completed with closure of midline incision and formation of a neoanus.

large enough to admit an index finger. According to these workers, a large tunnel was necessary in order to prevent stenosis or ischemia. Although the original abdominoperineal operation and its subsequent modifications were favored by many surgeons during the 1960s, they have been superseded by the sacroperineal or perineal approach, which offers a more precise placement of the bowel.

Posterior Sagittal Anoplasty[26]

For posterior sagittal anoplasty, the patient is placed in the prone jackknife position with the surgeon seated at the end of the table. A midsagittal incision is made through the skin from the midsacrum to the anterior margin of the proposed anal site, as determined by transcutaneous muscle stimulation. The midsagittal incision is deepened down to the sacrum and coccyx. The external sphincter fibers (striated muscle complex) are identified by repeated electrostimulation and are carefully split in the midline. By watching the two halves contract and attempting to keep them equal, this division is possible. The split halves are surprisingly flimsy in the neonate, being only 1 to 2 mm thick. Two bands of striated muscle fibers are identified: the horizontal superficial sphincter and the vertical fibers pulling forward and upward. If the coccyx is present, it is split and the dissection continued in the midline. The sacrococcygeal raphe, with the insertion of the levator ani, and the pelvic parietal fascia are opened. Right-angled forceps are inserted, and the rest of the striated muscle complex is divided in the midline. This division includes the puborectal and pubococcygal fibers.

The pelvic parietal fascia is incised and removed to expose the muscular wall of the rectum. The site of the fistula is often determined by palpating the catheter within the ureter. The bowel is opened as close as possible to the fistula, which is identified and circumcised. Above the fistula, at the level of the prostate, it is advisable to leave part of the anterior rectal wall adherent to the prostate until the dissection extends well above the prostate. At this level the plane of dissection is outside the bowel wall but dorsal to Denonvilliers' fascia. The prostate and seminal vesicles should not be exposed during the dissection in order to prevent damage to their nerve supply. Mobilization of the bowel should be only sufficient to reach the perineum in order to prevent future prolapse. If the bowel is short, all the tethering tissue, which includes vessels and possibly extrinsic nerves, is extensively divided after coagulation, as far cranially as is deemed necessary. The bowel, if dilated, is trimmed and tailored to fit the striated muscle complex (about a no.

10 Hegar in the infants and no. 12 Hegar in older children.)

The bowel can be tapered either anteriorly or posteriorly. I think it is more logical to taper on the anterior surface, as this has already been thinned or cut in being freed from the prostate and fistula. The posterior aspect is favored by some, because the suture line is more remote from the site of the fistula and recurrence is less likely. The tip of the bowel and fistula must be preserved, as a potentially functioning internal sphincter is present. The apex of the bowel should be regarded as an ectopic anus, rather than as a fistula. The striated muscle complex, which includes both the levator ani and sphincteric components, is repaired in layers. An attempt should be made to identify the area of the puborectal muscle and carefully to place a stitch, both to obtain angulation of the rectum to the anal canal and to complete the muscular sphincter around the anal canal. The repair is completed with 5-0 nonabsorbable sutures, by working from deep to superficial tissue; the repair should include the bowel wall. Sutures around the anus are left in place for 3 weeks. Calibration and dilatation of the anal opening is started and continued for 2 to 3 months before the diverting colostomy is closed.

There are many other variations of this operation, which are well summarized by de Vries (Fig. 21–10A to G).[27]

Sacroperineal Pull-Through

Stephens described the sacroperineal pull-through operation in 1953.[27a] The rectum can be mobilized from a purely perineal approach if the gas shadow of the distended rectum lies on or below the pubococcygeal line (Fig. 21–11). If it is higher than this line, a combined abdominosacroperineal approach may be necessary.

The patient is placed in the jackknife position, and a midline incision is made over the sacrococcygeal articulation, toward but not into the anal site. The coccyx is disarticulated at the sacrococcygeal junction by cutting the articular cartilage and extending the incisions for 1 cm laterally on each side to reach the gluteus maximus. The rectum is exposed in the midline above the levator ani, after the pararectal fascia is divided. Exposure of the rectourethral fistula may be best achieved by opening the rectum. Identifying, circumcising, and oversewing the fistula is most effectively done from within the bowel lumen. The opening in the rectal wall is closed following identification and closure of the rectourethral fistula. Because the tip of the fistula is actually an anus and may contain a functioning internal sphincter, no bowel should be

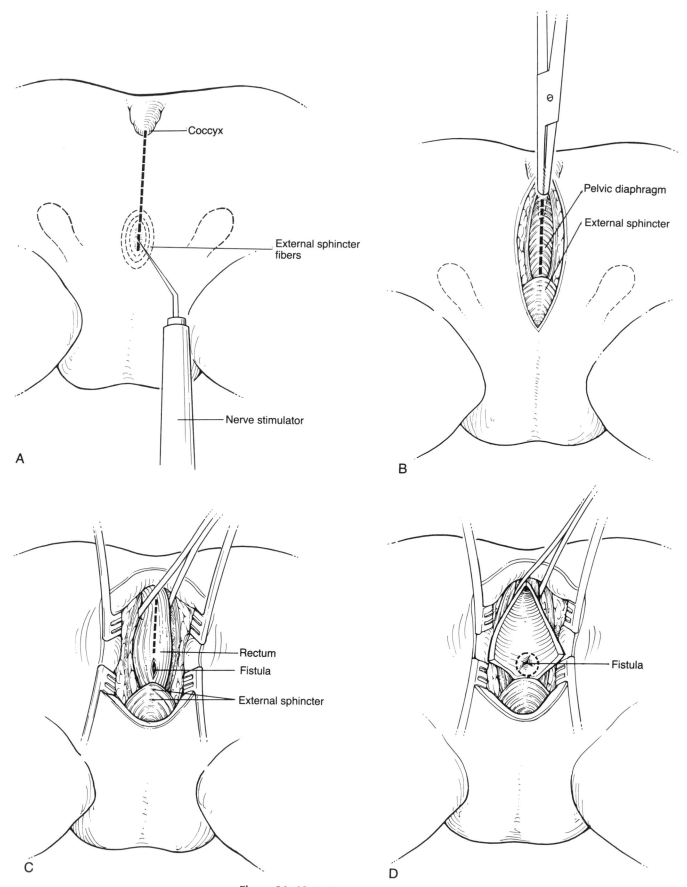

Figure 21–10 *See legend on opposite page*

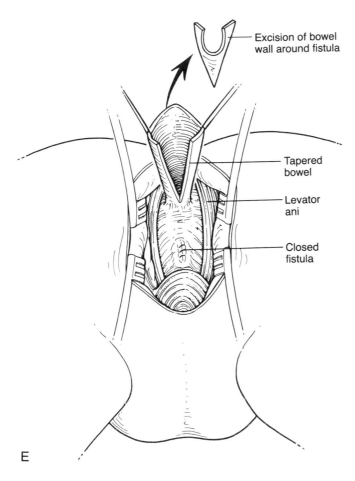

Excision of bowel wall around fistula

Tapered bowel

Levator ani

Closed fistula

E

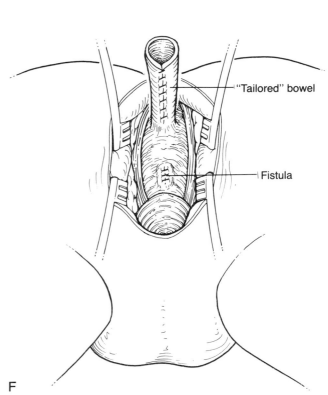

"Tailored" bowel

Fistula

F

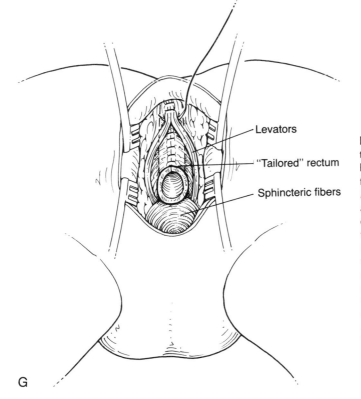

Levators

"Tailored" rectum

Sphincteric fibers

G

Figure 21–10. Posterior sagittal anoplasty. *A*, With the patient in the prone jackknife position the location of the anus is determined by transcutaneous muscle stimulation. A midline incision is made from the tip of the coccyx to the midpoint of the proposed anal site. *B*, The sacrococcygeal raphe with the insertion of the levator ani along with the pelvic parietal fascia is opened to the point of the external sphincter. *C*, The pelvic parietal fascia is incised and treated to expose the muscular wall of the rectum, which is mobilized. The bowel is opened as close as possible to the fistula, which is identified and circumcised. *D*, The fistula is circumcised, and the bowel is tapered either anteriorly or posteriorly. *E*, The tip of the bowel is preserved and tapered anteriorly or posteriorly following closure of the fistula. The bowel should be mobilized only enough to reach the perineum. The bowel is trimmed to fit the striated muscle complex (size 10–12 Hegar dilator). *F*, The bowel is tailored posteriorly and is dissected long enough to reach the proposed anal site. *G*, The levators are closed, and the tailored bowel is brought through the anal opening and sutured in place through the striated muscle complex as in Figure 21–9F.

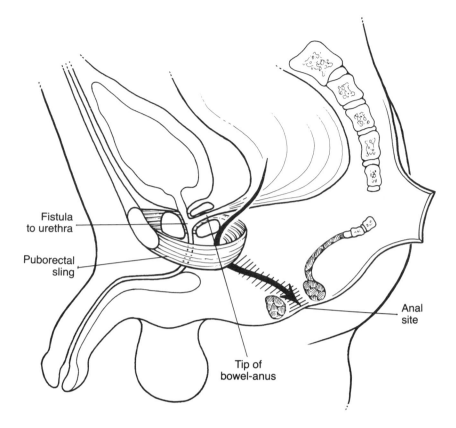

Figure 21–11. Schematic representation of sacroperineal pull-through. The coccyx is disarticulated at the sacrococcygeal junction; the rectum is exposed in the midline above the levator ani; and the fistula to the urethra is circumcised after the rectum is opened, and is oversewn from within the lumen of the bowel. The opening in the rectal wall is closed, and no bowel is excised. The puborectal sling is dilated just enough to accommodate the bulk of the new rectum. By using a nerve stimulator, the site of the anus is determined and opened by means of a cruciate incision. By keeping within the contracting sphincter this tunnel through the striated muscle complex can be developed. The channel is marked with a tape and gently dilated. The bowel is then brought down and sutured into position using interdigitation of the cruciate skin flaps with the tip of the bowel.

Fistula to urethra

Puborectal sling

Tip of bowel-anus

Anal site

excised. The puborectal sling is dilated just enough to accommodate the bulk of the new rectum.

The site of the anus is determined with a nerve stimulator and opened by means of a cruciate incision. By keeping within the contracting sphincter, the tunnel through the striated muscle complex can be developed. The channel is marked with a tape or a sling and is gently dilated. The bowel is then brought down and sutured into position by interdigitation of the cruciate skin flaps with the tip of the bowel.

Dilatation is started after 7 days and continued until the anus is soft and supple. Afterward, the colostomy is closed.

If the bowel is above the pubococcygeal line, a combined approach is necessary. The tunnel and anal canal are developed as described for the posterior sagittal anoplasty, from a sacrococcygeal approach, and the tunnel is marked with a tape or Paul's tubing. The patient is turned to a supine position, and the bowel and fistula are dissected from the abdomen via a midline infra-umbilical incision. The mobilization of the bowel from above reduces the chance of damaging the *nervi erigentes*. If the bowel will not reach the site of the anus easily, the inferior mesenteric artery is divided at its origin. If the bowel is very large and hypertrophied, it can be tapered. The previously identified tract is now used to pull the bowel down and

suture it into position. If a cruciate incision is made on the skin, these flaps can be raised and interdigitated with the bowel, thus producing a longer suture line that is less likely to stenose.

This technique was further modified by Kieswetter,[28] who combined it with the endorectal mucosectomy described by Romualdi and Soave.[29, 30] The theoretical advantages of this operation are minimal dissection in the pelvis and preservation of the puborectal muscle. The disadvantage is that if an internal sphincter exists at the tip of the fistula, this is left behind within the pelvis and is not available for the development of fecal continence.

Endorectal Rectoplasty

Rehbein adopted a technique for adults who have carcinoma of the rectum that was to minimize damage to the pelvic nerves or viscera.[31, 32] This operation involved dividing the rectum at the rectosigmoid and then carefully removing the mucosa to the site of the fistula. The bowel was then brought down to the perineum inside the seromuscular cuff. Several modifications followed in order to place the pulled-down bowel accurately within the puborectal muscle and external sphincter complex. Kieswetter combined the

Rehbein abdominal and Stephens sacrococcygeal approach in the hope of improving results. This method involves beginning with a sacral approach (in the jackknife position) to identify the puborectal muscle and to develop a tunnel just wide enough for the pulled-through bowel. A cruciate incision is made over the site of the proposed anus. The tunnel is marked with a Penrose drain up to the blind rectal pouch, and the sacrococcygeal incision is closed. The patient is then turned over to the lithotomy position, and the endorectal mucosectomy is completed from the abdomen. The rectum is divided about 8 to 10 cm from the blind end. The mucosa is dissected down to the fistula, which is oversewn, although closure of the fistula is not always necessary. A sound is passed upward within the Penrose drain, from the perineum, to indent the denuded seromuscular cuff near the site of the fistula. An incision is made to the sound at this point. The Penrose drain is grasped and pulled up, thus accurately delineating the tunnel. This tunnel is dilated with sounds to an appropriate size, in order to accommodate the colon. The sigmoid colon is then pulled down to the anal site. Four V-shaped wedges can be cut in the tip of the colon and the perianal skin flaps, which can be interdigitated. The cruciate incision has the advantage of creating a long suture line with less tendency for stenosis and brings up some perianal skin into the anal canal, which is vital for future sensation.

Yokoyama described a further modification in the attempt to preserve all the functioning muscle and sphincteric components without division of any muscle fibers.[17] The abdomen is opened, and the rectum is divided 10 cm above the peritoneal reflection. Endorectal stripping of the mucosa is carried out to within 2 to 3 cm of the fistula, and the mucosa is divided. A Penrose drain is sutured to the stump of mucosa. The Penrose drain and rectal stump are left in the pelvis, and the abdomen is closed temporarily. The baby is now turned into a jackknife position, and the rectum exposed via an extended sacroperineal approach. The Penrose drain and the stump of the rectum are retrieved into the sacroperineal wound. The remaining dissection of the mucosa to the fistula and ligation of the fistula are completed. At this point the thickened orifice of the internal sphincter should be visible. With a stimulator a track is defined within the center of the puborectal muscle, external sphincter, and anal site. The Penrose drain is pulled through this tract, which is then dilated from within the Penrose drain to Hegar size no. 11. The baby is once again turned and the abdomen reopened. The colon is pulled through while the Penrose drain serves as a guide. Although this operation is an attractive alternative, its disadvantages are the frequent change of position and the high risk of contamination and infection.

Anterior Perineal Approach

Mollard, in a combined abdominoperineal approach, identified the sphincter complex (puborectal) from the anterior aspect via a U-shaped perineal flap based posteriorly.[33] The site of the anus, which will be placed in the center of the U, is first identified by electrostimulation. By keeping close to the urethra or vagina, and gently dissecting aside the encircling fibers of the puborectal muscle, the site of the fistula is reached anterior to the puborectal muscle. The abdomen is now opened, and the rectum is divided above the peritoneal reflection. The mucosa of the rectum is freed by endorectal stripping from the seromuscular coat to the level of the fistula, which is ligated with catgut. A small swab is pushed against the fistula from below in the previously defined tract, and the rectal cul-de-sac is opened from above by cutting onto the swab. The channel is marked with a Penrose drain and dilated with Hegar dilators to a size just large enough to accommodate the colon. A cruciate incision is made over the site of the anus, and the colon is pulled through this passage and sutured into position. The bowel wall in the anal canal should be secured to the puborectal muscle. The acute anorectal angle is well maintained by this operation. Mucosal prolapse remains a problem, as in other pull-through operations.

Nixon and Aluwihare perform a similar operation from the perineum without the need for any abdominal mobilization.[19, 34] The principle is to bring skin flaps up to the fistula rather than to mobilize the fistula and pull it down to the perineum, because the fistula is considered an ectopic anus. A sound is placed in the colostomy and pushed down to identify the fistula. Nixon first described this operation in 1967.[35] He later modified it by using a kite-shaped incision to create a skin-lined anal canal.

Cloaca

A cloacal malformation is one in which the intestinal, genital, and urinary tracts join to form a common channel. These are very complex anorectal anomalies with a number of variations. They are thought to occur as a result of an early embryologic insult, which prevents differentiation of the cloaca into the urogenital and gastrointestinal tracts. There are frequent concomitant anomalies in the cardiovascular, renal, and skeletal systems because of an early embryologic insult at the time of critical organogenesis. The anatomy in each patient must be carefully evaluated, and treatment must be individualized.

The uterus may be obstructed by a long common channel or, in patients with urogenital sinus anomalies, by an atresia of the vagina. As a result of maternal estrogen secretion, the vagina and uterus may become grossly distended, sometimes sufficiently to cause severe respiratory distress in the newborn that requires urgent abdominal decompression. When an anus is present on the perineum and a single opening represents the vagina and urethra, the hydrometrocolpos can be treated by an incision into the distended vagina, followed by a finger into the vagina with downward pressure onto the perineum between the anus and "urethra." An incision is made into the vagina from the perineum, and the vagina is sutured to the perineum. This allows the previous urogenital sinus to act as the urethra and the hydocolpos to drain via the perineum. The urinary tract may also be abnormal and obstructed, requiring decompression via a cystostomy or ureterostomy. If no anus is present, drainage of all three tracts by cystostomy, vaginostomy, and colostomy may be necessary prior to any reconstruction.

This operation is a formidable surgical challenge and requires a highly skilled and patient surgeon for total simultaneous correction of all anomalies. The principle of the repair is to separate the rectum from the vagina, and the vagina from the urethra. This approach can be successfully undertaken via an extended posterior sagittal anorectoplasty. The ease and success of the operation are dependent on the type of anomaly present and on the length of the urethra and vagina. The rectum is freed from the vagina and usually has sufficient length to be brought to the perineum within the striated sphincter complex. The most difficult part of the operation is separation of the thin tissue between the urethra and anterior vaginal wall. Once this has been achieved, the vagina can be freed sufficiently to reach the perineum. The remaining urogenital sinus tissue is used to fashion a new urethra around a catheter, and the reconstruction of the perineum is completed.

COMPLICATIONS IN ANORECTAL ANOMALIES

The following is a summary of the major complications likely to occur after surgery in anorectal anomalies.

Gastrointestinal Complications

Stricture. Strictures may occur at the mucocutaneous junction, at the anal canal, or within the pelvis. In some cases the entire pelvis is "frozen" as a result of fibrosis. The stricture may be attributable to ischemia, infection, or excessive tapering of the bowel, especially in the posterior sagittal pull-through operation.

Prolapse. The prolapse is usually that of full-thickness bowel wall. The child suffers from an unacceptable cosmetic appearance and from a distressing mucus leak and bleeding. The possible cause is excessive mobilization of the colon during the pull-through operation. Fixation of the colon to the puborectal muscle reduces the chance of prolapse.

Constipation. Constipation is a frequent complication. Stricture, secondary megarectum (ectasia), and possible aganglionosis need to be excluded in its management.

Colostomy Complications. Any of the following may occur: stenosis, prolapse, retraction, fistula, obstruction, sucrose intolerance, and even death.

Genitourinary Complications

Urethra. Stricture may result from instrumentation or catheterization. It is often difficult to insert a catheter into the bladder because of the distortion of the posterior urethra by the fistula. Complete division of the urethra has occurred if a catheter is not passed preoperatively and the urethra is mistaken for the fistula. Tenting and narrowing of the posterior urethra during ligation of the fistula may result in stricture. Leaving too much of the fistula results in a urethral diverticulum with infection and stone formation. A recurrent rectourethral, rectovaginal, or rectocutaneous fistula may form as a result of infection or breakdown of the repair.

Prostate, Seminal Vesicles, and Vas Deferens. All these structures are at risk during the dissection of the rectoprostatic fistula. It is safer to open the bowel, "circumcise" the fistula, and sacrifice the portion of the anterior wall of the rectum, which is closely adherent to the prostate, while dissecting cranially until a plane of separation is reached above the prostate. The vasa deferentia and seminal vesicles should not be exposed during the dissection to avoid their damage.

Bladder. The most common bladder complications are neurogenic ones. The dissection in the sacral or sagittal approach must remain in the midline; otherwise the parasympathetic nerves are liable to injury. This approach is especially true near the fistula.

Hydrocolpos or hydrometrocolpos occurs in the neonate with a cloacal deformity when the outflow is obstructed by vaginal atresia or by excessive contraction of the puborectal muscle. The mucoid secretion is secondary to maternal estrogen stimulation and can be massive enough to cause respiratory distress.

Muscular Complications

The delicate muscles of the pelvic diaphragm or external sphincter, especially in the neonate, are liable to damage by tearing and overstretching. This may result in poor function and control if the bowel is not within the muscle sling or if there is severe fibrosis in the pelvis. The muscle planes must be identified by using an electrostimulator and dilated only enough to admit the smallest diameter of the bowel. The distended bowel may be reduced in size by deflation, plication, or tapering.

Metabolic Complications

Hyperchloremic acidosis is a well-recognized complication of urine draining into a large rectoprostatic fistula. This may occur regardless of whether a colostomy has been performed, as urine enters and is absorbed from the distal rectum. It is preferable to disconnect the fistula from the urinary tract at the earliest opportunity. Extensive prenatal calcification within the lumen of the colon is an occasional *interesting* observation. This appears because of an admixing of meconium and urine and in radiographs may be mistaken for meconium peritonitis.

REOPERATIONS

Even in skilled hands, the results of operations for anorectal anomalies are disappointing with regard to fecal continence or near-normal bowel function. The cause of this is multifactorial. Failure may result from the type of anomaly originally treated or from the other anomalies present. Poor results after an operation need to be assessed by several criteria. Is the present incontinence the result of a complication of a proper operation in the first instance, or was the first operation improper?

It is often difficult to decide when the operation is a failure and that a secondary procedure is necessary as an attempt to restore some degree of continence.

Age of Patient in Relation to Fecal Control

Some state that they can assess fecal control by the age of 18 months. Four to five years may be a more reasonable age at which to observe the results of active bowel emptying and training before reoperation is considered. Biofeedback training, which can start only when the child is able to cooperate intelligently at about the age of 7 years, is also worth attempting before performing secondary surgery.[36] However, if one knows that an incomplete or an imperfect opera-

tion was done in the first instance, there is no reason to delay secondary surgery.

Following a cutback operation, if the parents cannot accept the anterior position of the anus, a posterior transplant anus can be accomplished at any age.

A careful neurologic and urologic assessment must be done before operation is considered. Any neurologic or urologic defect detected may be congenital or iatrogenic from the previous operation. A gross neurologic defect probably does not warrant further reconstructive surgery, but rather a permanent colostomy. The principle of most secondary operations is the repair of the pelvic musculature. This can be achieved by repair of the levator muscles, muscle grafts to surround or strengthen the missing sphincter, free muscle grafts, and free and flap smooth muscle transplantation.

Secondary Anal Transplant

The anal cutback or Y-V plasty may be unsatisfactory for cosmetic or functional reasons. If the anal canal curls sharply forward and toward the vulva (rather than down and back), when the child strains at stool, the expulsion force tends to be directed downward with bulging of the perineum but without resultant evacuation of the fecal mass. In certain cultures the state of the hymen is vital for a successful marriage, and the close proximity of the anus and vagina with no perineal body is unacceptable. The anus can be transplanted backward into the normal site by means of a limited sagittal exposure without the need for a colostomy. This operation can be done at any age once the decision for secondary surgery has been made.

Secondary Repair of Levators

Stephens and Smith described a midline posterior sagittal approach as a secondary procedure to correct fecal incontinence in patients previously operated on with anorectal anomalies.[18] The approach differs little from the current posterior sagittal rectoplasty. The aim of the operation was either to reroute the rectum if it had initially been misplaced, or to repair the levator ani and puborectal muscle, if these fibers had been torn at the original operation. The operation can be undertaken any time after about 3 years of age. The bowel is carefully prepared and emptied. A colostomy is not necessary unless the bowel wall is damaged at operation.

In the jackknife position a midline incision is made over the coccyx and encircling the anus. A sound or stiff catheter should be placed in the urethra or vagina. The anus is closed temporarily with a pursestring suture, which can be used for traction. By strictly following the midline and utilizing an electrostimulator to identify the muscles, the levator is opened, starting high up beneath the sacrococcygeal articulation. If the puborectal fibers had been previously damaged, the rectum is freed totally up to the urethra or vagina. The fibers are then repaired posteriorly, ensuring restoration of the anorectal angle and compression of the rectum. If the bowel was originally misrouted after mobilization of the rectum, the fibers of the puborectal muscle are easily seen and the bowel can be rerouted anteriorly. The anus is restored to its original site or to a more appropriate position if it was grossly misplaced. The position of the anus is verified by electrostimulation. The wound is closed with drainage. The rectum is kept deflated with a rectal tube and frequent saline irrigations. The patient is kept on a low-residue diet for a week and dilatations started at about 10 to 14 days. Kottmeier also frees the attachments of the levator sling laterally and posteriorly from the coccyx.[37] The levator is then plicated to increase the anorectal angle.

Free Autogenous Muscle Transplant

Hakelius demonstrated that a striated muscle such as a palmaris longus, if denervated for 2 weeks prior to removal and transplanted as a free graft, was capable of subsequent function.[38] The muscle is placed as a U-sling around and in contact with the puborectal muscle. Reinnervation takes place over a period of about 9 months. This operation can be carried out only in a nonscarred pelvis. If the muscle is prestretched by more than 15% in order to obtain an acute anorectal angle, the muscle fibers do not survive. Grotte and colleagues, in 1984, reported 21 patients; 10 achieved normal continence, 9 were "socially satisfactory," and 2 failed.[39]

Free and Flap Smooth Muscle Transplantation

In adults, Schmidt used a portion of ascending colon denuded of its mucosa to act as a cuff around a colostomy.[40] He claimed a continent colostomy in 300 patients treated in this manner. Subsequent manometric studies by Holschneider showed no physiological sphincter; the external pressure created by the free graft was causing obstruction to the bowel, which needed to be evacuated by enemata.[41–43] Holschneider and Hecker, because of the poor results obtained by Schmidt's free smooth muscle graft, developed a flap reverse smooth muscle plasty.[41] The operation can be performed as either a primary or a secondary procedure. When the colon is pulled through the striated muscle complex, the mucosa is resected from the colon for several centimeters. The seromuscular cuff is turned back 180 degrees, prestretched 120%, and sutured to the serosa of the pulled down colon. The colon and cuff are then returned within the puborectal tunnel to just above the pelvic floor.

Gracilis Muscle Transplant

Pickrell described the original procedure of using the gracilis muscle with its neurovascular bundle to serve as a sphincter.[44] Several modifications have since been described.[42, 45–47]

The principle of the operation is that the muscle should be long enough to surround the anus with muscle and not tendon. There must be one good neurovascular bundle in the proximal one third of the muscle. The tendon should be fixed with minimal tension to the opposite ischial tuberosity. A colostomy is not necessary.

The muscle is freed from its bed by means of an incision over the tibial attachment, and a second incision frees the muscle up to the neurovascular bundle. The muscle is tunneled subcutaneously to surround the anal canal, and the tendon is firmly attached to the contralateral tuberosity. Postoperatively the patient is taught to contract the gracilis without contracting the other abductor muscles.

Holschneider reported improvement in the continence of 28 of 56 patients following a gracilis muscle transplant.[43]

Secondary Procedures for Prolapse

A frequent and distressing complication of most of the early pull-through operations has been rectal prolapse. This is a full-thickness prolapse of the whole bowel wall, which requires treatment because the children suffer from a continuous loss of bloody mucus. The complication is not frequent in the more recent posterior sagittal rectoplasties, as the bowel is often tapered and sutured to surrounding muscle fibers during the repair. Simple trimming of the redundant bowel is not satisfactory, and some form of local skin flap rearrangement is needed. Several procedures are available. Nixon described an anoplasty that he performed at the primary operation in the neonate.[35] Two kite-shaped incisions are made, anterior and posterior to the anal site. The intermediate skin flaps are raised and joined to the end of the bowel. By closing the edges of the kite incisions the flaps are drawn upward to form a skin-lined anal canal. More elaborate rotational skin flaps can be constructed of skin from the thigh and scrotum.[48]

Freeman described a unique operation in which the patient's own foreskin (the majority of these patients are males) is made into a skin-lined anal canal, after the redundant prolapsed colon is excised.[49] The operation is performed in two stages. The redundant colon is dissected upward for 2 to 3 cm into the anal canal. The circumcised foreskin, which forms a cylinder, is slipped over the colon with the raw surface facing outward. The colon is split into four quadrants, which are loosely sutured to the perineum. The pressure from the colon ensures contact of the foreskin to the anal canal. After 2 weeks the excess colon is trimmed into the anal canal and sutured to the upper margin of the foreskin graft. The operation is performed without a colostomy. Dilatations are needed postoperatively until the anus is soft and supple. This operation provides a skin-lined anal canal, which later develops sensation and cures the prolapse and mucoid leak. The cosmetic result is satisfactory.

CONSTIPATION

Constipation is a common and worrisome complication in patients with anorectal anomalies. In the management of these patients it is assumed that all the common causes of constipation have been excluded. These causes include a faulty diet, overanxious parents, stressful potty training, poor and inadequate toilet facilities at school, hypothyroidism, hyperparathyroidism and hypercalcemia, cystic fibrosis, lead poisoning, and drug ingestion. Slow colonic transit time should be ruled out, especially in females. The remaining cause of the constipation is therefore usually some *local* pathology.

Primary and Secondary Ectasia

In most anorectal anomalies, and especially in those with a small fistula or no fistula or communication, the terminal bowel is grossly dilated. This dilation is limited to the rectum; if more of the bowel is involved, primary ectasia is present. If there is any degree of anal obstruction, the rectum can become hugely dilated and act as a terminal reservoir with overflow and incontinence. Histologic studies of the bowel wall showed cells of normal size and number in the primary group and an increase in size and number in the older children.[50]

In the posterior sagittal rectoplasty the bowel is trimmed drastically to fit the size of the predefined vertical fibers of the external sphincter. This trimming reduces the size of the ectasia and may lead to severe stenosis, which may necessitate many months of dilatation for correction. It is often these patients who present with problems, because the parents stopped dilatation too soon, thinking the children were progressing well. In the secondary or acquired group, the situation is often resolved by vigorous emptying of the bowel, enemata, or suppositories. In both male and female patients with low anomalies, intractable constipation is much more common than expected. A careful examination and a defecating proctogram reveal the mechanical disadvantage when the child strains at stool. The expulsion force is directed downward in the perineum, behind the puborectal muscle, with marked descent of the perineum and failure of the evacuation. These children improve after a secondary transplant of the anus or a Y-V anoplasty, if there is any degree of stenosis.

If severe scarring or stricture formation has occurred because of ischemia or infection, reoperation to bring down normal bowel is necessary. The association of aganglionosis (Hirschsprung's disease) and imperforate anus remains unsettled. It has been found in up to 3% of resected specimens primarily, but it may also occur as a result of ischemia during the pull-through operation. If the constipation remains intractable, a biopsy of the anal canal should be carried out to exclude an associated aganglionosis; if aganglionosis is present, myomectomy or further resection may be necessary.

Anismus or Sphincter Disobedience

There is a group of children without visible anorectal anomalies who suffer from intractable constipation. These children do not appear to be able to bear down or relax the puborectal muscle. Suspicion is raised on rectal examination when the child appears to pull up the perineum, rather than to push down onto the finger when instructed. Confirmation is possible by means of electromyographic studies, observed inability to defecate rectal balloons,[57] or defecating proctograms.[52] The child is unable to straighten the anorectal angle or to shorten the anal canal. The patient benefits from forceful anal stretching alone or stretching followed by anorectal myomectomy. A total of 87 patients were studied, and 22 of 28 responded to stretching alone. Sixteen initially responded to stretching, but as they experienced relapse anorectal myomectomy was carried out; an "excellent" or "marked" improvement was observed in 14.[53]

Retrorectal Tumors as a Cause of Constipation

In the Currarino triad, affected children often present with intractable constipation because of severe anal canal stenosis. As a digit cannot be inserted, the presacral mass is often overlooked for some time. Similarly, a rectal duplication cyst or a pelvic sacrococcygeal teratoma may cause constipation because of its size. Once the diagnosis has been established, a midposterior sagittal approach is recommended for identifying and removing the tumor.

EDITORIAL COMMENT

The editors realize that the relatively uncommon congenital anorectal anomalies will usually not be treated by most general or colorectal surgeons who practice in the Western World. Nevertheless, this detailed presentation concerning these anomalies was included for both theoretical and practical reasons. All surgeons dealing with colorectal disease should have an inherent interest in these problems and should be knowledgeable regarding their clinical syndromes, classifications, and operative treatments.

In addition to the concept of knowledge for knowledge's sake, there are compelling practical reasons for inclusion of these anomalies. The surgeon may be called upon for advice and treatment regarding an adult who suffered such an anomaly at birth. It is, therefore, obvious that an intelligent opinion can be rendered only on the basis of some familiarity with the disease state and the prior treatment.

In rural areas, a surgeon may be called upon to perform a colostomy on a neonate with a congenital anomaly or even to perform some of the simpler procedures for "low" lesions.

Some surgeons from the Western World periodically serve in the military or for charitable organizations. In these settings, they may be called upon to offer definitive advice or even treatment. Therefore, we consider this presentation appropriate and essential.

---

1. Potts WJ. The Surgeon and the Child. Philadelphia: WB Saunders, 1959.
2. Smith D. In: Anorectal Malformations in Children: Update 1988. March of Dimes New York: Alan R. Liss, Inc, 1988, p 240.
3. Smith D. In: Anorectal Malformations in Children: Update 1988. March of Dimes. New York: Alan R. Liss, Inc, 1988, pp 238–240.
4. Smith D. In: Anorectal Malformations in Children: Update 1988. March of Dimes. New York: Alan R. Liss, Inc, 1988, pp 211–222.
5. Ashcraft RW, Holder TM. Congenital anal stenosis with a presacral teratoma. Case report. Ann Surg 1965;162:1091–1095.
6. Haab O. Beitrage zu den angenborenen Fehlern des Auges. Albrecht Von Graefes. Arch Klin. Exp Ophthalmol 1878;24:257.
6a. Opitz JM, Kaveggia EG. Studies of malformation syndromes in man XXXIII: An X-linked recessive syndrome of multiple congenital anomalies and mental retardation. Zeitschrift Kinder 1974;117:1.
7. Ives EJ. Thalidomide and anal anomalies. Can Med Assoc J 1962; 87:670.
8. el-Haddad M, Corkery JJ. The anus in the newborn. Paediatrics 1985;76:927–928.
9. Leape LL, Ramenofsky ML. Anterior ectopic anus: A common cause of constipation in children. J Pediatr Surg 1978;13:627–630.
10. Reisner SH, Sivan Y, Nitzan M, Merlob P. Determination of anterior displacement of the anus in newborn infants and children. Pediatrics 1984;73:216–217.
11. Wangenstein OH, Rice CO. Imperforate anus: A method of determining the surgical approach. Ann Surg 1930;92:77.
12. Narashima RLL, Prasad GR, Katariya S, et al. Prone cross table view lateral view: An alternative to the invertogram in imperforate anus. Am J Roentgenol 1983;140:227–229.
13. Muragasu JJ. A new method of roentgenological demonstration of anorectal anomalies. Surgery 1970;68:706–712.
14. Willital GH. Advances in the diagnosis of anal and rectal atresia by ultrasonic-echo scan. J Pediatr Surg 1971;6:454–457.
15. Mezzacappa PM, Price AP, et al. MR and CT demonstration of levator sling in congenital anorectal anomalies. J Comput Assist Tomogr 1987;11:273–275.
16. Tam PK, Chan FL, Saing H. Direct sagittal T scan: A new diagnostic approach for surgical neonates. J Pediatr Surg 1987;22:397–400.
17. Yokoyama J, Ikawa H, Katsumata K. Abdomino-extended sacroperineal approach in high-type anorectal malformation—and a new operative method. Z Kinderchir 1985;40:151–157.
18. Stephens FD, Smith ED. Ano-rectal Malformations in Children. Chicago: Year Book Medical Publishers, 1971.
19. Aluwihare AP. Challenges in imperforate anus: I—Primary perineal recto-urethroanoplasty for anatomical and functional correction in males with supralevator anomalies. Ann Acad Med Singapore. 1987;16:511–515.
20. Freeman NV, Burge DM, Sedgewick EM, Soar G. Anal evoked potentials. Z Kinderchir 1980;31:22–29.
21. Freeman NV, Bulut M. "High" anorectal anomalies treated by early "neonatal" operation. J Paediatr Surg 1986;21:218–220.
22. Browne DB. Some congenital deformities of the rectum, anus, vagina and urethra. Ann R Coll Surg Engl 1951;8:173.
23. Nixon HH. Operative management of low anomalies in the female. In: Anorectal Malformations in Children: Update 1988. New York: Alan R. Liss, Inc, 1988, p 310.
24. Templeton JM, O'Neill JA. Anorectal malformations. In: Welch KT, Randolph JG, Ravitch MM, et al, eds. Pediatric Surgery. 4th ed. Chicago: Year Book Medical Publishers, 1986, p 1028.
25. Rhoades JE, Piper RL, Randall JP. A simultaneous abdominal and perineal approach in operations for imperforate anus with atresia of the rectum and rectosigmoid. Ann Surg 1948;127:552.
26. Penà A, de Vries PA. Posterior sagittal anorectoplasty: Important technical considerations and new applications. J Pediatr Surg 1982;17:796–811.
27. de Vries P, Dorairajan T, Guttman FM, et al. Operative management of high and intermediate anomalies in males. In: Stephens FD, Smith ED, eds. Anorectal Malformation in Children. An Update 1988. March of Dimes Birth Defects Foundation. New York: Alan R. Liss, pp 316–401.
27a. Stephens FD. Congenital imperforate rectum, rectourethral rectovaginal fistulae. Aust NZ J Surg 1953;22:161–166.
28. Kieswetter WB. Imperforate anus. II. The rationale and technique of the sacro-perineal operation. J Pediatr Surg 1967;2:106.
29. Romualdi P. A new technique for the treatment of some anorectal malformations. Arch Klin Chir 1960;296:371.
30. Soave F. Hirschsprung's disease: A new surgical technique. Arch Dis Child 1964;39:116.
31. Rehbein F. Operation for anal and rectal atresia with rectourethral fistula. Chirurgie 1959;30:417.
32. Babcock WW. Radical single stage extirpation of the large bowel for cancer of the large bowel, with retained functional anus. Surg Gynecol Obstet 1947;85:1.
33. Mollard P, Marechal JM, Jaubert de Beaujeu M. Surgical treatment of high imperforate anus with definition of the puborectalis sling by the anterior perineal approach. J Pediatr Surg 1978;13:499–504.
34. Nixon HH. Anorectal agenesis: Neonatal correction by a minimal mobilization inversion proctoplasty. Br J Surg 1986;73:933.
35. Nixon HH. A modification of the proctoplasty for rectal agen-

esis. Pamietrik I-ss Zjazdu Naukowego Polskiego Towarzystwa. Chirurgow Dzieciecyck, Warzawa 5–7, x.

36. Langemeijer R.A.Th.M. Home biofeedback training [poster demonstration]. Presented at British Association of Paediatric Surgeons XXXVII Annual International Congress, Glasgow, Scotland, 1990.

37. Kottmeier PK. A physiological approach to the problem of incontinence through the use of the levator ani as a sling. Surgery 1966;60:1262.

38. Hakelius L, Gierup J, Grotte G, Jorulf H. A new treatment for anal incontinence in children: Free autogenous muscle transplantation. J Pediatr Surg 1978;13:77–82.

39. Grotte G, Hakelius L, Trykberg T, Rasmundsson T. Nine years of free autogenous muscle transplantation for anal incontinence in children. Z Kinderchir 1984;(Suppl 1)39:80–82.

40. Schmidt E. Die chirurgische Behandlung der analen Inkontinenzmittels frei transplatiereter autologen korperagener Darmmuskulatur. Chirurg 1978;49:320.

41. Holschneider AM, Hecker WC. Smooth muscle reverse plasty. A new method to treat anorectal incontinence in infants with high anal and rectal atresia. Results after gracilis plasty and free muscle transplantation. Prog Pediatr Surg 1984;17:131–145.

42. Holschneider AM, Lahoda F. Elektromyographische und electromenometrische Untersuchugen zur gracilis plastik nach Pickrell. Z Kinderchir 1974;14:288.

43. Holschneider AM, Amano S, Urban A, et al. Free and reverse smooth muscle plasty in rats and goats. Dis Colon Rectum 1985;28:786–794.

44. Pickrell KL, Georziade N, Crawford H, et al. Construction of a rectal sphincter and restoration of anal continence by transplanting the gracilis muscle. Ann Surg 1952;135:853–862.

45. Brandesky G, Holschneider AM. Operations to improve faecal incontinence. Prog Pediatr Surg 1976;9:105–114.

46. Hartl M. A modified technique of gracilis plastic. Paediatr U Paedol 1972;(Suppl 2):99–107.

47. Holle J, Freilinger G, Mamoli B, et al. Neve wege zur chirurgischen Rekonstrucktion der analen Sphintermusckulstur. Wien Med Wochenschr 1975;125:734.

48. Millard DR, Rowe MI. Plastic surgical principles in high imperforate anus. Plast Reconstr Surg 1982;69:399–409.

49. Freeman NV. Foreskin anoplasty. Dis Colon Rectum 1984;27:309–317.

50. Brent L, Stephens FD. Primary rectal ectasia. A quantitive study of smooth muscle cells in normal and hypertrophied bowel. In: Rickham PP, Hecker W, Prevot J. Progress in Paediatric Surgery. Berlin: Urban and Schwarzenberg, pp 41–62.

51. Loenig-Baucke VA. Sensitivity of the sigmoid colon and rectum in children treated for chronic constipation. J Pediatr Gastroenterol Nutr 1984;3:454–459.

52. Aubert D, Destuynder O, Caetoano D, et al. Le syndrome urorectal par incordinationabdomino-levatorienne chez l'infant. Chir Pediatr 1987;28:48–51.

53. Freeman NV. Intractable constipation in children treated by forceful anal stretch and anorectal myomectomy: Preliminary communication. J Proc Roy Soc Med 1984;(Suppl 3) 77:6–8.

Hirschsprung's Disease

CHAPTER 22

Lewis Spitz

In 1691 Rieysch recorded the first documentation of megacolon at necropsy in a 5-year-old girl. Hirschsprung, in 1896, accurately defined the clinicopathologic features of congenital megacolon, but his attention was directed toward the dilated segment, which he believed was a true congenital abnormality. In 1938 Klingman believed that the condition resulted from an overactive parasympathetic nerve supply, and claims were made that lumbar sympathectomy produced good results.

Swenson, in 1948, recognized for the first time that the primary disease was in the distally contracted colon, rather than in the dilated hypertrophied colon. The true nature of the abnormal colonic innervation was finally described independently by Zuelzer in 1948, Whitehouse in 1948, and Bodian in 1949.

PATHOLOGY

The classic macroscopic appearance of megacolon in Hirschsprung's disease consists of a fairly normal-caliber distal bowel that extends proximally into the dilated, thick-walled, hypertrophied, and functionally obstructed bowel. The cone-shaped area between the dilated and collapsed intestine is referred to as the "transition zone."

The histopathology of Hirschsprung's disease consists of an absence of ganglion cells associated with an increase in nerve trunks in the distally affected colon. The absence of ganglion cells affects both the intermuscular (Auerbach) plexus and the submucosal (Meissner) plexus. There is also an increase in acetylcholinesterase activity of the parasympathetic nerve fibers in the lamina propria and muscularis mucosa and in the circular muscle fibers.

In approximately 75% of patients, the abnormality is confined to the rectosigmoid area. In 5% to 10% of patients, the aganglionosis extends throughout the entire colon and involves a varying length of small intestine.

CLINICAL FEATURES

Incidence. The incidence of Hirschsprung's disease is 1 in 5,000 live births. The condition affects all races. For the rectosigmoid disease, there is a male preponderance of 4 to 1, which lowers as the length of the involved colon increases. The incidence of total colonic aganglionosis is equally distributed between males and females.

Hereditary Factors. The risk of recurrence for patients with short-segment disease is about 2%, but this risk increases to 12.5% in patients with long-segment disease.

Associated Anomalies. Two conditions feature prominently in association with Hirschsprung's disease: Down's syndrome (trisomy 21) is present in 5% of patients, and urologic anomalies in 3% of patients. Other conditions that occur in patients with Hirschsprung's disease more frequently than explained by mere coincidence include pyloric stenosis, malrotation, Meckel's diverticulum, and anorectal anomalies.

CLINICAL PRESENTATION

Infancy

The cardinal feature of Hirschsprung's disease is failure to pass meconium within the first 24 hours of birth.

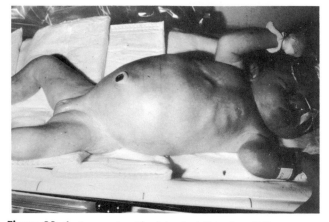

Figure 22–1. A neonate with abdominal distention. Failure to pass meconium within the first day of life should alert the clinician to suspect Hirschsprung's disease.

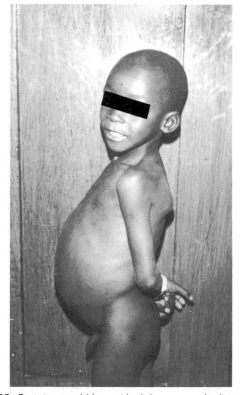

Figure 22–2. A 5-year-old boy with abdomen grossly distended as a result of untreated Hirschsprung's disease. He had bowel evacuations every 2 to 3 weeks. Note the thin limbs indicative of poor general nutritional status.

This symptom was present in 94% of patients in Swenson's series of 501 patients. Passage of meconium may be stimulated by a digital rectal examination, insertion of a rectal thermometer, or a saline rectal washout. The delayed passage of meconium is generally accompanied by other features of intestinal obstruction, such as bilious vomiting, abdominal distention (which may be severe enough to cause respiratory embarrassment by elevation and splinting of the diaphragms), and hyperactive bowel sounds. Rectal examination may induce the explosive evacuation of large volumes of liquid, foul-smelling stool when the examining finger is withdrawn from the anus. The infant with untreated Hirschsprung's disease shows evidence of failure to thrive (Figs. 22–1 and 22–2).

Enterocolitis, characterized by profuse diarrhea containing blood and mucus in association with abdominal distention and bilious vomiting, is the dreaded complication of Hirschsprung's disease. It generally occurs in the untreated infant, but it may be present in the first week of life or may even occur after apparently successful surgical correction. The accompanying fluid and electrolyte losses may be so severe and may occur so rapidly that the infant manifests signs of hypovolemic shock. The cause of the enterocolitis has not been definitely identified, but infection *(Clostridium difficile)*, immunologic deficiency (neutrophil function, mucin production), and obstructive stagnation all have been implicated. Treatment of the enterocolitis consists of emergency management of the hypovolemia, fluid and electrolyte correction, and relief of the intestinal obstruction by rectal washouts with small volumes of warm saline, which are repeated until the patient is relieved of the abdominal distention.

Older Child

The older child presents with chronic intractable constipation. There may be gross abdominal distention and evidence of failure to thrive manifested by loss of weight and emaciated limbs. Stool evacuations occur at irregular intervals, often a few weeks apart. Stool consistency varies from hard and pelletlike to soft, voluminous, and foul-smelling. Soiling is not generally a feature, although it did occur in 3% of patients in Swenson's series. Waves of peristalsis may be seen coursing across the upper abdomen. The rectum is usually empty on digital examination.

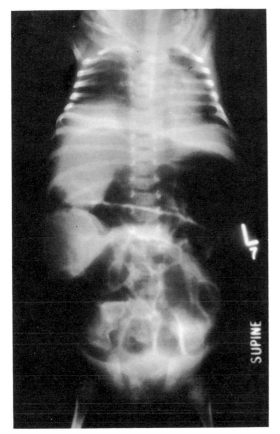

Figure 22–3. Plain radiograph of the abdomen and chest in a neonate with Hirschsprung's disease. There is gross dilatation of the transverse colon, but it is generally difficult to distinguish large intestine from small intestine on the plain radiograph at this young age.

DIAGNOSTIC STUDIES

A high index of clinical suspicion and an awareness of the significance of delayed passage of meconium in the neonate will facilitate early diagnosis and treatment and, one hopes, reduce the incidence of enterocolitis. The diagnostic modalities available include radiographic, manometric, and histopathologic investigations.

Radiography

The plain abdominal radiograph shows dilated loops of intestine with or without air-fluid levels. In the infant it is difficult to distinguish large bowel from small bowel on the plain radiograph. The absence of air in the pelvis should alert the clinician to carry out further investigations to elucidate the cause of the obstruction (Figs. 22–3 and 22–4).

A barium contrast study is the next logical investigation. The procedure is carried out using 50% weight for volume barium solution without prior preparation of the colon. Rectal examination should not be performed immediately prior to the barium enema examination, as it may obscure a short segment of aganglionosis.

A small soft rubber catheter is inserted just within the anal canal, and the buttocks are strapped together to avoid leakage of contrast material. With the infant in the lateral position, the barium solution is slowly injected into the rectum. Filling of the bowel continues until an obviously dilated area is visible. At that point the instillation of contrast material is stopped and the catheter withdrawn. Additional radiographs in the supine, oblique, and prone positions are taken. In patients for whom the diagnosis remains doubtful, delayed films are taken 12 to 24 hours later.

The diagnostic criteria for barium contrast examination are as follows:

Disparity in Size. The funnel-shaped transition between the narrow aganglionic segment and the dilated proximal bowel is highly suggestive of Hirschsprung's disease. This feature may be appreciated only on the delayed films. It is often stated that the disparity in size is an unreliable criterion in the neonatal period, because there has been insufficient time for the dilatation to develop. This contention is fallacious, as experienced radiologists establish a positive diagnosis in over 80% of patients (Fig. 22–5).

Irregularity in Contour. The aganglionic segment reveals irregular contractions, which are manifest as deep sawtooth filling defects or as fine marginal serrations. The irritability and irregular contraction waves

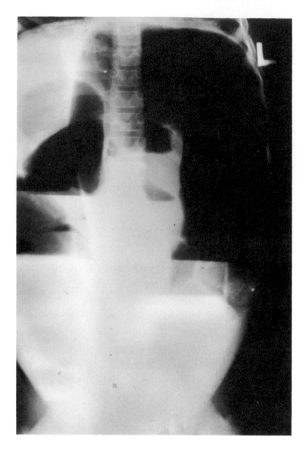

Figure 22–4. Plain erect abdominal radiograph in a 9-year-old child with untreated Hirschsprung's disease. There are gross dilatation of the large intestine with long air-fluid levels and evidence of fluid within the rectum in the pelvic region.

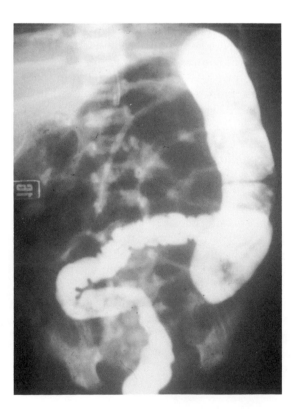

Figure 22–5. Barium enema in an infant with Hirschsprung's disease. The rectum is small and contracted, and the wall shows evidence of spasm and irritability. The transition into the relatively dilated descending colon is clearly demonstrated.

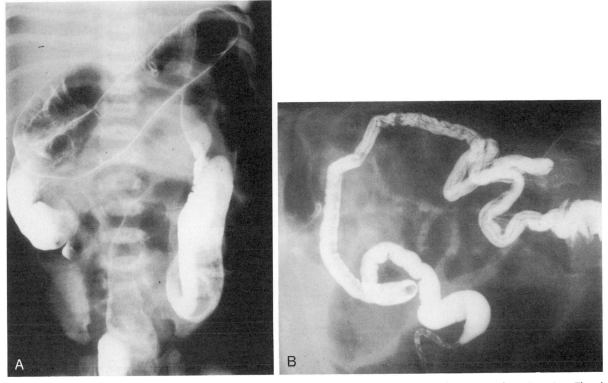

Figure 22–6. Barium enema in total colonic aganglionosis varies considerably. *A*, A relatively normal-appearing large intestine. The clue to the diagnosis is failure to evacuate the contrast material spontaneously within 24 hours following the investigation. *B*, A microcolon with distended small intestine in the background.

of the aganglionic segment are best visualized during fluoroscopic examination.

The radiographic appearance of total colonic aganglionosis varies from a uniformly narrow contracted colon to a virtually normal-appearing large intestine. In the latter case, failure to achieve significant evacuation of contrast material on the delayed 24-hour film should be regarded as highly suspicious for Hirschsprung's disease (Fig. 22–6*A* and *B*).

Manometry

The hallmark of the manometric diagnosis of Hirschsprung's disease is failure of relaxation of the internal sphincter muscle in response to proximal distention of the rectum. A balloon mounted on a catheter device is inserted into the rectum, and two or more recording channels are located in the anal canal. Distention of the rectal balloon normally results in reflex relaxation of the internal sphincter. This reflex may be poorly developed in the early neonatal period, which results in false-positive readings. However, Holschneider reported 96% accuracy, and Schuster 100% accuracy by using this method of diagnosis.

Histopathology

The histopathologic diagnosis of Hirschsprung's disease relies on the absence of ganglion cells in the myenteric (Auerbach) and submucosal (Meissner) nerve plexuses. In addition, there are large nerve trunks and a greatly increased number of parasympathetic nerve fibers. The accuracy of diagnosis is facilitated by histochemical techniques that stain specifically for acetylcholinesterase, an enzyme found in large quantities in parasympathetic nerve fibers.

Full-thickness biopsy of the rectal wall is no longer necessary for the histopathologic diagnosis. The suction biopsy technique introduced by Campbell and Noblett in 1969 has superseded the full-thickness biopsy. Suction biopsy specimens consisting of mucosa and submucosa can be obtained without either anesthesia or sedation (Fig. 22–7).

Suction biopsies are performed at three levels from the anal verge: 2, 3, and 5 cm. The 2- and 5-cm biopsy specimens are submitted for histochemical stains, and the 3-cm biopsy is examined by conventional hematoxylin and eosin stains. Frozen-section examination of the 3-cm biopsy may be carried out if a rapid diagnosis is required. Multiple serial sections of all specimens

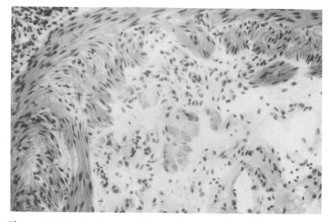

Figure 22–7. Suction rectal biopsy, hematoxylin and eosin (H & E) stain. This reveals the presence of normal ganglion cells in the submucosa. Hirschsprung's disease is excluded as a diagnosis.

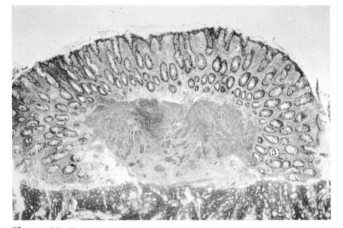

Figure 22–8. Suction rectal biopsy, H & E stain. There are no ganglion cells in the submucosal plexus of Meissner. There are prominent nerve fibers that are diagnostic of Hirschsprung's disease.

are examined. The criteria of the morphologic diagnosis are as follows:

1. Absence of ganglion cells in the submucosa (Fig. 22–8)

2. Presence of large nerve trunks in the submucosa

3. Increase in acetylcholinesterase activity in the parasympathetic nerve fibers in the muscularis mucosa and the lamina propria (Fig. 22–9A and B)

Complications from suction biopsy are rare. Transient hemorrhage and infection may rarely occur. Failure to adhere to a meticulous technique may result in full-thickness biopsy, particularly when excessive pressure is applied to the biopsy instrument. In approximately 5% of patients, the biopsy specimen is inadequate for accurate diagnosis; even in these patients, the demonstration of increased acetylcholinesterase activity in the lamina propria may be sufficient for diagnosis.

TREATMENT

The immediate aim of treatment, once the diagnosis of Hirschsprung's disease has been definitely established, is to relieve the intestinal obstruction. Relief may be achieved by regular colonic washouts or by fashioning a temporary loop colostomy. The stoma must be fashioned in normally functioning intestine. This can be guaranteed only by confirming the presence of ganglion cells, done by submitting a seromuscular biopsy at the proposed site of the colostomy for frozen-section histopathologic examination. Details of the technique for performing the colostomy are shown further on. An immediate definitive pull-through procedure has been advocated by some surgeons, but most prefer to delay definitive operation until the infant is 4 to 9 months of age (Fig. 22–10).

Infants presenting with enterocolitis are often critically ill because of massive fluid and electrolyte losses. Emergency colostomy under these circumstances should be avoided until the infant is hemodynamically stable. These infants require intensive resuscitation, including circulatory fluid volume expansion (plasma 20 ml/kg given intravenously as rapidly as possible) and correction of acid-base imbalance and fluid and electrolyte deficiencies. Antibiotics are administered parenterally as well as enterally. Vancomycin is currently the antibiotic of choice, chiefly because of its anticlostridial action.

In addition, gentle rectal washouts with small volumes of warm isotonic saline achieve decompression of the obstructed bowel and reduce the danger of

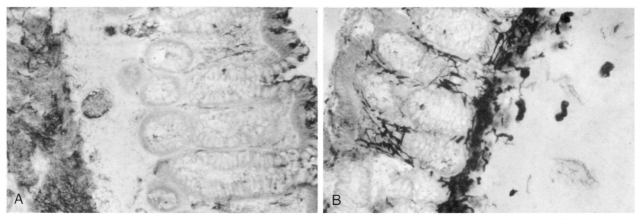

Figure 22–9. Suction rectal biopsy, acetylcholinesterase stain for nerve fibers. *A,* Normal appearance with relatively few fibers in the submucosa and almost no fibers in the lamina propria. *B,* Hirschsprung's disease showing a greatly increased density of fibers in the submucosa and prominent nerve fibers in the lamina propria.

perforation. Administration of 1 or 2 liters of isotonic saline may be required before adequate decompression is achieved and clear returns of infused saline are obtained. Tap water should never be used for the washouts, as absorption of the hypotonic water from the rectum may lead to circulatory overload and water intoxication.

Complications of colostomy in infancy and childhood are not uncommon. Minor complications include excoriation of the skin and ulceration and bleeding of the exposed mucosa, which may lead to iron-deficiency anemia. Prolapse of the stoma is a fairly common occurrence and may affect either limb, although it more commonly involves the distal colon. Stenosis of the proximal stoma may result in an excessive output with accompanying peristomal skin excoriation. Unfortunately, fashioning a colostomy does not guarantee against episodes of enterocolitis, which may occur even after definitive surgery. Each episode of enterocolitis should be treated aggressively with fluid and electrolyte restoration, antibiotic chemotherapy, and colonic decompression with saline evacuations.

DEFINITIVE TREATMENT

Details of the three most commonly performed operative procedures—Swenson, Duhamel, and Soave operations—are illustrated further on. Each procedure has inherent advantages and disadvantages, but the overall results are roughly equivalent (Table 22–1). The most important determinants of outcome are the experience and expertise of the surgeon. *There is no justification for a general surgeon to perform the occasional pull-through procedure when the expertise of a pediatric surgeon is available.*

Preoperative Preparation

The patient is admitted to the hospital for colonic washouts a day or two before surgery. These are performed with saline solution until the bowel selected for the pull-through procedure is completely cleared of all content. Only clear fluids given orally are per-

Table 22–1. COMPARISON OF SURGICAL TECHNIQUES

	Swenson	Duhamel	Soave
Advantages	Elimination of aganglionic segment	Technical ease in avoiding pelvic dissection	Avoidance of extensive pelvic dissection
Disadvantages	Technical difficulty	Retention of anterior aganglionic wall; potential pouch impaction	Retention of aganglionic muscular cuff of rectum
Complications			
Early			
Anastomotic leak	10%	7%	5%
Stenosis	8%	9%	12%
Late			
Constipation	10%	7%	10%
Incontinence	12%	7%	3%
Diarrhea or enterocolitis	12%	6%	6%

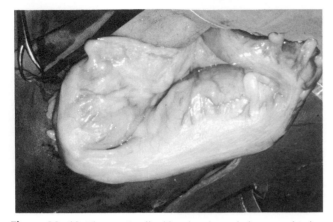

Figure 22–10. The proximally dilated and greatly hypertrophied colon in a 5-year-old child with untreated Hirschsprung's disease. Ganglion cells were present in an extramucosal biopsy of this part of the large bowel.

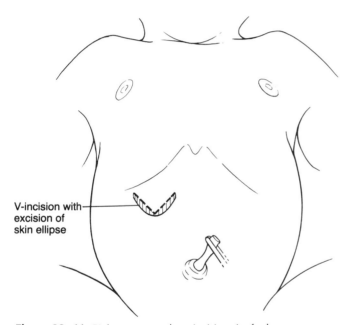

V-incision with excision of skin ellipse

Figure 22–11. Right upper quadrant incision site for loop colostomy. The incision is a V-shaped incision with excision of a skin ellipse.

mitted on the day before surgery. Metronidazole and an aminoglycoside or a broad-spectrum cephalosporin are administered prophylactically on induction of anaesthesia and again 6 hours postoperatively.

The patient is placed in the lithotomy position on the operating table. This position permits simultaneous access to the abdomen and perineum. An indwelling urethral catheter decompresses the bladder during the operation and during the first 3 to 5 postoperative days. The anal sphincter is dilated to facilitate the operative approach and to paralyze the sphincter during the early postoperative period. The abdomen, perineum, and upper thighs are prepared with an antiseptic solution (e.g., povidone-iodine).

Operative Procedures

Colostomy

A V-shaped incision is made in the right upper quadrant of the abdomen, extending through the subcutaneous fat to the external oblique aponeurosis. Small ellipses of skin on either side of the V are excised to avoid compressing the exteriorized bowel (Fig. 22–11). The V-shaped flap is elevated to expose the external oblique aponeurosis, which is incised transversely along the length of the incision. This incision is carried down to the peritoneum, which is likewise incised along the length of the incision (Fig. 22–12). The transverse colon is identified within the peritoneal cavity by the presence of the longitudinal taenia coli and the attachment of the greater omentum. The right transverse colon is delivered out of the incision and is prepared as a loop colostomy. A seromuscular biopsy is taken at the site of the proposed colostomy to ensure the presence of normal ganglion cells. This specimen is submitted for immediate frozen-section histopathologic examination (Fig. 22–13).

The omentum is detached from the area of colon selected for the colostomy. An opening is made in the mesocolon, through which the apex of the V-flap of skin is passed to act as a skin bridge, which prevents retraction of the stoma. The apex of the V is sutured to the skin with three interrupted full-thickness sutures (Fig. 22–14).

After the colon is attached to the anterior abdominal wall with a few interrupted seromuscular sutures, the colon is opened longitudinally, the wall is everted, and the open colostomy is sutured circumferentially to the skin edges with interrupted 5–0 polyglycolic acid sutures.

Swenson Procedure

For the Swenson procedure, a seromuscular biopsy specimen of the colon is obtained to confirm the

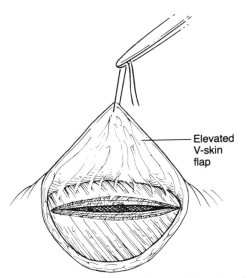

Figure 22–12. Construction of loop colostomy. Elevation of skin flap.

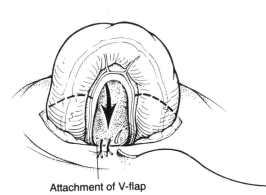

Figure 22–13. Construction of loop colostomy. The V-flap is brought through the mesenteric defect in the loop colostomy and attached to the inferior portion of the incision so as to form a skin bridge to guard against retraction.

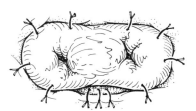

Figure 22–14. Construction of loop colostomy. The colostomy is matured by interrupted sutures.

presence of normal ganglion cells. If these are absent, further biopsies are taken until the lowest level of normally ganglionated bowel is identified. The rectum is mobilized, and the ureters are identified and preserved. The rectum is mobilized down into the pelvis, and the numerous short vessels in the immediate proximity of the rectal wall are ligated and divided. In this way, the nerve supply to the bladder is preserved. The dissection is continued to the level of the perineum, that is, below the pelvic musculature (Fig. 22–15).

Sponge-holding forceps are inserted through the anus into the rectum, and the wall of the bowel grasped by the forceps. The rectum is now intussuscepted out through the anus, while the anal canal is everted, until the level of resection determined by the biopsy specimen is reached. It is often necessary to ligate and divide the main trunk of the inferior mesenteric vessels in order to accomplish this maneuver (Fig. 22–16).

The everted rectum is transected obliquely to leave a cuff of anorectum measuring 0.5 cm posteriorly and 1.5 cm anteriorly from the dentate line. The proximal bowel is divided just above the ganglionic biopsy site (Fig. 22–17).

Bowel continuity is restored by a single-layer full-thickness anastomosis utilizing 4–0 or 5–0 Dexon sutures. The completed anastomosis is returned into the pelvis by reducing the "intussusception" (Fig. 22–18).

Duhamel Procedure

For the Duhamel procedure, the lowest level of ganglionic bowel is determined by frozen-section examination of the seromuscular biopsy. The areolar tissue in the midline posterior to the rectum is opened and the retrorectal dissection carried down to the level of the dentate line. The rectum is mobilized to the pelvic diaphragm while the numerous vessels adjacent to the rectum are ligated and divided (Fig. 22–19).

The proximal bowel is then divided below the level of the ganglionic biopsy site, and the end is closed with a pursestring suture of 1–0 silk. An incision is made in the posterior wall of the rectum at or just above the dentate line and extending through half the circumference of the rectum (Fig. 22–20).

Stay sutures of 4–0 silk are placed at either side of the incision in the posterior rectal wall and on the anterior and posterior flaps. A long artery clamp is passed up into the pelvis from below and through the posterior rectal incision, and the proximal colon is pulled through the retrorectal tunnel into the incision in the posterior rectal wall (Fig. 22–21).

The end of the pull-through colon is divided at the level of the ganglionic biopsy site, and an anastomosis is performed between the end of the colon and the

Text continued on page 564

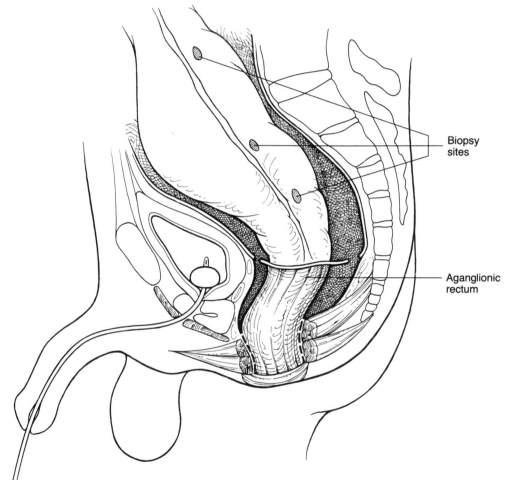

Biopsy sites

Aganglionic rectum

Figure 22–15. The Swenson operation. A sagittal section of the pelvis indicates the sites of serial biopsy samples that are taken to determine the level of ganglionated bowel.

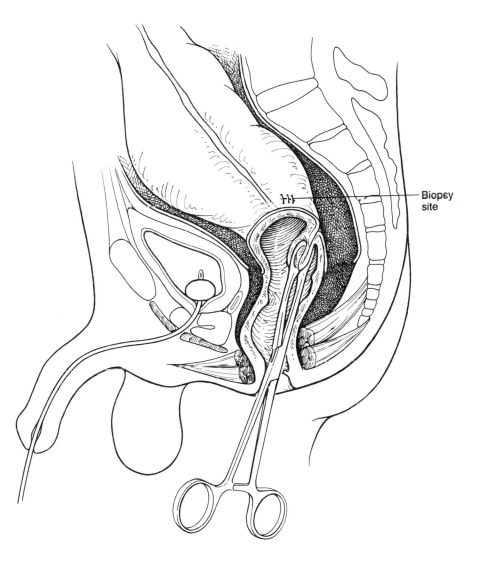

Biopsy site

Figure 22–16. The Swenson operation. Ring forceps are introduced through the anus to grasp the rectal wall so as to intussuscept the rectocolonic segment through the anus.

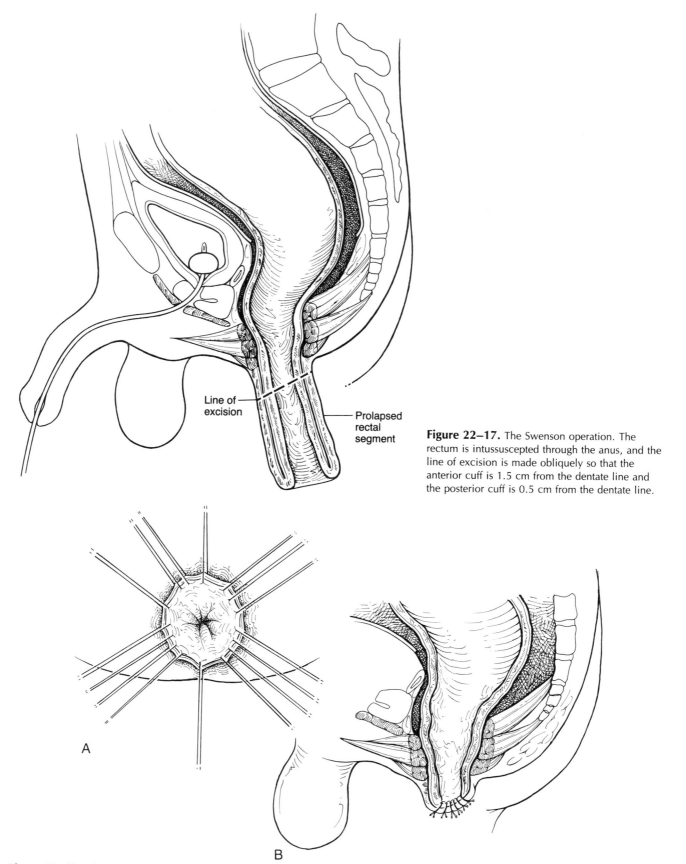

Line of excision

Prolapsed rectal segment

Figure 22–17. The Swenson operation. The rectum is intussuscepted through the anus, and the line of excision is made obliquely so that the anterior cuff is 1.5 cm from the dentate line and the posterior cuff is 0.5 cm from the dentate line.

A

B

Figure 22–18. The Swenson operation. A, Bowel continuity is restored by a single-layer full-thickness anastomosis between the ganglionated colon and the anorectal canal. B, A sagittal section showing the completed anastomosis of the ganglionated colon to the transected rectum at the dentate line.

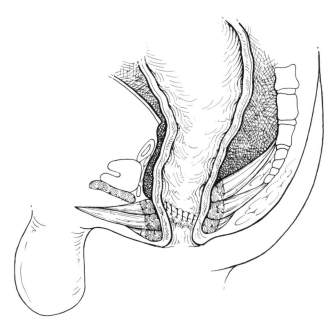

Figure 22–19. The Swenson procedure. The intussuscepted bowel in which the anastomosis has been completed externally is returned into the pelvis. The completed anastomosis is shown as an oblique line, because the anterior wall of the rectum is longer than the posterior wall.

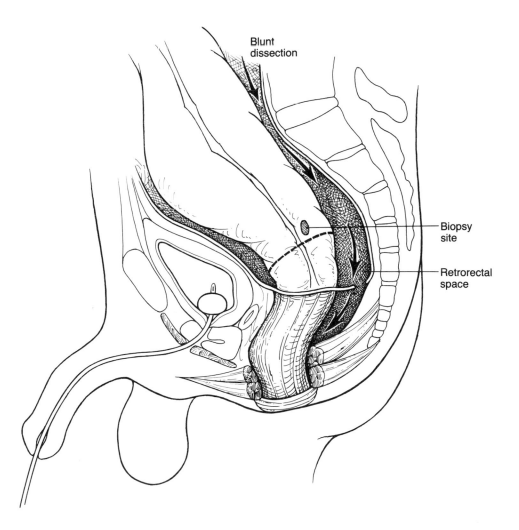

Figure 22–20. The Duhamel operation. The colon and rectum are mobilized in the retrorectal space down to the level of the dentate line at the puborectal sling.

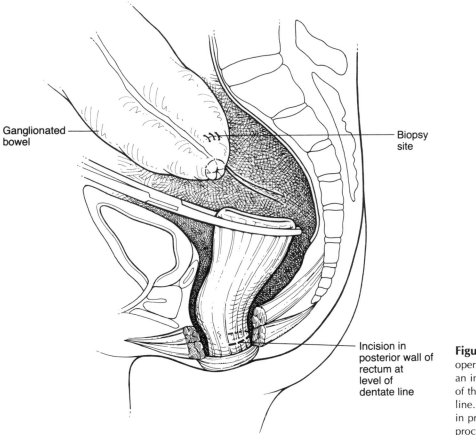

Figure 22–21. The Duhamel operation. The rectum is transected, and an incision is made in the posterior wall of the rectum at the level of the dentate line. The ganglionated bowel is closed in preparation for the pull-through procedure.

posterior wall of the rectum circumferentially by using interrupted 4–0 polyglycolic acid sutures. The GIA stapler is inserted from below with one blade in the rectum and the other in the pull-through colon. The common wall comprising the posterior rectal wall and the anterior colonic wall is stapled and divided to fashion a neorectum consisting of anterior aganglionic rectal wall and posterior ganglionic colonic wall (Fig. 22–22).

The rectum is divided as low in the pelvis as is possible to eliminate an anterior rectal pouch; alternatively, the rectum may be divided slightly higher above the peritoneal reflection, and the common wall divided by the GIA stapler with the open end of the rectum anastomosed in an end-to-side fashion to the pull-through colon (Martin modification) (Figs. 22–23 to 22–26).

Soave Procedure

The level of the pull-through is determined by frozen-section examination of the seromuscular biopsies from the proximal bowel. A longitudinal seromuscular incision is made through a convenient taenia coli, and the mucosal layer is exposed. By a combination of blunt and sharp dissection, a tube of mucosa is freed circumferentially from the underlying muscle layer. The mu-

cosal tube is dissected down to the perineum; the mucosa is freed from the seromuscular layer while meticulous hemostasis is maintained by coagulating the numerous intraluminal blood vessels. An incision extending down to the level of the dentate line is made in the seromuscular cuff. From the perineal end, a circumferential incision is made at the level of the dentate line through the mucosal layer in order to join the mucosal tube fashioned from above. The mucosal tube and the attached proximal seromuscular layer are pulled through the anus to the level of the predetermined ganglionic biopsy site. The pulled-through colon is transected at this level (Figs. 22–27 to 22–29).

An end-to-end anastomosis is constructed by using a single layer of interrupted 4-0 polyglycolic acid sutures between the full thickness of the end of the pulled-through colon and the mucosal layer of the rectum at the level of the dentate line. The seromuscular cuff of the rectum is sutured to the wall of the pulled-through colon with a few interrupted 4-0 polyglycolic acid sutures (Fig. 22–30).

Postoperative Complications

Early complications include anastomotic leaks and strictures at the anastomotic site. Leaks are more

Text continued on page 571

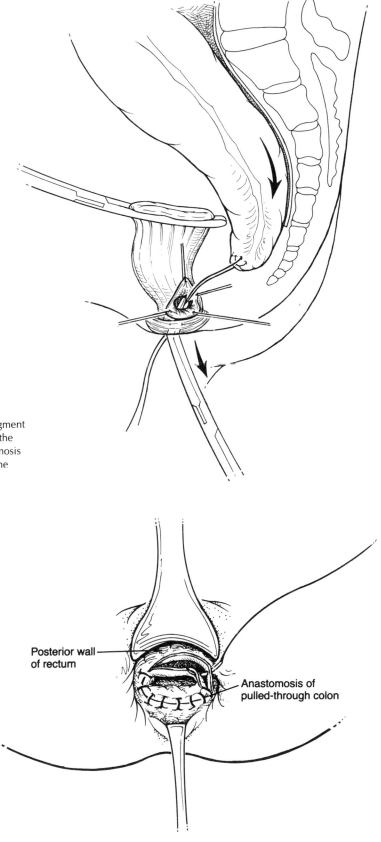

Figure 22–22. The Duhamel operation. The ganglionated segment of the bowel is brought into the retrorectal space and through the posterior incision in the rectum at the dentate line. An anastomosis is fashioned between the end of the ganglionated bowel and the incised rectum.

Posterior wall of rectum

Anastomosis of pulled-through colon

Figure 22–23. The Duhamel operation. A view of the anastomosis and the neorectum in the Duhamel procedure, as viewed through the anus.

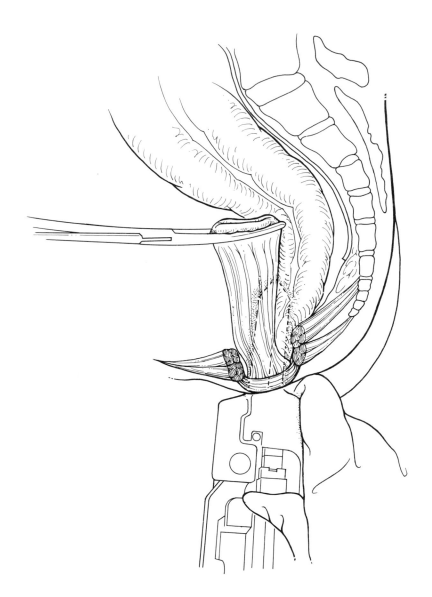

Figure 22–24. The Duhamel operation. The common wall comprising the posterior rectal wall and the anterior colonic wall is stapled and divided to fashion a neorectum consisting of anterior aganglionic rectal wall and posterior ganglionic colonic wall. Note that one limb of the stapler device is in the rectum, and the other end is in the colonic segment.

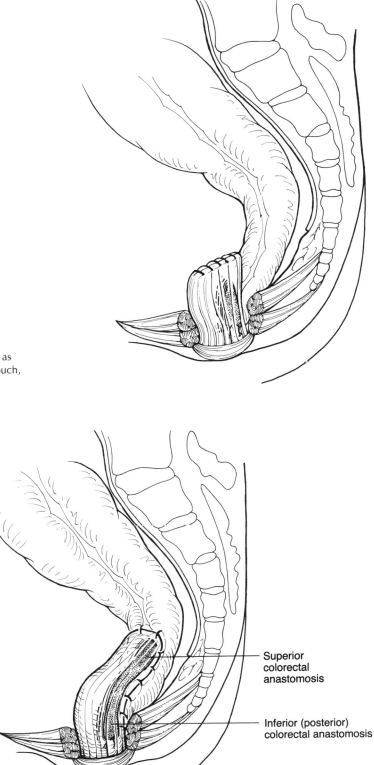

Figure 22–25. The Duhamel operation. The rectum is divided as low in the pelvis as is possible to eliminate an anterior rectal pouch, and the rectum is closed.

Superior colorectal anastomosis

Inferior (posterior) colorectal anastomosis

Figure 22–26. The Duhamel operation. An alternative is the Martin modification of the Duhamel procedure, in which the rectal stump is anastomosed to the ganglionated colon to eliminate the anterior rectal pouch.

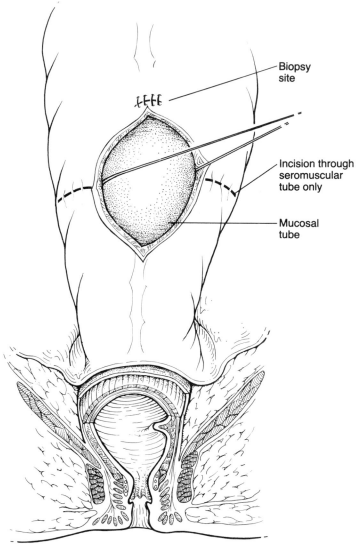

Biopsy site

Incision through seromuscular tube only

Mucosal tube

Figure 22–27. The Soave operation. A composite drawing indicating the site of the biopsy, which showed normal ganglionated bowel. The incision is made through the seromuscular coat of the rectum in order to construct a circumferential mucosal tube.

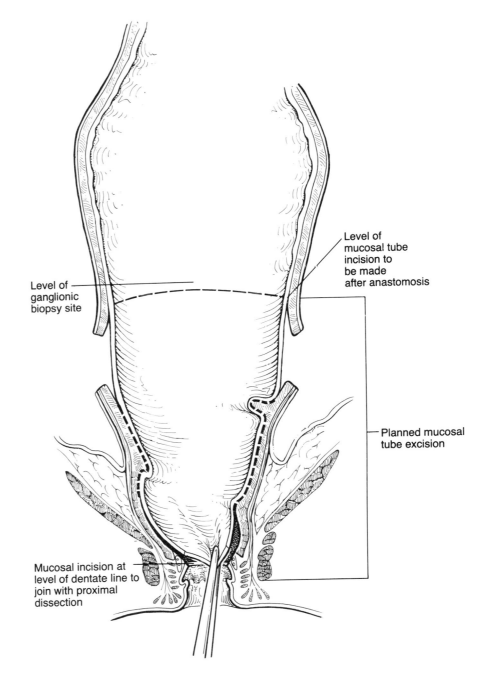

Level of
mucosal tube
incision to
be made
after anastomosis

Level of
ganglionic
biopsy site

Planned mucosal
tube excision

Mucosal incision at
level of dentate line to
join with proximal
dissection

Figure 22–28. The Soave operation. The mucosectomy is being completed in the rectum and carried up to the level of ganglionated bowel. The ganglionated bowel will be brought to the dentate line through the muscular cuff of rectum.

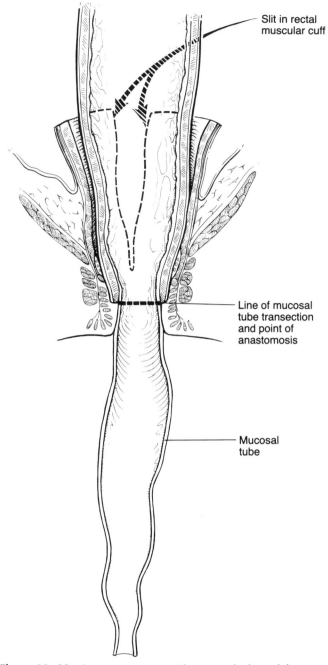

Slit in rectal
muscular cuff

Line of mucosal
tube transection
and point of
anastomosis

Mucosal
tube

Figure 22–29. The Soave operation. The mucosal tube and the attached proximal seromuscular layer are pulled through the anus to the level of the predetermined ganglionic biopsy site. The pulled-through colon is transected at this level. An incision has been made in the seromuscular cuff of the rectum down to the level of the dentate line.

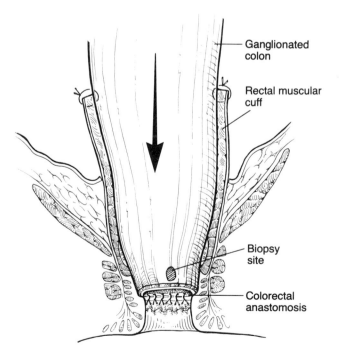

Ganglionated
colon

Rectal muscular
cuff

Biopsy
site

Colorectal
anastomosis

Figure 22–30. The Soave operation. The completed anastomosis is shown in sagittal section. The colorectal anastomosis between the anorectal canal and the ganglionated colon is completed. The ganglionated colon has been brought through the muscular cuff of the rectum.

commonly seen after the Swenson procedure, whereas strictures are most frequently encountered after the Soave operation. The morbidity associated with anastomotic leakage may be limited by the routine use of a "covering" proximal colostomy or ileostomy in the patient with long-segment disease. The frequency of anastomotic strictures is generally reduced by regular dilatations.

The incidence of postoperative enterocolitis varies from 2% to 15% and averages about 10% for all procedures. The enterocolitis occurs even after "successful" pull-through procedures in which ganglionic intestine constitutes the most distally utilized bowel. Postoperative enterocolitis appears to be more frequent after operation for total colonic aganglionosis. The treatment of each episode of enterocolitis is similar to that for preoperative enterocolitis: nasogastric decompression, correction of fluid and electrolyte imbalance, antibiotics (especially vancomycin), and gentle saline rectal washouts to decompress the bowel.

Attacks of enterocolitis may be associated with fecal stasis due to hypertonicity of the internal sphincter or due to an anastomosis fashioned to be slightly more proximal than recommended. The latter applies particularly to the Swenson procedure. The frequency of these attacks may be lessened by a forceful anal stretch or by a partial sphincterotomy.

EDITORIAL COMMENT

The details of the various operations proposed for the remedy of Hirschsprung's disease in infancy and childhood have been included to familiarize the student of surgery with these techniques and to fulfill general educational purposes. Hirschsprung's disease is a relatively rare condition; thus, only a few surgeons have the experience and expertise to undertake correction of these malformations. Operations for definitive correction should be undertaken only by experienced pediatric surgeons who are well familiar with the techniques and complications and who have the ability to render the appropriate postoperative care.

Nevertheless, the informed surgeon who understands the nature of the disease entity and the probability of the operations to be eventually performed may be able to serve the patient in the immediate perinatal period by undertaking appropriate diagnostic procedures and, when necessary, appropriate fecal diversion in emergency or even life-saving situations.

BIBLIOGRAPHY

Berdon WE, Baker DH. The roentgenographic diagnosis of Hirschsprung's disease in infancy. Am J Rotentgenol 1965;93:432.

Bill AH, Chapman ND. The enterocolitis of Hirschsprung's disease. Its natural history and treatment. Am J Surg 1962;103:70.

Bodian M, Stephens FD, et al. Hirschsprung's disease and idiopathic megacolon. Lancet 1949;1:6.

Boley SJ. New modification of the surgical treatment of Hirschsprung's disease. Surgery 1964;56:1015.

Boley SJ. An endorectal pull-through operation with primary anastomosis for Hirschsprung's disease. Surg Gynecol Obstet 1968;127:353.

Cass D. Hirschsprung's disease: An historical review. Prog Pediatr Surg 1986;20:199.

Coran AG, Weintraub WH. Modification of the endorectal procedure for Hirschsprung's disease. Surg Gynecol Obstet 1976;143:277.

Duhamel B. A new operation for the treatment of Hirschsprung's disease. Arch Dis Child 1960;35:38.

Ehrenpreis Th. Megacolon in the newborn. A clinical and roentgenological study with special regard to the pathogenesis. Acta Chir Scand 1946;94:112.

Hirschsprung H. Stuhltragheit Neugebornener infolge Dilatation und Hypertrophie des Colons. Jahresbericht Kinderheilkd 1888;27:1.

Holschneider AM, ed. Hirschsprung's Disease. Stuttgart: Hippokrates Verlag, 1982.

Holschneider AM, et al. Clinical and electromanometrical investigations of postoperative continence in Hirschsprung's disease. Z Kinderchir 1980;29:39.

Ikeda K, Goto S. Total colonic aganglionosis with or without small bowel involvement: An analysis of 137 patients. J Pediatr Surg 1986;21:319.

Lake BD, Puri P, et al. Hirschsprung's disease: An appraisal of histochemically demonstrated acetylcholinesterase activity in suction rectal biopsies as an aid to diagnosis. Arch Pathol Lab Med 1978;102:244.

Lister J. Hirschsprung. The man and the disease. J R Coll Surg Edinb 1977;22:377.

Martin LW, Caudill DR. A method for elimination of the blind rectal pouch in the Duhamel operation for Hirschsprung's disease. Surgery 1967;62:951.

Nixon HH. Hirschsprung's disease: Progress in management and diagnostics. World J Surg 1985;9:189.

Noblett HR. A rectal suction biopsy tube for use in the diagnosis of Hirschsprung's disease. J Pediatr Surg 1969;4:406.

Polley TZ, Coran AG. Hirschsprung's disease in the newborn. An 11-year experience. Pediatr Surg Int 1986;1:80.

Polley TZ, Coran AG, Wesley JR. The definitive management of Hirschsprung's disease with the endorectal pull-through procedure. Pediatr Surg Int 1986;1:90.

Polley TZ, Coran AG, Heidelberger KP, Wesley JR. Suction rectal biopsy in the diagnosis of Hirschsprung's disease and chronic constipation. Pediatr Surg Int 1986;1:84.

Soave F. Hirschsprung's disease: Technique and results of Soave's operation. Br J Surg 1966;53:1023.

Swenson O, Bill AH. Resection of rectum and rectosigmoid with preservation of sphincter for benign spastic lesions producing megacolon. Surgery 1948;24:212.

Swenson O, Sherman JO, et al. The treatment and postoperative complications of congenital megacolon: A 25-year follow-up. Ann Surg 1975;182:266.

Teitelbaum DH, Qualman SJ, Caniano DA. Hirschsprung's disease. Identification of risk factors for enterocolitis. Ann Surg 1988;207:240.

Vane DW, Grosfeld JL. Hirschsprung's disease. Experience with the Duhamel operation in 195 cases. Pediatr Surg Int 1986;1:95.

Weitzman JJ. Management of Hirschsprung's disease with the Swenson procedure with emphasis on long-term follow-up. Pediatr Surg Int 1986;1:100.

Whitehouse F, Kernohan JW. Myenteric plexus in congenital megacolon. Arch Int Med 1948;82:75.

Zuelzer WW, Wilson JL. Functional intestinal obstruction on a congenital neurogenic basis in infancy. Am J Dis Child 1948;75:40.

Anorectal Disease in Children

CHAPTER 23

Hernan M. Reyes

RECTAL PROLAPSE

Rectal prolapse occurs frequently in infants and children between the ages of 1 and 3 years and shows no racial or sexual predilection. With few exceptions, it is a self-limited disease with an acute onset precipitated by marked straining from diarrhea or constipation and requiring simple reduction and dietary regulation. Unlike in adults, operative correction in children is rarely necessary.[1-6]

Excessive straining secondary to nonspecific diarrhea appears to be the predominant cause of rectal prolapse in the pediatric patient. Constipation from any cause, psychosocial problems, and faulty toilet training may also play a significant role in pathogenesis. It is not unusual for rectal prolapse to develop in cystic fibrosis patients because of their frequent episodes of steatorrhea. On rare occasions, prolapse due to constipation has been observed in patients with Hirschsprung's disease. No doubt, rectal prolapse would occur more frequently in the absence of early surgical intervention to relieve the functional obstruction of congenital megacolon.

Certain anatomic features, such as a low pelvic peritoneal reflection and shallow sacral concavity in an infant, are predisposing factors in the pathogenesis of rectal prolapse. Additional causative factors are deficient fat and fascial support of the rectum from malnutrition, weakness of the pelvic musculature from meningomyelocele, and the association of increased intra-abdominal pressure frequently observed in exstrophy of the urinary bladder. Furthermore, changes related to the operative correction of an imperforate anus or the related anatomic deficiencies of the levator ani muscle and the rectal muscle complex are likely to be factors in the development of rectal prolapse. Al-

though rare, rectal polyps may be a predisposing factor for rectal intussusception and rectal prolapse.

Despite early conjectures to the contrary, most cases of rectal prolapse in infants and children involve the mucosal layer of the rectum, which stretches and separates from the muscular coat. Repeated episodes of mucosal prolapse during each bowel movement eventually weaken the attachments of the rectum at the pelvic floor, stretch and weaken the internal and external sphincters, and dilate the puborectal hiatus; the last results from increased laxity of the puborectal musculature with failure to maintain proper angulation of the rectum during defecation. This process eventually leads to a full-thickness rectal prolapse.

The exceptions to these theories of pathogenesis are the pre-existence of a primary anatomic defect or a neurologic abnormality with associated weakness of the pelvic musculature, such as meningomyelocele, malnutrition, postsurgical changes following correction of Hirschsprung's disease and imperforate anus, exstrophy of the urinary bladder, and Ehlers-Danlos syndrome. In these conditions rectal procidentia occurs de novo, and surgical correction is more likely to be necessary than in the common variety of mucosal rectal prolapse.

Cystic Fibrosis and Rectal Prolapse

The incidence of rectal prolapse in patients with cystic fibrosis ranges from 11% to 23%. In a study of 605 patients with cystic fibrosis reported by Stern and associates, 112 (18.5%) had rectal prolapse.[2] In 48 (43%) the onset of rectal prolapse preceded the diagnosis of cystic fibrosis. The delay in diagnosis of the systemic lesion in the study was 1 month to 17 years with a mean of 3.5 years. In this series rectal prolapse led to the physician's correct diagnosis of cystic fibrosis in only nine patients. Although steatorrhea, poor growth pattern, wasting, family history of cystic fibrosis, history of meconium plug syndrome, and digital clubbing led to the correct diagnosis of cystic fibrosis, the only presenting symptoms in the remainder were loose stools or diarrhea; this led to failure to make the correct diagnosis of the primary disease.

The acute onset of rectal prolapse in an infant or child with no known predisposing condition should be investigated for cystic fibrosis, even in the absence of other symptoms of that disease. This should be done because of the common association of these two conditions and the devastating complications of delay in the diagnosis of cystic fibrosis.[3]

Diet regulation, enzyme replacement therapy, and manual reduction of the prolapse are usually successful treatments for these patients. Unfortunately, rectal prolapse in a patient with cystic fibrosis who is already on replacement therapy has been observed to be more refractory to nonoperative measures. Surgical correction is limited to patients who suffer from considerable pain and discomfort or to those in whom manual reduction of the prolapse is difficult. The natural history of rectal prolapse in most patients with cystic fibrosis is a gradual reduction in the frequency of prolapse with eventual disappearance of the condition.

Rectal Prolapse and Incontinence

Incontinence in association with rectal prolapse is usually a result of the primary condition causing the prolapse. Rectal prolapse per se does not appear to produce incontinence in the pediatric patient.

Treatment

Most patients with rectal prolapse respond to conservative therapy.

Treatment for Diarrhea. The cause of diarrhea must be properly evaluated. Appropriate treatment, including liquids, tea, and antidiarrheal drugs, almost always leads to spontaneous cessation of the rectal prolapse.

Treatment for Constipation. Mineral oil, stool softener, high-fiber diet, and concentrated preparation of a highly efficient dietary fiber to promote bulk are helpful in treating the patient with constipation. Chronic habitual constipation must be treated aggressively with daily enemas, if there is no response to stool softeners and gentle laxatives. If the treatment is to be effective, it must be continued until voluntary bowel movements are regularly successfully achieved.

Reduction. Rectal prolapse should be reduced manually using mild sedation with barbiturates or chloral hydrate. It is uncommon for a rectal prolapse to remain irreducible. Changes signifying strangulation are an indication for aggressive reduction under general anesthesia. Taping both buttocks together following reduction does not appear to be essential to prevention of recurrence.

Pancreatic Enzyme Replacement. Pancreatic enzyme replacement is a major therapeutic measure in patients with cystic fibrosis.

Treatment for Local Cause. Eradication of any local cause, such as a rectal polyp, should be instituted. Local causes such as ulcerative colitis require treatment of the primary disease.

Surgical correction is advocated under the following conditions:

1. Recurrent prolapse with mucosal ulceration

2. Failure to reduce the prolapse, despite adequate sedation

3. Recurrent rectal prolapse associated with severe pain and discomfort, despite intensive medical treatment

4. Failure of conservative management

5. Full-thickness rectal prolapse in patients with meningomyelocele, exstrophy of the bladder, and postsurgical changes following pull-through operations for imperforate anus and Hirschsprung's disease.

Because more than 50 operative procedures are advocated in the medical literature for the treatment of rectal prolapse, the most common and effective surgical procedures are briefly described here and analyzed for ease or complexity, inherent morbidity, and effectiveness in preventing recurrence.

INJECTION PROCEDURES

Currently, two injection procedures are described in the literature, which appear to be effective in correcting rectal prolapse and preventing its recurrence.

The first is the injection of phenol in oil into the submucosal layer of the rectum in four quadrants, 7 to 8 cm above the anal verge, which was described by Wyllie in 1979 (Fig. 23–1).[7] Although this treatment has considerable merit for the management of rectal prolapse of the mucosal variety, there is doubt about its effectiveness in patients with full-thickness rectal prolapses. This is because, in concept, the effect of the injection is limited to producing inflammation and adhesions between the mucosal layer and the muscular coat. Despite this skepticism, 91 of 100 patients treated with this technique responded favorably after receiving one injection. In the nine other patients, all of whom had associated systemic disease responsible for the rectal prolapse, a second injection was sufficient to prevent further recurrence. The cases reported had a follow-up of 2 to 16 years after treatment.

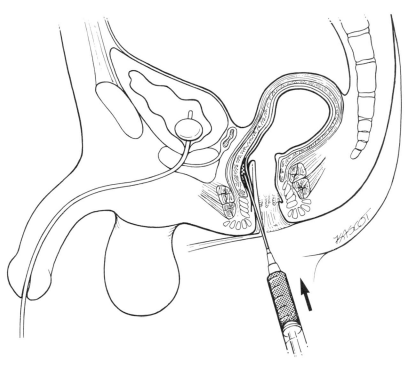

Figure 23–1. Submucosal injection treatment. Under general anesthesia, using direct vision and a speculum, one transanally injects 2 ml of 5% phenol in oil in the submucosal layer circumferentially at 4 to 5 sites 8 cm above the anal verge.

The injection treatment advocated by Kay and Zaachary consists of a perirectal injection of a 30% normal saline solution (Fig. 23–2).[8] The intention is to promote an inflammatory process with fibrosis and adhesions, and thereby to provide fixation of the rectum and to prevent recurrence of a full-thickness rectal prolapse. Of 51 cases reported, 11 required a second injection; in 3 others a third injection was necessary to prevent further prolapse.

THIERSCH OPERATION

The Thiersch operation is preferred by many surgeons in the treatment of poor-risk elderly patients because of its simplicity and because it can be performed while the patient is under local anesthesia (Fig. 23–3).[9] In a modification of this operation for the pediatric patient, reported by Stern, the anal sling consisted of one to three strands of Mersilene encased in Silastic.[2] This sling is placed perianally, beneath the subcutaneous layer of the external sphincter muscle, and inserted through four radially placed stab incisions 2 cm from the anal verge. The anal opening is constricted to the size of an 8 to 10 Hegar dilator. Major drawbacks of this procedure are the high incidence of infections, possible breakage of the sling, and problems with bowel movements, including impaction, tenesmus, and incomplete evacuation of stool. In a series of five pediatric patients who underwent a sling procedure, early removal of the sling was necessary in two because of infection, with recurrence of the rectal prolapse in one.

LOCKHART-MUMMERY OPERATION

The Lockhart-Mummery procedure consists of packing the retrorectal space with mesh gauze following a dissection carried out through a posterior perianal incision to a depth of 8 to 10 cm.[10] The packing is gradually removed in 8 to 10 days. Of 17 patients who were refractory to conservative measures, 8 were treated with this procedure, and in 7 there was no recurrence. In one patient, prolapse recurred, even after a second operation. In this patient, the prolapse gradually resolved 3 months after the second operation.

The major disadvantage of this operation is the requirement that the retrorectal pack be left in place for at least 8 to 10 days in order to achieve its goal of promoting adhesions to stabilize the rectum. It is our opinion, as well as that of the workers who advocated this procedure, that a less-complicated operation, such as an injection treatment, should remain the primary choice for the correction of rectal prolapse that is unresponsive to medical treatment. At our institution, other surgical procedures are preferred to the Lockhart-Mummery operation.

CAUTERIZATION TREATMENT

In 1982 Hight and associates described linear cauterization for treatment of rectal prolapse.[11] The prolapsed rectal mucosa is cauterized with a ball-tip electrocautery device. This is done in a linear fashion, including the inner and outer layers of the prolapsed mucosa and extending to the submucosa in four quadrants. In

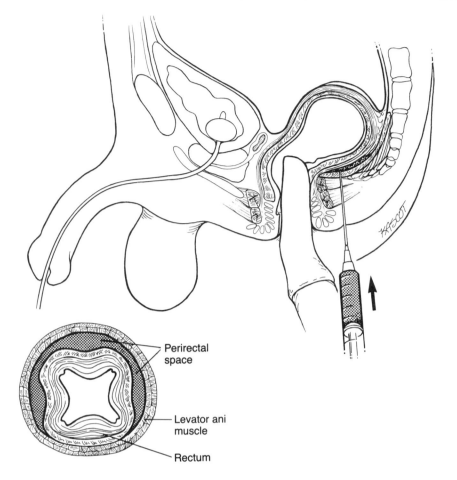

Perirectal space

Levator ani muscle

Rectum

Figure 23–2. Perirectal injection treatment. With the patient in the supine position and the left index finger in the anal canal, a spinal needle is introduced slowly through the perianal skin 2 cm away from the anal orifice to a distance of 5 to 8 cm above the anorectal junction. Next, 3 to 5 ml of 30% saline is injected into the left lateral perirectal region. A test dose of 1 ml is initially injected to ensure that the needle is not in the rectal wall. A similar procedure is followed, with injection of the same volume of hypertonic saline to the posterior and right lateral perirectal regions.

the male patient, care must be exercised not to place the anterior linear cauterization in the midline in order to avoid deep periurethral inflammation and injury to the bladder neck. This treatment protocol was utilized for 73 patients who failed nonoperative measures. In 67 children the prolapse was corrected, and no recurrence was observed. In five others, a second cauterization was required to correct the disease. The single failure was in a child who previously had a failed injection treatment and anal sphincteroplasty. This patient ultimately required an extensive anterior suspension of the rectum to relieve the symptoms.

QUADRANT MUCOSAL STRIPPING AND MUSCLE PLEATING

This operative procedure was reported by Momoh in 1986 for 21 patients whose rectal prolapse was refractory to conservative measures.[12] Following bowel preparation, the operative procedure consisted of excising 1- to 1.5-cm–wide strips of mucosa longitudinally in four quadrants by using electrocautery and beginning just above the dentate line to the apex of the prolapsed bowel. At each denuded quadrant, a continuous suture of 2-0 silk was placed longitudinally through the submucosa and muscular layers. When the two ends of

the sutures were tied, the prolapsed bowel was pleated. After the sutures were completed, the pleated prolapsed bowel was reduced.

In 14 of the patients, it was thought that the prolapse was a full-thickness one, and in 7 patients the prolapse was considered to be mucosal. The single recurrence in this series resolved following manual reduction of the prolapsed pleated bowel. The author claims that this procedure is relatively simple, safe, and reliable, and effective in the prevention of recurrence without special preoperative or postoperative care. Most patients were operated on as outpatients.

Complex operations that incorporate resection or plication of the rectum include fixation of the rectum and repair or plication of the sphincter mechanism (levator sling and anorectal muscle complex), or development of a skin flap for anal canal reconstruction. The complex operations are generally reserved for recurrent prolapse following simpler operations and for prolapse in patients with exstrophy of the bladder or meningomyelocele or that resulting from pull-through operations for Hirschsprung's disease or imperforate anus. The levator repair and posterior suspension technique described by Ashcraft and coworkers involves narrowing the levator hiatus posteriorly

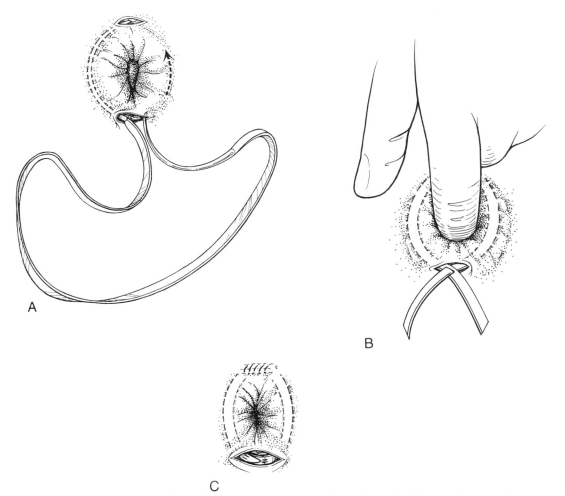

Figure 23–3. Thiersch repair. A double-armed Mersilene suture (5-mm) is passed on either side of the anus from anterior to posterior in the ischiorectal fossa through a small incision in the anterior and posterior positions 1 cm outside the anal verge. The two ends of the suture are tied snuggly against a size 12 Hegar dilator in the anal canal, and the knot is buried posteriorly.

and anchoring the rectum in its normal position at the puborectal arch with fixation by sutures between the rectum and the cut edge of the sacrum.[13] Total correction was achieved in a small number of patients. A report by Pearl and associates[14] advocates utilizing the technique, described by Pena and De Vries,[15] for the definitive correction of imperforate anus through a posterior sacrococcygeal approach.

The technique for correction of rectal prolapse consists of identifying and transecting the levator ani muscle complex in the midline posterior to the rectum, plicating the rectum to normal size for a length of 3 to 4 cm over a Hegar dilator, and incorporating the posterior plicated rectum to the closure of the levator ani muscle complex. Although a properly repaired levator ani and muscle complex would not ordinarily lead to incontinence, a poorly done operation may lead to that complication. If the primary problem of rectal prolapse is not initially associated with incontinence, as is the case in most pediatric patients, a

complex operation with the potential to produce this complication is unacceptable.

Mucosal or full-thickness rectal prolapse occurring postoperatively following pull-through operations for imperforate anus is frequent and leads to soiling, occasional bleeding, and pain. The ideal corrective operation in this setting should be one that provides a skin-lined anal canal to prevent recurrence and stricture formation. The operative procedure described by Millard and Rowe,[16] with a two-skin-flap anoplasty and modified by Caouette-Laberge and colleagues[17] to a three-skin-flap procedure, is an excellent operation for the primary correction of rectal prolapse that follows a pull-through operation for imperforate anus. The technique consists of resecting the distal 2 cm of colon from the mucocutaneous junction of the anus. Multiple skin flaps are developed, which are then interposed between the distal end of the resected colon and the perianal skin.

In the last 20 years, our most frequently performed

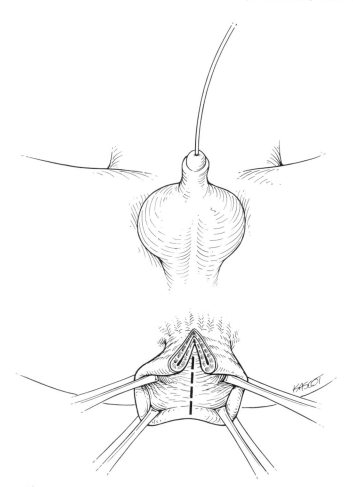

Figure 23–4. Limited perineal proctectomy and anoplasty. When the patient is under general anesthesia and following dilation of the anal canal, the entire prolapsed segment is everted through the anal opening with Allis forceps. The prolapsed segment is divided, full thickness, at the midline anteriorly and posteriorly with electrocautery to 1 cm above the anal verge. The divided segments in the midline are approximated, full thickness, with 2-0 Vicryl sutures.

operation for the surgical correction of rectal prolapse has been a limited perianal proctectomy and anoplasty (Fig. 23–4). Despite the lack of enthusiasm by others for this operation because of the possibility of stricture formation, we have been pleased with our results. We have not observed any recurrences or stenosis.

The patient is admitted on the night before the operation, and, depending on the age of the child, bowel preparation with either a cleansing saline enema or a polyethylene glycol solution (GoLYTELY) given by means of a nasogastric tube is instituted. At operation, the patient is placed in a lithotomy position and the anal canal is dilated and generously prepared with a gauze soaked with povidone-iodine (Betadine) solution. The prolapse is grasped by Allis forceps in four quadrants, and a full-thickness incision is made using an electrocautery device; the incision is placed anteriorly and posteriorly at the six o'clock and twelve o'clock positions, 5 mm from the mucocutaneous junction and through both layers of the prolapse. The apex of the incised margins at the mesocutaneous junction is approximated in one layer with 2-0 Vicryl sutures. The rest of the prolapsed rectum is excised circumferentially by means of electrocautery, alternating excision and full-thickness one-layer suture approximation (Fig. 23–5). The anal canal is then packed with petroleum jelly (Vaseline)–covered gauze and removed 12 hours later.

Oral liquids are started immediately and followed by a soft diet 3 days postoperatively. Hot sitz baths are utilized daily until the wound is completely healed. Finger dilatation of the anal canal is performed daily starting 1 week after the operative procedure until complete healing is achieved and narrowing of the anal opening is not observed.

FISTULA-IN-ANO

Although the etiology of fistula-in-ano in infants and children may be somewhat different from that of the disorder in adults, it is a surgical condition that requires urgent management. This disease of infancy appears to result from a congenital abnormality of the anal glands and the anal crypts. Parks, Duhamel, and Kleinhaus independently alluded to such a concept.[18–20] Shafer and associates postulated that the developmental anomaly predisposing one to the formation of fistula-in-ano in infancy results from a thick, irregular dentate line with deep crypts of Morgagni.[21] This abnormality leads to trapping of bacteria and cryptitis, which develop into perianal abscess and fistula-in-ano.

Conversely, Fitzgerald postulates that the anal glands are abnormal in affected patients and that these glands may spontaneously discharge their secretions

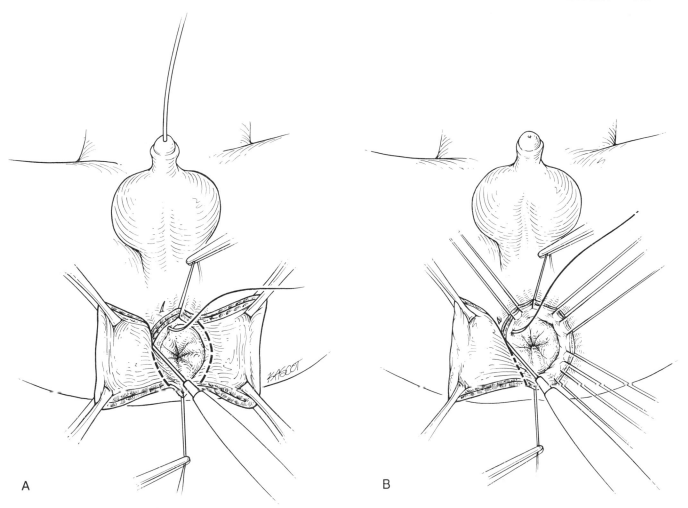

Figure 23–5. *A* and *B*, The prolapsed segment is then resected, full thickness, with electrocautery, excising both lateral segments circumferentially and approximating the bowel at full thickness with 2-0 Vicryl sutures.

directly to the skin surface, even in the absence of a concomitant infection.[22] This theory is based on his observation that fistula-in-ano occurs in infants younger than 18 months of age, whereas perianal abscess almost always appears after 2 years of age. He is convinced that a circulating hormone or excessive androgen production may play a significant role in the development of this lesion. This concept is reinforced by the observation that almost all fistula-in-ano occurs in male patients (more than 90%). The hormone theory may explain the multiplicity of the lesions found in about 17% to 20% of the patients.

Another observation in some infants is the multiplicity of fistula-in-ano with separate tracts but without the complex tracts seen in adults. The external opening of the fistula in relation to the anal opening is frequently in the anterolateral and lateral positions, with equal distribution on the right and left sides. Furthermore, the fistulous tract appears contiguous to the closest crypt and for the most part is superficial,

traversing only the subcutaneous layer of the external sphincter muscle.

The appropriate surgical correction consists of unroofing the entire length of the fistula, including its contiguous abnormal deep crypts, by using an electrocautery device. Shafer further advocates unroofing all abnormal deep crypts behind the dentate line to prevent recurrence. In a large series of patients, he and his associates claim to have identified the association of from 2 to 13 abnormal crypts in their patients with fistula-in-ano.

On the basis of our experience, we conclude that electrodesiccation of the base of the fistula and excision of its margins are essential in the management of the condition. The entire length of the fistula can be identified readily by using a size 00 or 000 lacrimal duct probe. With gentle pressure to the probe, the contiguous crypt of Morgagni can be identified in most cases.

If no direct communication of the fistula with the

crypt is identified, the fistula is simply unroofed to the distal end of the probe. A separate examination is done behind the dentate line, with identifying and unroofing of the abnormal crypts.

Postoperatively, the patient is given a regular diet. Our practice is to give the infant a stool softener for 1 week and hot sitz baths after each bowel movement. Packing the anal canal postoperatively is not essential, and antibiotics are not routinely administered to these patients. Generally, healing takes place within 2 weeks, and if the operation is properly performed, recurrence is uncommon.

PERIANAL INFECTIONS

Perianal infection in infants and children is a significant problem and must be addressed in any discussion of perianal disease. The three conditions included in this discussion are (1) perianal cellulitis, (2) condyloma acuminatum (human papillomavirus) anogenital infections, and (3) perianal excoriation and secondary infection following pull-through operations.

Perianal Cellulitis

This condition represents the cutaneous manifestation of group A β-hemolytic streptococcal infection that occurs in adults and children.[23, 24] It is seen more frequently in children, because group A streptococci rank among the most common pathogenic bacteria of childhood. The infectious process is so subtle that it is often unrecognized, and in many instances undiagnosed. Treatment by the local application of nonspecific antibiotics and antifungal and steroid ointments usually fails.

The characteristic lesions are painful erythematous and pruritic ones found in the perianal region. They are associated with small fissures covered by a small layer of a whitish purulent discharge.

Cultures disclose the correct diagnosis, and appropriate treatment is instituted. This lesion is most likely transmitted by direct host-to-host contact and by airborne dissemination. The mainstay of treatment is oral penicillin for 2 weeks. All lesions must be healed and cultures negative before the treatment is discontinued.

Allergy to penicillin or only partial response to this drug is an indication for erythromycin therapy. Erythromycin is given orally at a suggested dosage of 40 mg per kilogram of body weight per day, for the ethylsuccinate form of the drug, for 10 days. However, the duration of treatment must be dictated by the complete eradication of perianal lesions and negative culture findings for the streptococcal organism.

Condyloma Acuminatum (Human Papillomavirus) Anogenital Infection

Anogenital warts in infants and children are generally caused by the human papillomavirus, predominantly types 6, 11, 16, and 18.[25] Although transmission of infection by nonsexual means is possible and includes perinatal exposure, poor hygiene, and shared bathing, the current concept is that all or almost all anogenital warts, which include condyloma acuminatum and verruca vulgaris, are sexually transmitted.[26] Any infant or child with anogenital warts should be investigated thoroughly for a history of sexual abuse or physical findings that indicate child abuse, such as vaginal scarring, large vaginal orifice, dilated anal canal, laxity of the external anal sphincter, other infections that are sexually transmitted or associated with sexual activity, and other stigmata of child abuse, such as multiple skeletal fractures in different stages of healing and cigarette burns distributed over the body.

Before therapy is instituted, a detailed examination of the anogenital area under general anesthesia must be done. This evaluation should include vaginoscopy and anoscopy. Although localized lesions can be readily treated with local application of podophyllin, more extensive lesions must be excised by electrocautery. Surgical excision must be repeated on a weekly schedule until all lesions are eradicated. Other forms of treatment include topical fluorouracil, immunotherapy, and the experimental use of alfa-N1 interferon.[26] In our experience, the only successful treatment has been the excision by electrocoagulation.

Postoperatively, a Foley catheter is inserted if periurethral lesions were excised, and it must be left in place for at least 72 hours. Local anesthetic ointment can be applied as necessary and daily hot sitz baths given after each bowel movement until healing is complete. To prevent recurrence, all lesions must have been excised by electrocautery and the source of reinfection removed. The patient should also be re-examined at least once every 3 months until the offending source of infection is eradicated.

One report describes an extensive anogenital wart in a 17-month-old infant with acquired immunodeficiency syndrome–related complex (ARC) refractory to all forms of known or experimental treatment. This finding suggests that in children this lesion can be a manifestation of human immunodeficiency virus (HIV) infection and that effective treatment may be problematic.[27]

Perianal Excoriation and Secondary Infection Following Pull-Through Operations

Chemical irritation of the perianal skin by intestinal contents following pull-through operations for imperforate anus or Hirschsprung's disease is a frequent occurrence. The lesion begins as an erythematous change in the skin followed by excoriation, denudation of the superficial skin layer, and frank ulceration with secondary infection. Uncontrolled, secondarily infected lesions may proceed to abscess formation and septicemia. These lesions tend to occur despite aggressive local application of antibacterial, antifungal, or steroid ointments.

The application of aluminum paste or zinc oxide to the perianal region immediately after a pull-through operation and after an ileoanal anastomosis for ulcerative colitis or total colonic Hirschsprung's disease appears to provide protection from this condition. If application is done repeatedly and liberally, perianal excoriations may be prevented. Any drained intestinal contents must be immediately washed off the surface of the skin by a normal saline solution, and a cake of the aluminum paste or zinc oxide must be frequently applied to the perianal skin. We have also utilized karaya powder or ointment in the perianal skin, which appears to be effective in the prevention of perianal skin irritation and infection.

A child with full-blown perianal skin irritation, especially when excoriations or ulcerations are present, should be treated as an inpatient. Culture specimens are initially obtained, and the perineum is washed completely after each bowel movement. A combination of aluminum paste and karaya powder is applied liberally on the involved skin, and the area is placed under a heat lamp. During the active phase, oral feedings must be limited to clear liquids, and intravenous fluids may be started to complement the oral intake. As a rule, most of these lesions heal within 10 days. More severe lesions may require weeks, or even months, before healing is complete.

Hospitalization should be limited to the acute phase; when the lesions start to clear, the patient can be discharged with a strong admonition that diapers should not be worn at any time and that stools or urine draining to the perianal skin should be washed off immediately. The treatment with aluminum paste and karaya powder should also be continued until all lesions are healed. If active bacterial infection is present, the appropriate antibiotic may be given orally. Fungal infections must be treated by the local application of an antifungal drug.

Hayashi and associates presented their experience in the treatment of peristomal and perianal excoriations with topical sucralfate in the form of either a powder or an emollient applied every 6 hours to maintain a visible layer.[28] They found this drug to have no systemic or toxic effects. It was a safe and effective treatment for this condition. It is also soothing and subjectively reduces the patient's discomfort. The presence of a fungal infection, however, still requires antifungal drug therapy.

Sucralfate can be used to prevent development of perineal excoriations from chemical irritation of the intestinal contents following a pull-through operation for Hirschsprung's disease, ulcerative colitis, polyposis, and imperforate anus. We have chosen this form of treatment for a few patients who have developed excoriations following these operations. Our experience duplicates that of the original investigators. The mechanism by which sucralfate promotes healing of this condition is unknown.

REFERENCES

1. Fowler R. The anatomy and treatment of rectal prolapse in childhood. Aust Paediatr J 1967;3:90–98.
2. Stern RC, Izant RJ Jr, Boat TF, et al. Treatment and prognosis of rectal prolapse in cystic fibrosis. Gastroenterology 1982;82:707–710.
3. Zempsky WT, Rosenstein BJ. The cause of rectal prolapse in children. Am J Dis Child 1988;142:338–339.
4. Leape LL. Other disorders of the rectum and anus. In: Welch KJ, et al, eds. Pediatric Surgery. Chicago: Year Book, 1986, pp 1038–1046.
5. Wassef R, Rothenberger DA, Goldberg SM. Rectal prolapse. Curr Probl Surg 1986;23:398–451.
6. Holder TM, Ashcraft KW. Acquired anorectal lesions. In: Holder TM, Ashcraft KW, eds. Pediatric Surgery. Philadelphia: WB Saunders, 1980, pp 429–432.
7. Wyllie GG. The injection treatment of rectal prolapse. J Pediatr Surg 1979;14:62–64.
8. Kay NRM, Zaachary RB. Treatment of rectal prolapse in children with injection of 30 percent saline solution. J Pediatr Surg 1970;5:334–337.
9. Corman ML. Rectal prolapse: Surgical techniques. Surg Clin North Am 1988;68:1255–1265.
10. Qvist N, Rasmussen L, Klaaborg KE, Hansen LP, Pedersen SA. Rectal prolapse in infancy: Conservative versus operative treatment. J Pediatr Surg 1986;21:887–888.
11. Hight DW, Hertzler JH, Philippart AI, Benson CD. Linear cauterization for the treatment of rectal prolapse in infants and children. Surg Gynecol Obstet 1982;154:400–402.
12. Momoh JT. Quadrant mucosal stripping and muscle pleating in the management of childhood rectal prolapse. J Pediatr Surg 1986;21:36–38.
13. Ashcraft KW, Amoury RA, Holder TM. Levator repair and posterior suspension for rectal prolapse. J Pediatr Surg 1977;12:241–245.
14. Pearl RH, Ein SH, Churchill B. Posterior sagittal anorectoplasty for pediatric recurrent rectal prolapse. J Pediatr Surg 1989;24:1100–1102.
15. Pena A, De Vries PA. Posterior sagittal anorectoplasty: Important technical considerations and new applications. J Pediatr Surg 1986;21:887–888.

16. Millard Dr, Rowe MI. Plastic surgical principles in high imperforate anus. Plast Reconstr Surg 1982;69:399–409.

17. Caouette-Laberge L, Yazbeck S, Laberge J-M, Ducharme J-C. Multiple-flap anoplasty in the treatment of rectal prolapse after pull-through operations for imperforate anus. J Pediatr Surg 1987;22:65–67.

18. Parks AG. Pathogenesis and treatment of fistula-in-ano. Br Med J 1961;5224:463–469.

19. Duhamel J. Anal fistulae in childhood. Am J Protocol 1975; 26:40–43.

20. Kleinhaus S. Rectum and anus: Miscellaneous anal disorders. In: Ravitch MM, Welch KJ, Bensen CD, et al, eds. Pediatric Surgery. Chicago: Year Book, 1975, pp 1078–1079.

21. Shafer AD, McGlone TP, Flanagan RA. Abnormal crypts of Morgagni: The cause of perianal abscess and fistula-in-ano. J Pediatr Surg 1987;22:203–204.

22. Fitzgerald RJ, Harding B, Ryan W. Fistula-in-ano in childhood: A congenital etilogy. J Pediatr Surg 1985;20:80–81.

23. Rehder PA, Eliezer ET, Lane AT. Perianal cellulitis: Cutaneous group A streptococcal disease. Arch Dermatol 1988;124:702–704.

24. Farmer G. Perianal infection with group A streptococcus. Arch Dis Child 1987;62:1169–1170.

25. Vellejos H, Del Mistro A, Kleinhaus S, et al. Characterization of human papilloma virus types in condylomata acuminata in children by situ hybridization. US Can Acad Pathol 1987;56:611.

26. Herman-Giddens MC, Gutman LT, Berson NL, The Duke Child Protection Team. Association of coexisting vaginal infections and multiple abusers in female children with genital warts. Sex Transm Dis 1988;15:63–67.

27. Laraque D. Severe anogenital warts in a child with HIV infection. N Engl J Med 1989;320:1220–1221.

28. Hayashi AH, Lau HYC, Gillis DA. Management of resistant peristomal and perineal excoriation with topical sucralfate. Presented at the Poster Session of the APSA Annual Meeting, May 19–22, 1990.

Tumors of the Perineum and Perirectal Region

C H A P T E R 2 4

Dennis W. Shermeta

The sacrococcygeal teratoma is the most common noninflammatory perineal tumor of the pediatric population. This rare tumor, also known as a sacrococcygeal germ cell tumor, leads a list of even rarer masses tabulated and referenced by Werner and Taybi (Table 24–1).[1]

Techniques for operative removal of the sacrococcygeal tumor would be applicable for most of the other unusual masses. A unique characteristic of the sacrococcygeal tumor is its gradual but inevitable conversion from a benign to a malignant form. This potentially lethal change requires urgent diagnosis and extirpation of the mass. To minimize the risk of malignant conversion and dissemination, early operation is performed on the very small pelvic and perineal structures of the neonate. Such surgery in the neonatal period is usually curative, but it unquestionably demands a total excision. The need for preservation of all non-neoplastic structures should be emphasized, because some of these structures provide the means for achieving future anorectal continence, a capability greatly valued by our society.

From 80% to 90% of all sacrococcygeal tumors are exophytic and easily diagnosed at the time of delivery (Fig. 24–1). As its name implies, this teratoma arises from the anlage of the coccyx. These tumors must arise early in the development of the fetus, because many grow to a size and weight that equal or exceed those of the fetus. Because of the tumor's massive size, it is necessary to be aware of the diagnosis prenatally. Fetal ultrasound and elevated alpha-fetoprotein from amniocentesis are diagnostic tools reliable in establishing early diagnosis. Planned delivery by cesarean section provides the least-traumatic route of presentation. The risk of vascular injury during vaginal delivery with subsequent near or complete exsanguination of the newborn establishes the cesarean section as the safest and most effective method of delivery.

Once an atraumatic delivery is accomplished, a period of stabilization in the neonatal intensive care unit is necessary. Lethal associated anomalies rarely occur; however, my experience includes one female infant with concomitant esophageal atresia and tracheoesoph-

Table 24–1. CLASSIFICATION OF PRESACRAL MASSES

I. Congenital	IV. Osteocartilaginous
1. Anterior meningocele	1. Aneurysmal bone cyst
2. Chordoma	2. Chondroma
3. Dermoid and developmental cysts	3. Chondrosarcoma
4. Ectopic kidney	4. Giant cell tumor
5. Hamartoma	5. Osteogenic sarcoma
6. Neurenteric cyst	6. Osteoma
7. Teratoma	V. Miscellaneous
II. Neurogenic	1. Fibroma
1. Ependymoma	2. Fibrosarcoma
2. Ganglioneuroma	3. Hemangioendothelioma
3. Neuroblastoma	4. Hematoma
4. Neurofibroma	5. Leiomyoma
5. Neurilemoma	6. Leiomyosarcoma
6. Neurinoma	7. Lipoma
7. Paraganglioma	8. Lymphoma
III. Inflammatory	9. Metastatic tumor
1. Abscess	10. Ovarian tumor
2. Granuloma	
3. Osteomyelitis of sacrum	
4. Ulcerative colitis	

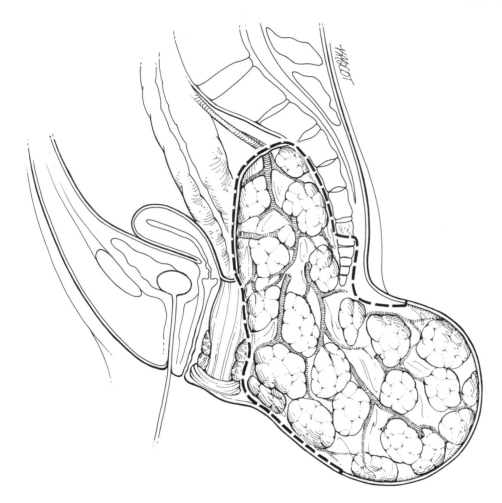

Figure 24–1. Schematic representation of typical exophytic sacrococcygeal teratoma in sagittal view with proposed plan of resection.

ageal fistula. The sacrococcygeal tumor was relatively small and, although diagnosed by prenatal ultrasound, was not considered a cause of the classic signs and symptoms of the esophageal atresia, which had been diagnosed preoperatively. Correction of the esophageal atresia and tracheoesophageal fistula preceded the removal of the sacrococcygeal tumor by 2 weeks. Other unrelated anomalies have been reported with sacrococcygeal tumors, and treatment for the life-threatening ones have routinely taken precedence.

In the intensive care setting, it is advisable to evaluate the hemodynamic status as well as hemoglobin and hematocrit levels. Some infants have an undetected hemorrhage of significant volume or a long-term hemoglobin depletion, both of which require resuscitation before operation. Because hemorrhage at the time of operation is the most commonly reported complication, it is good practice to begin the surgical procedure with a normal vascular volume.

An experience with a neonate whose exophytic tumor exceeded fetal weight illustrates an additional concern. This infant's lower extremities were scissored around the tumor mass and exhibited poor muscle tone. Following excision of the tumor, there was poor movement of both lower extremities as well as significant rectal prolapse. Diagnostic studies at 6 months, including magnetic resonance imaging, revealed a residual tumor mass in the region of the cauda equina that displaced the sacral nerve roots upward. Lumbosacral laminectomy allowed removal of a mature tumor mass, which appeared to have grown through the neural foramina. Total excision required sacrifice of a significant portion of the levator musculature. A piece of 1-mm Gore-Tex soft tissue patch was used for reconstruction. No further prolapse occurred.

The surgical procedure begins with a suitably warmed operating theater and a generous supply of type-specific cross-matched red blood cells. A central venous catheter should be placed with at least one additional peripheral conduit. A urinary catheter and nasogastric tube are also utilized. Following the induction of general anesthesia, the endotracheal tube should be firmly affixed to the infant's head. This step is taken in preparation for placing the infant in a prone position, with rolls under the chest and abdomen. Large sacrococcygeal tumors are best positioned by assigning one assistant the task of keeping the tumor mass in an upright and central location (Fig. 24–2).

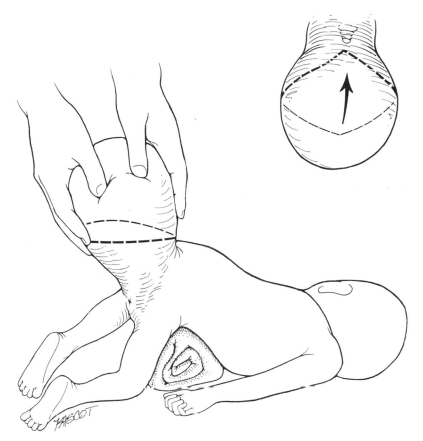

Figure 24–2. Ideal line of resection with retained skin sufficient to close defect after resection of tumor mass.

Waterproof drapes are placed around the field to prevent fluids from soaking beneath the patient and contributing to hypothermia. The skin incisions are outlined in ink; the resultant skin flaps are usually elevated by the bulk of tumor, and generous skin flaps facilitate the eventual closure.

Once the skin is incised, the tumor is usually encountered immediately. Most sacrococcygeal tumors are a conglomerate of multiple masses—some cystic, others solid. In order to preserve pelvic muscles, it is necessary to dissect in the interface between tumor and muscle. The dissection is initially done circumferentially, but as soon as possible, the dissection at the cephalic side of the field should be deepened to allow exposure of the coccyx and distal sacrum. The sacrococcygeal junction is carefully divided to allow identification and double ligation of the middle sacral artery and vein, directly beneath the transected coccyx (Fig. 24–3). Once these vessels are ligated, most of the remaining dissection should cause little blood loss.

An exception to this procedure occurs in the older patient whose tumor has spread to occupy most of the pelvis or has undergone malignant degeneration. Such tumors are usually friable, necrotic, and infiltrating. Devascularization of such a pelvic mass may require initial bilateral suprainguinal incisions for retroperitoneal exposure and ligation of the internal iliac arteries.

Vascular control can be life-saving and in these circumstances should be achieved before the pelvic dissection is initiated.

By using the coccyx as a handle, one can slowly and meticulously elevate the remainder of the tumor from the pelvis. Particular care is taken to prevent breaking any of the cystic nodules. If a nodule is punctured, the probability of leaving behind a small portion of the wall is greatly increased, which leads inevitably to recurrence.

Because the sacrococcygeal tumor begins at the coccyx, it grows outward laterally beneath the gluteal musculature, stopping on either side at the ischial tuberosity. The outward growth of tumor mass causes significant stretching and thinning of the gluteal muscles. The thin layer of tissue that separates the muscle from the tumor must be preserved by careful dissection.

Perhaps the most important structure that is almost totally destroyed by the larger tumors is the pubococcygeal ligament. When the deeper muscles of anorectal continence alter the rectal angle, this structure provides support for the musculature and maintains alignment of the external anal orifice (Fig. 24–4). During dissection, the ligament should be recognized and tagged for subsequent reattachment to the periosteum of the sacrum. Failure to reconstruct this posterior anchor

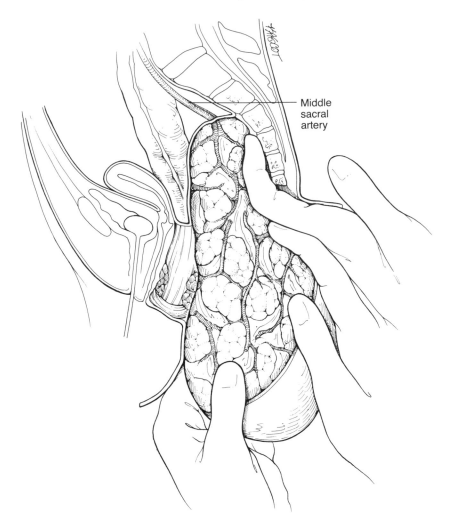

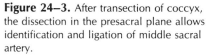

Figure 24–3. After transection of coccyx, the dissection in the presacral plane allows identification and ligation of middle sacral artery.

point can lead to significant constipation in later life from anterior displacement of the anorectal orifice.

Dissection of the tumor from its anterior boundary should be performed only after identification of the position of the thickened rectal muscle wall, which represents the puborectal muscle and the thin posterior wall of the rectum itself. The rectum is frequently compressed forward by the tumor mass to such a degree that it does not admit the fifth finger. Lateral release of the tumor attachments allows forward displacement of the tumor mass and facilitates insertion of the fifth finger into the rectum. With this finger in the rectum, the tumor may be easily and safely removed, regardless of lateral displacement caused by tumor growth. In addition, identification of the rectum with respect to the tumor protects the vagina, in the female, and the urethra, in the male, against injury.

The final and often most difficult part of the dissection is the upward extension into the presacral space. The tumor may extend well above the limits of the true pelvis, displacing the peritoneal reflection upward and the bladder anteriorly. These displacements may expose the ureters to potential injury. Once the tumor has been circumferentially freed from all structures in the perineum, downward traction usually allows blunt separation from the peritoneum superiorly. This is a crucial part of the surgical dissection, because much of it is done blindly by the surgeon's finger. Great care must be exercised to ensure that no small remnant of tumor remains. If there is any question about maintaining continuity in the dissection, a heavy silk suture should be placed at that point and the remainder of the tumor resected. After the perineal wound is closed, the patient should be turned to a supine position and the pelvic area explored from above, locating the marking suture and excising residual tumor to complete the total resection.

Closure of the perineal wound follows a three-step procedure. First, the levator ani muscle is loosely joined in the midline to reconstruct the floor of the pelvis. Second, reconstruction or, if necessary, fabrication of the anococcygeal raphe or ligament, as pre-

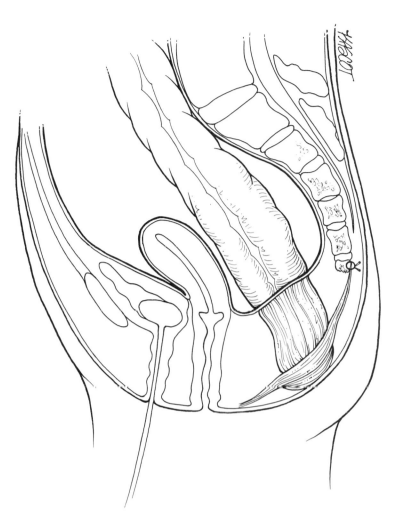

Figure 24–4. After removal of the tumor mass the structures of the pelvis and perineum should be allowed to assume the normal position. The posterior attachment of the anorectal canal must be reconstructed with a suture.

viously described, is completed. Third, the skin flaps are loosely applied in an inverted V configuration. Drainage is not necessary in a dry field, although oozing from raw muscle edges may mandate some form of drainage of the newly created ischiorectal space. Adjuvant treatment with broad-spectrum antibiotics is routinely utilized in both the neonate and the older infant or child.

If entry into the rectum occurs during the dissection, a proximal diverting colostomy should be carried out after the tumor resection is completed. This ensures proper healing of the pelvic soft tissue and anorectal canal.

The results, even for infants born with gigantic sacrococcygeal tumors, have been uniformly gratifying both cosmetically and functionally. Anorectal continence is present in all patients by their third or fourth year. Follow-up in my series, as well as in several published reports,[2, 3] indicates an excellent disease-free state for most infants with mature teratomas. Infants with immature histologic components have a recurrence rate between 15% and 30%.

In addition to resection, tumors of the embryonal carcinoma variety have been aggressively treated with radiotherapy and chemotherapy. Vincristine, actinomycin D, cytotoxin, and newer antisarcoma drugs have been given in large doses. Such aggressive multimodal therapy has resulted in improved long-term disease-free states.

The analysis of current and future multimodality therapies is beyond the scope of this chapter. By following the guidelines outlined here, resection remains the primary therapeutic modality to ensure total removal of the tumor and coccyx.

REFERENCES

1. Werner JL, Taybi H. Presacral masses in childhood. Am J Roentgenol 1970;109:403–410.
2. Altman RP, Randolph JG, Lilly JR. Sacrococcygeal teratoma: American Academy of Pediatrics Surgical Section Survey—1973. J Pediatr Surg 1974;9:389–398.
3. Noseworthy J, Lack EE, Kozakewich HPW, et al. Sacrococcygeal germ cell tumors in childhood: An updated experience with 118 patients. J Pediatr Surg 1981;16:358–364.

SECTION VI

LAPAROSCOPY

Laparoscopy for the Diagnosis and Treatment of Diseases of the Colon and Rectum

C H A P T E R   2 5

Jonathan M. Sackier

The enthusiasm that accompanied the introduction of laparoscopic cholecystectomy has led to the application of this endoscopic approach to many other surgical conditions. Not the least of these are the diseases affecting the large bowel. This chapter includes a discussion of laparoscopy of the appendix as well as of the colon and rectum.

To the casual observer it would seem that laparoscopy was comparatively new to the surgical community. However, the first laparoscopy—or celioscopy, as it was originally known—was performed almost simultaneously at the beginning of the twentieth century by Ott in Petrograd[1] and Kelling in Dresden.[2] These procedures were carried out in animals, and it was Jacobaeus in Stockholm who carried out the first human operation.[3] The German hepatologist Kalk conceived the dual trocar technique, which allowed for the introduction of other instruments. Kalk also described the laparoscopic appearance of liver disease.[4]

A number of technical innovations were required in order to advance laparoscopy to its current status. These include the introduction of carbon dioxide as the insufflation agent by Fervers in 1933,[5] the design of the hollow sprung needle (initially for pneumothorax) by Janos Veress of Hungary in 1938,[6] and the development of the Hopkins Rod Lens system in London in the 1960s.[7]

An American surgeon, Ruddock, initially popularized laparoscopy, but his enthusiasm for the technique was not shared by others.[8] Berci and Cuschieri declared the method to be of value to practicing surgeons, but they too were largely ignored.[9]

Operative laparoscopy owes much to gynecologists Patrick Steptoe in England[10] and Kurt Semm in Germany,[11] who greatly advanced the technique. Surgeons were more amenable to video laparoscopy, when it was introduced, because it eliminated the discomfort of working through a monocular eyepiece.

Laparoscopic cholecystectomy was probably first performed in the experimental model by Cuschieri in swine[12] or Filipi in dogs.[13] The first clinical cases may well have been performed by Phillipe Mouret of Lyon, France,[14] although Muhe from Germany has claimed this honor.[15] Many reports rapidly ensued, and numerous surgeons were soon practicing the technique.[16–19]

General surgeons practicing therapeutic laparoscopy soon began to focus less on only the gallbladder fossa and more on treating common bile duct stones,[20, 21] coping with perforated duodenal ulcers,[22] and treating peptic ulcer disease in the elective setting.[23] Laparoscopic appendectomy had already been described,[24] but it had not gained popularity because surgeons—who remove most appendices—were not performing laparoscopy routinely.

Apocryphal reports circulated a wide range of other procedures carried out by the minimally invasive technique. After 1991, reports appeared in the peer-reviewed medical literature.

This chapter details the basic techniques and equipment required for laparoscopic colon and rectal surgery, addresses issues of training, and covers the role of laparoscopy for diagnostic as well as therapeutic purposes. Finally a number of concerns about the procedure are discussed.

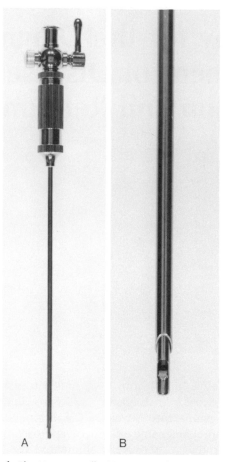

A　　　B

Figure 25–1. The Veress needle *(A)* consists of a sprung hollow, blunt, inner obturator held *(B)* within a sharp trocar.

BASIC TECHNIQUES AND INSTRUMENTATION

In order to perform any laparoscopic operation, it is vital to create a "working space." The formation of this pneumoperitoneum is one of the most important steps of the operation. There are basically two techniques: the Veress needle, or closed, induction and the Hasson, or open, technique.

Veress Needle, or Closed, Induction

In the Veress needle induction, a small incision is made at the site of election, the abdominal wall is raised, and the abdominal wall is punctured with the needle (Fig. 25–1). The blunt inner cannula springs back out of the trocar once a space—ideally the peritoneum—has been entered. The usual site of entrance of this needle is below the umbilicus, because it is the thinnest part of the abdominal wall, where all layers are in close apposition. If the presence of a scar suggests adhesions, either iliac fossa at the lateral border of the rectus abdominis or hypochondrium is chosen.

Once the needle is positioned, saline should be injected slowly and aspirated at least twice. If the needle is in the peritoneal cavity, the saline will enter easily and nothing should be aspirated. If the needle is in a blood vessel its position should be changed, because to insufflate in this position risks a fatality. If intestinal content is retrieved, the needle should be repositioned, the laparoscopy continued, and the damage assessed. Saline retrieval implies that the needle is in the preperitoneal space, and, once again, it should be reintroduced. The position of the needle can be confirmed by performing the "hanging drop test," in which a drop of saline is placed at the top of the needle, the abdominal wall is raised, and the saline is seen to fall into the abdomen with respiration.

Hasson, or Open Laparoscopy, Technique

Some perform the Hasson technique routinely, maintaining that it is safer than the needle technique; however, if all the safety measures already described are followed, and if the clinician is experienced, this is probably not the case. I prefer to use this technique selectively when (a) the history, examination, or investigation suggests the presence of intra-abdominal adhesions; (b) the Veress needle introduction has been attempted and has failed; or (c) the patient has a para-umbilical hernia that requires simultaneous repair. Here, a small infra-umbilical incision, either vertical or para-umbilical, is made, and the linea alba is isolated between two stay sutures. A blunt-tipped trocar is introduced after the peritoneum has been incised and is secured with the two suture "wings" on the device (Fig. 25–2). Insufflation begins directly through the cannula with no need for a Veress needle.

Insufflator

Therapeutic laparoscopy requires high-flow insufflators capable of maintaining a pneumoperitoneum with rates up to 10 l/min. These devices have a number of controls that include a display demonstrating volume of gas available, a flow rate adjustment, a preset pressure adjustment, a current pressure, and an indicator of volume infused (Fig. 25–3). It is usual to establish an operating pressure of around 15 mm Hg. Once this pressure has been reached insufflation ceases; it starts again only when pressure is lost through exchange of instruments, absorption of gas, or introduction of other trocars.

Initially, the flow rate should not exceed 1.5 l/min; a higher rate increases the risk of diaphragmatic rupture[26] and cardiac dysrhythmia. If the needle has been misplaced inside a blood vessel, the lower flow rate gives the anesthesiologist an opportunity to detect the rising arterial carbon dioxide tension (PCO_2) and to alert the surgeon.[27] One is able to infuse possibly up to 3 l/min through a Veress needle. At these high flow rates, death may ensue before one has an opportunity to correct the situation.

One should be familiar with the technique of changing gas tanks from the back of the insufflator and replacing faulty gaskets. In preparation, a wrench, spare cylinder, and gasket should always be available in the operating room.

There has been much discussion about the choice of insufflating gas, and most investigators agree that air is no longer suitable. Carbon dioxide is ideal because it does not support combustion, is readily available, and is inexpensive. However, there are drawbacks to carbon dioxide because it lowers the pH and arterial oxygen tension (PO_2) and raises PCO_2. The anesthesiologist should be aware of the chosen gas and should make the necessary adjustment to ventilatory parameters. The laparoscopist should be alert to the fact that carbon dioxide causes vasodilatation, which may mimic peritonitis and may be severe enough to cause vascular collapse.

Research on the use of inert gases, such as helium, is progressing.[28] It will be of interest to learn whether they confer any advantages. Because of concerns about the effects of gases, a number of authors have proposed a mechanical U-shaped device, which is passed in and out of the abdomen after initial pneumoperitoneum

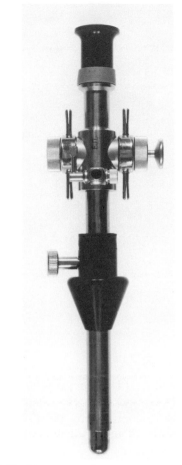

Figure 25–2. The Hasson open laparoscopy cannula. The gas-seal olive, suture wings, and blunt obturator are demonstrated.

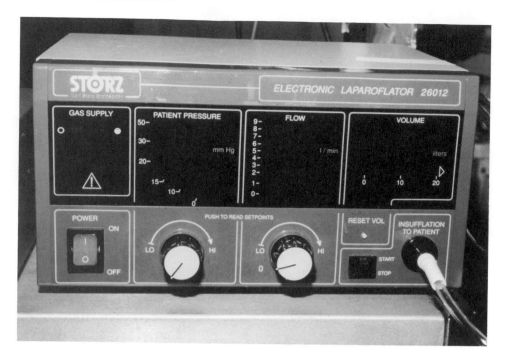

Figure 25–3. The insufflator has gauges for preset pressure, flow rate, and volume of infused gas.

has been induced.[29, 30] This device totally replaces the pneumoperitoneum and also acts as an exhaust mechanism for smoke generated by the dissecting equipment. The passage of time will demonstrate whether this is a true advance.

Trocar

The word "trocar" is derived from the French meaning, literally, "three-sided," and to be punctilious one would apply the word only to the sharp inner part of the trocar-cannula assembly. The cannula is the hollow tube through which instruments are then introduced. However, in common parlance trocar has come to mean the entire assembly. These are available in both reusable and disposable forms and in a variety of sizes. The most commonly used trocars are sizes 10 to 11 mm, which accommodate the telescope and large instruments, and size 5 mm for grasping instruments.

One must ensure that reusable trocars have been sharpened before each use, because sharpness limits the amount of force required to introduce the trocar.[31] Undoubtedly, the most important aspect of trocar introduction is attention to detail: the trocar tip should not be directed toward the aorta, and two hands should be used, one ensuring that the trocar cannula assembly is not inadvertently advanced too far.

Telescope

For most purposes the 10-mm Hopkins Rod Lens system telescope is ideal. The 30-degree forward oblique viewing scope is advantageous in that it provides five different views of the structure: straight on, from the right and left, and from above and below. Before the telescope is introduced, the light source and camera should be attached, and the lens should be treated to prevent fogging due to condensation. One may apply an antifogging agent or heat the telescope to above body temperature.

Light Source

The light source should be a 300-watt xenon variety, and it is misleadingly called a "cold" light source. It is vital, when the light source is attached to the telescope outside the body, that it not be permitted to rest on the sterile field, for the heat may ignite paper drapes. The cables that attach the light source to the telescope are of two types: fluid- and fiber-filled. The former are preferable because they transmit about 30% more light, leading to a higher-quality image.

Camera

The available cameras are either single-chip, with a daisy wheel to provide a color image, or triple-chip, with one pixel for each primary color. All have a focusing ring and a ring for attachment to the telescope, and some have a "zoom," which merely limits the size of the image, hence magnifying it. Some camera control units are equipped with an automatic iris, which prevents the problem of glare when the telescope is brought too close to the part of the anatomy under consideration. All have a system of "white balancing," whereby the camera is programmed to "recognize" white. Any discrepancy in the color balance on the screen should be adjusted at the television in order to give a true representation.

Accessory Trocars

Once the telescope has been introduced and a diagnostic laparoscopy has been performed, it is necessary to introduce additional trocars. First, one should choose the appropriate site. Ideally, this is at a 90-degree angle to the line of sight between the telescope and the object under consideration. Bringing instruments toward the camera generates problems with depth of field, and if instruments are brought into the abdomen parallel with the camera, the tips will not be visible and the surgeon will tend to "sword fight" with the laparoscope. One should also ensure that the point of insertion is neither too far away, meaning that the instrument will not reach the site, nor too close, as the trocar will interfere with the action of the tip of the instrument. Having decided on the ideal position, the surgeon must ensure that no vital viscera underlie the point of insertion and that there are no large vessels in the abdominal wall, which may be demonstrated by transillumination. All accessory trocars must always be brought into the abdomen under direct vision; a visceral or vascular injury at this point is preventable. In order to help maintain a constant pneumoperitoneum, it is useful to bifurcate the gas line and thereby attach a second tube to one of the accessory cannulas. This is necessary during long procedures.

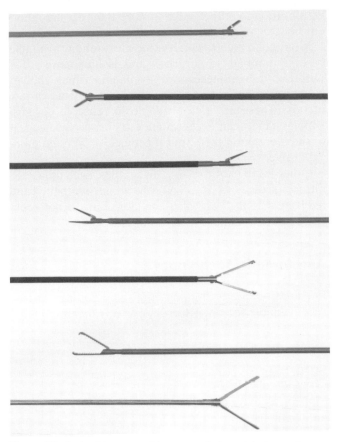

Figure 25–4. A wide range of laparoscopic bowel instruments are available, including needle holders, bowel clamps, and grasping forceps.

Accessory Instruments

The wide range of available instruments includes toothed and nontoothed, and locking and nonlocking graspers. For intestinal surgery, bowel clamps are required and are available with well-known formats, including Allis, Babcock, and Glassman tips. Needle holders are available in the 5- and 3-mm sizes with either right-angle or coaxial design (Fig. 25–4). Devices for placing a pursestring suture include the modified Judd forceps[32] and specially designed appliers,[33] which are far less time-consuming than hand-suturing.

Energy Sources

Much attention has been paid to methods of dividing tissue in the laparoscopic cholecystectomy literature. Again, knowledge of the technology and attention to detail probably affect success more than do any inherent benefits or faults of the system.

Monopolar electrocautery, the most readily available type, is familiar to surgeons and is inexpensive.[34, 35] Disposable handpieces are available, which deliver irrigation, suction, and coagulation with a wide variety of tips. These are also available in reusable designs. Bipolar electrocautery is said not to possess the dangers of the monopolar form, but it is much slower and more expensive.[36]

Other more exotic dissection sources, such as laser,[37] ultrasonic dissector (CUSA),[38] harmonic scalpels,[39] and hydrodissection,[40] are also available but do not seem to possess any inherent advantages.

Anastomotic Techniques

For anastomotic techniques, the same equipment that was available for open surgery has now been modified for laparoscopy.

Suturing

Suturing is extremely demanding of the surgeon's time and patience and requires a high degree of skill and dedication.[41, 42] A high level of coordination is required to "choreograph" the hand movements. Needle design is a key consideration, and the ski-shaped needles are my preference.

Stapling

End-to-end stapling devices have been implemented laparoscopically, and the linear stapler-cutter has been developed in 30- and 60-mm forms. Clip appliers have been fashioned in either single-shot reusable form with metal or absorbable clips or disposable form with metal clips.

Biofragmentable Anastomotic Ring

The biofragmentable anastomotic ring, a modification of the Murphy Button, has been covered elsewhere in this volume.[43, 44] A delivery system has been modified for application to laparoscopic surgery.[45]

Other modalities, such as tissue glues[46] and laser welding,[47] may eventually be used in laparoscopic colon surgery.

Documentation

It is essential to document laparoscopic operations for the purpose of teaching residents and colleagues and for presentation at scientific meetings, especially in the early days of the technique. Additionally, medicolegal issues make documentation necessary. It is valuable for surgeons to review their operations and to learn from the experience.

The choice of video format is based on personal preference and is dictated by the intended use of the videotape. The $\frac{3}{4}$-inch U-matic provides the best image quality and allows for later editing, but the tape is large and expensive. The standard VHS format is more readily available but is also bulky to store. The smaller 8-mm cassettes provide excellent image quality and solve the problem of storage.

Static images may be captured in a variety of fashions, but undoubtedly the best quality is achieved by placing a 35-mm single-lens reflex camera on the end of the telescope; this is time-consuming and increases the peril of breaking the sterile field. The Mavigraph System (Sony Corporation, Park Ridge, New Jersey) directly produces Polaroid images from the video screen and makes a valuable addition to the patient's chart and for the referring physician. A number of digital capture units are available but costly, although the quality of the images is superb. The choice of equipment is mitigated by the surgeon's requirements, regardless of whether they are merely for the case sheet or for future publications and lectures.

TRAINING

Until all laparoscopic procedures become common practice and part of residency programs, a knowledge deficit will continue to exist, which necessitates specially designed training modules.[48] Laparoscopic colonic procedures require more technical ability than does cholecystectomy, and it is to be hoped that no surgeon would embark on an operation before being confident of performing it safely and efficaciously. The spectrum of training that was available for laparoscopic cholecystectomy in the past illuminates the training for these more complex operations.

Some surgeons believed that a one-day course in cholecystectomy on one rabbit constituted full and proper training for extracting a human gallbladder under laparoscopic guidance. Other courses were more stringent. They recommended carrying out at least two laparoscopic cholecystectomies in the porcine model, working as first operator in a group of three. One performed at least two more procedures as first assistant and as camera operator.[49] This by no means represented the beginning or end of training. The sensible surgeon would first become experienced with diagnostic laparoscopy, take a course, continue working in the experimental laboratory, hone technical skills, and rely on a skilled laparoscopic cholecystectomy surgeon to assist and proctor during the first few cases.[50] Continuous peer review is a vital component of any laparoscopic program, so that problems may be immediately identified and corrected.

The efforts of the American Society of Colon and Rectal Surgeons[51] and the Society of American Gastrointestinal Endoscopic Surgeons (SAGES) are to be commended.[52] These two societies have initiated registers that will doubtless yield valuable data in matters affecting patient safety.

For the surgeon who wishes to advance from cholecystectomy to the more complex operations, the porcine model will be found to be unsuitable, as the pig has a spiral colon that renders dissection difficult.[53] However, the small intestine can be used to practice suturing and stapling. For the purpose of learning colon anastomosis, the canine model is preferred, although the freely mobile nature of the mesentery reduces the challenge of its resection.[54]

PATIENT PREPARATION

Merely changing the route of entry into the abdominal cavity does not alter the preoperative workup—if anything, it is more thorough than for conventional surgery. First, the patient should be fully informed about the nature of the laparoscopic intervention and should be involved in a full and frank discussion of the additional risks, although in competent hands they are extremely small.[55] The consent form should always include the open alternative to laparoscopy, because conversion is sometimes required, especially with more complex operations.

When taking the patient's history, one should note any cardiorespiratory problems, as these may influence the safety of pneumoperitoneum. The patient should also be asked about previous operations as a clue to intra-abdominal adhesions, which, as previously mentioned, influence the placement of cannulas. If the patient has a history strongly suggestive of hiatal hernia, this should be investigated. Similarly, if the patient has a history of an inguinal hernia, special attention should be directed toward the groins during the examination. Taking drugs that may interfere with coagulation, such as aspirin, should be noted, because hemorrhage is more difficult to control laparoscopically.

Obviously, a thorough physical examination is vital. The position of scars should be noted to ensure that they correspond to the patient's history. If an indirect inguinal hernia is present, it should be protected perioperatively with a truss to avoid the embarrassing complication of scrotal emphysema. It is now possible to perform inguinal herniorrhaphy under laparoscopic visualization,[56] although this procedure remains investigational, and one would not wish to place prosthetic material in the peritoneal cavity while performing an open colonic procedure. The patient's umbilicus should be checked for hernia, which could be repaired at the time of laparoscopy. If organomegaly exists, one should mark the position of the enlarged organ on the abdomen with a felt-tip pen before the operation in order to avoid accidental puncture with the Veress needle or trocar.

Investigations will include the routine preoperative workup, and a coagulation profile should always be performed. Additional cardiorespiratory evaluations may be performed as indicated by the patient's history and examination. If the patient does have a history strongly suggestive of a hiatal hernia, gastroscopy should be considered to confirm or refute the diagnosis. A hiatal hernia may represent a threat to respiratory status during induction of pneumoperitoneum, and the surgeon should be aware of this situation. If the patient does have abdominal scars and ultrasound is indicated for another reason, it may be worthwhile to employ the technique of adhesion mapping described by Siegel et al.[57] Adhesion mapping is based on the observation that the viscera will slide with respiration relative to the abdominal wall, and the technique will help the surgeon locate, and thereby avoid, adherent loops of bowel.

The final preparations for the operation are much like those for an open operation with a few important additions. The raised intra-abdominal pressure impedes venous return, thereby increasing the likelihood of deep venous thrombosis. For this reason I routinely use sequential compression stockings, and they should be applied before the operation begins. Because of the risks of gastric and bladder puncture, it is wise to decompress these organs with nasogastric and Foley catheters, which may be removed at the end of the operation. Antibiotics are administered as indicated for open operation.

DIAGNOSTIC LAPAROSCOPY

Diagnostic laparoscopy may conveniently be divided into elective and emergency situations as they pertain to the large bowel.

Elective Laparoscopy

Oncology

Laparoscopy is a valuable adjunct in the assessment of the patient with cancer.[58] The technique has several functions:

1. It can be employed for the initial diagnosis and to stage the case, at which time biopsies may be taken from the serosa of the bowel, omentum, and liver.

2. It can be used to plan operative therapy by detecting unsuspected widespread metastases, which may alter the surgical approach (see further on). Definitive procedures can also be carried out with the laparoscope.

3. It can aid in follow-up of patients after chemotherapy, immunotherapy, and other adjunctive treatments.[59] At this time a "second-look" laparoscopy may be performed with peritoneal washings as well as biopsies.

4. It can be used to investigate the patient with a rising carcinoembryonic antigen (CEA) who has no demonstrable radiographic evidence of recurrence. Often such patients have widespread peritoneal carcinomatosis, which is easily seen with a laparoscope.

Abdominal Pain

Patients often will present with chronic abdominal pain with a history suggestive of a colonic origin. The possible diagnoses are endometriosis and congenital adhesive bands. Both are amenable to laparoscopically assisted treatment.

Inflammatory Bowel Disease

Laparoscopy may be utilized to gauge the extent of Crohn's disease or ulcerative colitis, and a suitable stoma site may be selected during the procedure. This obviously avoids a major laparotomy incision in this unfortunate group of patients. It has been suggested that laparoscopy leads to fewer adhesions,[60] which is a benefit to these patients, who often will have multiple operations throughout their lives.

Emergency Laparoscopy

Trauma

Laparoscopy has been helpful in the evaluation of blunt and penetrating abdominal trauma.[61–64] In blunt trauma it may be an alternative to diagnostic peritoneal lavage and computed tomography (CT) and may have advantages over both, in that if blood is seen in the peritoneal cavity, one can assess whether the source of hemorrhage is ongoing. In deceleration accidents, mesenteric tears are sometimes seen and may be fully assessed with the laparoscope.

For penetrating trauma, one can assess with the laparoscope whether a knife has penetrated the peritoneum when concern exists about colonic puncture. Laparoscopy to investigate gunshot wounds is less obvious and is probably limited to small-caliber weapons in obese patients when the entrance and exit wounds suggest an oblique extraperitoneal path.[65] Occasionally with rectal foreign bodies, it is necessary to perform abdominal manipulation, and the laparoscope allows the surgeon to assess whether the foreign body has penetrated the serosal surface and whether such manipulations may be feasible, thereby avoiding laparotomy.

Diverticulitis

By using the classification developed by Hinchey and associates it is possible to identify cases of peridiverticulitis in which the disease does not communicate with the remainder of the peritoneal cavity.[66] These patients do not require emergency operations, although if the abscess bursts mere drainage may suffice. As is discussed further on, therapeutic options are feasible in these situations.

Obstruction

In many situations obstruction would be deemed a contraindication to laparoscopy, because the distended loops of bowel may make the examination difficult. However, for the experienced laparoscopist, and in carefully selected patients, it may prove to be of value. In one such situation, the patient with volvulus may be decompressed colonoscopically, the diagnosis confirmed laparoscopically, and the treatment effected at the same time.

Right Iliac Fossa Pain

There is often a dilemma in diagnosis of young women who present with right iliac fossa pain with suspected acute appendicitis.[67] If laparotomy is performed and the cause is found to be pelvic inflammatory disease, an unnecessary incision has been made without benefit to the patient; the procedure will lead to the formation of adhesions that may adversely affect fertility. However, foregoing operation in the presence of an inflamed appendix is also deleterious. Diagnostic laparoscopy enables the surgeon to obtain an early diagnosis and to undertake therapy. In the presence of pelvic inflammatory disease, swabs for culture may be retrieved and copious lavage carried out. Managing the inflamed appendix laparoscopically is discussed further on.

THERAPEUTIC LAPAROSCOPY

Laparoscopic Appendectomy

This procedure was first carried out in the early 1980s by Kurt Semm,[24] but for the reasons noted in the introduction to this chapter, it did not receive wide popularity. More recent series have demonstrated that it is valuable in treating pregnant patients (in whom diagnosis is often difficult)[68] and children[69]—indeed, in treating patients in all groups.[70] The results must be critically evaluated, because the benefits are not as clearly apparent as those for laparoscopic cholecystectomy.

Probably laparoscopic appendectomy is most valuable in the young female patient who presents with abdominal pain of which the diagnosis is in doubt. If an inflamed appendix is seen at laparoscopy, removal is appropriate. If pelvic inflammatory disease is noted, it is wise to leave the appendix alone and thereby to avoid adding enteric bacteria to the flora. If a normal appendix is seen and no other abnormality is noted, the same philosophy that would apply in the presence of a Lanz or gridiron incision results: to remove the appendix.

Technique

For laparoscopic appendectomy, the patient is placed supine on the operating table. The surgeon stands to the patient's left, and a monitor is placed at the patient's right. After induction of the pneumoperitoneum and insertion of an 11-mm trocar at the umbilicus, further working trocars are introduced: one in the left iliac fossa and another in the right hypochondrium. After a general laparoscopy is performed and the diagnosis confirmed, the appendix is elevated with an atraumatic grasping forceps through one of the accessory trocars. The mesentery may be secured with bipolar electrocautery, laser, clips, intracorporeal or extracorporeal ties, or the linear stapler-cutter.

Especially in patients in whom the tip of the appendix is necrotic, it is helpful to apply a pre-tied Roeder loop to the tip of the appendix and to use this as a grasper. The base of the appendix may be secured with two more loops, and one other loop is applied on the side to be removed. Alternatively, the linear stapler-cutter may be employed, but a 12-mm trocar is needed in the right hypochondrial position to accommodate it.

The base of the appendix should not be fulgurated with electrocautery, for to do so risks transmission of the current into the narrowed areas, where clips or loops are present, which may lead to their falling off. It is not necessary to invert the stump, as was clearly demonstrated with open appendectomy.[71] The retrieved appendix may be brought out in the 5-mm reducer (appendix extractor) or placed in a plastic bag to prevent contamination of the abdominal wall. Copious lavage should be done, and the irrigant and purulent material should be sucked out. All cannulas should be removed and the pneumoperitoneum released; the operating room team members take care not to breathe in this potentially particle-laden gas, by using the suction tube to collect it. The abdominal wall is closed in layers, the Foley catheter and nasogastric tube removed, and the patient treated as for open appendectomy.

RECTOPEXY

Rectopexy has been discussed in detail elsewhere in the book, and only the points of relevance to the laparoscopic approach are discussed here. The surgeon works from both left and right sides of the patient, and the television screen should be placed at the patient's feet, thereby ensuring that the surgeon's eyes and hands, the organ under consideration, and the television screen are all in one line of sight. The laparoscope is placed through an umbilical portal, and accessory trocars are introduced, one in each iliac fossa. With electrocautery the peritoneum is scored over the rectum and down each side of the sacrum. By using a combination of electrocautery, clips, scissors, and blunt dissection, the plane between the rectum and sacrum is developed. Rectopexy may be performed with either sutures or prosthetic material, according to the techniques described by Ripstein,[72] or in Britain, by means of the Ivalon sponge technique proposed by Wells.[73]

It seems likely that this operation will be a valuable addition to the surgeon's armamentarium for managing the elderly patient with prolapse of the rectum.

CECOPEXY

Cecopexy was alluded to earlier, in the discussion of diagnosis. Cecal volvulus is a challenging problem, and its management has been the subject of much debate.[74-76] By means of the laparoscopic approach, it is possible to fashion a cecostomy, for which it is an improvement over blind percutaneous introduction, to fix the cecum with a series of sutures from the taenia coli to the parietal peritoneum,[77] or to resect the right colon. This is covered further on.

In order to carry out cecopexy, it is vital to learn techniques of laparoscopic suturing for tying either intracorporeal or extracorporeal knots.[41, 42]

STOMA

An ileostomy or colostomy may be fashioned with the laparoscope.[78] It is beyond the scope of this chapter to give an exhaustive description of the indications for either procedure, and only laparoscopic techniques are given.

Ileostomy

After the laparoscopy is completed with the telescope in the umbilical position, the site of election for ileostomy is chosen, probably in the right iliac fossa. A 5-mm trocar is introduced in the right hypochondrium, and another at the putative site of the stoma. Bowel-grasping forceps introduced through the hypochondrial and iliac cannulas are used to select the appropriate loop of bowel. The peritoneum is scored with scissors, if necessary, to provide mobility. The mesentery may be incised and a cotton tape passed into the abdomen through the iliac fossa portal, looping the bowel and thereby allowing it to be withdrawn through the incision, where it is secured to the skin in the usual fashion. With the laparoscope, one may survey the internal aspect of the stoma to check for the correct position and to arrest any hemorrhage.

Colostomy

The same techniques utilized for ileostomy are appropriate here. However, a large 20-mm-diameter trocar-cannula provides an excellent route for bringing either a loop stoma or an end-stoma to the skin. In the loop stoma, a rubber drain is passed into the abdomen and used to retract the prepared loop.

COLON RESECTION

Broadly speaking, there are two types of operations: laparoscopy-assisted colectomy[79] and total laparoscopic colectomy.[80] In the former, the mobilization is performed under laparoscopic visualization, and the prepared specimen is brought out through a small incision, for resection and anastomosis. The laparoscope can thus be used for final inspection of the abdomen, and it minimizes manipulation with the peritoneal cavity exposed. In total laparoscopic colectomy, the specimen is withdrawn through the anus; this is feasible only for low left-sided resections.

As for the other procedures, only aspects that are different from open surgery are detailed here. The surgeon's eyes and hands, the lesion, and the television screen must all be in a straight line. For a right-sided lesion, therefore, the surgeon stands to the patient's left and the television screen is on the patient's right side; the reverse is true for a left-sided resection. The patient should be in the lithotomy position to allow passage of a colonoscope that will aid in the localization of small mucosal lesions.

The general principle is the same as that for open resection. The proximal and distal points of the resection are chosen. The serosa of the bowel is scored or its position marked with a tape passed through the mesentery and around the bowel. This has the advantage of simultaneously providing retraction and occluding the bowel. Alternatively, the bowel may be immediately transected at this juncture with the linear stapler-cutter. For malignant lesions, it is necessary to follow the mesentery down to the origin of the feeding vessels. At this time it is vital, as in open surgery, to note the position of the ureters. This is more difficult in the laparoscopic operation, so it is useful to pass a lighted ureter probe with the aid of a cystoscope at the beginning of the operation.[81]

By turning down the laparoscope light, one can clearly see the position of the ureter. Occasionally, it may prove difficult to note the location of vessels in the mesentery, and there are two techniques to assist in this stage of the operation. A laparoscopic Doppler probe may be used to "hear" the blood flow. Alternatively, another laparoscope may be introduced through a more lateral cannula to transilluminate the mesentery.

Mesenteric vessels can be occluded with clips or with intracorporeal or extracorporeal ties. I find the latter preferable, as it is possible to assess with much more confidence the security of the knot one ties. In the laparoscopically assisted operation the anastomosis will be fashioned outside the abdomen and the mesenteric defect closed. After the bowel is returned to the abdomen, a final laparoscopic surveillance is carried out. Currently, this is the only effective way to perform right hemicolectomy. For left-sided operations, if the bowel has been stapled across, in order to retrieve the specimen one may make a small incision in the left flank or one may excise the staple line from the rectum and pass an instrument through the anus to retrieve the resected bowel. A plastic bag to hold the specimen prevents seeding. One would think that an open rectum would lead to immediate loss of pneumoperitoneum, but this is not the case, as the pressure seems to keep the bowel together until the specimen has been withdrawn. At withdrawal there is some loss of pneumoperitoneum, but this is quickly re-established.

In order to effect the colorectal anastomosis if the linear stapler-cutter has been implemented, an end-to-end anastomosis may be fashioned by dropping the anvil into the proximal bowel, which is brought to the skin through the large 20-mm cannula. Alternatively, a hand-sewn anastomosis may be selected, but this approach is time-consuming. The biofragmentable anastomotic ring (BAR) has also been used in the laparoscopically assisted procedure.[82] A technique has been developed to deliver the BAR through the anus in a fashion similar to the staple gun technique, which will allow for a totally laparoscopic pressure anastomosis.[45]

It has been possible to perform a totally laparoscopic abdominoperitoneal resection of the rectum by completing the mobilization down the sacral hollow and by performing the final mobilization only via an incision around the anus, as is done with the open operation.[83] A colostomy is brought out through a 20-mm cannula placed at the preselected stoma site. In fact, total abdominal colectomy with ileal pouch has also been reported,[84] but with the current generation of instruments, the time taken to perform this operation does not seem to justify the effort. Even in patients undergoing laparoscopy-assisted colectomy, there seems to be a significant advantage with early mobilization, feeding, and discharge, probably because of the reduced exposure of the internal milieu to the atmosphere. It is probable that reduced handling of the bowel contributes to a lower likelihood of ileus.

CONCERNS

The fact that we have been able to perform many of these operations, largely because of the array of instruments available to us, does not mean that we *should* practice these procedures. We must adhere to firmly established principles in all aspects of surgery. These principles are especially pertinent to colon resection; it is essential to maintain a field free of fecal contamination, achieve a sound anastomosis, and complete an operation with assurance that no other sites are "seeded" with "spilled" cancer cells.

Certainly, the benefits of laparoscopic surgery appear to be applicable to diseases of the colon and rectum.[85] However, a hospital stay should not be shortened by sacrificing any of the principles detailed above. Another area of concern is the escalating cost of delivering health care. The numerous disposable instruments used to carry out these procedures certainly increase the costs. Additionally, laparoscopic operations take longer, thereby limiting the availability of the operating room and surgeon. The information yielded by the ASCRS and SAGES registry will provide us with valuable data and enable us to decide whether these new procedures should be adopted. In this way, the high standard set by open surgery will be upheld.

EDITORIAL COMMENT

Since the time of its introduction by Cuschieri, the utilization of laparoscopic cholecystectomy has accelerated with a velocity equaled only by the use of surgical staples, personal computers, and VCRs. For better or for worse, laparoscopy is now firmly established as part of the surgeon's armamentarium. With a few notable exceptions, however, the phenomenal acceptance of operation by laparoscopy appears to have been, at least in part, commercially driven rather than a response to clinical or scientific data proving its efficacy or superiority.

It was inevitable that laparoscopic techniques would be extended to other areas of clinical endeavor. Laparoscopic pulmonary resection, retroperitoneal lymph node dissection, and appendectomy, for example, appear to have an accepted and established place in surgical technique. The future of laparoscopic herniorrhaphy is doubtful, and laparoscopic intervention for peptic ulcer disease remains sporadic.

For laparoscopic resections of the colon and rectum, one must retreat to the obvious question: "Should it be done merely because it *can* be done?" The enthusiasts have jettisoned their scalpels and hemostats while the critics condemn the concept rather than its applications. The editors are justifiably concerned that laparoscopic colectomies have the potential to be adopted as a fad (again driven by commercial considerations), rather than being accepted or rejected on the basis of clinical trials to determine their safety, effectiveness, end results (particularly in resections for cancer), cost, and, if adaptable, the various indications and contraindications.

The editors have included this presentation of laparoscopic colon surgery to acquaint the reader with the general principles of the technique, its current status, and the paucity of clinical data available. One may ask if this presentation should be the last chapter of this book, or the first chapter of a future text.

REFERENCES

1. Ott D: Die direkte Beleuchtung der Bauchhohle, der Harnblase, des Dickdarms und des Uterus zu diagnostichen Zwecken. Rev Med Tcheque (Prague) 1909;2:27–30.
2. Kelling G. Zur coelioskopie. Arch Klin Chir 1923;126:226–229.
3. Jacobeus HC. Kurze Ubersicht uber meine Erfahrungen Mit der Laparoskopie. Munch Med Wschr 1923;58:2017–2019.
4. Kalk H, Bruhl W. Leitfaden der Laparoskopie. Stuttgart: Thieme, 1951.
5. Fervers C. Die Laparoskopie mit dem Zystoskope. Medsche Klin 1933;29:1042–1045.
6. Veress J. Neues Instrument zue Ausfuhrung von Brust Oder Bauchpunktionen. Dt Med Wschr 1938;41:1480–1481.
7. Hopkins HH. Optical principles of the endoscope. In: Berci G, ed. Endoscopy. New York: Appleton Century Crofts, 1976, pp 3–27.
8. Ruddock JC. Peritoneoscopy surgery. Gynecol Obstet 1937;65: 523–539.
9. Berci G, Cuschieri A, eds. Practical Laparoscopy. London: 1986. Bailliere Tindall.
10. Steptoe PC. Laparoscopy in Gynaecology. Edinburgh: Churchill Livingstone Press, 1967.

11. Semm K. Endoscopic appendectomy. Endoscopy 1983;15:59–64.
12. Cuschieri A. Personal communication. University of Dundee, Scotland, 1989.
13. Filipi CJ, Fitzgibbons RJ, Salerno GM. Historical review: Diagnostic laparoscopy to laparoscopic cholecystectomy and beyond. In: Zucker KA, ed. Surgical Laparoscopy. St Louis: Quality Medical Publishing, 1991.
14. Cuschieri A, Berci G, Sackier JM, et al. Clinical aspects of laparoscopic cholecystectomy. In: Cuschieri A, Berci G, eds. Laparoscopic Biliary Surgery. London: Blackwell, 1990, pp 82–88.
15. Muhe E. Laparoskopische Cholezystektomie—Spatergebnisse Langenbecks. Arch Chir (Kongressbericht 1991) 1991;(suppl): 416–423.
16. Dubois F, Berthelots G, Levard H. Cholecystectomy par coelioscopie. Presse Med 1989;18:980–982.
17. Perissat J, Collet D, Belliard R. Gallstones: Laparoscopic treatment. Surg Endosc 1990;4:1–5.
18. Berci G, Sackier JM, Paz-Partlow M. A new endoscopic treatment for symptomatic gallbladder disease. Gastrointest Endosc Clin North Am 1991;1:191–203.
19. Perrisat J, Collet DR, Belliard R. Gallstones: Laparoscopic treatment, intracorporeal lithotripsy followed by intraoperative cholangiography during laparoscopic cholecystectomy—a personal technique. Endoscopy 1989;21:373.
20. Sackier JM, Berci G, Paz-Partlow M. Laparoscopic transcystic choledocholithotomy as an adjunct to laparoscopic cholecystectomy. Am Surg 1991;57:323–326.
21. Hunter JG. Laparoscopic transcystic common bile duct exploration. Am J Surg 1992;163:53–58.
22. Nathanson LK, Easter DW, Cuschieri A. Laparoscopic repair/peritoneal toilet of perforated duodenal ulcer. Surg Endosc 1990;4:232–233.
23. Mouiel J, Katkhouda N. Laparoscopic vagotomy in the treatment of chronic duodenal ulcer disease. In: Berci G, Cuschieri A, Sackier JM, eds. Problems in General Surgery. 1991;8:358–365.
24. Semm K. Endoscopic appendectomy. Endoscopy 1983;15:59–64.
25. Hasson HM. Open laparoscopy versus closed laparoscopy. A comparison of complication rates. Adv Planned Parenthood 1978;13:41–44.
26. Doctor HN, Hussain Z. Bilateral pneumothorax associated with laparoscopy: A case report of a rare hazard and review of the literature. Anesthesiology 1973;28:75–81.
27. Wittgen CM, Andrus CH, Fitzerald SD, et al. Analysis of the hemodynamic and ventilatory effects of laparoscopic cholecystectomy. Arch Surg 1991;126:997–1001.
28. Berci G. Personal communication. Cedars-Sinai Medical Center, Los Angeles, California, 1991.
29. Kitano S, Tomikawa M, Iso Y, et al. A safe and simple method to maintain a clear field of vision during laparoscopic cholecystectomy. Surg Endosc 1992;6:197–198.
30. Araki K, Yamamoto H, Doiguchi M, et al. Abdominal wall retraction during laparoscopic cholecystectomy. World J Surg. In press.
31. Corson SL, Batzer FR, Gocial B, Maislin G. Measurement of the force necessary for laparoscopic trocar entry. J Reprod Med 1989;44:282–284.
32. Bessler M, Treat MR. Laparoscopic Judd forceps for placement of purse-string sutures. Presented at the Society of American Gastrointestinal Endoscopic Surgeons (SAGES) Annual Scientific Session, Washington DC, April, 1992.
33. Sackier JM, Jessup G. A device for placing purse-string suture in laparoscopic surgery. Br J Surg. Submitted for publication.
34. Voyles CR, Meena AL, Petro AB, et al. Electrocautery is superior to laser for laparoscopic cholecystectomy [Editorial]. Am J Surg 1990;160:457.
35. Hunter JG. Laser or electrocautery for laparoscopic cholecystectomy? Am J Surg 1991;161:345–349.
36. Olsen DO, Corbitt JD, Edelman DS, et al. Clinical experience using a bipolar electrosurgical device for laparoscopic cholecystectomy. Surg Endosc 1992;6:104.
37. Reddick EJ, Olsen DO. Laparoscopic laser cholecystectomy. Surg Endosc 1989;3:131–133.
38. Wetter LA, Payne J, Kirschenbaum G, et al. The ultrasonic dissector (CUSA) facilitates laparoscopic cholecystectomy. Arch Surg. In press.
39. Amaral JF. Personal communication. Brown University, Rhode Island, 1991.
40. Nezhat C, Nezhat FR. Safe laser endoscopic excision or vaporization of peritoneal endometriosis. Fertil Steril 1989;52:149–151.
41. Soper NJ, Hunter JG. Suturing and knot tying in laparoscopy. Surg Clin North Am 1992;72:1139–1152.
42. Szabo Z. Laparoscopic suturing and tissue approximation. In: High Tech Surgery. Hunter JG, Sackier JM, eds. New York: McGraw-Hill, 1993.
43. Hardy TG, Pace WG, Maney JW, et al. A biofragmentable ring for sutureless bowel anastomosis: An experimental study. Dis Colon Rectum 1985;28:484–490.
44. Bubrick MP, Corman ML, Cahill CJ, et al. Prospective, randomized trial of the biofragmentable anastomosis ring. Am J Surg 1991;161:136–143.
45. Sackier JM, Jessup G, Easter DW. Laparoscopic colon and gastro-enteric anastomosis with the biofragmentable anastomotic ring. Surg Endosc. Submitted for publication.
46. Cuschieri A. Tissue approximation. Prob Gen Surg 1991;8:366–377.
47. Sauer JS, Hinshaw JR, McGuire KP. The first sutureless laser-welded, end-to-end bowel anastomosis. Lasers Surg Med 1989;9:70–73.
48. Sackier JM, Berci G, Paz-Partlow M. A new training device for laparoscopic cholecystectomy. Surg Endosc 1991;5:158–159.
49. Society of American Gastrointestinal Endoscopic Surgeons (SAGES). Guidelines on privileging and credentialling: Standards of practice and continuing medical education of laparoscopic cholecystectomy. Am J Surg 1991;161:324–325.
50. Sackier JM. Training and education in laparoscopic surgery. In: Cuschieri A, Berci G, eds. Laparoscopic Biliary Surgery. London: Blackwell Scientific, 1990.
51. Policy Statement American Society of Colon and Rectal Surgeons. Dis Colon Rectum 1992;35:5A.
52. Society of American Gastrointestinal Endoscopic Surgeons (SAGES). Surg Endosc 1992;6:82–83.
53. Getty R. The Anatomy of the Domestic Animals. Vol 2. Philadelphia: WB Saunders, 1975, pp 1281–1282.
54. Sackier JM. Training for minimal access surgery. Curr Pract Surg. In press.
55. Chamberlain GVP, Carron-Brown JA. Report of the working party of the confidential inquiry into gynaecological laparoscopy. London: Royal College of Obstetricians and Gynaecologists, 1978.
56. Berci G, Cuschieri A, Sackier JM. The laparoscopic management of inguinal hernias. Prob Gen Surg 1991;8:458–463.
57. Sigel B, Golub RM, Loiacano L, et al. Technique of ultrasonic detection and mapping of abdominal wall adhesions. Surg Endosc 1991;5:161.
58. Greene FL. Laparoscopy in malignant disease. Surg Clin North Am 1992;72:1125–1138.
59. Steis RG, Urba WJ, VanderMolen LA, et al. Intraperitoneal lymphokine-activated killer cell and interleukin-2 therapy for malignancies limited to the peritoneal cavity. J Clin Oncol 1990;8:1618–1629.
60. Luciano AA, Maier OB, Koch EI, et al. A comparative study of postoperative adhesions following laser surgery by laparoscopy versus laparotomy in the rabbit model. Obstet Gynecol 1989;74:220–224.
61. Gazzaniga AB, Slanton WW, Bartlett RH. Laparoscopy in the diagnosis of blunt and penetrating injuries to the abdomen. Am J Surg 1976;131:315.
62. Cuschieri A, Hennessy T, Stephens R, et al. Diagnosis of significant abdominal trauma after road traffic accidents: Preliminary results of a multicenter clinical trial comparing minilaparoscopy with peritoneal lavage. Ann R Coll Surg Engl 1988;70:153–155.
63. Du Priest RW Jr, Rodriguez A, Khaneja SC, et al. Open

diagnostic peritoneal lavage in blunt abdominal trauma victims. Surg Gynecol Obstet 1979;148:890–892.

64. Sackier JM. Laparoscopy in the emergency setting. World J Surg 1992;16:1083–1088.

65. Sosa JL, Sims D, Martin L, et al. Laparoscopic evaluation of tangential abdominal gunshot wounds. Arch Surg 1992;127:109.

66. Hinchey EJ, Schall PGH, Richards GK. Treatment of perforated diverticular disease of the colon. Adv Surg 1978;12:85–109.

67. Patterson-Brown S, Eckersley JRT, Sim AJW, et al. Laparoscopy as an adjunct to decision making in the acute abdomen. Br J Surg 1986;73:1022–1024.

68. Schreiber JH. Laparoscopic appendectomy in pregnancy. Surg Endosc 1990;4:100–102.

69. Valla JS, Limonne B, Valla V, et al. Laparoscopic appendectomy in children: Report of 465 cases. Surg Lap Endosc 1991;1:166–172.

70. Gotz F, Pier A, Bacher C. Modified laparoscopic appendectomy in surgery: A report of 388 operations. Surg Endosc 1990;4:6–9.

71. Engstom L, Fenyo G. Appendicectomy: assessment of stump invagination versus simple ligation: A prospective, randomized trial. Br J Surg 1985;72:971–972.

72. Ripstein CB. Surgical care of massive rectal prolapse. Dis Colon Rectum 1965;8:34–38.

73. Wells C. New operation for rectal prolapse. Proc R Soc Med 1959;52:602–603.

74. Howard RS, Catto J. Cecal volvulus, a case for nonresectional therapy. Arch Surg 1980;115:272–277.

75. Todd, GJ, Forde KA. Volvulus of the cecum: Choice of operation. Am J Surg 1979;138:632–634.

76. Ostergaard E, Halvorsen JF. Volvulus of the cecum. An evaluation of various surgical procedures. Acta Chir Scand 1990;156:629–631.

77. Shoop SA, Sackier JM. Laparoscopic cecopexy for cecal volvulus. Surg Endosc. Submitted for publication.

78. Lange V, Meyer G, Schardey HM, et al. Laparoscopic creation of a loop colostomy. J Lap Endosc Surg 1991;1:307–312.

79. Fowler DL, White SA. Laparoscopy assisted sigmoid resection. Surg Lap Endosc 1991;1:183–188.

80. Jacobs M, Berdeja JC, Goldstein HS. Minimally invasive colon resection (laparoscopic colectomy). Surg Lap Endosc 1991;1:144–150.

81. Sackier JM. Visualization of the ureter during laparoscopic colon resection. Br J Surg. Submitted for publication.

82. Sackier JM, Slutzki S, Wood CB, et al. Laparoscopic endocorporeal mobilization followed by extracorporeal sutureless anastomosis for the treatment of carcinoma of the left colon. Dis Colon Rectum. Submitted for publication.

83. Sackier JM, Berci G, Hiatt JR, Hartunian S. Laparoscopic abdominoperineal resection of the rectum. Br J Surg 1992;79:1207–1208.

84. Wexner SD, Johanson OB, Nogueras JJ, Jagelman OG. Laparoscopic total abdominal colectomy. Dis Colon Rectum 1992;35:651–655.

85. Sackier JM. Laparoscopy: Applications to colorectal surgery. Semin Colon Rectal Surg 1992;3:2–8.

I N D E X

Note: Page numbers in *italics* refer to illustrations;
page numbers followed by t refer to tables.

ISBN 0-7216-3366-8

9 780721 633664

90038